ICSA Book Series in Statistics

The ICSA Book Series in Statistics showcases research from the International Chinese Statistical Association that has an international reach. It publishes books in statistical theory, applications, and statistical education. All books are associated with the ICSA or are authored by invited contributors. Books may be monographs, edited volumes, textbooks and proceedings.

More information about this series at http://www.springer.com/series/13402

Zhen Chen • Aiyi Liu • Yongming Qu
Larry Tang • Naitee Ting • Yi Tsong
Editors

Applied Statistics in Biomedicine and Clinical Trials Design

Selected Papers from 2013 ICSA/ISBS Joint Statistical Meetings

Springer

Editors
Zhen Chen
National Institutes of Health
Rockville, Maryland, USA

Aiyi Liu
National Institutes of Health
Rockville, Maryland, USA

Yongming Qu
Lilly Corporation Center
Indianapolis, Indiana, USA

Larry Tang
George Mason University
Fairfax, Virginia, USA

Naitee Ting
Boehringer-Ingelheim
Ridgefield, Connecticut, USA

Yi Tsong
Food and Drug Administration
Silver Spring, Maryland, USA

ISSN 2199-0980 ISSN 2199-0999 (electronic)
ICSA Book Series in Statistics
ISBN 978-3-319-12693-7 ISBN 978-3-319-12694-4 (eBook)
DOI 10.1007/978-3-319-12694-4

Library of Congress Control Number: 2015934689

Springer Cham Heidelberg New York Dordrecht London

Printed on acid-free paper

Springer is part of Springer Science+Business Media (www.springer.com)

This symposium volume is dedicated to
Dr. Gang Zheng for his passion in statistics

Preface

The 22nd annual Applied Statistics Symposium of the International Chinese Statistical Association (ICSA), jointly with the International Society for Biopharmaceutical Statistics (ISBS) was successfully held from June 9 to June 12, 2013 at the Bethesda North Marriott Hotel & Conference Center, Bethesda, Maryland, USA. The theme of this joint conference was "Globalization of Statistical Applications," in recognition of the celebration of the International Year of Statistics, 2013. The conference attracted about 500 attendees from academia, industry, and governments around the world. A sizable number of attendees were from nine countries other than the USA. The conference offered five short courses, four keynote lectures, and 90 parallel scientific sessions.

The 29 selected papers from the presentations in this volume cover a wide range of applied statistical topics in biomedicine and clinical research, including Bayesian methods, diagnostic medicine and classification, innovative clinical trial designs and analysis, and personalized medicine. All papers have gone through normal peer-review process, read by at least one referee and an editor. Acceptance of a paper was made after the comments raised by the referee and editor were adequately addressed.

During the preparation of the book, a tragic event occurred that saddened the ICSA community. Dr. Gang Zheng of the National Heart, Lung, and Blood Institute (NHLBI) of the National Institutes of Health (NIH) lost his battle with cancer on January 9, 2014. An innovative and influential statistician, Dr. Zheng was also a dedicated permanent member of the ICSA, a member of many ICSA committees, including the ICSA Board of Directors from 2008 to 2010. We would like to dedicate this entire volume to Dr. Gang Zheng, a great colleague and dear friend to many of us!

The completion of this volume would not have been possible without each of the contributing authors. We thank them for their positive responses to the volume, their willingness to contribute, and their persistence, patience, and dedication. We would also like to thank many referees for spending their valuable time to help review the manuscripts. Last, but not least, we thank Hannah Bracken of Springer for her wonderful assistance throughout the entire process of completing the book.

Zhen Chen
Aiyi Liu
Yongming Qu
Larry (Liansheng) Tang
Naitee Ting
Yi Tsong

In Memoriam: Gang Zheng (May 6, 1965–January 9, 2014)

Nancy L. Geller and Colin O. Wu

(Reprinted from Statistics and Its Interface 7: 3–7, 2014, with permission)

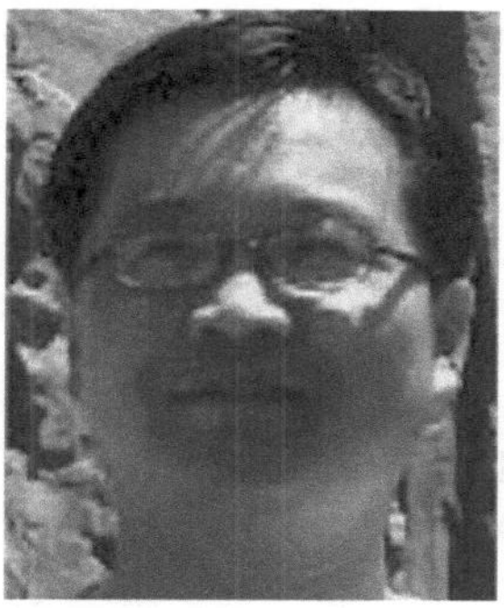

Dr. Gang Zheng

The statistical community was deeply saddened by the death of our colleague, Gang Zheng, who lost his battle with head and neck cancer on Thursday, January 9th. Gang received his BS in Applied Mathematics in 1987 from Fudan University in Shanghai. After serving as a teaching assistant at the Shanghai 2nd Polytechnic University, he emigrated to the USA in 1994 and received a master's degree in mathematics at Michigan Technological University in 1996. He then gained admission to the Ph.D. program in statistics at The George Washington University and received his Ph.D. in 2000.

Immediately, he joined the Office of Biostatistics Research at the National Heart, Lung, and Blood Institute (NHLBI) of the National Institutes of Health (NIH), where he remained until his death. From his interview seminar in early 2000, it was clear that the topic of his thesis, Fisher information and its applications, was an area in which he could pursue research for many years. What was not obvious then was how prolific his research would become.

Over the past 13 years since he got his Ph.D., Gang collaborated with many researchers in developing statistical methods, including his colleagues at NHLBI, statisticians from other NIH institutes, and statistical faculty from universities in the USA and other countries. He was one of the most productive researchers in biostatistics and statistics at NIH.

N. L. Geller (✉) · C. O. Wu
Office of Biostatistics Research, National Heart, Lung and Blood Institute, 6701 Rockledge Drive, Bethesda, MD 20892–7913, USA
e-mail: gellern@nhlbi.nih.gov

C. O. Wu
e-mail: wuc@nhlbi.nih.gov

Gang developed new statistical procedures, which were motivated from his consultations at NHLBI, and published methodology papers, in which principal investigators (PIs) of NHLBI or NHLBI-funded studies became his co-authors. One example is Zheng et al. (2005), in which he developed new methods for sample size and power calculations for genetic studies, taking into account the randomness of genotype counts given the allele frequency (the sample size and power are functions of the genotype counts). Dr. Elizabeth Nabel, the former director of NHLBI, and her research fellow were co-authors on that paper. Another example is his consultation with Multi-Ethnic Study of Atherosclerosis (MESA) and Genetic Analysis Workshop (GAW16) with his colleagues Drs. Colin Wu, Minjung Kwak, and Neal Jeffries. The studies contain data with outcome-dependent sampling and a mixture of binary and quantitative traits; for example, the measurements of a quantitative trait of all controls were not available. He developed a simple and practical procedure to analyze pleiotropic genetic association with joint binary (case-control) and continuous traits (Jeffries and Zheng 2009; Zheng et al. 2012; Zheng et al. 2013).

Most of Gang's research focused on three subject areas: (1) robust procedures and inference with nuisance parameters with applications to genetic epidemiology; (2) inference based on order statistics and ranked set sampling; and (3) pleiotropic genetic analysis with mixed trait data. Although he only started working on the last subject area in late 2012, he had already jointly published four papers in genetic and statistical journals (Li et al. 2014; Yan et al. 2013; Wu et al. 2013; Xu et al. 2013), and these results built a foundation for evaluating genetic data from combined big and complex studies.

His first paper in genetics dealt with applying robust procedures to case-control association studies (Freidlin et al. 2002). This paper has been cited over 160 times, according to the ISI Web of Science (Jan, 2014). It has become the standard robust test for the analysis of genetic association studies using a frequentist approach. The SAS JMP genomics procedure outputs the p-value of a robust test of Freidlin et al. (2002) (JMP Life Science User Manual 2014). Stephens and Balding (2009) mentioned the lack of an analogous robust test of Freidlin et al. (2002) for a Bayesian analysis. In 2010, an R package, RASSOC, for applying robust and usual association tests for genetic studies was developed by him and his co-authors (Zang et al. 2010).

In addition to novel applications of existing robust procedures to case-control genetic association studies, he developed several new robust procedures for genetic association studies. In Zheng and Ng (2008), he and his co-author used the information of departure from Hardy-Weinberg proportions to determine the underlying genetic model and incorporated genetic model selection into a test of association. Other robust procedures that he developed include Zheng et al. (2007) on an adaptive procedure, Joo et al. (2009) on deriving an asymptotic distribution for the robust test used by the Wellcome Trust Case-Control Consortium (The Welcome Trust Case Control Consortium (WTCCC) 2007), and Kwak et al. (2009) on robust methods in a two-stage procedure, so that the burden of genotyping can be reduced. Gang and his collaborators wrote an excellent tutorial on robust methods for linkage and association studies with the three most common genetic study designs (Joo et al. 2010). Kuo and Feingold (2010) discussed several robust procedures developed by Gang and his collaborators, including Freidlin et al. (2002) and Zheng and Ng (2008), and compared the power of robust tests with other tests under various situations. So and Sham (2011) reviewed and discussed many robust procedures developed by Gang, and also extended some of his procedures by allowing adjustment for covariates.

Gang developed an adaptive two-stage procedure for testing association using two correlated or independent test statistics with K. Song and R.C. Elston (Zheng et al. 2007). His adaptive procedure was used by other researchers to design optimum multistage procedures for genome-wide association studies (e.g., Pahl et al. 2009; Won and Elston 2008). His use of two independent test statistics sequentially in Zheng et al. (2007) was also used by others as one of the methods to replicate genetic studies (Murphy et al. 2008; Laird and Lange 2009). Gang also wrote an important review article with R.C. Elston and D.Y. Lin on multistage sampling in human genetics studies (Elston et al. 2007).

In 2012, Dr. Zheng and his collaborators published a book entitled "Analysis of Genetic Association Studies" with Springer (Zheng et al. 2012). It has over 436 pages with 40 illustrations. In the preface it states that "... both a graduate level textbook in statistical genetics and genetic epidemiology, and a reference book for the analysis of genetic association studies. Students, researchers, and professionals will find the topics introduced in Analysis of Genetic Association Studies particularly relevant. The book is applicable to the study of statistics, biostatistics, genetics, and genetic epidemiology." Unlike other books in statistical genetics, Zheng et al. (2012) also covers technical details and derivations that most other books omitted. In 13 years, Gang made a vast number of important contributions to statistical genetics.

In his early research (originating from on his Ph.D. thesis but extended considerably), Gang made important and extensive contributions to the computation and applications of Fisher information in order statistics and ordered data. In Zheng (2001), he characterized the Weibull distribution in the scale-family of all life time distributions in terms of Fisher information contained Type II censored data and a factorization of the hazard function, which motivated further investigations by other researchers. For example, Hofmann et al. (2005) extended his results using the Fisher information contained in the smallest order statistic. In a discussion paper by N. Balakrishnan (2007), these results were also reviewed. Some of his work on Fisher information in order statistics has been extended to Fisher information in record values (e.g., Hofmann and Nagaraja 2003) and progressive censoring (e.g., Balakrishnan et al. 2008).

Gang studied where most Fisher information is located in samples from a location-scale family of distributions, and provided theory and insight which explain why the tail and middle portions of the ordered data are most informative for the scale and location parameters, respectively. This added insight into an area initiated by the late John Tukey in the later part of the 1960s. Interestingly, this is not true for the Cauchy distribution (Zheng and Gastwirth 2000, 2002). The latest version of the classical book "Order Statistics" 3rd ed. by H. A. David and H. N. Nagaraja (2003) added a new section on Fisher information in order statistics (Sect. 8.2), which cites six papers Gang wrote on Fisher information in order statistics.

Applying his results, Sen et al. (2009) proposed a novel study design for quantitative trait locus by oversampling the informative tails of the distribution identified in Zheng's papers. Ranked set sampling is a very useful alternative to random sampling, and still an active research area, but lacked applications beyond field studies or agriculture. Gang and his collaborators applied ranked set sampling to genetics association and linkage studies, which led to two important papers (Chen et al. 2003; Zheng et al. 2006). Their work motivated many further contributions from others, including David Clayton (Wallace et al. 2006) and Danyu Lin (Huang and Lin 2007).

A very important editorial contribution by Gang is his guest editorship for a special issue on statistical methods of genome-wide association studies for Statistical Science, co-edited with Prof. Jonathan Marchini and Dr. Nancy Geller (Zheng et al. 2009). The special issue, which was published in November 2009, consists of 12 contributions from leading statisticians in the area. An introduction of this special issue appeared in the March 2010 IMS Bulletin (Zheng et al. 2010). The three editors were responsible for writing the proposal to the Editors of Statistical Science, identifying suitable contributors, and getting their agreement to participate. The executive editor, David Madigan, of Statistical Science, assigned Dr. Zheng to be the editor to handle the review process for all the submissions, except his own.

From the time of his arrival, Dr. Zheng was a statistical consultant on the design and analysis of many NHLBI-sponsored studies of cardiovascular diseases and asthma. One important project was the genetic study of in-stent restenosis, which started in 2004. With his colleagues Drs. Jungnam Joo (now at Korean National Cancer Center) and Nancy Geller, he designed this study, which was later expanded to the first genome-wide association study (GWAS) carried out by NHLBI in 2005, before NHLBI started funding GWAS. The original paper was published in Pharmacogenomics (Ganesh et al. 2004). In this study, he determined statistical procedures for quality control and developed methods for the analysis of the data. His early research in GWAS earned him invitations to present his work at the 2007 JSM, at a seminar series of the Washington Statistical Society (2007), and at a seminar series at the Department of Biostatistics at the University of Pennsylvania (2008).

In 2004, Dr. Zheng became a statistical consultant for an NHLBI study: "A Case-Control Etiologic Study of Sarcoidosis" (ACCESS). A paper of ACCESS Research Group claimed that there was no association between immunoglobulin gene polymorphisms and sarcoidosis among African Americans (Pandey et al. 2002). A routine two-degree-of-freedom test built in SAS was applied by ACCESS investigators to analyze the data. He and his colleague developed a new efficiency robust procedure with constrained genetic models for the ACCESS data and re-analyzed the genetic association. They found that it was statistically significant with the new procedure. The improvement came after incorporating the constraints on the genetic models but the routine chi-squared test ignores the restriction of the genetic model space. This research brought attention not only from the original PIs but also from the Steering Committee and the Data Safety and Monitoring Board of ACCESS. After more than 6 months of discussions in several Steering Committee meetings and consultation with a medical researcher outside of ACCESS, also under the pressure and objection from the original authors, the Steering Committee members finally voted to clear submission of Dr. Zheng's research for publication, which appeared in Statistics in Medicine (Zheng et al. 2006). The ACCESS Research Group also decided to include this paper as an ACCESS publication. Dr. Lee Newman (Ex Officio of ACCESS and Professor of Medicine at Colorado School of Public Health) later invited Dr. Zheng to give a presentation based on his research findings.

When analyzing the data from his consultation for medical publications at NHLBI, Dr. Zheng not only developed more powerful statistical methods for the unique data, but also applied more appropriate tests to the data analysis. In one ongoing NHLBI intramural research to analyze association of candidate markers in osteoprotegerin with clinical phenotypes and its effects on cell biology in lymphangioleiomyomatosis, the original analyses were done by a staff scientist using some statistical tools built in Excel. Associations were tested using an allele-based test by comparing allele frequencies, and a genotype-based test by comparing genotype frequencies. Both results are reported. Although this is fine after correcting for multiple testing for two tests, Gang employed a method newly developed by him and his colleagues (Joo et al. 2009) to this dataset with the same allele-based and genotype-based tests, but instead of applying the Bonferroni correction for the two tests, he applied a more powerful approach to find p-values using the joint distribution of the two tests.

In addition to research contributions, Gang served as an associate editor of Statistics and Its Interface and co-edited several issues of the journal, the current one and an earlier one in honor of his thesis adviser Joe Gastwirth. He served as a referee for 43 journals and volumes, including JASA, Biometrics, Biometrika, Annals of Human Genetics, American Journal of Human Genetics, and Statistics in Medicine.

Gang's degree of productivity was extremely rare and unusually versatile. He was honored for his work by election in 2005 as Fellow of the International Statistical Institute. He also gave a large number of invited talks, demonstrating the appreciation of his work by others.

One might think that such a productive researcher would be highly competitive. In fact, the opposite was true for Gang. He was an intellectually generous and nurturing colleague. He mentored new members of the Office of Biostatistics Research at NHLBI both in research and collaboration. He also mentored predoctoral fellows and served as a Ph.D. advisor to six students (two in China and four at George Washington University). In each case, he published joint papers with these students. There was an old e-mail about one of them in which he said, "This is one of the things that makes me happy. This was a fine Ph.D. student. I gave him three topics for his Ph.D. thesis and he worked out five papers. I actually turned down authorship on the last two papers because I wanted him to come into my world and come out of it independently."

He has been equally generous to his other colleagues. We learned very quickly that if Gang asked you to collaborate with him on a research paper, to just say yes and be prepared to rearrange your own priorities so that you had time to work on it immediately, for the paper he was proposing would get written quickly, with or without your input. Indeed, Gang collaborated with almost all of his colleagues in the Office of Biostatistics Research. It was our pleasure to collaborate with him on nearly

20 papers between us. His efficiency and creativity were marvelous and inspiring. He was truly an intellectual leader in the Office of Biostatistics Research.

Gang also contributed admirably to the statistical profession by undertaking significant editorial responsibilities, serving on organizing and program committees of many meetings as well as organizing many sessions at various statistical meetings. He was also a member of the ASA Noether Award Committee. These activities illustrate Gang's generosity as a colleague and his dedication to the profession. Despite the setback of his illness, he continued to be highly productive and published seven new papers in 2013.

Gang's efficiency, creativity, and generosity were truly inspiring. Those of us who have been his colleagues and collaborators will always remember the experience. He will be sorely missed.

References

Balakrishnan, N. (2007). Progressive censoring methodology: an appraisal. *Test* **16**, 211–259. MR2393645

Balakrishnan, N., Burkschat, M., Gramer, E. and Hoffman, G. (2008). Fisher information based progressive censoring plans. *Computational Statistics and Data Analysis* **53**, 366–380. MR2649092

Chen, Z., Zheng, G., Ghosh, K. and Li, Z. (2005). Linkage disequilibrium mapping for quantitative trait loci by selective genotyping. *American Journal of Human Genetics* **77**, 661–669.

David, H. A. and Nagaraja, H. N. (2003). *Order Statistics, Third Edition*. Wiley, Hoboken, New Jersey. MR1994955

Elston, R. C., Lin, D. Y. and Zheng, G. (2007). Multi-stage sampling for genetic studies. *Annual Reviews of Genomics and Human Genetics* **8**, 327–342.

Freidlin, B., Zheng, G., Li, Z. and Gastsirth, J. L. (2002). Trend tests for case-control studies of genetic markers: Power, sample size and robustness. *Human Heredity* **53**, 146–152.

Ganesh, S. K., Skelding, K. A., Mehta, L., O'Neill, K., Joo, J., Zheng, G., Goldstein, J., Simari, R., Billings, E., Geller, N. L., Holmes, D., O'Neill, W. W. and Nabel, E. G. (2004). Rationale and study design of the CardioGene study: genomics of in-stent restenosis. *Pharmacogenomics* **5**, 949–1004.

Hofmann, G., Balakrishnan, N. and Ahmadi, J. (2005). Characterization of hazard function factorization by Fisher information in minima and upper record values. *Statistics and Probability Letters* **72**, 51–57. MR2126293

Hofmann, G. and Nagaraja, H. N. (2003). Fisher information in record data. *Metrika* **57**, 177–193. MR1969251

Huang, G. B. E. and Lin, D. Y. (2007). Efficient association mapping of quantitative trait loci with selective genotyping. *American Journal of Human Genetics* **80**(3), 567–576.

Jeffries, N. and Zheng, G. (2009). Evaluation of an optimal receiver operating characteristics procedure. *BMC Proceedings* **15**;3 Suppl 7:S56.

JMP Life Science User Manual (Genomics and Clinical) (2014). SAS Institute Inc., Cary, North Carolina.

Joo, J., Kwak, M., Ahn, K. and Zheng, G. (2009). A robust genome-wide scan statistic of the Wellcome Trust Case-Control Consortium. *Biometrics* **65**, 1115–1122. MR2756499

Joo, J., Kwak, M., Chen, Z. and Zheng, G. (2010). Efficiency robust statistics for genetic linkage and association studies under genetic model uncertainty. *Statistics in Medicine* **29**, 158–180. MR2751387

Kuo, C. L. and Feinberg, E. (2010). Letter to the Editor. *Genetic Epidemiology* **34**, 772.

Kwak, M., Joo, J. and Zheng, G. (2009). A robust test for two-stage design in genome-wide association studies. *Biometrics* **65**, 1288–1295. MR2756517

Laird, N. M. and Lange, C. (2009). The role of family-based designs in genome-wide association studies. *Statistical Science* **24**, 388–397. MR2779333

Li, Q., Hu, J., Ding, J. and Zheng G. (2014). Fisher's method combining dependent statistics using generalizations of the gamma distribution with applications to genetic pleiotropic associations. *Biostatistics* **15**, 284–295.

Murphy, A., Weiss, S. T. and Lange, C. (2008). Screening and replication using the same data set: testing strategies for family-based studies in which all probands are affected. *PLOS Genetics* DOI: 10.1371/journal.pgen.1000197.

Pahl, R., Schafer, H. and Muller, H. H. (2009). Optimal multistage designs – a general framework for efficient genome-wide association studies. *Biostatistics* **10**, 297–309.

Pandey, J. P., Frederick, M. and Access Research Group. (2002). TNF-α, IL1-β, and immunoglobulin (GM and KM) gene polymorphisms in sarcoidosis. *Human Immunology* **63**, 485–491.

Sen, S., Johannes, F. and Broman, K. W. (2009). Selective genotyping and phenotyping strategies in a complex trait context. *Genetics* **181**, 1613–1626.

So, H. and Shan P. C. (2011). Robust association tests under different genetic models, allowing for binary or quantitative traits and covariates. *Behavior Genetics* **41**, 768–775.

Stephens, M. and Balding, D. J. (2009). Bayesian statistical methods for genetic association studies. *Nature Reviews Genetics* **10**, 681–690.

The Welcome Trust Case Control Consortium (WTCCC). (2007). Genome-wide association study of 14,000 cases of seven common diseases and 3,000 shared controls. *Nature* **447**, 1753–1773.

Wallace, C., Chapman, J. M. and Clayton, D. G. (2006). Improved power offered by a score test for linkage disequilibrium mapping of quantitative-trait loci by selective genotyping. *American Journal of Human Genetics* **78**(3), 498–504.

Won, S. and Elston, R. C. (2008). The power of independent types of genetic information to detect association in a case-control study design. *Genetic Epidemiology* **32**, 731–756.

Wu, C. O., Zheng, G. and Kwak, M. (2013). A joint regression analysis for genetic association studies with outcome stratified samples. *Biometrics* **69**, 417–426. MR3071060

Xu, J., Zheng, G. and Yuan A. (2013). Case-control genome-wide joint association study using semiparametric empirical model and approximate Bayes factor. *Journal of Statistical Computing and Simulation* **83**, 1191–1209.

Yan, T., Li, Q., Li, Y., Li, Z. and Zheng, G. (2013). Genetic association with multiple traits in the presence of population stratification. *Genetic Epidemiology* **37**, 571–580.

Zang, Y., Fung, W. K. and Zheng, G. (2010). Simple algorithms to calculate asymptotic null distributions for robust tests in case-control genetic association studies in R. *Journal of Statistical Software* **33**(8).

Zheng, G. (2001). A characterization of the factorization of hazard function by the Fisher information under Type II censoring with application to Weibull distribution. *Statistics and Probability Letters* **52**, 249–253. MR1838212

Zheng, G. and Gastwirth, J. L. (2000). Where is the Fisher information in an ordered sample? *Statistica Sinica* **10**, 1267–1280. MR1804545

Zheng, G. and Gastwirth, J. L. (2001). On the Fisher information in randomly censored data. *Statistics and Probability Letters* **52**, 421–426. MR1841610

Zheng, G. and Gastwirth, J. L. (2002). Do tails of symmetric distributions contain more Fisher information about the scale parameter? *Sankhya Series B* **64**, 289–300. MR1993915

Zheng, G., Ghosh, K., Chen, Z. and Li, Z. (2006). Extreme rank selection for linkage analysis of quantitative trait loci using selected sib-pairs. *Annals of Human Genetics* **70**, 857–866.

Zheng, G., Joo, J., Ganesh, S., Nabel, E. and Geller, N. L. (2005). On averaging power for genetic association and linkage studies. *Human Heredity* **59**, 14–20.

Zheng, G., Marchini, J. and Geller, N. L. (2009). Introduction to the Special Issue: Genome-wide association studies. *Statistical Science* **24**, 387. MR2779332

Zheng, G., Marchini, J. and Geller, N. L. (2010). Genome-wide association studies. *IMS Bulletin* **39**(2), 10.

Zheng, G. and Ng, H. K. T. (2008). Genetic model selection in two-phase analysis for case-control association studies. *Biostatistics* **9**, 391–399.

Zheng, G., Song, K. and Elston, R. C. (2007). Adaptive two-stage analysis of genetic association for case-control designs. *Human Heredity* **63**, 175–186.

Zheng, G. and Tian, X. for ACCESS Research Group (2006). Robust trend tests for genetic association using matched case-control design. *Statistics in Medicine* **25**, 3160–3173. MR2252289

Zheng, G., Xu, J., Yuan, A. and Wu, C. O. (2013). Impact on modes of inheritance and relative risks using extreme sampling when designing genetic association studies. *Annals of Human Genetics* **77**, 80–84.

Zheng, G., Wu, C. O., Kwak, M., Jiang, W., Joo, J. and Lima, J. A. C. (2012). Joint analysis of binary and quantitative trait with data sharing and outcome-dependent sampling. *Genetic Epidemiology* **36**, 263–273.

Zheng, G., Yang, Y., Zhu, X. and Elston R. C. (2012). *Analysis of Genetic Association Studies*. Springer, New York. MR2895171

Contents

Part VI Statistical Genomics and High-Dimensional Data Analysis

Contributors

Y. Mo Mount Sinai Hospital,, New York, NY, USA

Koko Asakura National Cerebral and Cardiovascular Center, Suita, Osaka, Japan

Veerabhadran Baladandayuthapan Department of Biostatistics, UT MD Anderson Cancer Center, Houston, TX, USA

Chakib Battioui Eli Lilly and Company, Indianapolis, USA

Pierre-Jérôme Bergeron Department of Mathematics and Statistics, University of Ottawa, Ottawa, ON, Canada

M. E. Boye Eli Lilly and Company, Indianapolis, IN, USA

Y. Cai Department of Applied Mathematics and Statistics, State University of New York, Stony Brook, NY, USA

Joseph C. Cappelleri Pfizer Inc, Groton, CT, USA

Martin O. Carlsson Pfizer Inc, New York, NY, USA

Ivan S. F. Chan Merck & Co. Inc., North Wales, PA, USA

Ivan S.F. Chan Late Development Statistics, Merck Research Laboratories, Upper Gwynedd, PA, USA

M.-H. Chen Department of Statistics, University of Connecticut, Storrs, CT, USA

Ming-Hui Chen Department of Statistics, University of Connecticut, CT, USA

George Y.H. Chi Janssen R & D, LLC, Raritan, NJ, USA

Dipak K. Dey Department of Statistics, University of Connecticut, Storrs, CT, USA

Jianing Di Janssen R & D, LLC, San Diego, CA, USA

Ying Ding Department of Biostatistics, University of Pittsburgh, Pittsburgh, USA

Alex Dmitrienko Quintiles, Inc, Durham, NC, USA

Kim-Anh Do Department of Biostatistics, UT MD Anderson Cancer Center, Houston, TX, USA

Gaohong Dong Biometrics & Statistical Sciences, Novartis Pharmaceuticals Corporation, East Hanover, NJ, USA

Scott R Evans Harvard School of Public Health, Boston, Massachusetts, USA

Yang (Joy) Ge Merck Research Laboratory, Merck & Co., Inc., North Wales, PA, USA
2013 ICSA/ISBS Joint Statistical Conference, Bethesda, MD, USA

A. Lawrence Gould Merck Research Laboratories, North Wales, PA, USA

Gerry Gray Division of Biostatistics, Center for Devices and Radiological Health, Food and Drug Administration, Silver Spring, MD, USA

Toshimitsu Hamasaki National Cerebral and Cardiovascular Center, Suita, Osaka, Japan

Alan Hopkins Theravance, Inc, South San Francisco, CA, USA

J. G. Ibrahim Department of Biostatistics, University of North Carolina, Chapel Hill, NC, USA

Michael Krams Janssen R & D, LLC, Titusville, NJ, USA

Lynn Kuo Departement of Statistics, University of Connecticut, Storrs, CT, USA

Pei Li CRDM Clinical Research and Reimbursement, Medtronic, Mounds View, MN, USA

Qian H. Li National Institute of Health, National Center for Complementary and Alternative Medicine, Bethesda, Democracy Blvd., Suite 401MD, USA

Wenqing Li Global Biostatistical Science, Amgen Inc., Thousand Oaks, CA, USA

Yu-Ping Li Theravance, Inc, South San Francisco, CA, USA

W. Liao New York Genome Center, New York, NY, USA

Ilya Lipkovich Quintiles, Inc, Durham, NC, USA

Danping Liu Biostatistics and Bioinformatics Branch, Division of Intramural Population Health Research, Eunice Kennedy Shriver National Institute of Child Health & Human Development, Bethesda, MD, USA

G Frank Liu Merck & Co. Inc., North Wales, PA, USA

Ming Lu Janssen R & D, LLC, Spring House, PA, USA

Nelson Lu Division of Biostatistics, Center for Devices and Radiological Health, Food and Drug Administration, Silver Spring, MD, USA

Yinghua Lu Risk Lighthouse LLC, Atlanta, GA, USA

Bani K. Mallick Department of Statistics, Texas A & M University, TX, USA

Mounir Mesbah Université Pierre et Marie Curie, Paris, France

M. Q. Zhang Department of Molecular & Cell Biology, Center for Systems Biology, The University of Texas at Dallas, Richardson, TX, USA

MOE Key Laboratory of Bioinformatics and Bioinformatics Division, Center for Synthetic and System Biology, TNLIST, Department of Automation, Tsinghua University, Beijing, P. R. China

Gengsheng Qin Georgia State University, Atlanta, GA, USA

Lei Shen Eli Lilly & Company, Indianapolis, IN, USA

Lei Shen Eli Lilly and Company, Indianapolis, USA

W. Shen Eli Lilly and Company, Indianapolis, IN, USA

H.D. Hollins Showalter Eli Lilly & Company, Indianapolis, IN, USA

Takashi Sozu Kyoto University School of Public Health, Kyoto, Japan

Shu-Chih Su Merck & Co. Inc., North Wales, PA, USA

Ewa Sucha Department of Mathematics and Statistics, University of Ottawa, Ottawa, ON, Canada

Tomoyuki Sugimoto Hirosaki University, Aomori, Japan

Xiao Sun Late Development Statistics, Merck Research Laboratories, Upper Gwynedd, PA, USA

Huaming Tan Clinical Statistics, Global Innovative Pharma Business, Pfizer Inc., Groton, CT, USA

Ye Tan Pfizer Inc, New York, NY, USA

Liansheng Larry Tang Department of Statistics, George Mason University, Fairfax, VA, USA

Naitee Ting Boehringer Ingelheim Pharmaceuticals, Inc, Ridgefield, CT, USA

Daniel Wang Janssen R & D, LLC, CA, USA

Ming-Dauh Wang Eli Lilly and Company, Indianapolis, IN, USA

Whedy Wang Theravance, Inc, South San Francisco, CA, USA

Xiaohui Wang Department of Mathematics, University of Texas-Pan American, Edinburg, TX, USA

Ziwen Wei Merck & Co., Inc., Rahway, NJ, USA

Steven A. Willke The Ohio State University, Columbus, OH, USA

Russell D. Wolfinger JMP Life Sciences, SAS Institute Inc, Cary, NC, USA

H. Xing Department of Applied Mathematics and Statistics, State University of New York, Stony Brook, NY, USA

Yunling Xu Division of Biostatistics, Center for Devices and Radiological Health, Food and Drug Administration, Silver Spring, MD, USA

Huyuan Yang Takeda Pharmaceuticals International Co., Cambridge, MA, USA

Ying Yang Food and Drug Administration Center for Devices and Radiological Health, Silver Spring, MD, USA

Xuan Ye Department of Statistics, George Mason University, Fairfax, VA, USA

Jaime Younger Toronto General Research Institute, University Health Network, Toronto, ON, Canada

Ching-Ray Yu Pfizer Inc, New York, NY, USA

Lilly Q. Yue Center for Devices and Radiological Health, US Food and Drug Administration, Silver Spring, MD, USA

D. Zhang Department of Statistics, Gilead Sciences, Inc., Foster City, CA, USA

Xin Zhao Janssen R & D, LLC, Fremont, CA, USA

Yanli Zhao Late Development Statistics, Merck Research Laboratories, Upper Gwynedd, PA, USA

MedImmune/Astrazeneca, Gaithersburg, MD, USA

Yichuan Zhao Department of Mathematics and Statistics, Georgia State University, Atlanta, GA, USA

Haochuan Zhou CyberSource, M3-5NW Foster City, CA, USA

Xiao-Hua Zhou Department of Biostatistics, University of Washington, Seattle, WA, USA

Northwest HSR & D Center of Excellence, VA Puget Sound Health Care System, Seattle, WA, USA

Richard C. Zink JMP Life Sciences, SAS Institute Inc, Cary, NC, USA

Kelly H. Zou Pfizer Inc, New York, NY, USA

Part I
Bayesian Methods In Biomedical Research

Chapter 1
An Application of Bayesian Approach for Testing Non-inferiority Case Studies in Vaccine Trials

G. Frank Liu, Shu-Chih Su and Ivan S. F. Chan

Abstract Non-inferiority designs are often used in vaccine clinical trials to show a test vaccine or a vaccine regimen is not inferior to a control vaccine or a control regimen. Traditionally, the non-inferiority hypothesis is tested using frequentist methods, e.g., comparing the lower bound of 95 % confidence interval with a pre-specified non-inferiority margin. The analyses are often based on maximum likelihood methods. Recently, Bayesian approaches have been developed and considered in clinical trials due to advances in Bayesian computation such as Markov chain Monte Carlo (MCMC) methods. Some of the advantages of using Bayesian methods include accounting for various sources of uncertainty and incorporating prior information which is often available for the control group in non-inferiority trials. In this chapter, we will illustrate the use of Bayesian methods to test for non-inferiority with real examples from vaccine clinical trials. Consideration will be given to issues including the choice of priors or incorporating results from historical trial, and their impact on testing non-inferiority. The pros and cons on using Bayesian approaches will be discussed, and the results from Bayesian analyses will be compared with that from the traditional frequentist methods.

1.1 Introduction

The purpose of a non-inferiority test is to show that a test treatment is "similar" to an active control for which effectiveness has been established. It is known that non-inferiority cannot be concluded from a non-rejection of a null hypothesis of superiority between test treatment and active control (Blackwalder 1982). To test

G. F. Liu (✉) · S.-C. Su · Ivan S. F. Chan
Merck & Co. Inc., 351 -N Sumneytown Pike,
North Wales, PA 19454, USA
e-mail: guanghan_frank_liu@merck.com

Ivan S. F. Chan
e-mail: ivan_chan@merck.com

Shu-Chih Su
e-mail: shu-chih_su@merck.com

Z. Chen et al. (eds.), *Applied Statistics in Biomedicine and Clinical Trials Design*,
ICSA Book Series in Statistics, DOI 10.1007/978-3-319-12694-4_1

for non-inferiority, we need to show that the effect of the test treatment is within a certain pre-specified amount of the effect of the active control. This pre-specified quantity, called the non-inferiority margin, has to be determined and agreed upon by the sponsor and regulatory agencies.

For a continuous response, suppose θ_T and θ_C are the treatment effects for test and control, respectively. Assuming a large value represents a better efficacy, a non-inferiority hypothesis can be formulated as follows:

Null hypothesis $H_0 : \theta_T - \theta_C \leq -\delta$ versus

Alternative hypothesis $H_1 : \theta_T - \theta_C > -\delta$

where $-\delta$ is a pre-specified non-inferiority margin. This fixed margin is often chosen such that by rejecting the null hypothesis, we can conclude that the test treatment will preserve certain amount of the treatment effect of the control, or the effect of the test treatment is not worse than the active control by the amount of δ. It may be difficult and sometimes controversial on how to choose the margin, but in general, the margin should be a negligible difference in clinical benefit between the two treatment groups. There are many researches and discussions on how to choose a non-inferiority margin in the literature. Some general guidelines and related references can be found in the regulatory guidance documents for non-inferiority studies (EMEA 2005 and US FDA 2010).

The non-inferiority hypothesis is conventionally tested using frequentist methods, where *p* value and confidence intervals for treatment difference (test treatment minus control) are calculated based on the observed data from the study. Some commonly used frequentist methods for non-inferiority tests can be found in Wang et al. (2006). For example, maximum likelihood methods are commonly used to obtain the estimate of the treatment difference and its 95 % confidence interval. The null hypothesis is rejected if the lower bound of the confidence interval for the treatment difference is greater than the pre-specified non-inferiority margin, $-\delta$. In the frequentist methods, prior information besides the current study is not utilized.

Recently, Bayesian approaches have been developed and considered in clinical trials due to advances in Bayesian computation such as Markov chain Monte Carlo (MCMC) methods. With a non-informative prior, the Bayesian approaches often produce similar results as that from the frequentist methods. One of the important advantages for Bayesian methods is the ability to incorporate prior information which is often available for the control group in non-inferiority trials. Gamalo et al. (2011) showed that the incorporation of prior information through the use of Bayesian methods may improve the power for non-inferiority tests. Here, we will illustrate the use of Bayesian methods to test non-inferiority with two real examples from vaccine clinical trials.

This chapter is organized as follows: Section 1.2 describes the vaccine studies and frequentist statistical methods and results. Section 1.3 presents Bayesian approaches including how to construct the prior distributions from a historical study, and discusses the impact of the choice of prior on the analysis results. Section 1.4 provides conclusions and discussions.

1.2 Vaccine Studies and Results from Frequentist Methods

We consider two vaccine clinical trials. To maintain some confidentiality, we will simply call them study I and study II without disclosing the names of studies and the test vaccine. Both studies are phase III double-blind, randomized multicenter trials to evaluate the safety, tolerability, and immunogenicity of a test vaccine administered concomitantly versus non-concomitantly with an influenza virus vaccine (in study I), or with PNEUMOVAX^{TM} 23 (in study II).

In each of these studies, subjects were randomly assigned to either the concomitant use group (receiving the test vaccine and the concomitant vaccine together) or non-concomitant use group (receiving the test vaccine and the concomitant vaccine separately, approximately a month apart). We will consider the non-concomitant group as the control group in the following discussions. Antibody titers were measured at baseline and approximately 4 weeks postvaccination. One of the primary objectives was to show that the antibody response to the test vaccine in the concomitant use group was non-inferior to that in the control group. The statistical hypothesis is H_0: GMT1/GMT2 ≤ 0.67 versus H_1: GMT1/GMT2 > 0.67, where GMT1 and GMT2 are the geometric mean titer (GMT) for the test vaccine in concomitant use group and that in the control group, respectively. The value of 0.67 is the pre-specified non-inferiority margin, which corresponds to a no more than 1.5-fold decrease in the GMT of the concomitant use group compared with the control group (Kerzner et al. 2007). In the statistical analyses, a natural log transformation was applied to the antibody titer. Therefore, the non-inferiority test was based on treatment mean difference in log antibody titer with a fixed margin of log(0.67).

1.2.1 *Traditional Frequentist Methods*

In the original trial designs, both studies were analyzed using a frequentist approach. For the primary analysis, a constraint longitudinal data analysis (cLDA) model proposed by Liang and Zeger (2000) was used. The model included natural log transformed baseline and postvaccination antibody titers as response variables. The covariates in the analysis model included treatment indicator, age at randomization, visit, and treatment by visit interaction. For study I, an indicator for region (USA vs. EU) was also included to designate the sites in the USA and European countries.

The cLDA model assumes that baseline and postvaccination values have a joint multivariate normal distribution. An unstructured covariance matrix was used to account for within subject correlation between baseline and postvaccination responses. The baseline means were constrained to be the same between two treatment groups in this cLDA model, which is reasonable due to randomization. Specifically, suppose Y_{i0} and Y_{i1} are the log titers observed at baseline and postvaccination for subject i, then the cLDA model under a bivariate normal distribution may be formulated as

$$\begin{aligned}
&\begin{pmatrix} Y_{i0} \\ Y_{i1} \end{pmatrix} \sim N\left(\begin{pmatrix} \mu_{i0} \\ \mu_{i1} \end{pmatrix}, \Sigma\right) \\
&\mu_{i0} = \beta_0 + \beta_1{}^*age_i + \beta_2{}^*region_i \\
&\mu_{i1} = \beta_0 + \beta_1{}^*age_i + \beta_2{}^*region_i + \gamma_0 + \gamma_1{}^*trt_i
\end{aligned} \tag{1.1}$$

where age_i represents the age of subject at randomization, trt_i represents the treatment indicator (1 for the concomitant group and 0 for the control group), $region_i$ represents the region indicator (1 for the USA and 0 for Europe), and Σ is an unstructured covariance matrix. The factor region is used for study I only. To make parameterization simpler, we used the centralized values for age and region in the analysis. So β_0 is the mean baseline response for study population, γ_0 is the change from baseline at postvaccination for control group, and γ_1 is the treatment difference between treatment and control group. All these parameters are on the log-transformed titer scale.

This cLDA model will compare the postvaccination antibody titers between the two treatment groups while adjusting for baseline antibody titer in the presence of incomplete data. In the event that there were no missing data, the estimated treatment difference from the cLDA model would be identical to that from a traditional analysis of covariance (ANCOVA) model (Liu et al. 2009). This cLDA model can be fit using the MIXED procedure in statistical analysis system (SAS Institute Inc. 2012).

1.2.2 Analysis Results from Frequentist Method

Suppose $\hat{\gamma}_1$ and $(\hat{\gamma}_{1L}, \hat{\gamma}_{1U})$ are the point estimate and 95 % confidence interval for γ_1, then we will claim non-inferiority if the lower bound of the 95 % confidence interval (CI) is larger than the non-inferiority margin, i.e., $\hat{\gamma}_{1L} > \log(0.67)$, or the lower bound CI of the GMT ratio, i.e., $\exp(\hat{\gamma}_1)$, is greater than 0.67.

Table 1.1 presents the analysis results for both studies based on the cLDA model. The conclusions from the analyses are that: Study I met the non-inferiority criterion and concluded that the antibody response induced by the test vaccine when administered concomitantly with influenza vaccine was similar (non-inferior) to that induced by the test vaccine administered alone. However, study II did not meet the non-inferiority criterion, which indicated that the antibody response in the concomitant use group would be inferior to that in the non-concomitant use group.

It will be interesting to investigate how Bayesian analysis may help and/or alter the analysis results for these two vaccine trials. Here, we apply Bayesian methods retrospectively for illustration in these two studies, recognizing that the frequentist cLDA model was the pre-specified analysis method in the protocol.

1.3 Bayesian Approach

1.3.1 Non-informative Prior

We first consider a non-informative prior for all parameters in the cLDA model (1.1). To have better mixture in the MCMC sampling, we use conjugate prior distributions for all parameters. That is, for location parameters $\beta_0, \beta_1, \beta_2, \gamma_0,$ and γ_1, we use normal priors with a mean of 0 and a large variance to reflect uncertainty (variance = 10,000 is used in the analysis models presented below). For the variance matrix Σ, we use an inverse Wishart prior with a degrees of freedom of 2 and a very small precision parameter (0.0001 is used in the analysis models below).

The results from 5000 MCMC samples (SAS PROC MCMC with the number of MCMC iterations (nmc) = 50,000 and thin = 10 options; SAS Institute Inc. 2012) are presented in Table 1.2. It can be seen that the results are almost identical to that from the frequentist method (Table 1.1). This is as expected because the posterior distribution under the non-informative prior is essentially the likelihood function. So the estimates and credible intervals from the Bayesian analysis would be very similar to that from the frequentist analysis.

1.3.2 Prior Based on Historical Data

At the time these two trials were conducted, a historical placebo controlled trial was completed in which the test vaccine was given non-concomitantly with other vaccines. Therefore, the antibody responses from this historical trial can provide good prior information for the control group in study I and study II.

Based on the historical trial, we construct prior distributions for the baseline mean β_0, the change from baseline at postvaccination γ_0 for the control group, and the variance covariance matrix Σ for the log titers at baseline and postvaccination. Using the data from the historical trial, we obtained

$$\begin{aligned} \beta_0 &\sim N(mean = 5.6400, sd = 0.04051), \\ \gamma_0 &\sim N(mean = 5.228, sd = 0.02937), \\ \Sigma &\sim invWishart\left(df = 2, S = \begin{pmatrix} 1.91 & -1.50 \\ -1.50 & 2.27 \end{pmatrix}\right). \end{aligned} \tag{1.2}$$

Table 1.1 Non-inferiority analysis results from cLDA models

Study	$\hat{\beta}_0(SE)$	$\hat{\gamma}_0(SE)$	GMT ratio (CI)	Conclusion[a]
I	5.557 (0.041)	0.833 (0.041)	0.93 (0.84, 1.03)	Similar
II	5.134 (0.045)	1.059 (0.052)	0.70 (0.61, 0.80)	Not similar

SE standard error, *cLDA* constraint longitudinal data analysis, *GMT* geometric mean titer, *CI* confidence interval

[a]Similar (i.e., non-inferior) if the lower bound CI is greater than 0.67

Table 1.2 Non-inferiority analysis results from Bayesian models with different prior

Prior	$\hat{\beta}_0(SE)^a$	$\hat{\gamma}_0(SE)^a$	GMT Ratio (CI)[a]	Conclusion[b]
Study I				
Non informative (a = 0, b = 0)	5.557 (0.041)	0.833 (0.040)	0.93 (0.84, 1.03)	Similar
Informative (a = 1, b = 1)	5.640 (0.029)	0.625 (0.024)	1.11 (1.01, 1.21)	Similar
Power prior (a = 0.98, b = 0.12)	5.611 (0.029)	0.763 (0.036)	0.97 (0.88, 1.08)	Similar
Power prior (a = 0.52, b = 0.03)	5.591 (0.033)	0.805 (0.040)	0.94 (0.85, 1.04)	Similar
Study II				
Non informative (a = 0, b = 0)	5.134 (0.045)	1.060 (0.053)	0.70 (0.61, 0.80)	Not similar
Informative (a = 1, b = 1)	5.478 (0.031)	0.610 (0.026)	0.92 (0.82, 1.04)	Similar
Power prior (a = 0.06, b = 0.03)	5.184 (0.043)	0.996 (0.051)	0.72 (0.63, 0.83)	Not similar
Power prior (a = 0.02, b = 0.01)	5.151 (0.044)	1.035 (0.052)	0.71 (0.62, 0.81)	Not similar

The parameters a and b for power priors are defined in formula (1.3)
SE standard error, *CI* credible interval
[a]Posterior mean, SE, and credible interval
[b]Similar (i.e., non-inferior) if the lower bound CI is greater than 0.67

Because the historical trials were conducted with subjects in different ages and regions, no prior information is available for $\beta_1$and β_2. There is no prior information for the concomitant use group. Thus, we use non-informative prior for β_1, β_2, and γ_1. The results from 5000 MCMC samples (SAS PROC MCMC with nmc = 50,000 and thin = 10 options) are presented in Table 1.2.

With the informative prior, the conclusion for study I is similar to that from the frequentist method or the Bayesian method with non-informative prior. It can be seen that the estimated GMT ratio and its 95 % credible interval are numerically larger than those from the frequentist method, which implies that the power for testing non-inferiority would be higher after incorporating the prior information.

For study II, the conclusion from the Bayesian analysis with informative prior is different from that using the frequentist method or Bayesian method with non-informative prior. The non-inferiority criterion is met as the lower bound of the 95 % credible interval for the GMT ratio is greater than 0.67.

The quite different results based on informative prior distributions made us to further investigate on how the prior distribution constructed from the previous study significantly altered the results. It may imply that the prior information overwhelms the evidence from the current study data. To examine the impact of prior distributions, we plotted the prior density functions of β_0 and γ_0 obtained from the historical study, and compare that to the density functions obtained from the current study data (likelihood function).

Figure 1.1 plots the informative prior density-obtained from the historical trial and the likelihood function–from study I. For β_0, it shows that these two curves have a good amount of overlap, which implies that the prior distribution from historical trial is compatible with the current study data on the log-transformed baseline titers. However, the informative prior density for γ_0, the change from baseline in log-titers, is totally separated from the likelihood function, which implies that the specified prior may not have good compatibility with the current study data.

Figure 1.2 gives a similar plot for study II. The informative prior density functions for both β_0 and γ_0 show clear incompatibility with the current study data. Using the historical results as the informative prior may have big impact on the Bayesian analysis in this case. This may explain the significant difference of the Bayesian analysis results from the frequentist analysis results.

Note that there were some differences between the historical study and the current studies I and II. First, the antibody titers were measured at about 6 weeks postvaccination in the historical trial while they were measured at about 4 weeks postvaccination in studies I and II. So the mean changes from baseline in the studies I and II were higher than that in the historical study (see Figures 1.1B and 1.2B). For study I, the subjects were aged 50 or above, while the subjects were aged 60 or above in study II and in the historical trial. The historical trial was conducted in the USA alone, while study I was conducted in the USA and European countries, and study II was conducted in Canada, Australia, and European countries. All these and other unidentified factors may contribute to the differences in the responses. We should consider the potential differences from the historical trial in constructing prior distributions, so the resulted prior distributions can be more compatible with the current studies.

1.3.3 Power Prior

Several methods have been proposed in the literature to construct prior distributions with discounting from historical data, including meta-analytic approach (Neuenschwander 2011), power prior (Ibrahim and Chen 2000), and commensurability priors (Hobbs et al. 2011). Here, we consider a power prior approach because there is only one historical study for these case studies. Specifically, the power prior for β_0 and γ_0 is taken as

$$\begin{aligned} \beta_0 &\sim f(\beta_0|D_0)^a \\ \gamma_0 &\sim f(\gamma_0|D_0)^b \end{aligned} \tag{1.3}$$

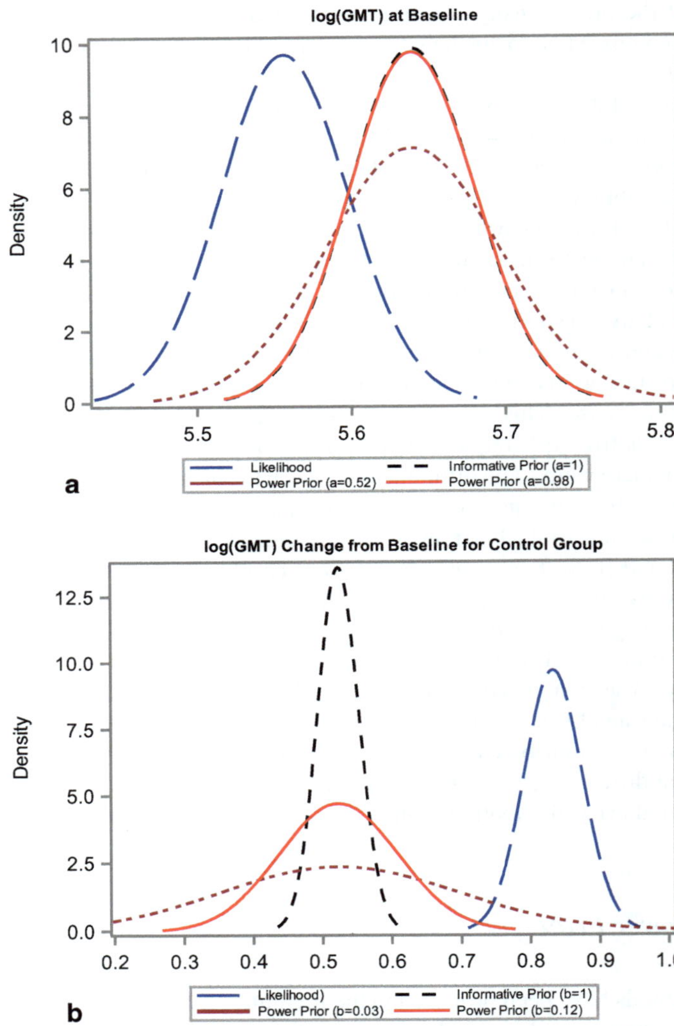

Fig. 1.1 Likelihood versus prior density plots for study I

where $f(\beta_0|D_0)$ and $f(\gamma_0|D_0)$ are the prior density functions for β_0 and γ_0 obtained from the historical data D_0. For the two case studies mentioned above, we have

$$f(\beta_0|D_0) \sim N(mean = 5.6400, sd = 0.04051)$$

$$f(\gamma_0|D_0) \sim N(mean = 0.5228, sd = 0.02937).$$

The power parameters, $0 \leq a \leq 1$ and $0 \leq b \leq 1$, are selected to control how much discount will be applied to the prior density directly obtained from the historical data. When $a = 0$ or $b = 0$, the power prior corresponds to a non-informative prior. When

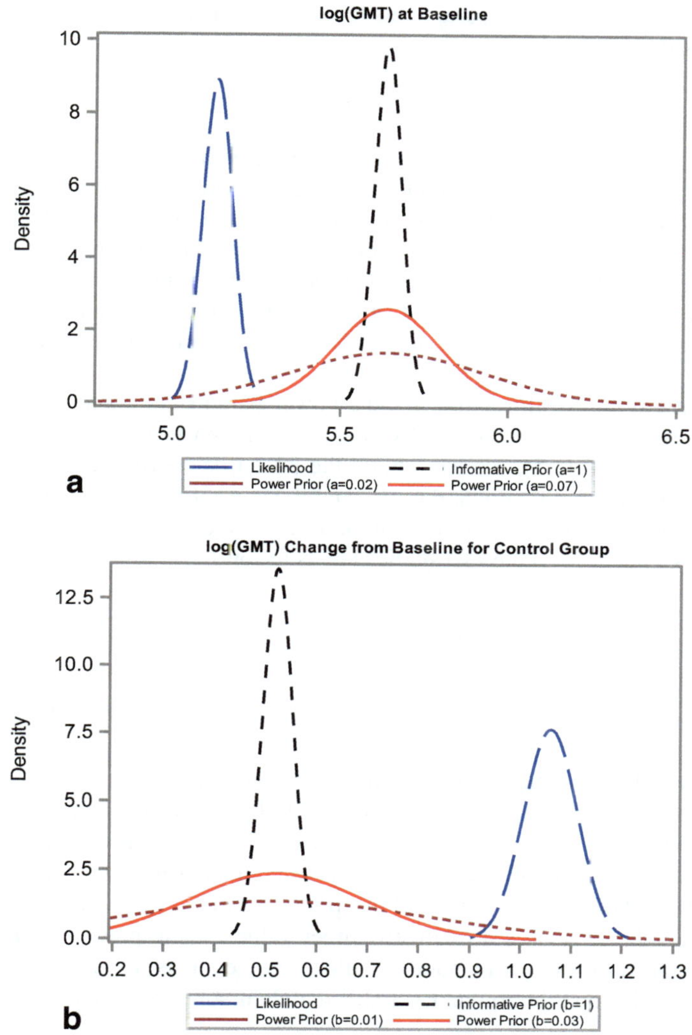

Fig. 1.2 Likelihood versus prior density plots for study II

a = 1 or b = 1, the power prior corresponds to using the entire likelihood from the historical data (i.e., the informative prior in Figures 1.1 and 1.2).

It is challenging to determine the optimum power parameters to discount the amount of previous data in constructing the prior for the current study. Chen et al. (2011) proposed to use a beta prior for the power parameter. For example, the joint prior for β_0 and a can be

$$f(\beta_0, \mathrm{a}|D_0) \sim f(\beta_0|D_0)^a a^{\omega-1}(1-a)^{\upsilon-1} \tag{1.4}$$

where ω and υ are the hyper-parameters for power parameter a. Similarly, for γ_0 and b, we consider

$$f(\gamma_0, b|D_0) \sim f(\gamma_0|D_0)^b b^{\kappa-1}(1-b)^{\psi-1} \tag{1.5}$$

where κ and ψ are the hyper-parameters for power parameter b.

However, there is no simple clinical interpretation for this random power parameter model, which poses further challenge in application to clinical trials. It has been suggested to consider multiple values for the power parameters in order to evaluate the sensitivity of the analyses to their values (e.g., Ibrahim et al. 2003; De Santis 2006). Here, we obtain certain fixed values for the power parameters based on the posterior distributions of a and b using the joint prior distribution modeling (1.4) and (1.5).

Without any prior information for the power parameters a and b, we assumed a non-informative prior beta(1,1) distribution for a and b. Using the joint density functions (1.4) and (1.5), we can obtain the posterior distributions for the power parameters giving the historical data D_0 and the current study data from study I or study II. The estimated posterior mean and 95 % credible intervals for the power parameters a and b from the two studies are as follows:

Study	Mean (CI) for a	Mean (CI) for b
I	0.521 (0.055, 0.974)	0.034 (0.0023, 0.118)
II	0.021 (0.0017, 0.068)	0.010 (0.0007, 0.033)

We considered two scenarios for choosing power parameters: one is to take the mean values and another is to select the upper bound of the credible interval. The former uses the central values from the posterior distribution as possible choices, which may still be conservative. This is because the estimated mean value may tend to discount the historical data to make the resulting prior distribution like that of the current study data. The later uses a relatively larger value for the power parameter (i.e., less discounting) which corresponds to allow more contribution from the historical data to the prior distribution and yet still maintain some minimum credibility for compatibility.

Figures 1.1 and 1.2 provide a visual display for the power prior distributions under these two scenarios for studies I and II, respectively. We can see that the power prior density with the power parameters at their mean value does have more overlap with the likelihood density of the current study, while the density with the power parameters at their upper credible interval value still provides certain amount of overlap with the likelihood density.

The Bayesian analysis results under these two power prior parameter scenarios are provided in Table 1.2. In general, the conclusions from these two power prior models are the same as that from the frequentist method. As expected, the results using the power parameter at the mean level are very close to that of the frequentist method. When we take the power parameter at the upper credible interval, the results numerically show more evidence of non-inferiority for study I, which again implies that the power may be higher after incorporating prior information in the Bayesian analysis. For study II, the results from different power parameters are fairly similar because the power parameters were very small in both scenarios. This also indicates that the data in study II may be quite different from the historical trial.

Considering that the study design and data collection in study I was more similar to that of study II, we also looked at the Bayesian analysis for study II using the control group data from study I to construct the prior. We first used the joint power prior models (1.4) and (1.5) as we did above but here the priors

$$f(\beta_0|D_0) \sim N(mean = 5.5573, sd = 0.0412)$$

$$f(\gamma_0|D_0) \sim N(mean = 0.8330, sd = 0.04125)$$

were taken from the results of the control group in study I. From the posterior distributions, we have the estimated mean and 95 % credible interval for the power parameters a: 0.035 (0.002, 0.120) and b: 0.204 (0.011, 0.807), respectively. If we take the upper bound values, i.e., a = 0.12 and b = 0.81, to construct the power priors in the Bayesian analysis, we obtain the Bayesian analysis results: $\hat{\beta}_0 = 5.222$, $\hat{\gamma}_0 = 0.919$, and estimated GMT ratio = 0.772 with a 95 % CI = (0.683, 0.872). Because the lower bound CI is greater than 0.67, this analysis shows the non-inferiority criterion is met for study II.

1.4 Conclusions and Discussions

A Bayesian approach provides an alternative method for testing non-inferiority. As compared to the frequentist methods, the Bayesian analysis can incorporate prior information, which is often available for control groups in non-inferiority studies. With non-informative priors, the results from Bayesian analysis are very similar to that from the frequentist methods. When informative prior is constructed from historical trials and applied to the non-inferiority test, the impact may depend on the consistency of the historical data with the current study data. A power prior may be considered to discount the historical data in constructing the prior distribution. We illustrate the application of Bayesian methods and compared the results with frequentist methods in two vaccine studies.

The results from the two studies showed that:

1. For study I, the estimated GMT ratios with the informative prior are closer to 1.0 compared to that from the frequentist method or Bayesian method with non-informative prior. Therefore, the Bayesian analysis with informative prior strengthened the non-inferiority test. Overall, the results are robust and the conclusions for the non-inferiority testing are the same with different choices of prior distributions.
2. For study II, however, the conclusion varied depending on the choice of prior distribution. Using the informative prior from the entire historical study data without discounting, the Bayesian analysis concluded non-inferiority for this study. However, the frequentist analysis or the Bayesian analysis with non-informative prior

or power prior (with several selected power parameters) cannot conclude a non-inferiority for the study. If we used the control group in study I to construct a power prior, the non-inferiority for study II can also be achieved. Therefore, the conclusion of the study II clearly depended on the choice of prior distribution.

These two examples show that Bayesian method has potential advantages when using informative prior constructed from previous completed trials. When the historical data for the control group are "consistent" with the current study data, the Bayesian analysis can improve testing power and show robust results. However, when there is a clear difference between the historical data and the current study data, the Bayesian analysis may conclude differently depending on the choice of prior. Therefore, the choice of prior distribution can be critical and can significantly impact the analysis results. In real clinical trials, it can be quite challenging to prespecify the informative prior because it is very difficult to assess consistency or compatibility assumptions before the study data are available.

Many factors may contribute to the difference between a historical trial and the current study under consideration. Some examples include study design, patient population, cohort effect, medical practice, etc. Because the consistency assumption is critical for Bayesian analysis, some visual display of the prior distribution densities and likelihood functions is recommended for assessing the consistency. When there are multiple historical trials, Neuenschwander et al. (2010) and Neuenschwander (2011) suggested assessing the between-trial heterogeneity to find a proper discounting of historical data in constructing prior distributions.

The power prior approach provides a reasonable tool to discount historical data for a prior distribution. As illustrated in the two examples in this chapter, it can be challenging to select a specific power parameter value. It is suggested to consider multiple values for the power parameters in order to evaluate the sensitivity of the analyses (e.g., De Santis 2006). To help selecting values for the power parameters, we considered a full Bayesian model proposed by Chen et al. (2011) including the power parameter as a random variable. The resulted posterior distribution of the power parameter provides some guidance for us to choose the values. To maximize the contribution from the historical data while still maintaining some minimum credibility for compatibility, a relatively larger value, such as the upper bound of the credible interval for the power parameter, may be used. Alternatively, the mean value for the power parameter could also be considered, which provides a more conservative analysis by taking less information from historical data into the construction of priors.

While Bayesian method may provide advantages, it still has many concerns. First, prespecify prior distributions for clinical trials is always challenging. Even if all settings between historical and current trials are very similar, there is no guarantee that the historical and current study data will have good agreement. Another concern on using Bayesian analysis in clinical trials is the overall versus independent evidence obtained from the trials. With informative prior from historical studies, the Bayesian analysis is similar to a meta-analysis which combines data from the historical and current studies for inference, while the frequentist method makes inference using the current study data only. Therefore, the Bayesian analyses for a few studies using the same historical data to construct prior may not be totally independent to each other. The details in this topic are out of the scope for this chapter (see Soon et al. 2013). Nevertheless, the Bayesian approach may serve as a reasonable sensitivity analysis rather than as a primary analysis method.

References

Blackwelder WC (1982) Proving the null hypothesis. Control Clin Trials 3:345–353
Chen M, Ibrahim J, Lam P, Yu A, Zhang Y (2011) Bayesian design of non-inferiority trials for medical devices using historical data. Biometrics 67:1163–1170
DeSantis F (2006) Power priors and their use in clinical trials. Am Stat 60:122–129
EMEA (2005) Guidance on the choice of the non-inferiority margin. European Medicines Agency, July 2005
FDA (2010) Guidance for industry non-inferiority clinical trials (draft guidance). U.S. Food and Drug Administration, March 2010
Gamalo M, Wu R, Tiwari R (2011) Bayesian approach to non-inferiority trials for proportions. J Biopharm Stat 21:902–919
Hobbs BP, Carlin BP, Mandrekar SJ, Sargent DJ (2011) Hierarchical commensurate and power prior models for adaptive incorporation of historical information in clinical trials. Biometerics 67:1047–1056
Ibrahim JG, Chen MH (2000) Power prior distributions for regression models. Stat Sci 15:46–50
Ibrahim JG, Chen MH, Sinha D (2003) On optimality properties of the power prior. J Am Stat Assoc 98:204–213
Kerzner B, Murray AV, Cheng E, Ifle R, Harvey PR, Tomlinson M, Barben JL, Rarrick K, Stek JE, Chung MO, Schodel FP, Wang WW, Xu J, Chan IS, Silber JL, Schlienger K (2007) Safety and immunogenicity profile of the concomitant administration of ZOSTAVAX and inactivated influenza vaccine in adults aged 50 and older. J Am Geriatr Soc 55:1499–1507
Liang K, Zeger S (2000) Longitudinal data analysis of continuous and discrete responses for pre-post designs. SankhyāSer B 62:134–148
Liu G, Lu K, Mogg R, Mallick M, Mehrotra D (2009) Should baseline be a covariate or dependent variable in analyses of change from baseline in clinical trials? Stat Med 28:2509–2530
Neuenschwander B (2011) From historical data to priors. Proceedings of Biopharmaceutical Section, Joint Statistical Meetings, American Statistical Association, Miami Beach, Florida, 3466–3474
Neuenschwander B, Capkun-Niggli G, Branson M, Spiegelhalter D (2010) Summarizing historical information on controls in clinical trials. Clin Trials 7:5–18
SAS Institute Inc. (2012) SAS/STAT@ 12.3 User's Guide, SAS, Cary, NC, USA
Soon G, Zhang Z, Tsong Y, Nie L (2013) Assessing overall evidence from noninferiority trials with shared historical data. Stat Med 32:2349–2363
Wang W, Mehrotra D, Chan I, Heyse J (2006) Stat considerations for non-inferiority/equivalence trials in vaccine development. J Biopharm Stat 16:429–441

Chapter 2
Bayesian Design of Noninferiority Clinical Trials with Co-primary Endpoints and Multiple Dose Comparison

Wenqing Li, Ming-Hui Chen, Huaming Tan and Dipak K. Dey

Abstract We develop a Bayesian approach for the design of noninferiority clinical trials with co-primary endpoints and multiple dose comparison. The Bayesian approach has the potential of power increase and hence sample size reduction due to the incorporation of the historical data and the correlation structure among multiple co-primary endpoints while it still maintains the family-wise type I error control without additional multiplicity adjustment. In this chapter, we compare the Bayesian method to the conventional frequentist method with or without Bonferroni multiplicity adjustment resulting from the multiple dose comparison. The proposed method is also applied to the design of a clinical trial, in which the study drug at a low dose level and at a high dose level is compared with the active control in terms of the bivariate co-primary endpoints.

2.1 Introduction

A noninferiority clinical trial is often designed to demonstrate that a test treatment is not worse than an active control or the current standard of care (SOC). Phase III confirmatory clinical trials are recently seen to be conducted via noninferiority trials in comparison with an active comparator for various reasons, including ethic compliance, comparison effectiveness, benefit and risk assessment. Details

---

W. Li (✉)
Global Biostatistical Science, Amgen Inc., 1 Amgen Center Dr., Thousand Oaks, CA 91320, USA
e-mail: Wenqingl@amgen.com

M. Chen · D. K. Dey
Department of Statistics, University of Connecticut, 215 Glenbrook Road, U-4120, Storrs, CT 06269, USA
e-mail: ming-hui.chen@uconn.edu

D. K. Dey
e-mail: dipak.dey@uconn.edu

H. Tan
Clinical Statistics, Global Innovative Pharma Business, Pfizer Inc., 445 Eastern Point Road, Groton, CT 06340, USA
e-mail: huaming.tan@pfizer.com

Z. Chen et al. (eds.), *Applied Statistics in Biomedicine and Clinical Trials Design*,
ICSA Book Series in Statistics, DOI 10.1007/978-3-319-12694-4_2

of medical reasons and the inherent issues of the conduction of a non-inferiority trial have been discussed extensively (CPMP 2000). A number of health authorities guidelines, including the draft guidance from the US Food and Drug Administration (FDA), have been released to guide the pharmaceutical industry to conduct non-inferiority trials (CPMP Working Party on Efficacy of Medicinal Products Note for Guidance III/3630/92-EN 1995, CHMP 2005, FDA Guidance for industry 2010, ICH Harmonised tripartite guideline 1998, ICH Harmonized tripartite guideline 2000).

There is a substantial literature on both the frequentist design and the Bayesian design for a simple noninferiority clinical trial to compare a test treatment with a control in terms of one primary endpoint, including Liu and Chang (2011) and Chen et al. (2011). Often there is only one primary endpoint involved in the hypothesis testing in a clinical trial. But sometimes multiple endpoints are simultaneously tested in a trial even though the formulation of hypotheses may be different depending on the study objectives, the study design, and the nature of multiplicity. Several corresponding statistical methods have been proposed. Sugimoto et al. (2012) present a convenient formula for sample size calculation in clinical trials with multiple co-primary continuous endpoints. Laska et al. (1992) extend the well-known optimality of the *min* test in the univariate case to the multivariate case and apply to superiority hypothesis testing on multiple endpoints. Kong et al. (2004) adopt the *min* test to non-inferiority hypothesis testing for multiple endpoints following a multivariate normal distribution.

The clinical trial with multiple co-primary endpoints is a special case of the one with multiple endpoints, in which all endpoints are equally important clinically. The conventional frequentist approach for a clinical trial with multiple co-primary endpoints is via the intersection–union testing (IUT; Eaton and Muirhead 2007). Recently, new statistical approaches have been developed to achieve a higher power while the family-wise type I error rate is still controlled. For example, Chuang-Stein et al. (2007) propose an approach based on the notion of controlling the average type I error rate over a restricted null space rather than over the conventional full null space. The other Bayesian approaches include Gonen et al. (2003) and Scott and Berger (2006). While most clinical trials compare two treatments, some trials compare three or more medications, multiple doses of medications, or medical devices against each other or against the standard treatment, which often leads to the multiplicity issue. If the global hypothesis involves multiple comparisons, an appropriate multiplicity adjustment method is required in order to control the family-wise type I error rate. Dmitrienko et al. (2010) give a comprehensive review on the multiple testing procedures widely used in clinical studies, including procedures based on univariate *p* values (e.g., Bonferroni, Holm, fixed-sequence, Simes, Hommel, and Hochberg procedures), parametric procedures, and resampling-based procedures. A noninferiority clinical trial involving multiple dose levels for a study drug is often designed to demonstrate the noninferiority of the study drug under at least one dose level; hence, it is a typical multiple testing problem and an appropriate multiplicity adjustment method is required in a frequentist design. By now, there is a rich literature on the frequentist design of a noninferiority trial with multiple tests, including Ng (2003), Hung and Wang (2004), Tsong and Zhang (2007), and Röhmel and Pigeot (2010).

In this chapter, we develop a Bayesian approach for noninferiority clinical trials with co-primary endpoints and multiple dose comparison by incorporating historical data. One of the advantages of the Bayesian approach is that it has the potential of increasing power and reducing sample size due to the incorporation of historical data and the correlation structure among the multiple co-primary endpoints. Another advantage of the proposed Bayesian approach is to control the family-wise type I error automatically without an additional multiplicity adjustment. The Bayesian method is also demonstrated and compared with the conventional frequentist method with or without Bonferroni multiplicity adjustment via the design of a clinical trial.

The rest of the chapter is organized as follows. A motivation example of a noninferiority clinical trial with co-primary endpoints and multiple dose comparison is described in Sect. 2.2. In Sect. 2.3, firstly the statistical settings of the noninferiority clinical trial with co-primary endpoints and multiple dose comparison are introduced. Then the conventional frequentist approach is briefly reviewed, and the Bayesian method using the commonly used conjugate prior and the power prior with fixed power parameter(s) to incorporate historical data for the control group is proposed and described. In Sect. 2.4, the proposed Bayesian method is applied to the noninferiority clinical trial described in Sect. 2.2 in comparison with the conventional frequentist method. Finally, the chapter ends with the conclusion and discussion in Sect. 2.5.

2.2 Design of a Noninferiority Clinical Trial with Two Co-primary Endpoints and Multiple Dose Comparison

An experiment agent is currently in mid to the late-stage development as a treatment of signs and symptoms of benign prostatic hyperplasia or hypertrophy (BPH). BPH is a chronic and progressive condition that adversely affects health-related quality of life (HRQoL) by interfering with normal daily activities and sleep patterns. The International Prostate Symptom Score (IPSS) ranging from 0 to 35, also known as the American Urologic Association Symptom Score (AUA-SS), is collected in a questionnaire. The change of IPSS from the baseline score (denoted by ΔIPSS thereafter) is one of the primary endpoints for all drug trials in the treatment of BPH. Although it is not mandatory, the change from baseline maximum urinary flow rate (denoted by ΔQmax thereafter) is recommended as another co-primary endpoint by European regulatory authority. In addition, the smaller ΔIPSS is and the bigger ΔQmax is, the better the treatment effect of the test drug is.

A non-inferiority clinical trial design demonstrating that at least one dose regime of 15 mg QD or 30 mg QD of the experiment compound is non-inferior to the active comparator, Tamsulosin, the SOC for BPH, is explored to support further development of the experiment compound.

Based on the above consideration, a hypothetical study will be a multicenter, double-blind, three-arm parallel trial. The patients will be on placebo for 4 weeks before they are randomized to one of the three arms: 15 mg QD and 30 mg QD of

Table 2.1 Summary statistics (n, mean ± standard deviation and correlation) of ΔIPSS and ΔQmax for Tamsulosin

Study	n	ΔIPSS	ΔQmax (ml/s)	Correlation coefficient between ΔIPSS and ΔQmax
1	244	−5.1±6.4	1.52±3.59	N/A
2	34	−7.03±5.84	1.68±4.08	−0.29

IPSS International Prostate Symptom Score

the experiment compound, and Tamsulosin 0.4 mg QD dose group, for 12 weeks. After the 12-week double-blind treatment period, the patients who are randomized to the experiment compound will remain on the same treatment, and the patients who are on Tamsulosin will be re-randomized at the end of 12-week treatment to one of the dose groups of the experiment compound for another 40 weeks to assess the safety and tolerability of the compound. The two co-primary endpoints are ΔIPSS and ΔQmax at the end of the 12-week double-blind treatment period.

Historical data are available from the two previous studies on Tamsulosin capsule 0.4 mg QD regime. The first study was a multicenter, randomized, double-blind, placebo-controlled, parallel group, phase III trial to evaluate the efficacy and safety of Tamsulosin for the treatment of patients with symptoms of moderate to severe BPH (Narayan and Ashutosh Tewari 1998). This study was conducted by Boehringer Ingelheim Pharmaceuticals, Inc. in 1993. The second study was a multicenter, randomized, double-blind, placebo-controlled, parallel group, phase II trial to evaluate the efficacy and safety of an experiment compound in the treatment of patients with lower urinary tract symptoms (LUTS), in which Tamsulosin was an active comparator (Tamimi et al. 2010). This study was conducted by Pfizer Inc. in 2007. Summary statistics for ΔIPSS and ΔQmax for the active comparator of Tamsulosin from these two studies are shown in Table 2.1. The pooled standard deviations (SD) for ΔIPSS and ΔQmax are 6.34 and 3.70 ml/s, respectively. In addition, clinically meaningful non-inferiority margins for ΔIPSS and ΔQmax are chosen to be 1 and −0.6 ml/s, respectively, to design the noninferiority trial. The historical data in Table 2.1 is incorporated in the Bayesian design developed in the subsequent sections.

2.3 Methodology

2.3.1 Assumption and Notation

We assume that there are three treatments in a clinical trial, including the study drug at a high dose level, the study drug at a low dose level, and the (active) control treatment, denoted by the h, l, and c (treatment) groups, respectively. The objective of the study is to show non-inferiority of the study drug at a (high or low) dose level compared to the control group.

Let $\{y_{gi}, i = 1, 2, \ldots, n_g\}$ be a J-dimensional random sample of size n_g collected for the gth group. Furthermore, given μ_g and Σ, we assume that y_{gi} follows a multivariate normal $N_J(\mu_g, \Sigma)$ distribution, where μ_g is the mean vector for the gth group, and Σ is the common variance covariance matrix for all the groups with the dimension of $J \times J$. Let $\theta = (\mu_h, \mu_l, \mu_c, \Sigma)$ denote the collection of parameters.

Without loss of genercsity, we assume there are two co-primary endpoints, i.e., $J = 2$, where a smaller value of the first co-primary endpoint is better and a larger value of the second co-primary endpoint is better. Assume $\mu_g = (\mu_{g1}, \mu_{g2})'$, where μ_{g1} and μ_{g2} are the true means for the two co-primary endpoints for the gth group, respectively. The noninferiority hypotheses comparing the gth study drug group, $g = h, l$, with the control group can be formulated as H_{0g}: $\mu_{g1} - \mu_{c1} \geq \delta_{g1}$ or $\mu_{g2} - \mu_{c2} \leq \delta_{g2}$ versus H_{1g}: $\mu_{g1} - \mu_{c1} < \delta_{g1}$ and $\mu_{g2} - \mu_{c2} > \delta_{g2}$, where δ_{g1} and δ_{g2} are the noninferiority margins of the co-primary endpoints. Let $\delta_g = (\delta_{g1}, \delta_{g2})'$ for $g = h, l$. The noninferiority margins should be the same for both high and low doses in the comparison and, hence, we assume that $\delta_h = \delta_l = \delta$, where $\delta = (\delta_1, \delta_2)'$, in the subsequent sections. The objective of the study is to demonstrate non-inferiority of the study drug at a dose level after the noninferiority margin is chosen based on both clinical and statistical considerations.

We assume that $\{y_{gi}, i = 1, \ldots, n_g\}$, $g = h, l, c$, are independent across the groups. The likelihood function of the data can be written as

$$
\begin{aligned}
f(\theta|D) &\propto \Pi_{g=h,l,c}|\Sigma|^{-\frac{n_g}{2}} \exp\left(-\frac{1}{2}\sum_{i=1}^{n_g}(y_{gi} - \mu_g)'\Sigma^{-1}(y_{gi} - \mu_g)\right) \\
&= \Pi_{g=h,l,c}|\Sigma|^{-\frac{n_g}{2}} \exp\Big(-\frac{1}{2}tr\left(\sum_{i=1}^{n_g}(y_{gi} - \bar{y}_g\right)(y_{gi} - \bar{y}_g)'\Sigma^{-1} \\
&\quad + n_g(\mu_g - \bar{y}_g)(\mu_g - \bar{y}_g)'\Sigma^{-1})\Big),
\end{aligned}
$$

where $\bar{y}_g = (\sum_{i=1}^{n_g} y_{gi})/n_g$, and the data $D = \{(y_{gi}, y_{lj}, y_{ck}),\ i = 1, \ldots, n_h,\ j = 1, \ldots, n_l, k = 1, \ldots, n_c\}$.

2.3.2 *Preliminary: The Frequentist Design*

Under the multivariate normal assumption, $(\bar{y}_h, \bar{y}_l, \bar{y}_c, S)$ are the sufficient statistics, where S denotes the pooled matrix of sums of squares and cross products: $S = \sum_g (n_g - 1)S_g$, $g = h, l, c$, and $S_g = \left(\sum_{i=1}^{n_g}(y_{gi} - \bar{y}_g)(y_{gi} - \bar{y}_g)'\right)/(n_g - 1)$.

Let $\mathbf{W}_h = (n_h n_c/(n_h + n_c))^{1/2}(\bar{y}_h - \bar{y}_c - \delta)$, and $\mathbf{W}_l = (n_l n_c/(n_l + n_c))^{1/2}(\bar{y}_l - \bar{y}_c - \delta)$. Then $\mathbf{W}_h$ and S are independent, and $\mathbf{W}_l$ and S are independent, with $\mathbf{W}_h \sim N((n_h n_c/(n_h+n_c))^{1/2}(\mu_h - \mu_c - \delta), \Sigma)$, $\mathbf{W}_l \sim N((n_l n_c/(n_l+n_c))^{1/2}(\mu_l - \mu_c - \delta), \Sigma)$, and $S \sim \text{Wishart}(n, \Sigma)$, where $n = n_h + n_l + n_c - 3$.

In the conventional frequentist design, an appropriate multiplicity adjustment method due to the multiple dose comparisons must be adopted in order to control the family-wise type I error rate. Let α denote the desired overall one-sided significance level, and assume Bonferroni multiplicity adjustment is used to assign significance levels to comparisons of the study drug at the high and the low dose levels to the control group. Suppose that we consider the comparison of the study drug at either the high or the low dose level with the control group first. The standard test involves testing the two endpoints separately at the same significance level of $\alpha/2$ using the one-sided t tests, and rejecting the null hypothesis H_{0g} (in favor of the alternative hypothesis H_{1g}) if and only if the two separate t test statistics are significant. Specifically, let $\mathbf{W}_g = (W_{g1}, W_{g2})'$, $g = h, l$, and define $T_{g1} = W_{g1}(s_{11}/n)^{-1/2}$ and $T_{g2} = W_{g2}(s_{22}/n)^{-1/2}$, where s_{11} and s_{22} are the diagonal elements of S. T_{gd} has a standard t distribution with degrees of freedom of n when the dth element of $\mu_g - \mu_c - \delta$ is zero ($d = 1, 2$). The standard test rejects H_{0g} if and only if $\max_d T_{gd} \leq c_{\alpha/2}$, where $c_{\alpha/2}$ is the $(\alpha/2)$th quantile of the t distribution with degrees of freedom of n. Eaton and Muirhead (Eaton and Muirhead 2007) show that the standard test is an IUT and the size of the test is $\alpha/2$. Moreover, the standard test may be conservative because the two statistics T_{gd}, $d = 1, 2$, are assumed independent. The type I error rate approaches to $\alpha/2$ as the correlation coefficient of the two end points approaches to one.

Note that the assumption of the equal variance covariance for all groups could be relaxed if necessary. For example, Welch's t test (Welch 1947) is an adaptation of the Student's t test when the two samples have possibly unequal variances. Specifically, the test statistic is given by $T = (\bar{X}_1 - \bar{X}_2)(S_1^2/n_1 + S_2^2/n_2)^{-1/2}$, where $\bar{X}_i$, S_i^2, and n_i, $i = 1, 2$, are the ith sample mean, sample variance, and sample size, respectively. The degrees of freedom ν associated with the test can be approximated by

$$\nu = (S_1^2/n_1 + S_2^2/n_2)^2/[S_1^4/\{n_1^2(n_1 - 1)\} + S_2^4/\{n_2^2(n_2 - 1)\}].$$

2.3.3 The Proposed Bayesian Design

Following Chen et al. (2011), let $\pi^{(f)}(\theta)$ be the fitting prior and also let $\pi^{(s)}(\theta)$ be the sampling prior. The fitting prior is used to perform Bayesian analysis once data are collected. The sampling prior is the distribution for the parameters which we believe the future data would follow, and it is used to generate psuedo-data for the design evaluation, i.e., the type I error and power assessment. We assume the hypotheses: H_{0g}: $\eta_g(\theta) \geq \eta^*(\delta)$ versus H_{1g}: $\eta_g(\theta) < \eta^*(\delta)$, where $\eta^* = (\delta_1, -\delta_2)'$, $\eta_g(\theta) = (\mu_{g1} - \mu_{c1}, -(\mu_{g2} - \mu_{c2}))'$, the subscript $g = h$ is for the comparison between the high dose group of the study drug and the control group, and $g = l$ is for the comparison between the low dose group of the study drug and the control group.

Define the key quantity:

$$\beta_s = E_s\left[\mathbf{1}\{\cup_{g=h,l}\{P(\eta_g(\theta) < \eta^*(\delta)|D) \geq \gamma_g\}\}\right], \tag{2.1}$$

where $\mathbf{1}(\cdot)$ is the indicator function, and γ_g is a prespecified credible level in (0, 1), e.g., 0.95. It is reasonable to assume that $\gamma_h = \gamma_l = \gamma$ for our scenario since there is no differentiation for the high and low dose group comparisons with the control group in terms of γ_g. Therefore, we use the same credible level γ in β_s in the subsequent sections. The probability in (2.1) is calculated with respected to the posterior distribution of θ, given the data D and the fitting prior $\pi^{(f)}(\theta)$, and the expectation is taken with respect to the marginal distribution of the data under the sampling prior $\pi^{(s)}(\theta)$.

We use the same Bayesian sample size determination algorithm from (Chen et al. 2011). Let Θ_0 and Θ_1 denote the parameter spaces corresponding to the null and alternative hypothesis, respectively, and let $\bar{\Theta}_0$ and $\bar{\Theta}_1$ be the closure of Θ_0 and Θ_1. Further, let $\pi_0^{(s)}(\theta)$ be the sampling prior with support $\Theta_B = \bar{\Theta}_0 \cap \bar{\Theta}_1$ and let $\pi_1^{(s)}(\theta)$ be the sampling prior with support $\Theta_1^* \subset \Theta_1$. For given $\alpha_0 > 0$ and $\alpha_1 > 0$, we compute

$$n_{\alpha_0} = \min\{n : \beta_{s0} \leq \alpha_0\}; \quad n_{\alpha_1} = \min\{n : \beta_{s1} \geq 1 - \alpha_1\}, \tag{2.2}$$

where β_{s0} and β_{s1} in (2.2) are the β_s's in (2.1) by letting $\pi^{(s)}(\theta)$ be $\pi_0^{(s)}(\theta)$ and $\pi_1^{(s)}(\theta)$, respectively, and they are the Bayesian type I error and power, respectively. The Bayesian sample size is given by $n_B = \max\{n_{\alpha_0}, n_{\alpha_1}\}$. One possible choice of γ is 0.975, which is comparable to a significant level of 0.05/2 used for the individual hypothesis test under the frequentist design with multiplicity adjustment. Common choices of α_0 and α_1 include $\alpha_0 = 0.05$ and $\alpha_1 = 0.2$ so that in a Bayesian design with sample size n_B, the family-wise type I error rate is less than or equal to 0.05 and the power is at least 0.8. The choice of Θ_1^* is often related to the design margins δ_d's. For example, for a continuous endpoint, a typical choice of μ_{gd} in Θ_1^* for the noninferiority hypothesis testing is μ_{cd}.

Historical data can be incorporated via the different forms of the fitting prior, including the power prior with a fixed or random or mixture power parameter, the hierarchical prior, and the hierarchical commensurate and power prior. In this chapter, for simplicity, we consider the commonly used conjugate prior and the power prior with a fixed power parameter. Often the historical data are only available for the control group; hence, a noninformative fitting prior is assumed for the study drug.

2.3.4 *The Conjugate Prior*

The conjugate priors for the unknown parameters $\theta = (\mu_h, \mu_l, \mu_c, \Sigma)$ are given as

$$\Sigma \sim \text{Inv–Wishart}_{\nu_0}(\Lambda_0),$$
$$\mu_g|\Sigma \sim N(\mu_{g0}, \Sigma/\kappa_{g0}),$$

where ν_0, Λ_0, μ_{g0}, and κ_{g0} are known constants. The posterior distributions for (μ_g, Σ), $g = h, l, c$, are in the same families as the prior distributions but with updated parameters. Specifically, the marginal posterior distribution for μ_g is a multivariate

t distribution:

$$\mu_g|D \sim t_{\nu_n - J+1}\left(\mu_{gn}, \frac{\Lambda_n}{\kappa_{gn}(\nu_n - J + 1)}\right),$$

the marginal distribution of Σ is an Inverse–Wishart distribution:

$$\Sigma|D \sim \text{Inv–Wishart}_{\nu_n}(\Lambda_n),$$

and the conditional distribution of μ_g given Σ is a multivariate normal:

$$\mu_g|\Sigma, D \sim N(\mu_{gn}, \Sigma/\kappa_{gn}),$$

where $J = 2$, $\mu_{gn} = \frac{\kappa_{g0}}{\kappa_{g0}+n_g}\mu_{g0} + \frac{n_g}{\kappa_{g0}+n_g}\bar{y}_g$, $\kappa_{gn} = \kappa_{g0} + n_g$, $\nu_n = \nu_0 + n_h + n_l + n_c$, $\Lambda_n = \Lambda_0 + \sum_{g=h,l,c}\left\{S_{gn} + \frac{\kappa_{g0}n_g}{\kappa_{g0}+n_g}(\bar{y}_g - \mu_{g0})(\bar{y}_g - \mu_{g0})'\right\}$, and $S_{gn} = \sum_{i=1}^{n_g}(y_{gi} - \bar{y}_g)(y_{gi} - \bar{y}_g)'$.

Samples from the joint posterior distribution for (μ_g, Σ), $g = h, l, c$, can be obtained using the following procedure:

Step 1. Draw $\Sigma|D \sim \text{Inv–Wishart}_{\nu_n}(\Lambda_n)$
Step 2. Independently draw $\mu_g|\Sigma, D \sim N(\mu_{gn}, \Sigma/\kappa_{gn}), g = h, l, c$.

The following is a computation algorithm to compute the study type I error or power for given n_g, δ, γ, M (number of Monte Carlo samples), and N (number of simulations):

Step 1. Generate θ from the sampling prior, i.e., $\theta \sim \pi^{(s)}(\theta)$.
Step 2. Generate data from the multivariate normal distribution, i.e., $y_g \sim N(\mu_g, \Sigma)$, $g = h, l, c$.
Step 3. Generate M samples $\theta^{(m)}$, $m = 1, \ldots, M$, from the joint posterior distribution using the algorithm shown above.
Step 4. Compute $\hat{P}_g = M^{-1}\sum_{m=1}^{M}\mathbf{1}\{\eta_g(\theta^{(m)}) < \eta^*(\delta)\}$, and check whether $\hat{P}_g \geq \gamma$ or not.
Step 5. Repeat steps 1–4 N times, then calculate the proportion of $\{\cup_{g=h,l}\hat{P}_g \geq \gamma\}$ among those N times, which gives an estimate of β_s, i.e., the type I error or power.

For the sample size determination, we need to repeat the above procedure for other scenarios of different combinations of n_g's and then choose the optimal combination of n_g's as the desired sample size under which both the type I error and power satisfy the design requirement.

A Special Case: The Noninformative Prior. In order to facilitate the comparison between the Bayesian approach and the frequentist approach, it is desirable to specify a noninformative prior in the Bayesian approach. A commonly used noninformative prior is the multivariate Jeffreys prior, $\pi(\mu_g, \Sigma) \propto |\Sigma|^{-\frac{J+1}{2}}$, which is the limit of the conjugate prior as $\kappa_{g0} \to 0$, $\nu_0 \to -1$, and $|\Lambda_0| \to 0$, $g = h, l, c$. Consequently, the corresponding posterior distribution can be obtained by

$$\Sigma|D \sim \text{Inv–Wishart}_{n_h+n_l+n_c-1}(S_{hn} + S_{ln} + S_{cn}),$$

$$\mu_g|\Sigma, D \sim N(\bar{y}_g, \Sigma/n_g).$$

The computational algorithm to determine the sample size is exactly same as that described above except for the Monte Carlo sampling steps, where the samples of parameters are drawn from a different posterior distribution. In addition, the marginal distribution for μ_g is a multivariate t distribution:

$$t_{n_h+n_l+n_c-J}(\bar{y}_g, S_{gn}/(n_g(n_h+n_l+n_c-J))),$$

where $J = 2$.

2.3.5 *The Power Prior*

We extend the power prior of (Ibrahim and Chen 2000) to construct the fitting prior for μ_c and Σ. In general, we assume that there are a total of K sets of historical data available for the control group, denoted by $y_{c0k} = (y_{c0ki}, i = 1, 2, \ldots, n_{0k})'$, $k = 1, 2, \ldots, K$, where n_{0k} is the number of samples collected in the kth historical dataset. Furthermore, we let $y_{c0} = ((y_{c01})', (y_{c02})', \ldots, (y_{c0K})')'$ denote all the K historical datasets.

We consider the power prior with a fixed power parameter $\mathbf{a}_0$ for μ_c and Σ as

$$\pi(\mu_c, \Sigma|y_{c0}, \mathbf{a}_0)$$
$$\propto \prod_{k=1}^{K}\left[|\Sigma|^{-\frac{n_{0k}}{2}} \exp\left(-\frac{1}{2}\sum_{i=1}^{n_{0k}}(y_{c0ki}-\mu_c)'\Sigma^{-1}(y_{c0ki}-\mu_c)\right)\right]^{a_{0k}} \pi_0(\mu_c, \Sigma), \quad (2.3)$$

where $\mathbf{a}_0 = (a_{01}, \ldots, a_{0K})'$, $0 \le a_{0k} \le 1$, for $k = 1, \ldots, K$, and $\pi_0(\mu_c, \Sigma)$ is an initial prior. When $\pi_0(\mu_c, \Sigma) \propto |\Sigma|^{-(d+1)/2}$, i.e., the noninformative Jeffreys prior, (2.3) can reduce to the conjugate prior

$$\Sigma|y_{c0}, \mathbf{a}_0 \sim \text{Inv–Wishart}_{\nu_0}(\Lambda_0),$$
$$\mu_c|\Sigma, y_{c0}, \mathbf{a}_0 \sim N\left(\sum_{k=1}^{K}(a_{0k}n_{0k}\bar{y}_{c0k})/n_0(\mathbf{a}_0), \Sigma/\kappa_{c0}\right),$$

where

$$\Lambda_0 = \sum_{k=1}^{K} a_{0k}S_{0k} + \sum_{k=1}^{K}(a_{0k}n_{0k}\bar{y}_{c0k}\bar{y}_{c0k}')$$
$$-\sum_{k=1}^{K}(a_{0k}n_{0k}\bar{y}_{c0k})\sum_{k=1}^{K}(a_{0k}n_{0k}\bar{y}_{c0k})'/n_0(\mathbf{a}_0),$$

$S_{0k} = \sum_{i=1}^{n_{0k}}(y_{c0ki} - \bar{y}_{c0k})(y_{c0ki} - \bar{y}_{c0k})'$, $\bar{y}_{c0k} = \left(\sum_{i=1}^{n_{0k}} y_{c0ki}\right)/n_{0k}$, $\nu_0 = n_0(\mathbf{a}_0) - 1$, $\kappa_{c0} = n_0(\mathbf{a}_0) = \sum_{k=1}^{K} a_{0k}n_{0k}$. Then, the computational algorithms developed in Sect. 2.3.4 for the conjugate prior can be applied here correspondingly.

2.4 Application to the Design of a Non-inferiority Trial

In this section, we apply the proposed Bayesian approach to the design of the non-inferiority trial described in Sect. 2.2. We use simulations to investigate the performance of the proposed approach in terms of the type I error and power, and compare the Bayesian approach with the conventional frequentist approach with or without the Bonferroni multiplicity adjustment. We assume the data corresponding to the high dose group of the study drug, the low dose group of the study drug, and the control group have the distributions $y_{gi}|\mu_g, \Sigma \sim N_2(\mu_g, \Sigma)$, where μ_g is the mean vector for the gth group, Σ is the common variance covariance matrix for all groups, and $i = 1, 2, \cdots, n_g$. Let $\mu_g = (\mu_{g1}, \mu_{g2})'$, where μ_{g1} and μ_{g2} are the true means for the two co-primary endpoints, respectively, for the gth group. We choose the point mass sampling priors as commonly used in the frequentist trial design and trial analysis. That is, we let

$$\pi^{(s)}(\mu_g) = \begin{cases} 1 & \text{if } \mu_g = \mu_g^{(s)} \\ 0 & \text{otherwise} \end{cases} \quad \text{and} \quad \pi^{(s)}(\Sigma) = \begin{cases} 1 & \text{if } \Sigma = \Sigma^{(s)} \\ 0 & \text{otherwise,} \end{cases}$$

where $\mu_c^{(s)}$ and $\Sigma^{(s)}$ are prespecified values. The sample size is also allowed to change in the simulations, which can be used for the sample size determination during the design stage. The design strategy is to find a minimum total size n, i.e., $n = n_h + n_l + n_c$, so that the power is at least 80 % and the type I error is controlled at 5 %.

Figure 2.1 shows mean vectors of the two co-primary endpoints for the control group from the two historical data as well as the pooled mean vector. We assume that the mean vector for the co-primary endpoints for the control group for the future data is a linear combination of the mean vector from the first historical data, $\bar{y}_{c01} = c(-5.1, 1.52)'$, and the mean vector from the pooled historical data, $\bar{y}_{c0\cdot} = c(-5.34, 1.54)'$. That is, $\mu_c^{(s)}$ is chosen to be any point on the line interval of AC in Fig. 2.1. Moreover, $\Sigma^{(s)}$ is chosen to be that the variance components are the pooled variances for the two co-primary endpoints from the two historical trials, i.e., 6.34^2 and 3.70^2, respectively, and the correlation coefficient to be -0.29, estimated from the second historical study. The design value of $\mu_g^{(s)}$, $g = h, l$ is chosen according to the type I error or power evaluation.

Let $\delta = (\delta_1, \delta_2)' = (1, -0.6)'$. For the type I error evaluation, we simulate the data from the sampling priors with parameters of $\mu_h^{(s)} = \mu_c^{(s)} + \delta$, $\mu_l^{(s)} = \mu_c^{(s)} + \delta$, or $\mu_h^{(s)} = \mu_c^{(s)} + (\delta_1, 0)'$, $\mu_l^{(s)} = \mu_c^{(s)} + (\delta_1, 0)'$, or $\mu_h^{(s)} = \mu_c^{(s)} + (0, \delta_2)'$, $\mu_l^{(s)} = \mu_c^{(s)} + (0, \delta_2)'$, and define the type I error for the design as the maximum type I error. For the power evaluation, we let the sampling prior parameters be $\mu_h^{(s)} = \mu_c^{(s)}$, $\mu_l^{(s)} = \mu_c^{(s)}$, or $\mu_h^{(s)} = \mu_c^{(s)} + (\delta_1, 0)'$, $\mu_l^{(s)} = \mu_c^{(s)}$, or $\mu_h^{(s)} = \mu_c^{(s)} + (0, \delta_2)'$, $\mu_l^{(s)} = \mu_c^{(s)}$, or $\mu_h^{(s)} = \mu_c^{(s)} + (\delta_1, \delta_2)'$, $\mu_l^{(s)} = \mu_c^{(s)}$, and define the power for the design as the minimum power.

We use the power prior in Sect. 2.3.5 to incorporate the two historical data for the control group and use a power prior with an approximately noninformative prior

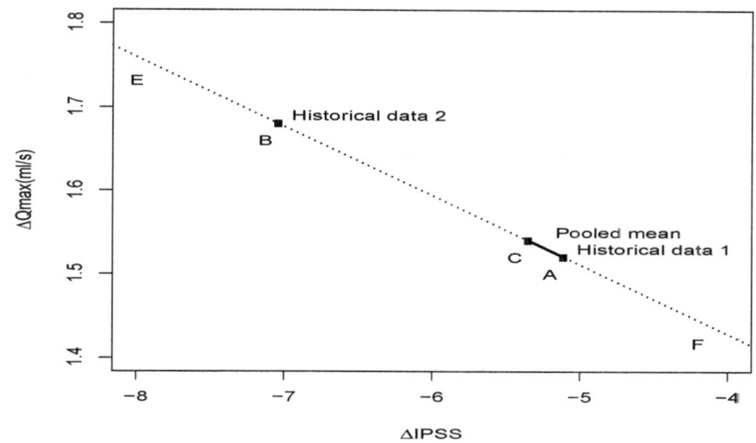

Fig. 2.1 The means of the two co-primary endpoints for the control group from the historical data, where points A, B, and C represent the mean vector of the two co-primary endpoints from the *historical data 1*, the *historical data 2*, and the *pooled historical data*, respectively

for the high and low dose groups. Specifically, we assume the fitting priors for μ_g, $g = h, l, c$, and Σ as

$$\Sigma_g^{(f)} \sim \text{Inv–Wishart}_{\nu_0}(\Lambda_0),$$
$$\mu_g^{(f)}|\Sigma \sim N(\mu_{g0}, \Sigma/\kappa_{g0}),$$

where $\nu_0 = n_0(\mathbf{a}_0) - 1$, $\Lambda_0 = \sum_{k=1}^{K} a_{0k} S_{0k} + \sum_{k=1}^{K} (a_{0k} n_{0k} \bar{y}_{c0k} \bar{y}'_{c0k}) - \sum_{k=1}^{K} (a_{0k} n_{0k} \bar{y}_{c0k}) \times \sum_{k=1}^{K} (a_{0k} n_{0k} \bar{y}_{c0k})'/n_0(\mathbf{a}_0)$, $S_{0k} = \sum_{i=1}^{n_{0k}} (y_{c0ki} - \bar{y}_{c0k})(y_{c0ki} - \bar{y}_{c0k})'$, $\bar{y}_{c0k} = \left(\sum_{i=1}^{n_{0k}} y_{c0ki}\right)/n_{0k}$, $\kappa_{c0} = n_0(\mathbf{a}_0) = \sum_{k=1}^{K} a_{0k} n_{0k}$, $\kappa_{h0} = \kappa_{l0} = 0.1$, $\mu_{c0} = \sum_{k=1}^{K} (a_{0k} n_{0k} \bar{y}_{c0k})/n_0(\mathbf{a}_0)$, $K = 2$. As κ_{h0} and κ_{l0} are very small, the choices of μ_{h0} and μ_{l0} would not matter much. For simplicity, we chose $\mu_{h0} = \mu_{l0} = \mu_c^{(s)}$.

As the sample correlation coefficient for the first historical trial was not reported, we use the following Bayesian approach to impute the sample correlation coefficient based on the two historical datasets. Suppose the variance–covariance matrix $\Sigma = \begin{pmatrix} \sigma_{11} & \sigma_{12} \\ \sigma_{12} & \sigma_{22} \end{pmatrix}$. Then, $S_{01} = (n-1)S_1 \sim \text{Wishart}_{n_{01}-1}(\Sigma)$, where S_1 denotes the sample variance covariance matrix for the two co-primary endpoints from the first historical trial, and $\text{Wishart}_{n_{01}-1}(\Sigma)$ denotes the Wishart distribution with $n_{01} - 1$ degrees of freedom and a positive definite 2×2 scale matrix Σ. Thus, the density function of S_1 is

$$p(S_1|\Sigma) \propto |\Sigma|^{-\frac{n-1}{2}} |(n_{01}-1)S_1|^{\frac{n_{01}-4}{2}} \exp\{-(1/2)tr((n_{01}-1)\Sigma^{-1}S_1)\}. \quad (2.4)$$

Suppose the sample variance–covariance matrix is written as $S_1 = \frac{S_{01}}{n_{01}-1} = \begin{pmatrix} s_{11} & s_{12} \\ s_{12} & s_{22} \end{pmatrix}$. For the first historical dataset, the off-diagonal elements of S_1 are unknown. We combine the two historical trials together to recover the missing sample correlation coefficient. Denote the sample correlation coefficient for the first historical data as $r_1 = s_{12}(s_{11}s_{22})^{-1/2}$. If we can derive the distribution of r_1 given Σ, s_{11}, and s_{22}, say, $f(r_1|\Sigma, s_{11}, s_{22})$, we can use the Bayesian sampling technique to draw r_1 based on the samples of Σ from the posterior distribution of $\Sigma | y_{c0}, \mathbf{a}_0$, and $f(r_1|\Sigma, s_{11}, s_{22})$.

For the case of two co-primary endpoints, the density of r_1 can be written explicitly as

$$
\begin{aligned}
f(r_1|\Sigma, s_{11}, s_{22}) &\propto (1-r_1^2)^{\frac{n_{01}-4}{2}} \\
&\times \exp\left\{ -\frac{(n_{01}-1)}{2} tr \left(\begin{pmatrix} \sigma_{11} & \sigma_{12} \\ \sigma_{12} & \sigma_{22} \end{pmatrix}^{-1} \begin{pmatrix} s_{11} & r_1\sqrt{s_{11}s_{22}} \\ r_1\sqrt{s_{11}s_{22}} & s_{22} \end{pmatrix} \right) \right\} \\
&= (1-{r_1}^2)^{\frac{n_{01}-4}{2}} \exp\left\{ -\frac{(n_{01}-1)}{2} \frac{\sigma_{22}s_{11} + \sigma_{11}s_{22} - 2\sigma_{12}\sqrt{s_{11}s_{22}}r_1}{\sigma_{11}\sigma_{22} - {\sigma_{12}}^2} \right\}.
\end{aligned}
$$

The normalizing constant of the above density can be computed numerically. However, this normalizing constant does not need to be evaluated if we use the Metropolis algorithm. We further take the Fisher transformation for r_1, i.e, let $z_1 = (1/2)\log\{(1+r_1)/(1-r_1)\}$, then sample z_1, and finally back-transform to r_1. Moreover, for the Bayesian approach, we allow γ to vary to examine how the choice of γ does impact the performance of the proposed approach. Specifically, we set γ to be either 0.97 or 0.975.

For the frequentist approach, within a specific high dose level or low dose level (of the study drug) comparison with the control, we consider the conventional IUT approach for the co-primary endpoints where no multiplicity adjustment is needed. We use the Bonferroni multiplicity adjustment to account for the multiplicity issue resulting from the two dose level (of the study drug) comparison with the control with the overall type I error rate of $\alpha = 0.05$. With the Bonferroni multiplicity adjustment method, a significant level of $\alpha/2$ is used for the individual hypothesis test of the comparison between the high (or low) dose level group of the study drug and the control group. At the same time, we also evaluate the frequentist approach without the multiplicity adjustment for comparison with the other approaches considered in this chapter.

The simulation results for $n_h = n_l = 800$, and $n_c = 500$ are reported in Table 2.2. The results in the top three panels are for $\mu_c^{(s)} = \bar{y}_{c0\cdot}$, and those in the bottom three panels are for $\mu_c^{(s)} = \bar{y}_{c01}$. We can see from Table 2.2 that among the frequentist approaches, the method without multiplicity adjustment inflates type I error for all scenarios while the method with Bonferroni multiplicity adjustment controls the type I error below 5 %. For the cases with noninformative priors, the Bayesian approach with $\gamma = 0.97$ controls the family-wise type I error rate, and it has a similar power

Table 2.2 Powers and type I errors for $n_h = n_l = 800$, and $n_c = 500$

			Bayesian approach		Frequentist approach	
		Power or	γ		Without	With
$\mu_c^{(s)}$	a_0	Type I error	0.97	0.975	adjustment	adjustment
$\bar{y}_{c0\cdot}$	1	Power	0.8424	0.8202	0.7888	0.6712
	1	Type I error	0.0326	0.0254	0.0792	0.0398
	0.5	Power	0.7698	0.7410	0.7740	0.6638
	0.5	Type I error	0.0388	0.0308	0.0798	0.0428
	0	Power	0.6738	0.6434	0.7896	0.6692
	0	Type I error	0.0462	0.0374	0.0784	0.0386
$\bar{y}_{c01}$	1	Power	0.7880	0.7616	0.7846	0.6704
	1	Type I error	0.0308	0.0232	0.0842	0.0440
	0.5	Power	0.7408	0.7108	0.7832	0.6666
	0.5	Type I error	0.0306	0.0252	0.0764	0.0356
	0	Power	0.6768	0.6444	0.7870	0.6698
	0	Type I error	0.0472	0.0392	0.0816	0.0426

as the frequentist approach. From Table 2.2, we also see that $\gamma = 0.975$ is overly conservative for type I error and $\gamma = 0.97$ is sufficient to ensure that the family-wise type I error is controlled at 5 %. Moreover, the Bayesian approach allows for the incorporation of the historical data from the pervious studies. The Bayesian approach with the informative fitting priors has a higher power compared with the approach with the noninformative priors, which leads to the potential sample size reduction. For the Bayesian approach with $\gamma = 0.97$, as a_0 increases from 0 to 1, the type I error is always controlled at 5 % and the power is maximized when $a_0 = 1$ and $\mu_c^{(s)}$ is in an appropriate range such as on the line interval of AC in Fig. 2.1. In this case, we fully borrow the historical data for the control group.

If the mean vector for the co-primary endpoints for the control group for future data is on the line interval of CE as shown in Fig. 2.1, little historical data or no historical data at all should be borrowed so that the type I error is still controlled. If the mean vector for the co-primary endpoints for the control group for future data is on the line interval of CF as shown in Fig. 2.1, the full historical data can be borrowed and the type I error is still under control. However, the closer to point F the mean vector is, the less power the study has, hence a larger sample size is needed for the study. Therefore, practically an appropriate narrower range for $\mu_c^{(s)}$ should be considered, such as the line interval of AC as in Fig. 2.1.

Finally, we examine the performance of the type I error and power under different total sample sizes (n's) by incorporating the two full historical data. The corresponding results are given in Table 2.3 and Fig. 2.2 under $a_0 = 1$ and $\mu_c^{(s)} = \bar{y}_{c0\cdot}$, and we see that the total sample size of $n = 2100$ is the minimal total sample size for the study, under which the type I error is at most 5 % and the power is at least 80 %.

Table 2.3 Powers and type I errors under $a_0 = 1$ and $\mu_c^{(s)} = \bar{y}_{c0}$.

n	$n_h = n_l$	n_c	Type I error	Power
1500	600	300	0.0242	0.6962
1800	700	400	0.0320	0.7670
2100	800	500	0.0326	0.8424
2400	900	600	0.0354	0.8982
2700	1000	700	0.0418	0.9264

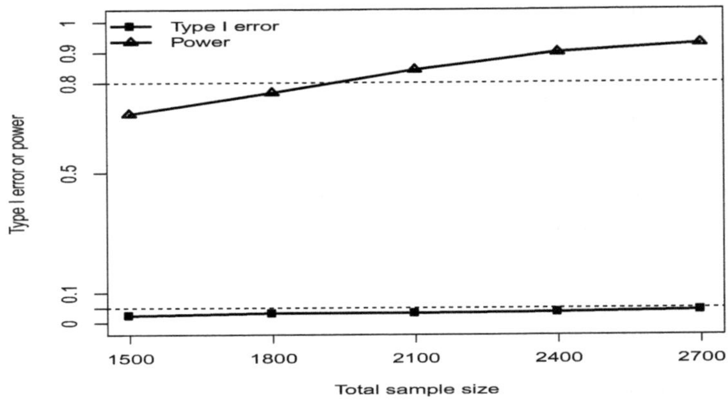

Fig. 2.2 Plot of the *power* and *type I error* versus the *total sample size* n under $a_0 = 1$ and $\mu_c^{(s)} = \bar{y}_{c0}$.

Furthermore, if we believe that $\mu_c^{(s)}$ can be any value on the line interval of AC as shown in Fig. 2.1, the corresponding type I error and power are given in Table 2.4 and Fig. 2.3, and we see that the total sample size of $n = 2400$ is the minimal total sample size for the study, under which the type I error is at most 5 % and the power is at least 80 %.

2.5 Discussion

In this chapter, we develop a Bayesian approach for non-inferiority clinical trials with co-primary endpoints and multiple dose comparison incorporating historical data. The proposed Bayesian approach can potentially increase the study power and reduce the sample size, due to the incorporation of historical data and automatically taking account of the correlation structure among the multiple co-primary endpoints while it controls the family-wise type I error rate. In addition, the Bayesian approach does not require any additional multiplicity adjustment method as it automatically controls the family-wise type I error compared with the conventional frequentist approach, and it also performs better than the conventional frequentist approach considered in this chapter regardless of the use of the informative prior or the noninformative prior. The Bayesian methodology can be used not only to choose an appropriate sample size at

Table 2.4 Powers and type I errors under $a_0 = 1$ and $\mu_c^{(s)} = \bar{y}_{c01}$

n	$n_h = n_l$	n_c	Type I error	Power
1500	600	300	0.0202	0.5986
1800	700	400	0.0236	0.7028
2100	800	500	0.0308	0.7880
2400	900	600	0.0314	0.8524
2700	1000	700	0.0330	0.9014

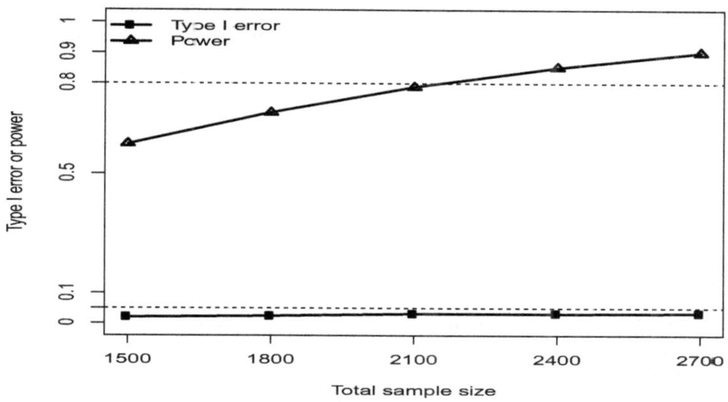

Fig. 2.3 Plot of the *power* and *type I error* versus the *total sample size n* under $a_0 = 1$ and $\mu_c^{(s)} = \bar{y}_{c01}$

the design stage but also to analyze the clinical trial data and facilitate the decision making. Using the historical data, the Bayesian analysis can be carried out and the probability $P_g \equiv P(\eta_g(\theta) < \eta^*(\delta)|D)$ can be computed and compared with γ for $g = h, l$. If $P_h \geq \gamma$ and $P_l < \gamma$, we can only claim that the study drug at the high dose level is not worse than the control group, but we cannot claim the non-inferiority for the study drug at the low dose level. One limitation of the proposed Bayesian approach is the choice of γ in order to control the family-wise type I error since the closed form expression of β_s in (2.1) in terms of γ is not available. However, for the case with two co-primary endpoints, $\gamma \geq 0.97$ may be sufficient to guarantee a family-wise type I error at 5 % as demonstrated in Sect. 2.4.

Other frequentist approaches have recently been developed for multiple dose comparisons to improve the performance of the frequentist design by allowing a more flexible and efficient α allocation at the first testing stage using the prior information. For example, in a fixed sequence procedure we can assign full α to the comparison of the study drug at the high dose level to the control group first because we know that in most therapeutic areas, the study drug at the high dose level tends to be more effective than that at the low dose level. Actually the similar prior information can be borrowed in the Bayesian approach to improve the performance of the Bayesian design via appropriate setting(s) of the key quantity β_s in (2.1) and/or the fitting priors.

For the same example, one might want to increase the power parameter in the fitting power prior for the study drug at the high dose level, if possible, i.e., incorporating more historical data for the high dose group. In addition, the comparison of the proposed Bayesian approach to more complex frequentist multiple testing procedures such as the partitioning method and the gatekeeping method (e.g., Liu et al. 2007; Dmitrienko et al. 2006; Xu et al. 2009) has not been carried out and discussed in this chapter since these frequentist procedures are design specific and more appropriate for other sophisticated multiple comparison scenarios and they are not necessarily more powerful for the scenarios considered in this chapter. Although only the conjugate prior and the power prior with fixed power parameters are considered in this chapter, the proposed Bayesian approach can be easily extended to other types of priors, such as hierarchical priors or power priors with random power parameters.

References

Chen M-H, Ibrahim JG, Lam P, Yu A, Zhang Y (2011) Bayesian design of non-inferiority trials for medical devices using historical data. Biometrics 67:1163–1170

Chuang-Stein C, Stryszak P, Dmitrienko A, Offen W (2007) Challenge of multiple co-primary endpoints: a new approach. Stat Med 26:1181–1192

CPMP (2000) Points to consider on switching between superiority and non-inferiority. http://www.emea.europa.eu/docs/en_GB/document_library/Scientific_guideline/2009/09/WC500003658.pdf

CHMP (2005) Guideline on the choice of the non-inferiority margin. http://www.emea.europa.eu/docs/en_GB/document_library/Scientific_guideline/2009/09/WC500003636.pdf

CPMP Working Party on Efficacy of Medicinal Products Note for Guidance III/3630/92-EN (1995) Biostatistical methodology in clinical trials in applications for marketing authorizations for medicinal products. Stat Med 14:1659–1682

Dmitrienko A, Offen W, Wang O, Xiao D (2006) Gatekeeping procedures in dose-response clinical trials based on the Dunnett test. Pharm Stat 5:19–28

Dmitrienko A, Tamhane AC, Bretz F (2010) Multiple testing problems in pharmaceutical statistics. Chapman & Hall, Boca Raton

Eaton ML, Muirhead RJ (2007) On a multiple endpoints testing problem. J Stat Plan Inference 137:3416–3429

FDA Guidance for industry (2010) Non-inferiority clinical trials. http://www.fda.gov/downloads/Drugs/GuidanceComplianceRegulatoryInformation/Guidances/UCM202140.pdf

Gonen M, Westfall PH, Johnson WO (2003) Bayesian multiple testing for two-sample multivariate endpoints. Biometrics 59:76–82

Hung HJ, Wang SJ (2004) Multiple testing of noninferiority hypotheses in active controlled trials. J Biopharm Stat 14:327–335

Ibrahim JG, Chen M-H (2000) Power prior distributions for regression models. Stat Sci 15:46–60

ICH Harmonised tripartite guideline (1998) Statistical principles for clinical trials (E9). http://www.ich.org/fileadmin/Public_Web_Site/ICH_Products/Guidelines/Efficacy/E9/Step4/E9_Guideline.pdf

ICH Harmonized tripartite guideline (2000). Choice of control group and related issues in clinical trials (E10). http://www.ich.org/fileadmin/Public_Web_Site/ICH_Products/Guidelines/Efficacy/E10/Step4/E10_Guideline.pdf

Kong L, Kohberger RC, Koch GG (2004) Type I error and power in noninferiority/equivalence trials with correlated multiple endpoints: an example from vaccine development trials. J Biopharm Stat 14:893–907

Laska NS, Tang D, Meisner MJ (1992) Testing hypothesis about an identified treatment when there are multiple endpoints. J Am Stat Assoc 87:825–831
Liu KJ, Chang KC (2011) Test non-inferiority and sample size determination based on the odds ratio under a cluster randomized trial with noncompliance. J Biopharm Stat 21:94–110
Liu Y, Hsu J, Ruberg S (2007) Partition testing in dose-response studies with multiple endpoints. Pharm Stat 6:181–192
Narayan P, Ashutosh Tewari A, Members Of United States 93-01 Study Group (1998) A second phase i11 multicenter placebo controlled study of 2 dosages of modified release Tamsulosin in patients with symptoms of benign prostatic hyperplasia. J Urol 160:1701–1706
Ng TH (2003) Issues of simultaneous tests for noninferiority and superiority. J Biopharm Stat 13:629–639
Röhmel J, Pigeot I (2010) A comparison of multiple testing procedures for the gold standard non-inferiority trial. J Biopharm Stat 20:911–926
Scott JG, Berger JO (2006) An exploration of aspects of Bayesian multiple testing. J Stat Plan Inference 136:2144–2162
Sugimoto T, Sozu T, Hamasaki T (2012) A convenient formula for sample size calculations in clinical trials with multiple co-primary continuous endpoints. Pharm Stat 11:118–128
Tamimi NAM, Mincik I, Haughie S, Lamb J, Crossland A, Peter Ellis P (2010) A placebo-controlled study investigating the efficacy and safety of the phosphodiesterase type 5 inhibitor UK-369,003 for the treatment of men with lower urinary tract symptoms associated with clinical benign prostatic hyperplasia. BJU Int 106:674–680
Tsong Y, Zhang J (2007) Simultaneous test for superiority and noninferiority hypotheses in active controlled clinical trials. J Biopharm Stat 17:247–257
Welch BL (1947) The generalization of student's problem when several different population variance are involved. Biometrika 34:28–35
Xu H, Nuamah I, Liu J, Lim P, Sampson A (2009) A Dunnett-Bonferroni-based parallel gatekeeping procedure for dose-response clinical trials with multiple endpoints. Pharm Stat 8:301–316

Chapter 3
Bayesian Functional Mixed Models for Survival Responses with Application to Prostate Cancer

Veerabhadran Baladandayuthapan, Xiaohui Wang, Bani K. Mallick and Kim-Anh Do

Abstract In this chapter, we propose a flexible approach to model functional measurements for survival outcomes. Often the class of models for functional observations are assumed to be linear, which may be too restrictive in some cases. We propose an alternative model, in which the simple linear mixed model has been modified by a more flexible semiparametric spline-based functional mixed model, wherein the usage of splines simplifies parameterizations and the joint modeling framework allows synergistic benefit between the regression of functional predictors and the modeling of survival data. We explicitly model the number and location of change points such that our formulation allows for an unknown set of basis functions characterizing the population-averaged and patient-specific trajectories. In addition, we propose a novel auxiliary variable scheme for a fully Bayesian estimation of our model, which not only allows dimension reduction of the parameter space but also allows efficient sampling from the conditional distributions. We illustrate our approach with a recent prostate cancer clinical trial study.

3.1 Introduction

Metastatic prostate cancer is the second most common cancer-related cause of death in North American men (Greenlee et al. 2000). Hormonal treatments such as androgen ablation (AA) have been preferred treatments for metastatic prostate cancer for more than 50 years. Such therapies work by altering the natural history of the disease by specifically disrupting the growth-promoting effects mediated by androgen

V. Baladandayuthapani (✉) K. Do
Department of Biostatistics, UT MD Anderson Cancer Center, Houston, TX 77030, USA
e-mail: veera@mdanderson.org

X. Wang
Department of Mathematics, University of Texas-Pan American, Edinburg, TX 78539, USA
e-mail: xhwang@utpa.edu

B. K. Mallick
Department of Statistics, Texas A & M University, College Station, TX 77840, USA

Z. Chen et al. (eds.), *Applied Statistics in Biomedicine and Clinical Trials Design*,
ICSA Book Series in Statistics, DOI 10.1007/978-3-319-12694-4_3

receptor signaling. Regardless of the mode of administration of AA, most patients with clinically detectable metastatic disease will eventually progress to androgen-independent prostate cancer (AIPC) with a median of 12–18 months (Eisenberger et al. 1986). After progression to AIPC, only symptoms are treatable and patients survive with a median of less than a year (Tannock et al. 1996). Despite major efforts, most studies with various cytotoxic drugs have provided little hint of the disease-altering activity for AIPC. However, in a recent phase II study at the University of Texas M.D. Anderson Cancer Center, a regimen based on chemotherapy demonstrated a survival advantage over historical results (Ellerhorst et al. 1997). This regimen of ketoconazole and doxorubicin alternating with vinblastine and estramustine, termed KA/VE, produced obvious palliation in the majority of treated patients.

Based on these results, a phase III trial (Millikan et al. 2008) was conducted at M.D. Anderson Cancer Center to compare conventional hormonal therapy (AA) to chemohormonal (CH) therapy combined with three 8-week cycles of KA/VE (AA + CH) in patients with metastatic androgen-driven prostate cancer. The hypothesis of interest was that early intervention of KA/VE to standard, sustained AA would delay the emergence of AIPC and ultimately prolong survival. The primary end point of interest was the time to progression to AIPC.

In addition to the time to progression, the longitudinal measurements of prostate-specific antigen (PSA) level from each patient over time were recorded. PSA, a glycoprotein produced by the prostate gland, is considered a useful biomarker for prostate cancer since significant positive correlation has been observed between the levels of PSA and the volume of the prostate (Catalona et al. 1991). Monitoring PSA levels has not only been established as a good diagnostic tool but is also considered an important indicator of response to treatment, with low levels indicating good prognosis. PSA measures are easy to collect via a routine laboratory assay of the blood samples. Thus, given the two sets of measurements: PSA profiles and time to progression (to AIPC), and since the measurements are inherently correlated, our main goal of this chapter is to investigate methods for the joint analysis of both end points.

In practice (and as in our case), the latent functional process is often unobservable due to measurement error and is not available at all times, especially when failure occurs. It is well known that conventional partial likelihood approaches for the Cox model cannot avoid biased inference by using imputation of the latent functional process, such as last value carried forward method (Prentice 1982), smoothing techniques (Raboud et al. 1993), and any other generic two-stage approaches (Bycott and Taylor 1998; Tsiatis et al. 1995). This invoked the consideration of using functional and event processes simultaneously via *joint modeling,* a subject that has recently attracted substantial interest (see Ibrahim et al. 2001; Tsiatis and Davidian 2004 for an overview).

Suppose the data are comprised of a vector of observations $\{T_i, \mathbf{L}_i, \mathbf{Y}(\mathbf{t}_i), \mathbf{t}_i \geq 0\}$ for the ith subject, where T_i is an event time (possibly censored), $\mathbf{L}_i$ is a vector of baseline covariates, and $\{\mathbf{Y}(\mathbf{t}_i), t_{i\ell} \geq 0, i = 1, \cdots, n, \ell = 1, \cdots, p_i\}$ is the functional marker trajectory for all times $t_{i\ell} \geq 0$, where p_i is the number of functional

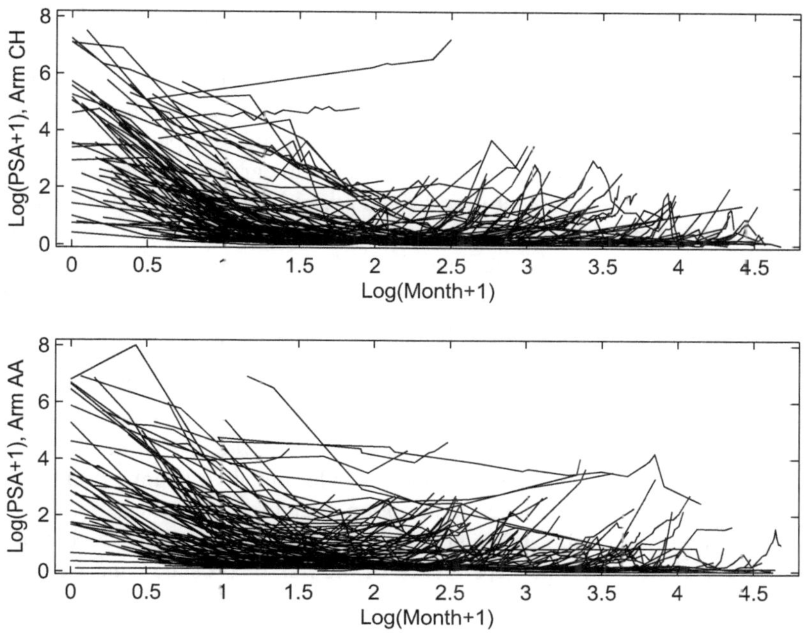

Fig. 3.1 Prostate-specific antigen (PSA) profiles for patients in arm androgen ablation (*AA*; upper panel) and arm chemohormonal (*CH*; lower panel)

measurements for subject i. One simple strategy is to introduce subject-specific random effects and then subsequently couple this model with a model on the survival process such as a proportional hazards model (Wulfsohn and Tsiatis 1997; DeGruttola and Tu 1994; Hogan and Laird 1997). A similar Bayesian method was explored by Faucett and Thomas (1996). Wang and Taylor (2001) introduced an integrated Orstein–Uhlenbeck (IOU) process into the functional modeling. Brown and Ibrahim (2003) started with a model similar to the ones in Wulfsohn and Tsiatis (1997) and Faucett and Thomas (1996) for their Bayesian semiparametric joint model; however, they used a quadratic form for the functional part and introduced a nonparametric specification for the distribution of the random effects, $\boldsymbol{\theta}_i$'s. Recent works include Zhang et al. (2009) proposing a semiparametric model based on Pólya trees and Guo and Carlin (2004) comparing separate and joint modeling of functional and event time data.

In most of these approaches, the form of the functional process or the *trajectory function* is assumed to be a simple parametric form. Although conceptually simple and easily implementable, this is a rather rigid assumption and may not hold in some cases such as the one we describe here. Figure 3.1 shows the overlapping PSA levels for the two treatment arms (AA and CH) posttreatment. The horizontal axes present the time (in logarithm of months) and the vertical axes present the log(PSA+1) measurements.

There are three key aspects of the PSA trajectories which need to be considered for any downstream analysis. First, there seems to be a definite overall pattern in the PSA trajectories for both treatment arms. The PSA levels decrease from time units 0 to 1, then stabilize and finally increase again (around 2.5) after the effect of treatment wears off. The patients have been normalized such that all patients receive their treatment at time 0. Thus, the profiles exhibit a nonlinear characteristic with definite change points at both the subject-specific and population levels—hence the need for flexible models for the functional process. Second, a further complication occurs since the number of PSA measurements for each patient are taken at different times, which causes them to be sparse and irregular. Third, there seems to be considerable heterogeneity among the patients in both treatment groups.

Due to these characteristics, the above mentioned parametric models might not be suitable for modeling such data. Specific to joint modeling of PSA and survival outcomes, Pauler and Finkelstein (2002) used a joint Bayesian model that consisted of piecewise linear functional model and Cox proportional hazard model. Their piecewise linear regression model adopted single unknown change point for each patient and implied independence assumption over functional measurements from the same patient. Ye et al. (2008) gave likelihood-based two-stage regression calibration methods to study the dependence of the risk of prostate cancer recurrence on the PSA level as well as time-independent covariates. Ye et al. (2008) provided a Bayesian-based joint modeling approach with added mixture structure to predict individual disease progression that results in either cure by treatment or susceptible to recurrence. The Ye et al. method models the PSA level with a nonlinear exponential decay and exponential growth model. We propose an alternative model in which the simple linear (or polynomial) model has been modified by a more flexible nonparametric model that cannot only capture nonlinear complex processes but also adopt unknown number of change points at both patient and population levels. We compare two different treatments, explore the effects of PSA level as well as several covariates on the survival outcome, and identify the PSA trajectory change points as patient disease progresses.

There has been an increasing interest in functional data analysis (FDA), analysis of data that are in the form of a (smooth) sample of curves or functions (Ramsay and Silverman 2005; Ngo and Wand 2004; Yao 2007; and Brown et al. 2005), in which the functions form the basic unit of data. Most functional data analyses focus on data which are frequently and regularly sampled across individuals and are not applicable here due to "sparseness and irregularity" of our data. We focus on methods for sparse functional data where not only the number and timing vary across subjects but also some subjects may be sampled at very few time points. Our mixed model uses a flexible spline basis; the usage of this basis simplifies the parameterizations and the joint modeling framework, thus allowing synergistic benefits between the regression of functional and survival data. Further, we explicitly model the number and location of change points such that our formulation allows for an unknown set of basis functions characterizing the population-averaged and patient-specific trajectories. We set up the spline-based model without the assumption of independence over functional measurements from the same patient. Meanwhile, the novelty of the proposed Bayesian model lies in its ability to draw information from the functional data as well as from the associated event time data by unifying the spline-based functional regression and survival models. In addition, we propose a novel auxiliary variable scheme for a fully Bayesian estimation of our model, which not only allows for dimension reduction of the parameter space but also allows for efficient sampling from the conditional distributions and greatly reduces the computational burden.

The rest of the chapter is organized as follows. Section 3.2 discusses our Bayesian joint hierarchical model, where we set up the functional regression model and the Cox proportional hazards model in an unified framework. Section 3.3 concerns elicitation of prior distributions for the proposed model. Section 3.4 compares our model with other joint models with parametric regression segments based on various model selection criteria. The novel proposed model is illustrated by a motivating example, prostate cancer data set, in Sect. 3.5. The chapter is concluded with a discussion in Sect. 3.6. All technical details are collected into the Appendix.

3.2 Probability Model

In this section, we propose a joint survival and functional model in which the functional curves are modeled nonparametrically via splines. In addition, we explicitly model the change points present in the profiles via a functional variable selection approach, which results in a more flexible and robust model. For ease of exposition, we assume a univariate functional outcome, although our method is easily generalizable to multiple functional outcomes, as we show in Sect. 3.6.

3.2.1 Regression Model for the Functional Covariates

Suppose our data construct for n subjects consists of the following: $\{\mathrm{T_i}, \mathrm{C_i}, \mathrm{L_i}, \mathbf{Y}_\mathrm{i}(\mathbf{t})\}$, where for the ith subject we observe a time-independent baseline covariates vector $\mathbf{L}_i$ of dimension m and time-dependent covariates $\mathbf{Y}_i(\mathbf{t})$ measured at time points $\mathbf{t}$. In addition, each individual has a lifetime $\mathrm{T_i}$ and a (right) censored time $\mathrm{C_i}$. Thus, one observes $T_i = \min(\mathrm{T_i}, \mathrm{C_i})$ and the failure indicator δ_i, defined as

$$\delta_i = \begin{cases} 1 & \text{if} \quad \mathrm{T_i} \leq \mathrm{C_i}, \\ 0 & \text{if} \quad \mathrm{T_i} > \mathrm{C_i}. \end{cases}$$

We further assume that the censoring mechanism is independent of all other survival and covariates information. For the functional covariate predictor $\mathbf{Y}_i(\mathbf{t})$, we posit the following functional regression model:

$$\mathbf{Y}_i(\mathbf{t}) = \boldsymbol{\mu}(\mathbf{t}) + \mathbf{b}_i(\mathbf{t}) + \boldsymbol{\epsilon}_i(\mathbf{t}) \quad 0 \leq t \leq T, \quad 1 \leq i \leq n,$$

where $\boldsymbol{\mu}(\bullet)$ is the overall mean profile and $\mathbf{b}_i(\bullet)$ is the ith subject's deviation from the mean profile, measured intermittently between times $[0, T]$ for an individual i with measurement error $\boldsymbol{\epsilon}_i(\bullet)$. We also assume that the error process $\boldsymbol{\epsilon}_i(\bullet)$ is independent of true functional process and follows a Gaussian process with mean zero and constant variance σ_ϵ^2. Other forms of correlations such as an autocorrelation process can be used for the errors, but to keep the exposition simple we do not consider that case here.

Our focus is on modeling $\boldsymbol{\mu}(\bullet)$ and $\mathbf{b}_i(\bullet)$ in a flexible manner. We achieve this via a basis function projection:

$$\boldsymbol{\mu}(\mathbf{t}) = \mathbf{X}(\mathbf{t})\boldsymbol{\beta}, \quad \mathbf{b}_i(\mathbf{t}) = \mathbf{X}(\mathbf{t})\boldsymbol{\beta}_i,$$

where $\mathbf{X}(\mathbf{t})$ is any generic basis function and the associated regression coefficients are denoted by $\boldsymbol{\beta}$ for the overall mean and $\boldsymbol{\beta}_i$ for subject i. In practice, we only observe the latent functional process on a finite number of time points $\mathbf{t}_i = (t_{i1}, \ldots, t_{ip_i})$ for the ith subject with p_i as the number of measurements, which varies from subject to subject. The discretized version of the model for the observed PSA measurements Y_{ij} for subject i and time t_{ij} is of the form:

$$Y_{ij} = Y_i(t_j) = \mathbf{X}(t_{ij})\boldsymbol{\beta} + \mathbf{X}(t_{ij})\boldsymbol{\beta}_i + \epsilon_{ij}, \tag{3.1}$$

where $\mathbf{X}(t_{ij})$ is the basis function evaluated at $t_{ij}, i = 1, \ldots, n, j = 1, \ldots, p_i$. There are various basis functions that one could potentially use for modeling the functional predictors, such as smoothing splines, B-splines, and wavelets, among others, depending on the application. For our model exposition, we use a truncated power series basis function (Ruppert et al. 2003) given its nice connections to mixed models (Ngo and Wand 2004).

Let dimension $K = 1 + p + K^*$, where p is the degree of the spline and K^* is the number of interior knots. We rewrite (3.1) in matrix notation as

$$\mathbf{Y}_i = \mathbf{X}_i\boldsymbol{\beta} + \mathbf{X}_i\boldsymbol{\beta}_i + \boldsymbol{\epsilon}_i, \tag{3.2}$$

where $\mathbf{Y}_i = (Y_{i1}, \ldots, Y_{ip_i})'$, $\mathbf{X}_i$ is the $p_i \times K$ basis matrix for the ith subject, $\boldsymbol{\beta} = (\boldsymbol{\beta}_1, \ldots, \boldsymbol{\beta}_K)'$ and $\boldsymbol{\beta}_i = (\boldsymbol{\beta}_{i1}, \ldots, \boldsymbol{\beta}_{iK})'$ are the K-dimensional regression coefficient vectors. The jth row of $\mathbf{X}_i$ can be written as

$$\mathbf{X}_{ij} = [1 \;\; t_{ij} \;\; t_{ij}^2 \;\; \cdots \;\; t_{ij}^p \;\; (t_{ij} - \mathrm{t}_1)_+^p \;\; \cdots \;\; (t_{ij} - \mathrm{t}_{K^*})_+^p],$$

where $\{\mathrm{t}_1, \cdots, \mathrm{t}_{K^*}\}$ are the interior knots. We assume that the subject level regression coefficients follow a Gaussian distribution, $\boldsymbol{\beta}_i \sim MVN(\mathbf{0}, \boldsymbol{\Omega})$, which are the random effects corresponding to the systematic deviation from the population mean $\boldsymbol{\beta}$ with a variance–covariance matrix $\boldsymbol{\Omega}$. This distribution implicity makes two key assumptions. First, it induces the same basis function and hence the same amount of smoothing for both the subject-specific and population level functions. This might seem a little restrictive in some sense, since the individual curves could be assumed to be more spatially heterogeneous than the population level curve. But for sparse functional data (as in our case), the assumption of the same degree of smoothness at both the population and subject level is a reasonable one given the low number of observations per individual. Second, conditional on the choice of basis function and treating the basis matrix as fixed, the model in (3.2) is essentially a semiparameteric random effects model, with the prior on $\boldsymbol{\beta}_i$ admitting the within-subject covariance $V(\mathbf{Y}_i) = \mathbf{X}_i' \boldsymbol{\Omega} \mathbf{X}_i + \sigma_\epsilon^2 \mathbf{I}_{p_i}$. Hence, the within-subject independence assumption is relaxed to allow within-subject correlation for the observed curve $\mathbf{Y}_i$.

Having posited the above model on the functional (PSA) profiles, conditional on the basis matrix $\mathbf{X}$, we can proceed with estimation using a variety of Bayesian or frequentist techniques. However, two related issues remain. First, the number and position of the knots or breakpoints need to be chosen, and second, conditional on the number of knots, the dimension of $\boldsymbol{\Omega}$, if left unstructured, is of dimension $K \times K$; thus, we need to estimate $K(K+1)/2$ unique parameters. From a practical and methodological point of view, it is useful to reduce dimensionality. This is essentially a model selection problem. Various approaches to solving this problem include using model selection procedures such as conditional predictive ordinate (CPO) or deviance information criteria (DIC), as proposed by Brown et al. (2005), or a fully Bayesian framework using free-knot spline methodology (Denison et al. 1998; Holmes and Mallick 2003). For our application, it is of interest to model the exact location and number of change points in the PSA profiles since drastic changes in PSA might directly impact on the survival of the patient. This is also evident in Fig. 3.1, where one notices a sharp drop in PSA levels initially and then an increase in PSA levels in the later stages of the disease.

We handle the problem of choosing the number of change points in a Bayesian framework via latent indicators (Smith and Kohn 1996; Thompson and Rosen 2008). Essentially, we start with a large pool of potential breakpoints and an associated latent indicator vector, which we denote as $\boldsymbol{\gamma}$. The elements of the latent indicator vector equal 1 if the corresponding change point is included in the model and 0 otherwise—this implies keeping or deleting one basis function in (3.2). Thus, conditional on $\boldsymbol{\gamma} = (\gamma_1, \ldots, \gamma_{K^*})$, where K^* is the number of the set of potential change points, our model in (3.2) can be written as

$$\mathbf{Y}_i = \mathbf{X}_{i,\gamma} \boldsymbol{\beta}_\gamma + \mathbf{X}_{i,\gamma} \boldsymbol{\beta}_{i,\gamma} + \boldsymbol{\epsilon}_i, \qquad \boldsymbol{\epsilon}_i \sim MVN(\mathbf{0}, \sigma_\epsilon^2 \mathbf{I}_{p_i}), \tag{3.3}$$

where each $\mathbf{X}_{i,\gamma}$ is the basis matrix corresponding to change points for the ith individual, and $\boldsymbol{\beta}_\gamma$ and $\boldsymbol{\beta}_{i,\gamma}$ are the corresponding regressed coefficients of size $1 + p + K_{i,\gamma}^*$, where p is the degree of the spline and $K_{i,\gamma}^*$ is the number of ones in the vector $\boldsymbol{\gamma}$ and within the span of the ith individual curve. Conditional on the latent indicator parameter $\boldsymbol{\gamma}$ (and basis function), model (3.3) is still essentially a Bayesian linear model for which an attractive conjugate prior distribution for parameters exists for efficient Gibbs sampling. Since this model is only a component of our joint functional survival model, we defer our discussion of appropriate priors to Sect. 3.3, after we present our joint modeling framework. Note that we have not included any covariate affecting the functional process in our model above; this is easy to handle in our framework by adding a term corresponding to the covariate in the regression model (3.3).

3.2.2 Joint Survival Model

Having specified our functional submodel above, we now proceed to model the relationship between the functional measures $\mathbf{Y}$ and event time T. We do so by constructing the likelihood in a prospective manner, $P(T, \mathbf{Y}) = P(T|\mathbf{Y})P(\mathbf{Y})$, rather than a retrospective manner using reverse factorization by conditioning on the survival process. The probability model for $P(\mathbf{Y})$ is as specified in (3.3). In this section, we describe how we characterize the distribution $P(T|\mathbf{Y})$.

We model the failure time via a proportional hazards model. Following Cox (1972, 1975), and under the conditions discussed by Kalbfleisch and Prentice (2002), we use the original Cox model formulation, in which the hazard depends on the (true) functional process $\mathbf{Y}_i(t)$ through its current value (and/or other time-dependent covariates) and time-independent covariates $\mathbf{L}_i$. The framework for characterizing associations among the functional and survival processes, as well as other covariates, is then given by

$$\begin{aligned} h(t) &= \lim_{dt \to 0} P\{t < T_i < t + dt | T_i \geq t, \mathbf{Y}_i^H(t), \mathbf{L}_i\} \\ &= h_0(t) \exp\{\boldsymbol{\theta}_1 \mathbf{Y}_i(t) + \boldsymbol{\theta}_2 \mathbf{L}_i\}, \end{aligned}$$

where the coefficients $(\boldsymbol{\theta}_1, \boldsymbol{\theta}_2)$ reflect the association of interest and $\mathbf{Y}_i^H(t) = \{\mathbf{Y}_i(u) : 0 < u < t\}$ is the history of the functional process $\mathbf{Y}_i$ up to time t. Note here that this implementation is complicated by two facts. First, the functional covariate is subject to measurement error and is observed only intermittently for each subject at $\mathbf{t}_i = (t_{i1}, \ldots, t_{ip_i})$. Second, and more important, plugging in the entire (smoothed) functional profile leads us to a high-dimensional integral in the likelihood:

$$\begin{aligned} f(T_i, \delta_i | \mathbf{Y}_i) = &\{h_0(T_i) \exp[\boldsymbol{\theta}_1 \mathbf{Y}_i(T_i) + \boldsymbol{\theta}_2 \mathbf{L}_i]\}^{\delta_i} \times \\ &\exp\left\{ - \int_0^{T_i} h_0(t) \exp[\boldsymbol{\theta}_1 \mathbf{Y}_i(t) + \boldsymbol{\theta}_2 \mathbf{L}_i] \mathrm{d}t \right\}. \end{aligned}$$

The high-dimensional integral in the likelihood does not have an analytical solution for the functional profile specified via a spline representation. Brown et al. (2005) use a trapezoidal rule to approximate the above integral. We present an exact Bayesian analysis via the use of auxiliary variables. To this effect, define a latent auxiliary variable w_i as

$$w_i = \boldsymbol{\beta}'_{\gamma(i)} \boldsymbol{\theta}_{1\gamma} + \mathbf{L}_i' \boldsymbol{\theta}_2 + e_i, \quad e_i \sim N(0, \tau^2), \tag{3.4}$$

where $\boldsymbol{\beta}_{\gamma(i)} = \boldsymbol{\beta}_\gamma + \boldsymbol{\beta}_{i,\gamma}$ represents the ith PSA trajectory, $\boldsymbol{\theta}_{1\gamma}, \boldsymbol{\theta}_2$ are the regression coefficient vectors corresponding to the time-dependent and time-independent covariate information, and e_i is an error term. The auxiliary variables summarize the time-dependent covariate effects via a simple projection. The functional submodel is then coupled with the survival model via these latent auxiliary variables by imputing the w_i into the proportional hazards model via the hazard function as:

$$h(t \mid \mathbf{Y}_i, \mathbf{L}_i) = h_0(t) \exp(w_i), \tag{3.5}$$

where $\mathbf{Y}_i$ is the ith individual time-dependent covariates vector, $\mathbf{L}_i$ is the time-independent covariates, and $h_0(t)$ is the baseline hazard function at time point t, free of the covariates.

The introduction of latent auxiliary variables not only eases the high-dimensional integration in the likelihood but also serves three purposes. The first concerns dimension reduction, wherein the information from the potentially high-dimensional regression coefficient $\boldsymbol{\beta}$ is passed along to the survival model via a simple projection into a lower dimensional subspace. Second, in adopting this Gaussian residual effect, many of the conditional distributions for the model parameters are now of a standard form, which greatly aids in the computations. To be specific, conditional on w_i's, model (3.3) is independent of the event time model (3.5) and can be written as a standard Bayesian linear regression on the basis space defined by $\mathbf{X}$, as we show in Sect. 3. The use of the residual component e_i is consistent with the belief that there may be unexplained sources of variation in the data, perhaps due to the lack of a linear relationship. Finally, the latent auxiliary variable formulation allows us to easily generalize our model to handle multiple functional covariates (Sect. 3.6).

We assume that the baseline hazard is a piecewise function as:

$$h_0(t) = \lambda_j \quad (s_{j-1} \leq t < s_j), \quad j = 1, \ldots, J. \tag{3.6}$$

In theory, increasing J approximates semiparametric methods. Other nonparametric priors (such as the gamma process and the beta process) can be easily incorporated within our framework. Based on (3.5) and (3.6), we write the cumulative hazard function for the ith individual as

$$\int_0^{T_i} h_0(t)\exp(w_i)\mathrm{d}t = \sum_{j=1}^{J} I(T_i > s_{j-1}) \int_{s_{j-1}}^{\min(s_j, T_i)} \exp(w_i)\lambda_j \mathrm{d}t,$$

where the indicator function $I(T_i > s_{j-1})$ yields 1 if the survival time is within or later than the jth interval and 0 otherwise.

3.3 Prior Distributions

The parameters and random variables to estimate in our model are

$$\mathcal{M} = \{\boldsymbol{\beta}, \sigma_\epsilon^2, \boldsymbol{\mu}_\gamma, \boldsymbol{\Omega}_\gamma, \boldsymbol{\gamma}, \boldsymbol{\theta}_\gamma, \tau^2, \boldsymbol{\lambda}\}.$$

We shall discuss each of the priors and distributions for the regression and survival models, respectively.

3.3.1 Priors for The Regression Model

We assign a Gaussian prior distribution, $MVN(\mathbf{0}, \boldsymbol{\Omega}_{i,\gamma})$, to the subject level regression coefficients $\boldsymbol{\beta}_{i,\gamma}$. Based on the fact that the ith curve may not span the complete set of selected change points, we use $\boldsymbol{\Omega}_{i,\gamma}$ to denote the subject-specific realizations of parameter $\boldsymbol{\Omega}_{\gamma}$ that respectively represent the population curve covariance corresponding to the latent variable $\boldsymbol{\gamma}$. In the implementation of our methodology for our particular example, the number of basis functions K is relatively small. At least in principle, we can then allow the covariance matrices $\boldsymbol{\Omega}_{\gamma}$ to be general. However, from both a practical and methodological point of view, it is crucial to lower the dimensionality of $\boldsymbol{\Omega}_{\gamma}$. There are a variety of approaches available to this end. For example, Shi et al. (1996) achieve parsimony using a principal component decomposition of the covariance matrix of random effects. In a different context, Daniels and Pourahmadi (2002) provide a Bayesian method based on Cholesky decomposition. Since in our application we work with truncated power series basis functions, dimension reduction has a natural form that exploits the mixed model representation of such basis functions (Ruppert et al. 2003; Baladandayuthapani et al. 2008). The essential idea is to take the coefficients at the knots to be independent while allowing the polynomial part to have an unstructured covariance matrix. Thus, if p is the degree of the regression splines and K_{γ}^{*} is the number of selected knots, then we take $\boldsymbol{\Omega}_{\gamma} = \text{diag}(\boldsymbol{\Sigma}, \sigma^2 \mathbf{I}_{K_{\gamma}^{*}})$, where $\boldsymbol{\Sigma}$ is an unstructured $p \times p$ matrix. Further, we specify a Gaussian prior distribution on the population level profile or the fixed effects, $\boldsymbol{\beta}_{\gamma}$, as $\boldsymbol{\beta}_{\gamma} \sim MVN(\mathbf{0}, \mathbf{c}\mathbf{I}_{\mathbf{K}_{\gamma}})$, where we set c to be 100, and $K_{\gamma} = 1 + p + K_{\gamma}^{*}$. We adopt an Inverse–Wishart prior distribution for $\boldsymbol{\Sigma}$ and an inverse-gamma prior distribution for σ^2. For the regression model (3.3), we assume an inverse-gamma prior distribution for the constant variance σ_{ϵ}^2.

The selected change points are identified by the vector $\boldsymbol{\gamma}$. We use a Bernoulli prior for each element of this indicator vector, $\gamma_k \sim \text{Bernoulli}(\pi_k)$, and let $\pi_k = \pi$ for all k. The hyperprior for the probability of being a change point is specified as a beta prior, $\pi \sim \text{Beta}(a_{\pi}, b_{\pi})$. Kohn et al. (2001) pointed out a flexible approach specifying beta prior hyperparameters according to a certain expectation or prior knowledge.

3.3.2 Priors for The Survival Model

We use conjugate prior distributions for the parameter pair $\boldsymbol{\theta}_{\gamma}$ and τ^2, defined as $\boldsymbol{\theta}_{\gamma} \sim MVN(\mathbf{0}, \tau^2 \mathbf{V}_{\gamma})$ and $\tau^2 \sim IG(a_{\tau}, b_{\tau})$, where $\mathbf{V}_{\gamma} = diag(\mathbf{h})$. The hyperprior for the vector $\mathbf{h} = \{h_{\ell}\}$ is specified elementwise as inverse-gamma distribution, $h_{\ell} \sim IG(c_{\ell}, d_{\ell})$. For the survival model, the prior distribution for a piecewise baseline hazard functions, $\boldsymbol{\lambda} = \{\lambda_j\}$ is $\lambda_j \sim IG(a_j, b_j)$, where a_j and b_j can be specified for each interval.

We proceed with the estimation of the above model setup via Markov chain Monte Carlo (MCMC) methods. The full conditional distributions are presented for the regression and survival models in the Appendix. We use the Gibbs sampler (Gelfand and Smith 1990) to obtain samples from the posterior distribution. Two parameters, w_i and γ_k, do not have close forms in their conditionals. Therefore, we use Metropolis–Hastings algorithm (Metropolis et al. 1953; Hastings 1970) to sample those two parameters.

3.4 Model Selection Criteria

For model selection and comparison, we use two comparison statistics: the DIC and the CPO (Gelfand et al. 1992). The DIC is the sum of the deviance estimated using posterior estimates of the parameters and twice the effective number of parameters (Spiegelhalter et al. 2002). A better fit will have a smaller DIC. The DIC for our joint models can be expressed as

$$DIC = 2\frac{1}{Q}\sum_{q=1}^{Q}\sum_{i=1}^{n} log f(T_i, \delta_i, \mathbf{Y}_i \mid \Theta^{(q)}) - \sum_{i=1}^{n} log f(T_i, \delta_i, \mathbf{Y}_i \mid \bar{\Theta}),$$

where $\Theta^{(q)}$ denotes the parameter samples at the qth iteration of the MCMC method and $\bar{\Theta}$ represents the means of the posterior samples. Chen et al. (2000) showed that a Monte Carlo approximation of the integral in the CPO calculation can be used. For our joint models, we have

$$\widehat{\mathrm{CPO}_i} = \left(\frac{1}{Q}\sum_{q=1}^{Q}\frac{1}{f(T_i, \delta_i, \mathbf{Y}_i \mid \Theta^{(q)})}\right)^{-1}.$$

Models with greater $\sum_{i=1}^{n} log(\widehat{\mathrm{CPO}_i})$'s indicate a better fit.

Computing DIC and $\sum_{i=1}^{n} log(\widehat{CPO_i})$ is straightforward based on the samples from the MCMC method and the joint likelihood function:

$$\begin{aligned} f(T_i, \delta_i, \mathbf{Y}_i) &= f(T_i, \delta_i \mid \mathbf{Y}_i) f(\mathbf{Y}_i) \\ &\propto \left[h_0(T_i)\exp(w_i)\right]^{\delta_i} \exp\left\{-\int_0^{T_i} h_0(u)\exp(w_i)du\right\} |2\pi\sigma_\epsilon^2 \mathbf{I}|^{-\frac{1}{2}} \\ &\times \exp\left\{-\frac{1}{2\sigma_\epsilon^2}(\mathbf{Y}_i - \mathbf{X}_{i,y}\boldsymbol{\beta}_y - \mathbf{X}_{i,y}\boldsymbol{\beta}_{i,y})'(\mathbf{Y}_i - \mathbf{X}_{i,y}\boldsymbol{\beta}_y - \mathbf{X}_{i,y}\boldsymbol{\beta}_{i,y})\right\}. \end{aligned}$$

3.5 Application to Prostate Cancer Data

We now consider a data set from a phase III trial of prostate cancer patients conducted at M.D. Anderson Cancer Center (Millikan et al. 2008). The clinical trial studied 286 patients with metastatic or locally advanced prostate cancer who were randomized and treated with either AA alone (arm AA) or chemo/hormonal therapy plus AA (arm CH) between August 1996 and March 2003. A complete medical history was obtained from each patient. All patients also underwent a physical examination. For each patient, we have a record of the time (in days) between the trial starting day and progression to AIPC or end of study, an indicator of censoring, which treatment the patient received, day of each visit measured from registration, and PSA level measured on that day. The functional laboratory results of PSA, the leading diagnostic marker for prostate cancer, is considered a predictor variable in our application. The failure time variable, the time to progression of AIPC, is a right-censored variable. Four time-independent covariates are also considered in the analysis. Their age at diagnosis, prior local treatment, stratification via bone volume, and pretreatment PSA doubling time (PSADT). For prior local treatment, patients either did or did not receive definitive treatment. Patients were also stratified as follows: high-volume bone or visceral disease, low-volume bone disease (one or two spots on bone scan), local/nodal disease with prior definitive local therapy, or local/nodal disease without prior definitive therapy. For simplicity, the three low-volume groups of patients were combined into one category yielding two categories: high-volume disease or low-volume disease. Since we have (intermittent) PSA measurements from the patients before therapy, we include pretreatment PSADT as a time-independent covariate in our survival model. It is a categorical variable stratified, as 0 if data are not available to determine a doubling time, as 1 if doubling time is less than 3 months, and as 2 if doubling time is greater than 3 months.

The number of PSA observations for each patient varied from 1 to 65. We use the data set after a screening procedure removes those patients with fewer than four observations. We transform the PSA levels into a log scale after adding 1. This transformation is usually done so that residuals satisfy the assumption of homoscedasticity and also to reduce the influence of outliers. We also transform the time axis, via a one-to-one function, onto a log scale after dividing by 30 (the change from day to month) and adding 1. Figure 3.1 depicts the overlapping PSA levels for 134 patients in arm AA (upper panel) and 132 patients in arm CH (lower panel). The sparsity of the profiles is suggested by the percentage of patients who have measurements at or spanning the particular time point. More than 50 % of patients do not have measurements before day 18 (equal to 0.47 in the unit of log(month+1)) and after day 1210 (equal to 3.72 in the unit of log(month+1)).

We use a quadratic truncated power series basis function (Ruppert et al. 2003) to model the subject and population PSA profiles. To construct the candidate pools of change points we use 11 equally spaced knots for each arm, since it suffices for this application. For the baseline hazard step function in the proportional hazards model, we include ten-step intervals starting from day 0 to the last day. For the proposed unified Bayesian model, we wish to impose proper but weak prior information. For inverse-gamma priors, we let the shape hyperparameter to be larger than 1, allowing existence of the expectation of the inverse-gamma distribution. For Inverse–Wishart priors, we choose to use the degrees of freedom that are the smallest integers such that the expectation of the distribution exists. The scale matrix is specified as the identity matrix. We employ the following hyperparameter settings: (a_σ, b_σ), (c_σ, d_σ), (a_τ, b_τ), (c_ℓ, d_ℓ), and (a_j, b_j) are specified as (2, 2), and $(\mathbf{A}, b)$ is specified as identity matrices and 4. The hyperparameter c is specified as 100 to produce a non-informative prior for $\boldsymbol{\beta}_\gamma$. We found that the results are insensitive to moderate modifications of these priors. For the hyperparameter pair (a_π, b_π), we use the method by Kohn et al.

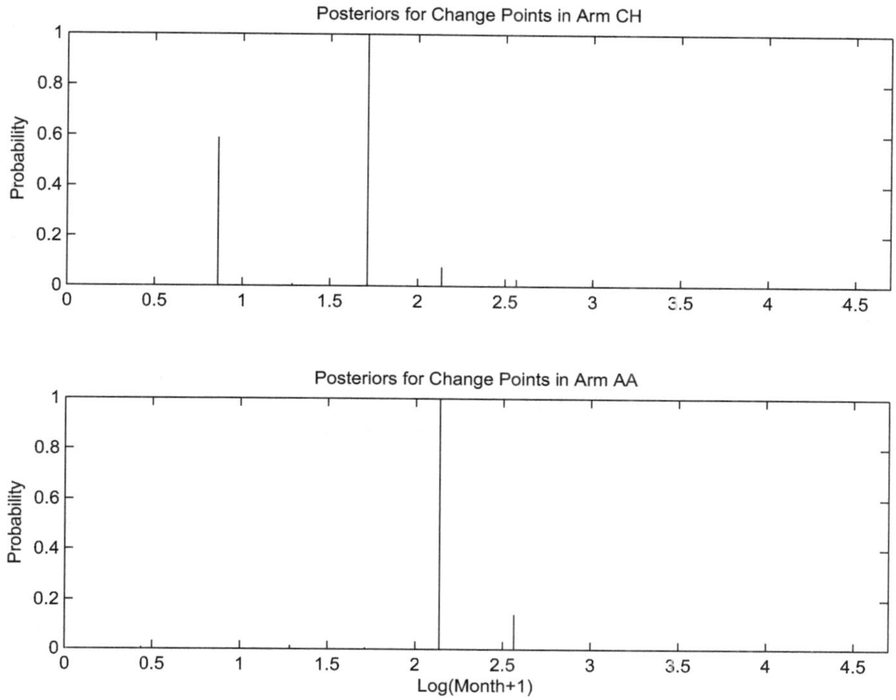

Fig. 3.2 The posterior probabilities of change points for arm chemohormonal (*CH*; *top panel*) and arm androgen ablation (*AA*; *bottom panel*). The vertical axes are the posterior probabilities and the horizontal axes are the location of the change points

(2001) to calculate the priors $a_\pi = 1.077$ and $b_\pi = 4.846$, with $E(K_y^*) = 2$ and $\text{std}(K_y^*) = 2$ so that the number of selected knots, K_y^*, is likely to range from 0 to 8. We run the MCMC chain for 60,000 iterations with 20,000 burn-in iterations. To verify the stability of the algorithm, we run several different chains with various starting knot vectors; the results show that the change point identification is quite stable. Figure 3.2 shows the posterior probabilities of 11 equally spaced change points for the treatment arms CH and AA.

Our results suggest that arm CH has two change points located at 0.86 (day 41) and 1.71 (day 136), while arm AA has one change point that is located at 2.14 (day 225) with posterior probabilities very close to 1. Thus, our model seems to correctly identify the change points of PSA trends for both arms, as suggested by Fig. 3.1. The PSA levels usually decrease sharply due to the effect of the therapy, since the therapy directly affects the prostate gland; but over time their effect wears off and the PSA levels remain constant before increasing and causes prostate cancer.

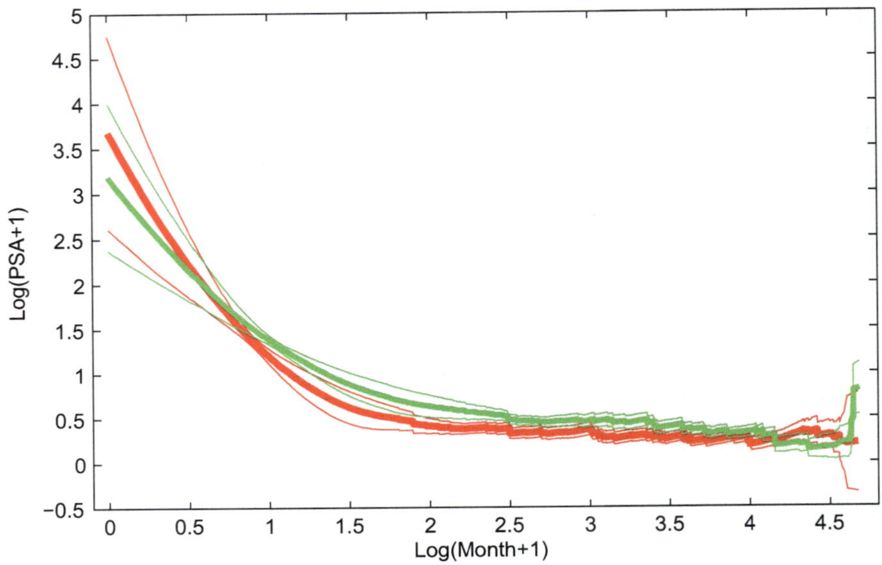

Fig. 3.3 Based on our proposed unified Bayesian model, the estimated trends of prostrate-specific antigen (*PSA*) levels for arm chemohormonal (CH; *red* line) and arm androgen ablation (AA; *green* line) with their 95 % credible intervals

Since it has been established that the volume of the prostate has a significant positive correlation with the level of PSA found by a blood test, we want to estimate the true trends of PSA levels over time for both arms. Figure 3.3 gives the estimated population-level PSA trajectory for both the arms along with the 95 % credible interval obtained using our proposed joint model, showing an L-shaped pattern.

The population profiles intersect for the most part except between time units 1–2. The difference in change points can explain the slight separation of the trends in the two arms, as depicted by Fig. 3.3. Because an increasing PSA level usually indicates prostate malfunction, we see the patients in arm AA deteriorating a bit at the end of the time period as compared to arm CH. We also see evidence that the drop in PSA levels is higher for arm CH than for arm AA. However, near the end of the study (with $\log(\text{month}{+}1) \geq 4.5$), the PSA difference between the two arms needs careful interpretation. This is because less than 10 % of patients have PSA observations at or spanning this period and some of those patients have extremely high PSA levels that may impose a larger influence on the estimation. Figure 3.4 shows the estimated individual PSA trajectories with 95 % posterior credible intervals for four randomly selected patients treated with CH.

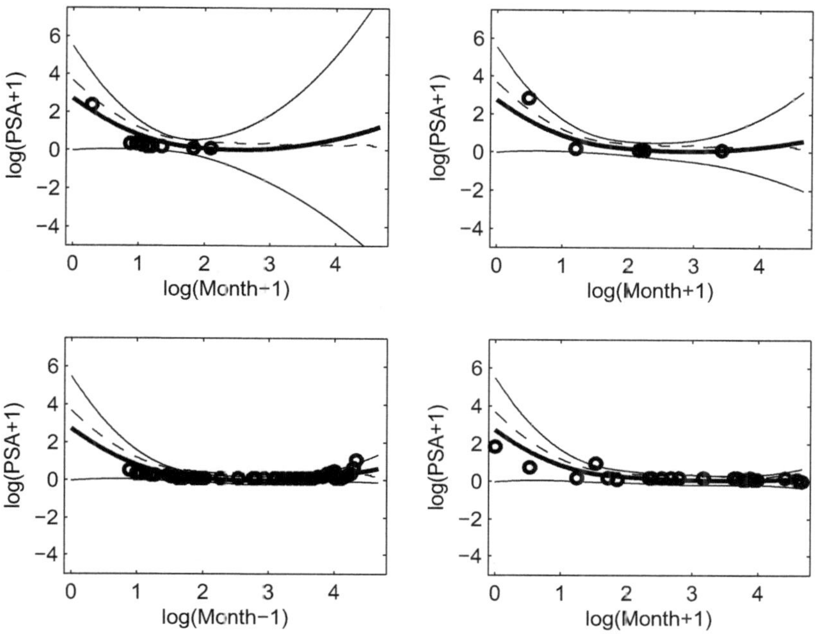

Fig. 3.4 Estimated individual prostrate-specific antigen (*PSA*) trajectories with 95 % posterior credible intervals for four patients treated in arm chemohormonal (CH). *Circles* are actual PSA measurements, *dashed* lines indicate the overall mean trend for arm CH

The figure reveals how we can borrow strength across subjects through our Bayesian model to estimate the PSA trajectories when there is little or no information. It is not surprising that the parts of the trajectories with little or no data have wider pointwise intervals.

For prostate cancer data, the effectiveness of treatment on time to AIPC is of interest. We apply our model to each of the two arms and compare the estimated time-to-event survival curves. The upper panel of Fig. 3.5 shows two superimposed survival curves based on our model and the Kaplan–Meier method with 95 % credible intervals for the two arms.

The lower panel depicts two superimposed cumulative hazard curves for the two arms based on our model, with 95 % credible intervals. The close approximation of estimated survival curves to the Kaplan–Meier curves indicates a fair fit of the model to the observed data. There is no apparent improvement for those in arm CH, but there is some evidence that arm CH may perform marginally better than arm AA because the estimated survival curve for arm AA is a little lower than the one for arm CH. On the other hand, the estimated time-to-AIPC expectancy is 1249 days for arm AA and 1527 days for arm CH. The 95 % credible bands are (881, 1768) and (1157, 2011) for arms AA and CH, respectively. The overlapping of the two credible bands

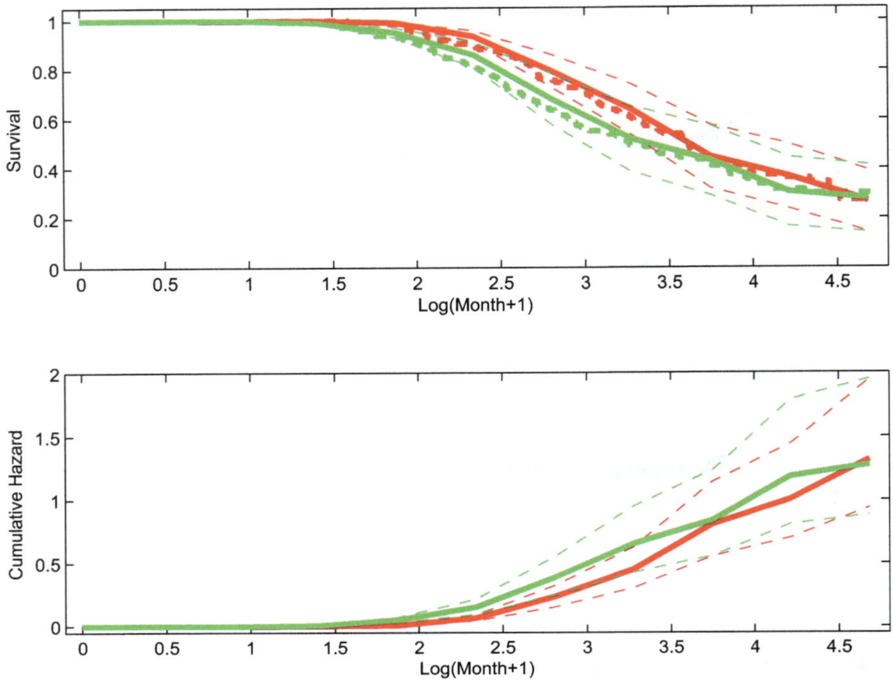

Fig. 3.5 Upper panel: Survival curves for arms androgen ablation (AA; *green* lines) and chemo-hormonal (CH; *red* lines), Kaplan–Meier curve (*thick dotted* line), our estimated survival curves (*solid* lines), and their 95 % credible intervals (*thin dashed* lines). Lower panel: Cumulative hazard curves for two arms and their 95 % credible intervals

means that there is no significant difference in time-to-AIPC expectancy between the two arms. The hazard curves exhibit a similar pattern.

In our model setup, the auxiliary variable w serves as a bridge parameter between the functional regression model and the survival model and captures the relationship between the functional predictor and the survival time. Figure 3.6 shows the box plots of the estimated w's and the observed PSA levels with high or low w's. The top two plots are for arm AA.

The top left plot overlaps ten observed PSA levels (*dotted* lines) that are for patients with the highest estimated w's, and ten other levels (*solid* lines) that are for patients with the lowest estimated w's. The mean observed survival time for the patients with the highest and lowest w's are 1.95 and 4.46, respectively. The separation of PSA levels for two groups of patients shows that long-survived patients have PSA levels that drop to very low levels and remain low after treatment, while short-survived patients have PSA levels that drop slightly yet bounce back quickly. Therefore, we conclude that the mostly nonzero w's reveal the validity of our joint model for these data based on the fact that the functional PSA levels have a (negative) effect on the progress to AIPC. The effect of informative scalar w is further illustrated by the top

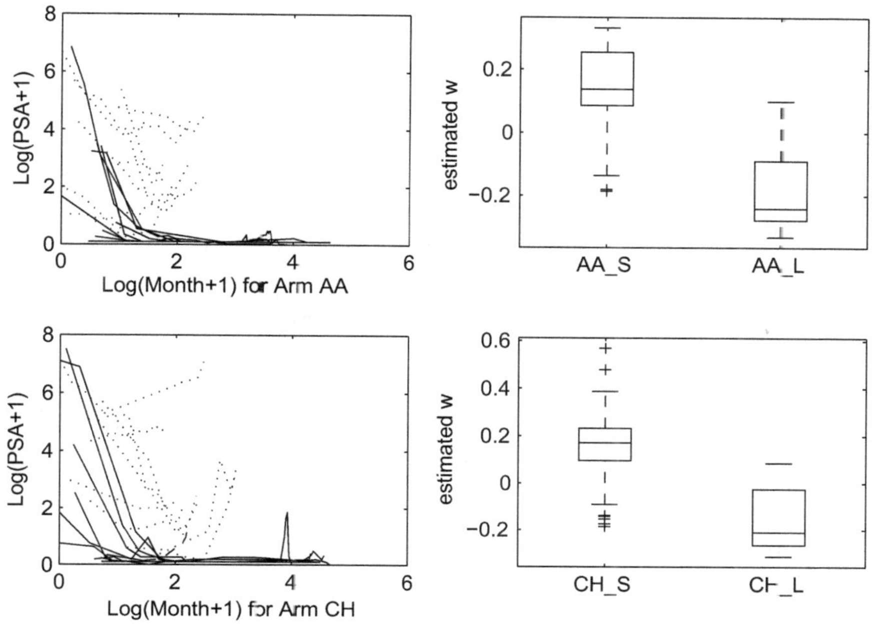

Fig. 3.6 Left: observed prostrate-specific antigen (*PSA*) trajectories for 20 patients. Ten patients with the highest estimated w's are plotted in *dotted* lines, and ten patients with the lowest estimated w's are plotted in *solid* lines. Right: box plots for posterior means of scalar w. For both arms, "_S" means patient's time to progression of androgen-independent prostate cancer (AIPC) is short than or equal to 32 months, and "_L" means patient's time to progression of AIPC is longer than 32 months

Table 3.1 The estimation of coefficients for time-independent covariates. The values in parentheses are the estimated standard deviations

	Age at *R*x	Definitive	Stratification	PSADT
Arm AA	−0.020(0.038)	−0.628(2.151)	0.595(1.984)	−0.569(1.308)
Arm CH	−0.056(0.033)	−1.397(1.733)	0.455(1.740)	−0.636(1.015)

PSADT prostrate-specific antigen doubling time, AA androgen ablation, CH chemohormonal

right plot in Fig. 3.6, where two box plots are stratified by long-term and short-term survivors according to the threshold of 32 months. We see that the w's are negatively associated with survival time. The bottom two plots in Fig. 3.6 are for arm CH, and the findings on w are the same as those for arm AA.

Table 3.1 gives the estimates of coefficients, which are the last four elements of vector $\boldsymbol{\theta}$, corresponding to the four time-independent covariates. The estimation shows that, for both arms, elder age at diagnosis, definitive treatment, low volume of stratification, and pretreatment PSADT longer than 3 months lead to lower hazards. However, there is only one significant covariate for arm CH: age at diagnosis.

Table 3.2 The model comparison measurements for both arms

	Model	DIC	$\sum_{i=1}^{n} \log(\widehat{\text{CPO}_i})$
Arm AA	Change point model	2362.7	−2652.7
	Quadratic model	2402.4	−2706.0
	Linear model	2616.3	−3033.6
Arm CH	Change point model	2129.5	−2405.5
	Quadratic model	2326.3	−2490.3
	Linear model	2859.9	−2951.0

AA androgen ablation, CH chemohormonal, DIC deviance information criteria

For comparison, we also consider two other models without the change points. The model setups are similar to that in Sect. 3.2, except that any term with the indicator vector $\boldsymbol{\gamma}$ is dropped. One model uses the linear basis:

$$\mathbf{X}_i^{Linear}(\mathbf{t}) = \begin{bmatrix} 1 & t_{i1} \\ \vdots & \vdots \\ 1 & t_{ip_i} \end{bmatrix},$$

and the other uses the quadratic basis

$$\mathbf{X}_i^{Quad}(\mathbf{t}) = \begin{bmatrix} 1 & t_{i1} & t_{i1}^2 \\ \vdots & \vdots & \vdots \\ 1 & t_{ip_i} & t_{ip_i}^2 \end{bmatrix}.$$

The model comparison measures DIC and $\sum_{i=1}^{n} \log(\widehat{\text{CPO}_i})$ are reported in Table 3.2 for both arms.

The change point model is a joint model using the change points selected by our proposed model (as shown in Fig. 3.2), two change points included for arm CH, and one change point included for arm AA. For both arms, the joint change point model is the best fit to the data with the largest CPO and smallest DIC. This result is consistent with the outcome in Fig. 3.2, where our flexible change point selection model identifies those significant change points.

3.6 Discussion

Motivated by the analysis of the data from a prostate cancer phase III clinical trial data, we present a joint modeling approach for functional and survival data using a nonparametric regression model and a proportional hazards model. Further, we allow random change points in the functional observations, both in terms of locations and number, to capture the important curvatures of the trajectory. This unified framework combines the information from both functional predictors and time to progression to generate reliable results for regression and survival analysis. Moreover, a novel auxiliary variable scheme for a fully Bayesian estimation of our model is proposed. This novel scheme reduces the dimension of the parameter space, and greatly eases the computations in Bayesian estimation. Our results indicate that this scheme aids in the understanding or interpretation of the linkage between the functional predictor and time to progression.

Our model can also benefit from several refinements and extensions. We propose to model the survival end point via Cox's proportional hazards model, mainly due to its ease of implementation and interpretability. Other survival models, such as accelerated failure time models and cure rate models, can easily be accommodated in our framework. In some situations one may want to consider the effect of time-independent covariates, such as age at diagnosis, on the progress of the disease. In the joint model, allowing interaction between $\boldsymbol{\theta}_1$ and $\boldsymbol{\theta}_2$ could address such concerns. Further, one may observe multiple functional predictors and may want to assess their impacts on survival. Suppose that for the ith individual we observe the κth functional covariate $\mathbf{Y}_{i\kappa}$, the basis matrix can be denoted by $\mathbf{X}_{i,\gamma_\kappa}$, and the fixed and random regressed coefficients can be denoted by $\boldsymbol{\beta}_{\gamma_\kappa}$ and $\boldsymbol{\beta}_{i,\gamma_\kappa}$. Then one can express the regression model as

$$\mathbf{Y}_{i\kappa} = \mathbf{X}_{i,\gamma_\kappa}\boldsymbol{\beta}_{\gamma_\kappa} + \mathbf{X}_{i,\gamma_\kappa}\boldsymbol{\beta}_{i,\gamma_\kappa} + \boldsymbol{\epsilon}_{i\kappa}, \qquad \boldsymbol{\epsilon}_{i\kappa} \sim MVN(\mathbf{0}, \sigma_\kappa^2 \mathbf{I}_{p_{i\kappa}}).$$

The information from multiple functional predictors can be easily absorbed into the survival segment via our novel proposed linear model for the auxiliary scalar w_i,

$$w_i = \sum_{\kappa=1}^{K} \mathbf{B}_{i,\gamma_\kappa}\boldsymbol{\theta}_{\gamma_\kappa} + e_i, \qquad e_i \sim N(0, \tau^2),$$

where $\mathbf{B}'_{i,\gamma_\kappa} = [(\boldsymbol{\beta}_{\gamma_\kappa} + \boldsymbol{\beta}_{i,\gamma_\kappa})', \mathbf{L}'_i]$. The rest of the model setup, including prior and posterior distributions, are analogous to the univariate case. Therefore, we conclude that the auxiliary scalar scheme is not only enabling feasible computing in the joint modeling framework but also exhibiting the potential for generalization to a more complex model.

Acknowledgments

We thank Dr. Randall Millikan from the University of Texas M.D. Anderson Cancer Center for supplying the prostate cancer data set as an application example of our proposed methodology. V. Baladandayuthapani was partially supported by NIH grant R01 CA160736. Both K-A Do and V. Baladandayuthapani were partially supported by the Cancer Center Support Grant (CCSG) (P30 CA016672). Dr. K-A Do was also partially supported by the University of Texas SPORE in prostate cancer National Institute of Health grant (P50 CA140388). The content is solely the responsibility of the authors and does not necessarily represent the official views of the National Cancer Institute or the National Institutes of Health.

3.7 Appendix

3.7.1 The Model Summary with Specified Prior Distributions

To summarize the hierarchical model setup, we define

$$
\begin{aligned}
\text{Random function } \mathbf{Y}_i &\sim MVN(\mathbf{X}_{i,\gamma}\boldsymbol{\beta}_{i,\gamma}, \sigma_\epsilon^2 \mathbf{I}_{p_i}),\\
\sigma_\epsilon^2 &\sim IG(a_\sigma, b_\sigma),\\
\boldsymbol{\beta}_{i,\gamma} &\sim MVN(\boldsymbol{\beta}_{\gamma_i}, \boldsymbol{\Omega}_{i,\gamma}),\\
\boldsymbol{\beta}_{\gamma_i} &= \mathbf{J}_i \boldsymbol{\beta}_\gamma,\\
\boldsymbol{\Omega}_{i,\gamma} &= \mathbf{J}_i \boldsymbol{\Omega}_\gamma \mathbf{J}_i' \text{ where } \boldsymbol{\Omega}_\gamma = \text{diag}(\boldsymbol{\Sigma}, \sigma^2 \mathbf{I}_{K_\gamma^*}),\\
\boldsymbol{\beta}_\gamma &\sim MVN(0, c\mathbf{I}_{K_\gamma}),\\
\boldsymbol{\Sigma} &\sim IW(\mathbf{A}, b),\\
\sigma^2 &\sim IG(c_\sigma, d_\sigma),\\
\gamma_k &\sim \text{Bernoulli}(\pi_k), \quad \text{where } \pi_k = \pi \text{ for all } k,\\
\pi &\sim \text{Beta}(a_\pi, b_\pi),\\
\text{Linear predictor } w_i &\sim N(\mathbf{B}_{i,\gamma}'\boldsymbol{\theta}_\gamma, \tau^2), \quad \text{where } \mathbf{B}_{i,\gamma}' = [\boldsymbol{\beta}_{i,\gamma}', \mathbf{L}_i'],\\
\boldsymbol{\theta}_\gamma, \tau^2 | \boldsymbol{\gamma}, \mathbf{V}_\gamma &\sim NIG(0, \mathbf{V}_\gamma, a_\tau, b_\tau), \quad \text{where } \mathbf{V}_\gamma = \text{diag}(\mathbf{h}),\\
h_\ell &\sim IG(c_\ell, d_\ell),\\
\text{Hazard function } h(t \mid \mathbf{Y}_i) &= h_0(t)\exp(w_i),\\
h_0(t) &= \lambda_j \ \ (s_{j-1} \le t < s_j),\\
\lambda_j &\sim IG(a_j, b_j),
\end{aligned}
$$

for $i = 1, \ldots, n$, $j = 1, \ldots, J$, $k = 1, \ldots, K$, and $\ell = 1, \ldots, (K_\gamma + m)$.

The fourth and fifth lines in the above model need special attention. Based on the fact that the ith curve may not span the complete set of selected change points, $\boldsymbol{\beta}_{\gamma_i}$ and $\boldsymbol{\Omega}_{i,\gamma}$ are the subject-specific realizations of parameters $\boldsymbol{\beta}_\gamma$ and $\boldsymbol{\Omega}_\gamma$, where they respectively represent the population curve and its covariance corresponding to the latent variable $\boldsymbol{\gamma}$. The relationship can be expressed via a rectangular indicator matrix $\mathbf{J}_i$ as $\boldsymbol{\beta}_{\gamma_i} = \mathbf{J}_i\boldsymbol{\beta}_\gamma$ and $\boldsymbol{\Omega}_{i,\gamma} = \mathbf{J}_i\boldsymbol{\Omega}_\gamma\mathbf{J}_i'$ with $\boldsymbol{\Omega}_\gamma = \text{diag}(\boldsymbol{\Sigma}, \sigma^2\mathbf{I}_{K_\gamma^*})$. For example, suppose there are five change points for the population curve, and the ith individual only spans the first two change points (i.e., does not have measurements beyond the third change point). Because the basis has the quadratic polynomial segment and the change points segment, the dimensions of $\boldsymbol{\beta}_\gamma$ and $\boldsymbol{\Omega}_\gamma$ will be 8 and 8 by 8. However, for the ith individual, the dimensions of $\boldsymbol{\beta}_{\gamma_i}$ and $\boldsymbol{\Omega}_{i,\gamma}$ are 5 and 5 by 5. Therefore,

$\boldsymbol{\beta}_{\gamma_i}$ is linked to $\boldsymbol{\beta}_{\gamma}$ via a 5 by 8 rectangular index matrix:

$$\mathbf{J}_i = \begin{bmatrix} 1 & 0 & 0 & 0 & 0 & 0 & 0 & 0 \\ 0 & 1 & 0 & 0 & 0 & 0 & 0 & 0 \\ 0 & 0 & 1 & 0 & 0 & 0 & 0 & 0 \\ 0 & 0 & 0 & 1 & 0 & 0 & 0 & 0 \\ 0 & 0 & 0 & 0 & 1 & 0 & 0 & 0 \end{bmatrix}. \quad (3.7)$$

The same $\mathbf{J}_i$ is used to link $\boldsymbol{\Omega}_{\gamma}$ and $\boldsymbol{\Omega}_{i,\gamma}$. These expressions with $\mathbf{J}_i$ enable the derivation of the posterior distributions below.

3.7.2 Posterior Distributions

The conditional distribution for the ith regressed covariates vector $\boldsymbol{\beta}_{i,\gamma}$ is updated using regression likelihood

$$\boldsymbol{\beta}_{i,\gamma} \mid \mathbf{X}_{i,\gamma}, \mathbf{Y}_i, \sigma_\epsilon^2, \boldsymbol{\Omega}_{\gamma}, w_i, \tau^2, \boldsymbol{\theta}_{\gamma}, \boldsymbol{\gamma} \sim MVN(\boldsymbol{\beta}^*_{i,\gamma}, \tau^2\boldsymbol{\Omega}^*_{i,\gamma}),$$

where $\boldsymbol{\Omega}^*_{i,\gamma} = (\tau^2(\boldsymbol{\Omega}^{-1}_{i,\gamma} + \mathbf{X}'_{i,\gamma}\mathbf{X}_{i,\gamma}/\sigma_\epsilon^2) + \boldsymbol{\theta}_{1i,\gamma}\boldsymbol{\theta}'_{1i,\gamma})^{-1}$ and $\boldsymbol{\beta}^*_{i,\gamma} = \boldsymbol{\Omega}^*_{i,\gamma} \times (\tau^2(\mathbf{X}'_{i,\gamma}\mathbf{Y}_i/\sigma_\epsilon^2 + \boldsymbol{\Omega}^{-1}_{i,\gamma}\boldsymbol{\mu}_{i,\gamma}) + (w_i - \mathbf{L}'_i\boldsymbol{\theta}_2)\boldsymbol{\theta}_{1i,\gamma})$. The notation $\boldsymbol{\theta}_{1i,\gamma}$ is the part of the coefficients corresponding to time-dependent covariates $\boldsymbol{\beta}_{i,\gamma}$, while $\boldsymbol{\theta}_2$ is the part of the coefficients corresponding to time-independent covariates $\mathbf{L}_i$ in later posteriors. The model variance σ_ϵ^2 is updated by

$$\sigma_\epsilon^2 | \boldsymbol{\beta}_{i,\gamma}, \mathbf{Y}_i, \mathbf{X}_{i,\gamma} \sim IG(a^*_\sigma, b^*_\sigma),$$

where $a^*_\sigma = a_\sigma + (\sum_{i=1}^n p_i)/2$ and $b^*_\sigma = b_\sigma + [\sum_{i=1}^n (\mathbf{Y}_i - \mathbf{X}_{i,\gamma}\boldsymbol{\beta}_{i,\gamma})'(\mathbf{Y}_i - \mathbf{X}_{i,\gamma}\boldsymbol{\beta}_{i,\gamma})]/2$. The indicator vector $\boldsymbol{\gamma}$ can be updated elementwise using the Metropolis–Hastings algorithm with marginal posterior $\gamma_k \mid \boldsymbol{\gamma}_{-k}, \mathbf{Y}_i, \mathbf{X}_{i,\gamma}, \sigma_\epsilon^2, \boldsymbol{\Sigma}, \sigma^2, \boldsymbol{\theta}_{\gamma}, \mathbf{V}_{\gamma}$ proportional to

$$\pi(\gamma_k)\pi(\boldsymbol{\theta}_\gamma)\pi(\mathbf{V}_\gamma)\left[\frac{|\boldsymbol{\Phi}^{-1}_\gamma|}{|c\mathbf{I}_\gamma|}\prod_{i=1}^n \frac{|\tau^2\mathbf{M}^{-1}_{i,\gamma}|}{|\boldsymbol{\Omega}_{i,\gamma}|}\right]^{1/2} \exp\left\{\frac{1}{2\tau^2}\sum_{i=1}^n \boldsymbol{\alpha}'_{i,\gamma}\mathbf{M}^{-1}_{i,\gamma}\boldsymbol{\alpha}_{i,\gamma}\right\}$$

$$\times \exp\left\{\frac{1}{2}\left(\sum_{i=1}^n \boldsymbol{\alpha}'_{i,\gamma}\mathbf{M}^{-1}_{i,\gamma}\boldsymbol{\Omega}^{-1}_{i,\gamma}\mathbf{J}_i\right)\boldsymbol{\Phi}^{-1}_\gamma\left(\sum_{i=1}^n \mathbf{J}_i\boldsymbol{\Omega}^{-1}_{i,\gamma}\mathbf{M}^{-1}_{i,\gamma}\boldsymbol{\alpha}_{i,\gamma}\right)\right\},$$

where $\boldsymbol{\alpha}_{i,\gamma} = \tau^2\mathbf{X}'_{i,\gamma}\mathbf{Y}_i/\sigma_\epsilon^2 + (w_i - \mathbf{L}'_i\boldsymbol{\theta}_2)\boldsymbol{\theta}_{1i,\gamma}$, $\mathbf{M}_{i,\gamma} = \tau^2(\mathbf{X}'_{i,\gamma}\mathbf{X}_{i,\gamma}/\sigma_\epsilon^2 + \boldsymbol{\Omega}^{-1}_{i,\gamma}) + \boldsymbol{\theta}_{1i,\gamma}\boldsymbol{\theta}'_{1i,\gamma}$ and $\boldsymbol{\Phi}_\gamma = (\sum_{i=1}^n \mathbf{J}'_i\boldsymbol{\Omega}^{-1}_{i,\gamma}\mathbf{J}_i) - \tau^2(\sum_{i=1}^n \mathbf{J}'_i\boldsymbol{\Omega}^{-1}_{i,\gamma}\mathbf{M}^{-1}_{i,\gamma}\boldsymbol{\Omega}^{-1}_{i,\gamma}\mathbf{J}_i) + (1/c)\mathbf{I}_{K_\gamma}$. It is worth to point out that the generation of a candidate $\boldsymbol{\gamma}$ is done by changing one element at a time in fixed sequencing order within each iteration. The conditional distribution for the informative scalar w_i follows the combination of information from both the regression and proportional hazards models. The likelihood of the PH model leads to its nonstandard form

$$w_i \mid T_i, \delta_i, h_0(t), \mathbf{B}_{i,\gamma}, \boldsymbol{\theta}_\gamma, \tau^2 \quad \propto \exp\left\{-\frac{(w_i^2 - 2w_i \mathbf{B}'_{i,\gamma}\boldsymbol{\theta}_{i,\gamma})}{2\tau^2}\right\}$$
$$\times\, [h_0(T_i)\exp(w_i)]^{\delta_i} \exp\left\{-\int_0^{T_i} \exp(w_i) h_0(t) du\right\},$$

which can be updated by a Metropolis step.

The following layer includes the regression coefficient as population mean $\boldsymbol{\beta}_\gamma$, which can be updated as

$$\boldsymbol{\beta}_\gamma \mid \boldsymbol{\beta}_{i,\gamma}, \boldsymbol{\Omega}_{i,\gamma} \sim MVN(\boldsymbol{\beta}^*_\gamma, c\mathbf{M}),$$

where $\mathbf{M} = (c\sum_{i=1}^n \mathbf{J}'_i \boldsymbol{\Omega}_{i,\gamma}^{-1} \mathbf{J}_i + \mathbf{I}_{K_\gamma})^{-1}$ and $\boldsymbol{\beta}^*_\gamma = c\mathbf{M}(\sum_{i=1}^n \mathbf{J}'_i \boldsymbol{\Omega}_{i,\gamma}^{-1} \boldsymbol{\beta}_{i,\gamma})$. The unstructured covariance matrix of the polynomial part for quadratic spline coefficients, $\boldsymbol{\Sigma}$, is updated as

$$\boldsymbol{\Sigma} | \boldsymbol{\beta}_\gamma, \boldsymbol{\beta}_{i,\gamma} \sim IW(\mathbf{A}^*, b^*),$$

where $\mathbf{A}^* = [\mathbf{A}^{-1} + \sum_{i=1}^n (\boldsymbol{\alpha}_{i1}\boldsymbol{\alpha}'_{i1})]^{-1}, \boldsymbol{\alpha}_i = \boldsymbol{\beta}_{i,\gamma} - \boldsymbol{\beta}_{\gamma_i} = [\boldsymbol{\alpha}'_{i1}, \boldsymbol{\alpha}'_{i2}]'$, and $b^* = b + n$. Here, the dimensions of $\boldsymbol{\alpha}_{i1}$ and $\boldsymbol{\alpha}_{i2}$ are 3×1 and $K^*_{\gamma_i} \times 1$. Linking to the covariance of the change points part for the quadratic spline coefficients, σ^2, is updated as

$$\sigma^2 \mid \boldsymbol{\beta}'_{i,\gamma}s, \boldsymbol{\beta}_\gamma \sim IG(c^*_\sigma, d^*_\sigma),$$

where $c^*_\sigma = c_\sigma + (\sum_{i=1}^n K^*_{\gamma_i})/2$ and $d^*_\sigma = d_\sigma + (\sum_{i=1}^n \boldsymbol{\alpha}'_{i2}\boldsymbol{\alpha}_{i2})/2$. The probability of being change point π can be updated as

$$\pi \mid \boldsymbol{\gamma} \sim Beta(a^*_\pi, b^*_\pi),$$

where $a^*_\pi = a_\pi + K_\gamma$ and $b^*_\pi = b_\pi + K + K_\gamma$. The common coefficient vector $\boldsymbol{\theta}$ in the linear predictor model is updated as

$$\boldsymbol{\theta}_\gamma \mid \mathbf{w}, \mathbf{B}, \tau^2, \mathbf{V}_\gamma \sim MVN(\boldsymbol{\theta}^*, \tau^2\mathbf{V}^*),$$

where $\mathbf{V}^* = (\mathbf{V}_\gamma^{-1} + \sum_{i=1}^n \mathbf{J}'_i \mathbf{B}_{i,\gamma} \mathbf{B}'_{i,\gamma} \mathbf{J}_i)^{-1}$ and $\boldsymbol{\theta}^* = \mathbf{V}^*(\sum_{i=1}^n w_i \mathbf{J}'_i \mathbf{B}_{i,\gamma})$. Here the definition of $\mathbf{J}_i$ is similar to its definition in (7.2) with a dimension adjustment to match $\mathbf{B}_{i,\gamma}$. The conjugate inverse gamma prior for variance τ^2 leads to its conditional distribution:

$$\tau^2 \mid \boldsymbol{\theta}_\gamma, \mathbf{V}_\gamma, \mathbf{w}, \mathbf{B} \sim IG(a^*_\tau, b^*_\tau),$$

where $a^*_\tau = a_\tau + (n + K_\gamma + m)/2$ and $b^*_\tau = b_\tau + [\boldsymbol{\theta}'_\gamma \mathbf{V}_\gamma^{-1} \boldsymbol{\theta}_\gamma + \sum_{i=1}^n (w_i - \mathbf{B}'_{i,\gamma}\boldsymbol{\theta}_{i,\gamma})^2]/2$.

The next layer includes scale parameters h_k, which is updated by

$$h_\ell \mid \boldsymbol{\theta}_\gamma, \tau^2 \sim IG(c_\ell^*, d_\ell^*),$$

where $c_\ell^* = c_\ell + 1/2$ and $d_\ell^* = d_\ell + \theta_\ell^2/2\tau^2$.

The parameters of baseline hazard step function $h_0(t)$, λ_j's, can be updated using the proportional hazards model:

$$\lambda_j \mid \mathbf{T}, \mathbf{w} \sim IG(a_j^*, b_j^*),$$

where $a_j^* = a_j + \sum_{i=1}^n \delta_i I(s_{j-1} \le T_i < s_j)$ and $b_j^* = b_j + \sum_{i=1}^n \big[I(T_i > s_{j-1}) \times \int_{s_{j-1}}^{\min(T_i, s_j)} \exp(w_i) \mathrm{d}u \big]$.

References

Baladandayuthapani V, Mallick BK, Young Hong M, Lupton JR, Turner ND, Carroll RJ (2008) Bayesian hierarchical spatially correlated functional data analysis with application to colon carcinogenesis. Biometrics 64:64–73

Brown ER, Ibrahim JG (2003) A Bayesian semiparametric joint hierarchical model for longitudinal and survival data. Biometrics 59:221–228

Brown ER, Ibrahim JG, DeGruttola V (2005) A flexible B-spline model for multiple longitudinal biomarkers and survival. Biometrics 61:64–73

Bycott P, Taylor J (1998) A comparison of smoothing techniques for CD4 data measured with error in a time-dependent Cox proportional hazards model. Stat Med 17:2061–2077

Catalona WJ, Smith DS, Ratliff TL, Dodds KM, Coplen DE, Yuan JJ, Petros JA, Andriole GL (1991) Measurement of prostate-specific antigen in serum as a screening test for prostate cancer. N Eng J Med 324:1156–1161

Chen M-H, Shao Q-M, Ibrahim JG (2000) Monte Carlo methods in Bayesian computation. Springer-Verlag, New York

Cox CR (1972) Regression models and life tables. J R Stat Soc, Ser B 34:187–202

Cox DR (1975) Partial likelihood. Biometrika 62:269–276

Daniels M, Pourahmadi M (2002) Bayesian analysis of covariance matrices and dynamic models for longitudinal data. Biometrika 89:553–566

DeGruttola V, Tu XM (1994) Modelling progression of CD4-lymphocyte count and its relationship to survival time. Biometrics 50:1003–1014

Denison DGT, Mallick BK, Smith AFM (1998) Automatic Bayesian curve fiting. J R Stat Soc B 60:333–350

Ding J, Wang JL (2008) Modeling longitudinal data with nonparametric multiplicative random effects jointly with survival data. Biometrics 64:546–556

Eisenberger M, O'Dwyer P, Friedman M (1986) Gonadotropin-hormone releasing hormone analogues: a new therapeutic approach for prostatic carcinoma. J Clin Oncol 4:414–424

Ellerhorst J, Tu S, Amato R, Finn L, Millikan R, Pagliaro L, Jackson A, Logothetis C (1997) Phase II trial of alternating weekly chemohormonal therapy for patients with androgen-independent prostate cancer. Clin Cancer Res 3:2371–2376

Faucett CJ, Thomas DC (1996) Simultaneously modelling censored survival data and repeatedly measured covariates: a Gibbs sampling approach. Stat Med 15:1663–1685

Greenlee R, Murray T, Bolden S, Wingo P (2000) Cancer statistics, 2000. CA Cancer J Clin 50:7–33

Gelfand AE, Smith AFM (1990) Sampling-based approaches to calculating marginal densities. J Am Stat Assoc 85:398–404

Gelfand AE, Dey DK, Chang H (1992) Model determination using predictive distribution with implementation via sampling based methods. In Bernardo JM, Berger JO, Dawid AP, Smith AFM (eds) Bayesian Statistics 4, 147–167. Oxford University Press, Oxford

Guo X, Carlin BP (2004) Separate and joint modelling of longitudinal and event time data using standard computer packages. Am Stat 58(1):16–24

Hastings WK (1970) Monte Carlo sampling methods using Markov chains and their applications. Biometrika 57:97–109

Hogan JW, Laird NM (1997) Mixture models for the joint distribution of repeated measures and event times. Stat Med 16:239–257

Holmes CC, Mallick BK (2003) Generalized nonlinear modeling with multivariate free-knot regression splines. J Am Stat Assoc 98:352–368

Hsieh F, Tseng YK, Wang JL (2006) Joint modelling of survival and longitudinal data: likelihood approach revisited. Biometrics 62:1037–1043

Ibrahim JG, Chen M-H, Sinha D (2001) Bayesian survival analysis. Springer-Verlag, New York

Kalbfleisch JD, Prentice RL (2002) The statistical analysis of failure time data, 2nd edn. Wiley, Hoboken

Kohn R, Smith M, Chan D (2001) Nonparametric regression using linear combinations of basis functions. Stat Comput 11:313–322

Metropolis N, Rosenbluth AW, Rosenbluth MN, Teller AH, Teller E (1953) Equation of state calculations by fast computing machines. J Chem Phys 21:1087–1092

Millikan R, Wen S, Pagliaro L, Brown M, Moomey B, Do K-A, Logothets C (2008) Phase III trial of androgen ablation with or without three cycles of systemic chemotherapy for advanced prostate cancer. J Clin Oncol 26:5936–5942

Ngo L, Wand MP (2004) Smoothing with Mixed Model Software. J Stat Softw 9:1–54

Pauler DK, Finkelstein DM (2002) Predicting time to prostate cancer recurrence based on joint models for non-linear longitudinal biomarkers and event time outcomes. Stat Med 21:3897–3911

Prentice R (1982) Covariate measurement errors and parameter estimation in a failure time regression model. Biometrika 69:331–342

Raboud J, Reid N, Coates RA, Farewell VT (1993) Estimating risks of progressing to AIDS when covariates are measured with error. J R Stat Soc A 156:343–406

Ramsay JO, Silverman BW (2005) Functional data analysis, 2nd edn. Springer-Verlag, New York

Ruppert D, Wand MP, Carroll RJ (2003) Semiparametric regression. Cambridge University Press, New York

Shi SR, Cote RJ, Yang C, Chen C, Xu HJ, Benedict WF, Taylor CR (1996) Development of an optimal protocol for antigen retrieval: a 'test battery' approach exemplified with reference to the staining of retinoblastoma protein (pRB) in formalin-fixed paraffin sections. J Pathol 179:347—352

Slasor P, Laird N (2003) Joint models for efficient estimation in proportional hazards regression models. Stat Med 22:2137–2148

Smith M, Kohn R (1996) Nonparametric regression using Bayesian variable selection. J Econ 75:317–343

Spiegelhalter DJ, Best NG, Carlin BP, van der Linde A (2002) Bayesian measures of model complexity and fit. J R Stat Soc, Ser B 64:583–639

Tannock I, Osoba D, Stockler M, Ernst D, Neville A, Moore M, Armitage G, Wilson J, Venner P, Coppin C, Murphy K (1996) Chemotherapy with mitoxantrone plus prednisone or prednisone alone for symptomatic hormone-resistant prostate cancer: a Canadian randomized trial with palliative end points. J Clin Oncol 14:1756–1764

Thompson W, Rosen O (2008) A Bayesian model for sparse functional data. Biometrics 64:54–63

Tsiatis AA, Degruttola V, Wulfsohn MS (1995) Modeling the relationship of survival to longitudinal data measured with error. Applications to survival and Cd4 counts in patients with AIDS. J Am Stat Assoc 90:27–37

Tsiatis AA, Davidian M (2004) Joint modeling of longitudinal and time-to-event data: an overview. Stat Sin 14:809–834

Wang Y, Taylor JMG (2001) Jointly modeling longitudinal and event time data with application to acquired immunodeficiency syndrome. J Am Stat Assoc 96:895–905
Wulfsohn MS, Tsiatis AA (1997) A joint model for survival and longitudinal data measured with error. Biometrics 53:330–339
Yao F (2007) Functional principal component analysis for longitudinal and survival data. Stat Sin 17:965–983
Ye W, Lin X, Taylor J (2008) Semiparametric modeling of longitudinal measurements and time-to-event data–two-stage regression calibration approach. Biometrics 64:1238–1246
Zhang S, Müller P, Do K-A (2009) A Bayesian semi-parameteric survival model with longitudinal markers. Biometrics 66(2):435–443

Chapter 4
Bayesian Predictive Approach to Early Termination for Enriched Enrollment Randomized Withdrawal Trials

Yang (Joy) Ge

Abstract When assessing chronic pain, in certain settings the enriched enrollment randomized withdrawal (EERW) design may offer advantages over traditional trial designs in characterizing the treatment effect in a clinically relevant way. The EERW design by definition includes two distinct phases: an enriched enrollment phase during which subjects initially receive open-label treatment with the test drug, and a double-blind randomized withdrawal phase during which apparent responders are randomized to receive test drug or placebo. The response rate during the enriched enrollment phase provides useful information on the effectiveness of the test drug, and interim monitoring of the response rate during the enriched enrollment phase can help terminate the trial early when evidence accumulates to demonstrate that the treatment is ineffective. This article reviews the method of Bayesian predictive probability for observing a sufficient magnitude of response rate at the end of enriched enrollment phase given the observed data at an interim look. The method is applied to derive futility stopping rules, and the sensitivity of the futility stopping rules is examined based upon the choice of prior distributions. The operating characteristics of these stopping rules are compared to those based on observed response rate using simulated examples.

4.1 Introduction

When designing clinical trials, one would like to show the benefit of the treatment if there truly is one, and to characterize the treatment effect. In a chronic pain study, the usual efficacy measure is subject-reported pain intensity scores, and treatment effect is characterized by the mean change from baseline in pain intensity scores. It is often difficult to demonstrate the beneficial effect of a drug in a traditional randomized study design, since it is conducted on a population, including subjects

Y. (Joy) Ge (✉)
Merck Research Laboratory, Merck & Co., Inc., Upper Gwynedd, PA, USA
Tel.: 267-305-1630
e-mail: joy_ge@merck.com

2013 ICSA/ISBS Joint Statistical Conference, Bethesda, MD, USA

351 N. Sumneytown Pike, UG1C-46, North Wales, PA 19454, USA

Z. Chen et al. (eds.), *Applied Statistics in Biomedicine and Clinical Trials Design*,
ICSA Book Series in Statistics, DOI 10.1007/978-3-319-12694-4_4

who are unlikely to respond to treatment. Inclusion of such nonresponders may prevent us from showing the drug benefit and from characterizing the treatment effect since the mean change from baseline will be calculated over both responders and nonresponders.

The enriched enrollment randomized withdrawal (EERW) design provides a solution to the challenge mentioned above by selecting a cohort of subjects who are likely to respond to and tolerate the test drug. Katz (2009) discussed the EERW trial design as a methodology for assessing the drug effect on analgesics pain, and Hewitt et al. (2011) discussed how enriched enrollment strategy increases assay sensitivity in a proof-of-concept (POC) study in neuropathic pain.

An EERW design for a chronic pain study is shown in Fig. 4.1. First, subjects will enter into a screening period during which a subject's pain intensity scores, on a scale from 0 to 10 (with 0 representing "no pain" and 10 representing "worst pain you can imagine"), will be recorded without taking any drug. Then those who meet the baseline entry criteria will continue into the single-blind active run-in period. The baseline entry criteria can be subjects must have daily pain intensity scores ≥ 5 and < 10 over the last 3 days prior to single-blind run-in period, as well as $\geq 75\,\%$ compliance with daily pain intensity score reporting. The single-blind run-in period is the enriched enrollment phase, during which subjects will take the active test drug and continue reporting daily pain intensity scores for 2 weeks. Next, at the end of the run-in period, pain improvement will be calculated as compared to the baseline of run-in, which defines "responders." For example, those with at least 20 or 30 % improvement as compared to run-in baseline scores will be identified as responders. Then responders will continue into the double-blind treatment period, which is the randomized withdrawal phase, to be randomized to receive test drug or placebo. The drug effect will be assessed by the "withdrawal" effect: If the drug is effective, a subject's pain experience shall be maintained (assuming a steady-state response) if randomized to the test drug group, but worsened or even return to the screening level if randomized to the placebo group; therefore, treatment effect is characterized by pain worsening in the placebo group relative to the test drug group.

It has been argued that the EERW design may cause the issue of generalizability. In December 2012, Food and Drug Administration (FDA) published a daft guidance: Enrichment Strategies for Clinical Trials to Support Approval of Human Drugs and Biological Products, which points out that enriched enrollment is the prospective use of any subject characteristic to select a study population in which detection of a drug effect (if one is in fact present) is more likely than it would be in an unselected population; and the selected responder population is in fact the population in which one would like to demonstrate the drug benefit and characterize treatment effect.

One potential issue with the EERW trial design is that the number of subjects who enter the enriched enrollment phase in order to achieve the desired number required for randomization is dependent upon the response rate. If the response rate during the enriched enrollment phase is much lower than expected, more subjects will need to be enrolled to achieve the number desired for randomization.

To minimize the number of subjects exposed to ineffective drugs, interim monitoring of the response rate during the enriched enrollment phase can be used to

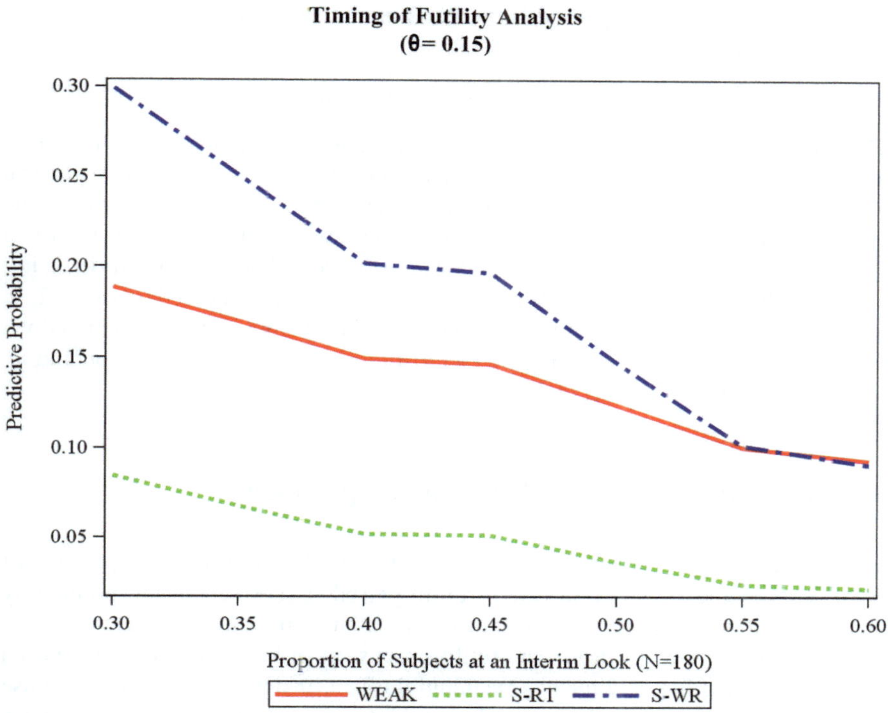

Fig. 4.1 Trial design of an enriched enrollment randomized withdrawal trial

terminate the trial early when evidence accumulates that suggests the treatment is ineffective, as compared to historical data assuming the same population. In an EERW trial, the active run-in enriched enrollment phase not only helps us identify responders but also provides useful information on the percentage of responders (i.e., drug effect): the smaller the proportion of subjects that respond to the test drug during the enriched enrollment phase, the less effective the drug. The futility rule can simply be based on the observed percentage of responders. If the observed percentage is lower than the prespecified futility bar, then the trial can be terminated early due to futility. However, given the relatively small sample sizes at interim looks, especially for POC studies with smaller sample sizes than phase IIb and phase III trials, the futility stopping rules based on observed response rate can be sensitive to outliers.

Bayesian methods have been a growing area of application in clinical trials. Gould (2005) described how the timing of interim evaluation based on predictive probability (PP) affects the ability to reach a decision to stop or continue. Dmitrienko and Wang (2006) reviewed Bayesian strategies with a focus on Bayesian PP for monitoring clinical trial data. Both reviewed the Bayesian methods for two-arm trial designs with normal continuous data as well as binary data. Herson (1979) discussed the early termination plans based on PP for phase II, single-arm trials with dichotomous outcome, by testing a simple null hypothesis on the Bernoulli parameter against a one-sided alternative:

$$H_0 : \theta = \theta_0; H_1 : \theta < \theta_0.$$

The same idea can be implemented in the early termination plan during the single-arm, enriched enrollment phase of an EERW trial. But unlike a phase II single-arm trial, significance level and power are not a concern for the interim monitoring of the enriched enrollment phase of an EERW study; therefore, in this chapter, a simplified Bayesian PP approach for interim monitoring is described without specifying a hypothesis. The method of the Bayesian predictive approach is discussed in Sect. 4.2. In Sect. 4.3, the introduced stopping rules based on the PP approach are illustrated via simulated examples, and operating characteristics are examined. Finally, concluding remarks are provided in Sect. 4.4.

4.2 Bayesian Predictive Probability Approach

To construct the PP method, consider an EERW trial with a total sample size of N subjects in the single-blind active run-in period. Let θ denote the probability that a subject will respond to the test drug, and assume individual subjects respond independently to the test drug. The futility bar is set to θ_0, which is dependent on information regarding a clinically meaningful effect, insight into the true response rate, or alternatives that exist on market. An interim analysis is conducted after n subjects have completed the run-in period, and X responders are observed among those n subjects. A reasonable question to ask is "Given X responders were observed out of the first n subjects, what is the probability of observing a response rate that would be greater than θ_0 at the end of the single-blind run-in period?" This probability is called the PP:

$$\text{Prob.(Response Rate} > \theta_0 | X \text{ responders were observed out of first } n \text{ subjects).}$$

If the PP is low, that is, given the interim results, it is unlikely to observe a response rate greater than θ_0 upon completion of the single-blind run-in period, then the trial can be stopped for futility.

Note that the criterion described above includes both the interim data and future observations. Let Y denote the number of responders observed out of $N-n$ new subjects after the interim look. Since Y is not observable at the interim look, calculation of PP will require replacing it with its predicted value. To construct the Bayesian framework for the calculation of PP, assume a priori that θ follows a β distribution $B(a,\ b)$. Given $X = x$ responders observed at the interim look, the posterior for θ is also a β distribution $B(a + x, n - x + b)$, and the predicted value of Y follows a β-binomial distribution, which is the predictive distribution for Y:

$$\Pr(Y = y|X = x) = \binom{N-n}{y} \frac{\Gamma(a+b)}{\Gamma(a)\Gamma(b)} \cdot \frac{\Gamma(a+y)\Gamma(b+N-n-y)}{\Gamma(a+b+N-n)}.$$

The Bayesian PP is given by summing over all possible future event counts that lead to a successful outcome upon completion of the single-blind run-in period, conditional on the data observed up to the interim look, i.e.,

$$\mathrm{PP} = \begin{cases} 1, x > N\theta_0 \\ \sum_{y=N\theta_0-x+1}^{N-n} \binom{N-n}{y} \frac{\Gamma(a+b)}{\Gamma(a)\Gamma(b)} \cdot \frac{\Gamma(a+y)\Gamma(b+N-n-y)}{\Gamma(a+b+N-n)}, x \le N\theta_0 \end{cases}.$$

As mentioned above, a futility stopping rule is constructed by comparing the computed PP to an appropriate threshold γ.

The next questions for consideration are: What is the timing of the first interim analysis? How does the choice of the prior affect PP? How does the choice of threshold γ impact futility stopping? Those questions will be explored in the next section.

4.3 Simulation Study

The proposed approach was applied via simulation to determine the optimal timing of futility analysis and to derive stopping rules.

For the simulations, a trial with $N = 180$ subjects is assumed to be enrolled in the single-blind active run-in period. The futility bar of the observed response rate is predetermined to be 20 %, i.e., $\theta_0 = 0.2$. The scenarios considered are:

- Stopping scenarios: true response rate $\theta = 0.10$ and 0.15
- Continuing scenarios: true response rate $\theta = 0.25$ and 0.30
- Borderline scenario: true response rate $\theta = 0.20$

Prior beliefs concerning the magnitude of the response rate, θ, have an impact on the performance of futility stopping rules. To examine the relationship between the assumed priors and the behavior of stopping rules, four types of priors are considered in this article: uniform, weak, strong right, and strong wrong, with strong right/wrong indicating correct/wrong prior belief of the magnitude of θ. Quantification of prior beliefs about θ is achieved through specifying parameters a and b in the β distribution:

- $a = 1$ and $b = 1$ for uniform prior
- a and b such that the mean of the prior distribution is equal to the prior belief of the true response rate, and the coefficient of variation is equal to 0.1 for the weak prior
- a and b such that the mean of the prior distribution is equal to the prior belief of the true response rate, and the coefficient of variation is equal to 0.05 for the strong prior

It is also of interest to study the impact of the criterion based on the choice of γ. Operating characteristics such as stopping probability and average sample size are examined under different choices of γ.

All results are based on 10,000 simulation runs per scenario. Please note that because the results are quite similar between scenarios $\theta = 0.10$ and 0.15, and between scenarios $\theta = 0.25$ and 0.30, the results for scenarios $\theta = 0.10$ and 0.30 are not displayed in this chapter.

4.3.1 Timing of Interim Analysis

Deciding to continue or terminate a trial based upon a small proportion of the planned sample size is challenging due to uncertainty about the true treatment effect. It is advisable to explore the PP under different prior beliefs as a function of the proportion of planned sample size to facilitate the decision on the timing and number of interim looks.

In Fig. 4.2, PP was calculated and plotted as a function of interim sample proportion. Data for the upper plot were simulated from a binomial distribution with $\theta = 0.15$, and for the lower plot, $\theta = 0.25$. The upper plot shows that a small threshold ($\gamma < 0.15$) and a small sample size at interim ($< 30\,\%$ of planned sample size) can lead to insensitivity of the stopping rule to a negative finding at interim, especially when the prior belief of θ is not strong or is wrong. A small threshold is not a concern when the true response rate is higher than the futility bar θ_0, as can be seen from the lower plot of Fig. 4.2.

In an EERW study, during the enriched enrollment phase, the trial will never be stopped for overwhelming efficacy and the focus is stopping for futility only; therefore, a small threshold is desirable ($\gamma < 0.3$). If stopping for efficacy is also desired in a single-arm study, then a larger threshold is needed. Plotting the PP as a function of interim sample proportion will provide help to determine the threshold for the efficacy stopping rule and for the timing of an interim analysis.

4.4 Operating Characteristics

The operating characteristics of the stopping rules based on observed response rate and based on Bayesian PP approach under different prior beliefs are examined for the EERW trial with two equally spaced interim looks during the run-in period, i.e., when 60 subjects and 120 subjects have completed the run-in period, respectively. The PP stopping threshold is investigated from 0.1 through 0.3.

Tables 4.1, 4.2, 4.3 display the results of stopping probabilities and average sample sizes for the stopping scenario ($\theta = 0.15$), borderline scenario ($\theta = 0.20$), and continuing scenario ($\theta = 0.25$), respectively.

It can be seen from Table 4.1 that a very small PP threshold ($\gamma < 0.2$) results in a lack of sensitivity of the corresponding futility stopping rule to negative interim findings, especially at earlier interim looks under uniform and weak priors. A larger PP threshold ($\gamma > 0.2$) increases the chance of stopping the trial early. Even though

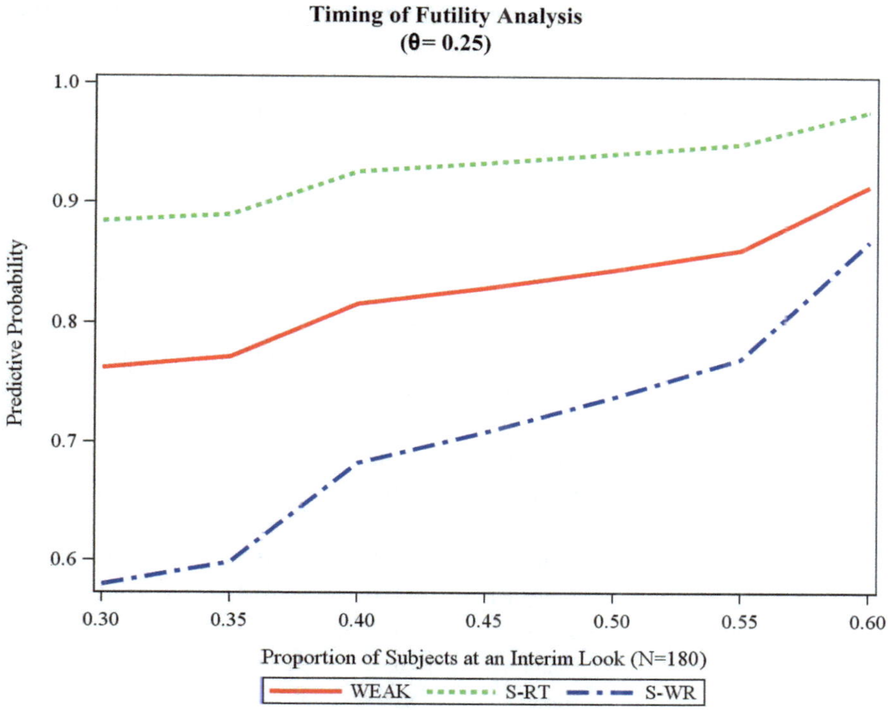

Fig. 4.2 Predictive probability under different prior distributions as a function of proportion of the planned sample size at an interim stage. Data were simulated with true response rates of 0.15 and 0.25 for the upper and lower plots, respectively. For the weak and strong right (S-RT) priors, the means of the prior distributions are equal to the true response rates, and the mean of the strong wrong (S-WR) prior distribution is set to 0.20

uniform and weak priors may fail to stop the trial at earlier interim looks, the chance of stopping the trial at later looks increases when evidence accumulates. Note that under strong wrong prior, the stopping rule exhibits a lower probability of terminating the trial. The performance is even worse than that based on observed response rate, and as a result, the average sample size is higher.

Table 4.2 implies that, when lacking evidence to determine trial continuation or termination, stopping rules based on Bayesian PP approach under uniform, weak, and strong right priors can decrease the chance of early futility termination compared to the rule based on observed response rate. Strong wrong prior belief does have an impact on the performance of stopping rules as a substantial amount of evidence needs to be accumulated at interim looks to overcome its impact.

As mentioned in Sect. 3.1, a small threshold is not a concern when the true response rate is higher than the futility bar θ_0, as confirmed by results from Table 4.3. Table 4.3 also suggests that when the true response rate is 25 %, i.e., only slightly higher than the futility bar, the stopping rule based on the observed response rate has a fairly

Table 4.1 Operating characteristics of stopping rules based on observed response rate and based on Bayesian PP (true response rate θ ue res)

			Operating characteristics		
	PP	Prior	Stopping probability (%)		Average
Approach	Threshold	Distribution	First IA	Second IA	Sample size
Observed	–	–	81.42	93.83	74.85
Bayesian	$\gamma = 0.10$	Uniform	0.00	71.53	137.08
		Weak	1.46	76.93	132.97
		Strong-RT	58.27	84.95	94.07
		Strong-WR	1.46	74.09	134.67
	$\gamma = 0.15$	Uniform	0.00	76.86	133.88
		Weak	30.08	81.78	112.88
		Strong-RT	81.42	90.14	77.06
		Strong-WR	9.41	80.03	126.34
	$\gamma = 0.20$	Uniform	0.00	81.09	131.35
		Weak	58.27	85.49	93.74
		Strong-RT	93.90	95.57	66.32
		Strong-WR	30.08	83.44	111.89
	$\gamma = 0.25$	Uniform	0.00	84.73	129.16
		Weak	88.95	91.88	71.50
		Strong-RT	96.89	97.42	63.41
		Strong-WR	44.65	86.51	101.30
	$\gamma = 0.30$	Uniform	0.00	84.93	129.04
		Weak	96.89	97.07	63.62
		Strong-RT	98.48	98.66	61.72
		Strong-WR	58.27	89.27	91.48

PP predictive probability, *strong-RT* strong right prior belief with mean equal to 0.15, *strong-WR* strong wrong prior belief with mean equal to 0.20, *IA* interim analysis

good chance (> 15 %) of terminating the trial, while the Bayesian approach, even under uniform, weak, and strong wrong priors, decreases the chance of early futility stopping.

4.5 Discussion

EERW design has gained more attention and acceptance in the pharmaceutical industry. There is precedence for regulatory acceptance of the EERW design for pivotal trials. The FDA draft guidance refers the approval of nifedipine for vasospastic angina

Table 4.2 Operating characteristics of stopping rules based on observed response rate and based on Bayesian PP (true response rate θ ue res)

			Operating characteristics		
	PP	Prior	Stopping probability (%)		Average
Approach	Threshold	Distribution	First IA	Second IA	Sample size
Observed	–	–	45.13	57.65	118.33
Bayesian	$\gamma = 0.10$	Uniform	0.00	22.12	166.73
		Weak	0.00	23.69	165.79
		Strong-RT	0.12	22.79	166.25
		Strong-WR[1]	87.08	87.10	75.49
		Strong-WR[2]	0.00	3.66	177.80
	$\gamma = 0.15$	Uniform	0.00	26.33	164.20
		Weak	0.00	28.40	162.96
		Strong-RT	1.36	28.23	162.25
		Strong-WR[1]	97.86	97.86	62.57
		Strong-WR[2]	0.00	5.49	176.71
	$\gamma = 0.20$	Uniform	0.00	31.19	161.29
		Weak	0.12	32.70	160.31
		Strong-RT	6.71	32.35	156.56
		Strong-WR[1]	98.99	98.99	61.21
		Strong-WR[2]	0.00	7.65	175.41
	$\gamma = 0.25$	Uniform	0.00	36.68	157.99
		Weak	1.36	37.52	156.67
		Strong-RT	12.89	37.62	149.69
		Strong-WR[1]	99.41	99.41	50.71
		Strong-WR[2]	0.00	10.14	173.92
	$\gamma = 0.30$	Uniform	0.00	36.91	157.85
		Weak	6.71	41.99	150.78
		Strong-RT	21.49	43.72	140.87
		Strong-WR[1]	99.78	99.78	60.26
		Strong-WR[2]	0.00	12.04	172.78

Strong-RT strong right prior belief with mean equal to 0.20, *strong-WR*[1] strong wrong prior belief with mean equal to 0.10, *Strong-WR*[2] strong wrong prior belief with mean equal to 0.30

as an example to illustrate the utility of the EERW design. The unique single-arm active run-in design of the enriched enrollment phase makes it possible to identify stopping rules to facilitate early detection of a futility signal and trigger an early trial termination when a very small treatment effect is demonstrated. This may help reduce subject exposure to an ineffective investigational product, and correspondingly

Table 4.3 Operating characteristics of stopping rules based on observed response rate and based on Bayesian PP (true response rate θ ue res)

Approach	PP Threshold	Prior Distribution	Operating characteristics Stopping probability (%) First IA	Second IA	Average Sample size
Observed	–	–	14.70	17.57	160.64
Bayesian	$\gamma = 0.10$	Uniform	0.00	2.50	178.50
		Weak	0.00	1.71	178.97
		Strong-RT	0.00	0.73	179.56
		Strong-WR	0.00	2.44	178.54
	$\gamma = 0.15$	Uniform	0.00	3.67	177.80
		Weak	0.00	2.45	178.53
		Strong-RT	0.00	1.18	179.29
		Strong-WR	0.14	3.76	177.66
	$\gamma = 0.20$	Uniform	0.00	4.95	177.03
		Weak	0.00	3.51	177.89
		Strong-RT	0.00	1.68	178.99
		Strong-WR	0.95	5.16	176.33
	$\gamma = 0.25$	Uniform	0.00	6.51	176.09
		Weak	0.00	4.52	177.29
		Strong-RT	0.00	2.19	178.69
		Strong-WR	2.27	6.83	174.54
	$\gamma = 0.30$	Uniform	0.00	6.61	176.03
		Weak	0.00	5.64	176.62
		Strong-RT	0.00	3.03	178.18
		Strong-WR	4.81	9.31	171.53

Strong-RT strong right prior belief with mean equal to 0.25, *Strong-WR* strong wrong prior belief with mean equal to 0.20

limit a sponsor's investment in an ineffective product. This chapter discusses the futility stopping rules based on the Bayesian PP: When the probability of observing a response rate higher than the prespecified futility bar at the end of the enriched enrollment phase given the interim findings is below a critical minimum value, the trial can be terminated for futility.

When planning the interim analyses, timing of interim analyses must be considered. Reaching a decision to terminate with less than 30 % of the planned sample size requires substantially negative findings, and still involves much uncertainty about the true treatment effect; therefore, early evaluation of data is not recommended to provide the basis for trial go/no go decisions.

A stopping rule based on Bayesian PP accounts for the trade-off between the relative strength of accumulated data and prior information. Although a decision about futility termination in practice will depend on only one prior, different prior distributions provide a way to balance the assumptions about the true response rate with the one actually observed when the interim analysis is carried out. The findings under different priors provide a useful perspective about the sensitivity of the stopping rule to the choice of priors. Strong priors give the prior more weight and would be expected to reduce the chance of early futility termination if the prior belief of the magnitude of true response rate is above the futility bar. Misspecified strong priors decrease the likelihood of terminating the trial in the face of negative interim findings, so the interim data would need to be very strongly negative to overcome the strong prior impact. Uniform and weak priors give the interim data more weight, and hence, unless the interim findings are particularly unpromising, make futility termination less likely when the interim occurs fairly early in the trial; however, termination of the trial for futility becomes more likely as interim negative findings accumulate.

There are various trade-offs in choosing γ. A weaker criterion (larger γ) allows the trial to stop for futility sooner, but this possibility must be balanced against the increased risk of terminating a truly effective treatment. A stronger criterion (smaller γ) causes the futility stopping rule to be less sensitive to negative interim findings, which decreases the likelihood of stopping the trial. The choice of γ does depend on considerations such as trial objective, prior beliefs, planned sample size, and futility bar, with a corresponding impact on the timing of the interim analysis, as discussed in Sect. 3.1.

References

Dmitrienko A, Wang MD (2006) Bayesian predictive approach to interim monitoring in clinical trials. Statist Med 25:2178–2195. doi:10.1002/sim.2204

FDA Guidance for Industry, Enrichment Strategies for clinical Trials to Support Approval of Human Drugs and Biological products. (Draft guidance) (2012). http://www.fda.gov/downloads/Drugs/GuidanceComplianceRegulatoryInformation/Guidances/UCM332181.pdf. Accessed 25 Mar 2013

Gould AL (2005) Timing of futility analyses for 'proof of concept' trials. Statist Med 24:1815–1835. doi:10.1002/sim.2087

Herson J (1979) Predictive probability early termination plans for phase II clinical trials. Biometrics 35:775–783

Hewitt DJ, Ho TW, Galer B, Backonja M, Markovitz P, Gammaitoni A, Michelson D, Bolognese J, Alon A, Rosenberg E, Herman G, Wang H (2011) Impact of responder definition on the enriched enrollment randomized withdrawal trial design for establishing proof of concept in neuropathic pain. Pain 152:514–521. doi:10.1016/j.pain.2010.10.050

Katz N (2009) Enriched enrollment randomized withdrawal trial designs of analgesics, focus on methodology. Clin J Pain 25:797–807

Part II
Diagnostic Medicine and Classification

Chapter 5
Estimation of ROC Curve with Multiple Types of Missing Gold Standard

Danping Liu and Xiao-Hua Zhou

Abstract In evaluating the diagnostic accuracy of a test, the gold standard might be missing because of high cost or harmfulness to the patient. The estimation of the diagnostic accuracy could be biased if the missingness is not handled appropriately. In this chapter, we propose a likelihood-based approach to jointly estimate the selection model and disease model when the missing data mechanism is a mixture of ignorable and nonignorable missingness. The receiver operating characteristic (ROC) curve and its area are estimated empirically using imputation and reweighting techniques. The proposed method extends the results of Liu and Zhou (2010, Biometrics, 66, 1119–1128), as the latter assumes a single source of nonignorable missingness. We perform simulation studies to compare the performance of the proposed method and the existing approaches in the literature. This methodology is motivated from and applied to a study in Alzheimer's disease (AD), where two reasons of missingness are modeled separately.

5.1 Introduction

A medical diagnostic test is often evaluated by its sensitivity, specificity or the receiver operating characteristic (ROC) curve. Many methods to estimate the ROC curve require the true disease status to be verified without error, which is called " gold standard." However, the gold standard could be subject to missingness, because of high cost or harmfulness to the patient. Deleting the subjects with missing gold standard results in biased estimates of the ROC curve, known as "verification bias."

D. Liu (✉)
Biostatistics and Bioinformatics Branch, Division of Intramural Population Health Research, *Eunice Kennedy Shriver* National Institute of Child Health and Human Development, Bethesda, MD 20892, USA
e-mail: danping.liu@nih.gov

X.-H. Zhou
Department of Biostatistics, University of Washington, Seattle, WA 98195, USA

Northwest HSR&D Center of Excellence, VA Puget Sound Health Care System, Seattle, WA 98108, USA
e-mail: azhou@uw.edu

Z. Chen et al. (eds.), *Applied Statistics in Biomedicine and Clinical Trials Design*, ICSA Book Series in Statistics, DOI 10.1007/978-3-319-12694-4_5

Under ignorable missingness, or missing at random (MAR) assumption, existing methods to adjust for the verification bias include but are not limited to Begg and Greenes (1983), Begg (1987), Zhou (1996), Zhou (1998), Rodenberg and Zhou (2000), Alonzo and Pepe (2005), and Liu and Zhou (2011). The verification of gold standard may also be associated with some unobserved covariates related to the missing disease status. Hence, the MAR assumption may not hold. The nonignorable (NI)verification bias was first discussed by Baker (1995), and later developed by Zhou (1998), Kosinski and Barnhart (2003), Zhou and Castelluccio (2003), Zhou and Castelluccio (2004). Rotnitzky et al. (2006) proposed a "doubly robust" estimator for the area under ROC curve (AUC), but they specified a NI parameter (the log odds ratio of verification for diseased vs. healthy subject). Liu and Zhou (2010) considered a likelihood-based approach to estimate the NI parameter. Then the empirical AUC estimators were constructed using imputation or reweighting techniques.

Modeling missingness mechanism by a selection model is a key step in many existing methods for ROC analysis. As the NI missingness assumption is not testable from the data without specifying a parametric model, a good understanding of the reason of missing data facilitates the selection model setup. All the above literature assume a single model of missingness, which is either ignorable or NI. However, missing data in practice may come from multiple sources. Different variables may account for each source of missingness, which may be either ignorable or NI. The mixture of ignorable and NI missingness was first discussed by Harel and Schafer (2009). They separately modeled the ignorable and NI missingness mechanism, and proposed a general framework of partially MAR and latently MAR models.

In this chapter, we assume the missing gold standard come from multiple sources, part of which are ignorable and part of which are not. When there are only two types of missingness, our setting of the selection models resembles the partially MAR model in Harel and Schafer (2009). But we also allow for more than two sources of missingness. We propose a two-step procedure to adjust for the verification bias: the first step estimates the verification probability and disease probability by maximizing the likelihood; the second step constructs empirical estimators for the AUC. This extends the results of Liu and Zhou (2010), in which the NI missingness was described by a single selection model. A more plausible missingness model would result in a more accurate estimator for the selection probability, and consequently a more accurate AUC estimator.

The methodology is motivated by the same Alzheimer's disease (AD) data set as in Liu and Zhou (2010). Since the gold standard of AD requires brain autopsy, it is automatically missing for the alive patients. Another reason of missingness may be that the the patients or their family opt not to have brain autopsy. Due to the fact that living people may have better health status and hence are less likely to have AD, the former type of missingness is probably NI, while the latter type can be assumed as ignorable. The data set includes the information of whether a patient is dead or not, so it could be used to improve the previous selection model in Liu and Zhou (2010).

The chapter is organized as follows. Section 5.2 discusses the framework of the selection models for the missingness mechanism, as well as the maximum likelihood estimator. We construct several empirical estimators for AUC in Sect. 5.3.

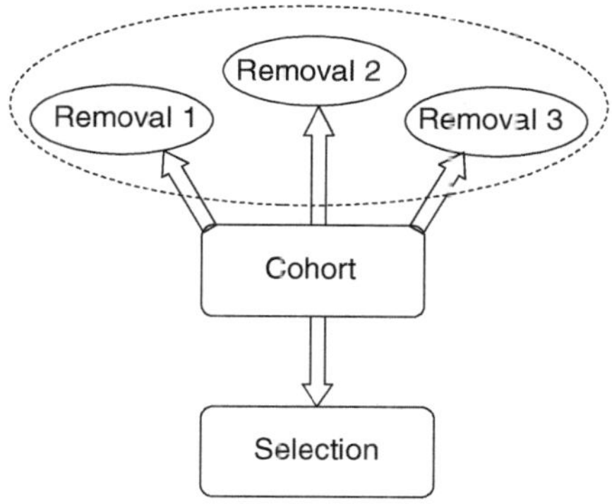

Fig. 5.1 Illustration of the simultaneous selection process—single source of missingness

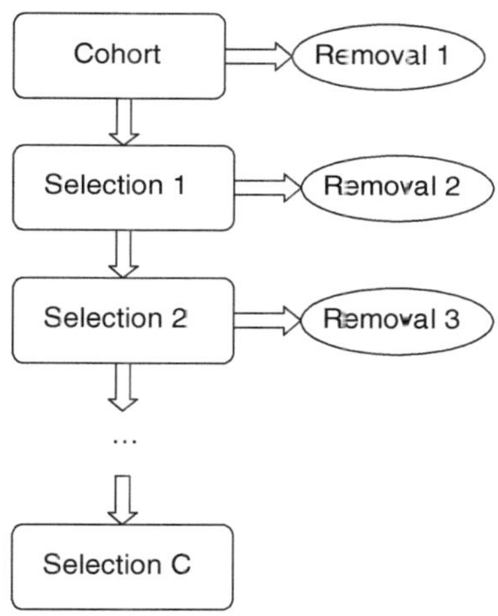

Fig. 5.2 Illustration of the sequential selection process in C steps—multiple sources of missingness

The simulation results are reported in Sect. 5.4, followed by analysis of the AD data set in Sect. 5.5. Finally, the concluding remarks are made in Sect. 5.6.

5.2 Multiple Types of Missingness

We assume that the disease verification process could go through C steps: at each step, a portion of the sample are selected to go through the next step, while the others are removed from gold standard verification. This process is illustrated in Fig. 5.2. As a comparison, the NI selection model in Liu and Zhou (2010) assumes that all the selection steps take place simultaneously, which is illustrated in Fig. 5.1. Therefore, the selection model in Liu and Zhou (2010) actually models the " overall" selection probability. In practical applications, different sources of missingness may indeed occur sequentially. For example, a survey may have NI unit nonresponse and ignorable item nonresponse (Harel and Schafer 2009), where the unit nonresponse apparently happens earlier. When there is no evident temporal order for the sources of missingness, the sequential assumption still provides a convenient way to model the missingness, by factoring out each of the sources.

Denote T_i, D_i, and X_i to be the test result, disease status and the covariates for the ith patient. Denote V_{ci} to be the selection indicator at the cth step ($c = 1, 2, \cdots, C$), with 1 indicating selection and 0 indicating removal. Denote W_{ci} to be the variables that are associated with the cth type of missingness, which may include covariates X_i, test result T_i, and their interactions. For notation simplicity, suppose there are only two types of missingness in D_i ($C = 2$). This could be easily extended to more than two types. The selection model is specified by the following conditional probabilities:

$$\pi_{1i} \equiv \Pr(V_{1i} = 1 | D_i, T_i, X_i) = \text{expit}(W_{1i}^T \beta_1 + \alpha_1 D_i), \quad (5.1)$$

$$\pi_{2i} \equiv \Pr(V_{2i} = 1 | D_i, T_i, X_i, V_{1i} = 1) = \text{expit}(W_{2i}^T \beta_2 + \alpha_2 D_i). \quad (5.2)$$

Note that $\Pr(V_{2i} = 1 | V_{1i} = 0) = 0$, which implies that, subjects removed in the first step cannot re-enter the verification sample. Then a total of three groups of verification status are defined by V_{1i} and V_{2i}: (1) verified sample ($V_{1i} = V_{2i} = 1$); (2) missing at step one ($V_{1i} = V_{2i} = 0$); (3) missing at step two ($V_{1i} = 1$, $V_{2i} = 0$). The NI parameters α_1 and α_2 could be 0, indicating the missingness at the first or the second step is ignorable. We can easily write out the " overall" verification probability:

$$\begin{aligned}\pi_i &\equiv \Pr(V_{1i} = V_{2i} = 1 | D_i, T_i, X_i) \\ &= \pi_{1i}\pi_{2i} \\ &= \text{expit}(W_{1i}^T \beta_1 + \alpha_1 D_i)\text{expit}(W_{2i}^T \beta_2 + \alpha_2 D_i).\end{aligned}$$

In addition, we also need to specify a disease model:

$$\rho_i \equiv \Pr(D_i = 1 | T_i, X_i) = \text{expit}(Z_i^T \gamma), \quad (5.3)$$

where Z_i is the design matrix of variables associated with the disease status.

Define

$$\begin{aligned}\pi_{1i}(d) &\equiv \Pr(V_{1i} = 1 | D_i = d, T_i, X_i) \\ \pi_{2i}(d) &\equiv \Pr(V_{2i} = 1 | D_i = d, T_i, X_i, V_{1i} = 1).\end{aligned}$$

For a subject with disease verification, we observe $V_{1i} = V_{2i} = 1$, D_i, T_i and X_i, and the contribution to the likelihood is

$$l_i = \rho_i^{D_i}(1 - \rho_i)^{1-D_i}\pi_{1i}\pi_{2i}.$$

For a subject missing at step one, we observe $V_{1i} = V_{2i} = 0$, T_i and X_i, and its contribution to the likelihood is

$$l_i = \rho_i(1 - \pi_{1i}(1))(1 - \pi_{2i}(1)) + (1 - \rho_i)(1 - \pi_{1i}(0))(1 - \pi_{2i}(0)).$$

For a subject missing at step two, we observe $V_{1i} = 1$, $V_{2i} = 0$, T_i and X_i. The likelihood contribution is

$$l_i = \rho_i \pi_{1i}(1)(1 - \pi_{2i}(1)) + (1 - \rho_i)\pi_{1i}(0)(1 - \pi_{2i}(0)).$$

Hence, the log likelihood is $L = \sum_i \log l_i$. Note that if $\alpha_c = 0$, $\pi_{ci}(1) = \pi_{ci}(0) = \pi_{ci}$, and the parameter β_c is separated with other parameters in the likelihood function. The estimated verification and disease probabilities, denoted by $\hat{\pi}_i = \hat{\pi}_{1i}\hat{\pi}_{2i}$ and $\hat{\rho}_i$, are then obtained by substituting the estimated parameters.

5.3 ROC Curve and Its Area

With the gold standard observed, the true and false positive rates at threshold s can be estimated as

$$TPR(s) = \frac{\sum_i I(T_i > s)D_i}{\sum_i D_i}$$

$$FPR(s) = \frac{\sum_i I(T_i > s)(1 - D_i)}{\sum_i (1 - D_i)}$$

The AUC is the probability of correctly ordering a case and a control's test result, which is estimated by the Wilcoxon statistic:

$$\hat{\nu} = \left\{ \sum_{i \neq j} I_{ij} D_i (1 - D_j) \right\} \Big/ \left\{ \sum_{i \neq j} D_i (1 - D_j) \right\}.$$

Similar to Alonzo and Pepe (2005), Liu and Zhou (2010), we replace the unobserved D_i with some estimated version.

The full imputation (FI) estimator replaces every D_i with the estimated disease probability $\hat{\rho}_i$ regardless of its missingness. Hence, the TPR(s), FPR(s), and AUC are given as follows:

$$TPR(s) = \frac{\sum_i I(T_i > s)\hat{\rho}_i}{\sum_i \hat{\rho}_i}, FPR(s) = \frac{\sum_i I(T_i > s)(1 - \hat{\rho}_i)}{\sum_i (1 - \hat{\rho}_i)},$$

$$\hat{\nu}_{FI} = \left\{ \sum_{i \neq j} I_{ij} \hat{\rho}_i (1 - \hat{\rho}_j) \right\} \Big/ \left\{ \sum_{i \neq j} \hat{\rho}_i (1 - \hat{\rho}_j) \right\}.$$

Denote $\rho_i^{(1)} \equiv \Pr(D_i = 1 | V_{1i} = 0, V_{2i} = 0, T_i, X_i)$ and $\rho_i^{(2)} \equiv \Pr(D_i = 1 | V_{1i} = 1, V_{2i} = 0, T_i, X_i)$ to be the disease probability given the verification indicator. Note that by Bayes rule,

$$\rho_i^{(1)} = \frac{\rho_i(1 - \pi_{1i}(1))(1 - \pi_{2i}(1))}{\rho_i(1 - \pi_{1i}(1))(1 - \pi_{2i}(1)) + (1 - \rho_i)(1 - \pi_{1i}(0))(1 - \pi_{2i}(0))}$$

$$\rho_i^{(2)} = \frac{\rho_i \pi_{1i}(1)(1 - \pi_{2i}(1))}{\rho_i \pi_{1i}(1)(1 - \pi_{2i}(1)) + (1 - \rho_i)\pi_{1i}(0)(1 - \pi_{2i}(0))}.$$

Both probabilities could be estimated by replacing $\rho_i, \pi_{1i}(d), \pi_{2i}(d)$ with their maximum likelihood estimators. The second approach, mean score imputation (MSI) only replaces the missing D_i's with $\hat{\rho}_i^{(1)}$ or $\hat{\rho}_i^{(2)}$, depending on the source of missingness for subject i. Let $D_{MSI,i} = I(V_{1i} = V_{2i} = 1)D_i + I(V_{1i} = V_{2i} = 0)\rho_i^{(1)} + I(V_{1i} = 1, V_{2i} = 0)\rho_i^{(2)}$, and $\hat{D}_{MSI,i}$ be the estimated version with $\rho_i^{(\cdot)}$ replaced by $\hat{\rho}_i^{(\cdot)}$. The estimated $TPR(s)$, $FPR(s)$, and AUC are

$$TPR(s) = \frac{\sum_i I(T_i > s)\hat{D}_{MSI,i}}{\sum_i \hat{D}_{\mathrm{MSI},i}}, FPR(s) = \frac{\sum_i I(T_i > s)(1 - \hat{D}_{MSI,i})}{\sum_i (1 - \hat{D}_{\mathrm{MSI},i})},$$

$$\hat{\nu}_{MSI} = \left\{\sum_{i \neq j} I_{ij}\hat{D}_{MSI,i}(1 - \hat{D}_{MSI,j})\right\} \Big/ \left\{\sum_{i \neq j} \hat{D}_{MSI,i}(1 - \hat{D}_{MSI,j})\right\}.$$

The third method is inverse probability weighting (IPW). We only make use of the verified subset ($V_{1i}V_{2i} = 1$), but weight each subject with inverse of the selection probability. The corresponding TPR, FPR, and AUC estimators are

$$TPR(s) = \frac{\sum_i I(T_i > s)\, V_i D_i / \hat{\pi}_i}{\sum_i V_i D_i / \hat{\pi}_i}, FPR(s) = \frac{\sum_i I(T_i > s)\, V_i\, (1 - D_i)/\hat{\pi}_i}{\sum_i V_i\, (1 - D_i)/\hat{\pi}_i},$$

$$\hat{\nu}_{IPW} = \left\{\sum_{i \neq j} I_{ij} \frac{I(V_{1i}V_{2i} = 1)D_i(1 - D_j)}{\hat{\pi}_i \hat{\pi}_j}\right\} \Big/ \left\{\sum_{i \neq j} \frac{I(V_{1i}V_{2i} = 1)D_i(1 - D_j)}{\hat{\pi}_i \hat{\pi}_j}\right\}.$$

The forms of the AUC estimators are analogous to those in Liu and Zhou (2010). The difference is in the likelihood function of the model parameters. Hence, the asymptotic variance of the AUC estimators can be proved using similar arguments as in the Theorem 3 of Liu and Zhou (2010). We briefly state the results here. Denote θ to be the parameters in the selection and disease models. The estimating function for the complate data is $U_{ij}^*(\nu, \theta) \equiv D_i(1 - D_j)(I_{ij} - \nu)$. The estimating functions for FI, MSI, and IPW estimators are

$$U_{ij}^{FI}(\nu, \theta) \equiv \rho_i(1 - \rho_j)(I_{ij} - \nu), \tag{5.4}$$

$$U_{ij}^{MSI}(\nu, \theta) \equiv D_{MSI,i}(1 - D_{MSI,i})(I_{ij} - \nu), \tag{5.5}$$

$$U_{ij}^{IPW}(\nu, \theta) \equiv \frac{I(M_i = M_j = 0)D_i(1 - D_j)}{\pi_i \pi_j}. \tag{5.6}$$

We denote these estimating functions by $U_{ij}(\nu, \theta)$ for the notation simplicity. Let

$$Q_i(\nu, \theta) \equiv E_j\left[U_{ij}(\nu, \theta) + U_{ji}(\nu, \theta)\right] + \left[E\frac{\partial}{\partial \theta}U_{ij}(\nu, \theta)\right] I(\theta)^{-1}\dot{l}_i(\theta),$$

where E_j is the expectation with respect to (V_j, D_j, T_j, X_j), $\dot{l}_i(\theta)$ is the ith subject's contribution to the score function, and $I(\theta) \equiv -E\frac{\partial}{\partial \theta}\dot{l}_i(\theta)$ is the information matrix for θ. Let

$$\hat{Q}_i \equiv n^{-1}\left[\sum_{j=1}^{n} U_{ij}(\hat{\nu},\hat{\theta}) + U_{ji}(\hat{\nu},\hat{\theta})\right] - n^{-1}\left[\sum_{i=1}^{n}\sum_{j=1,j\neq i}^{n} \frac{\partial}{\partial\theta}U_{ij}(\hat{\nu},\hat{\theta})\right] \times \left[\sum_{i=1}^{n}\frac{\partial}{\partial\theta}\dot{l}_i(\hat{\theta})\right]^{-1} \dot{l}_i(\hat{\theta}),$$

We have $\sqrt{n}(\hat{\nu}-\nu) \xrightarrow{d} N(0,\Omega)$, where $\Omega = \frac{var(Q_i(\nu,\theta))}{[\Pr(D_i=0)\Pr(D_i=1)]^2}$. The variance of the AUC estimator contains two sources of variabilities, one from using the U-statistic as an estimator of AUC, the other from estimating the disease and verification models. We note that the variance estimator is different from that of Liu and Zhou (2010), since the likelihood function and the estimated $\hat{\theta}$ are both different.

5.4 Simulation

In this section, we compare the finite sample performance of the proposed estimators with (1) the doubly robust (DR) estimator in Rotnitzky et al. (2006), and (2) the FI, MSI, and IPW estimators in Liu and Zhou (2010) under NI missingness assumption, denoted by NI method. Both DR and NI methods assume the one-step verification process.

We generate two covariates X_1 and X_2 from standard normal distribution and binary distribution, respectively, and the test result from uniform distribution $U(-1,1)$. The disease status is generated from a Bernoulli(ρ) distribution with

$$\rho \equiv \Pr(D=1|\,T,X_1,X_2) = \text{expit}(X_1 + 0.5X_2 + 2T).$$

Two types of missingness ($C = 2$) are simulated under the following cases A and B.

Case A: The first step verification V_1 is NI and the second step verification V_2 is ignorable:

$$\Pr(V_{1i}=1|\,D_i,T_i,X_i) = \text{expit}(1 + 0.8X_1 + 0.7X_2 + T + 1.2D),$$
$$\Pr(V_{2i}=1|\,D_i,T_i,X_i,V_{1i}=1) = \text{expit}(2 + 0.5X_1 + 0.2X_2 + 0.8T).$$

Case B: Both steps of verification, V_1 and V_2, are ignorable:

$$\Pr(V_{1i}=1|\,D_i,T_i,X_i) = \text{expit}(1.6 + 0.8X_1 + 0.7X_2 + T),$$
$$\Pr(V_{2i}=1|\,D_i,T_i,X_i,V_{1i}=1) = \text{expit}(2 + 0.5X_1 + 0.2X_2 + 0.8T).$$

The sample size was taken to be 5000. In both cases, we modeled the first step verification with a NI selection model, and the second step with an ignorable model. The simulation was repeated for 500 times. The results are shown in Table 5.1. We

Table 5.1 Comparison of the proposed method with the NI and DR methods for estimating AUC

			Bias	SD	SE	RMSE	Coverage (%)
Case A	Proposed	FI	−0.16	8.72	8.78	8.80	94.6
		MSI	−0.36	8.51	8.49	8.92	93.4
		IPW	−0.23	9.20	9.16	9.35	95.0
	NI	FI	−0.45	9.10	9.02	9.69	93.6
		MSI	−0.60	8.66	8.55	9.73	91.6
		IPW	−0.82	9.77	9.64	11.50	90.0
	DR	$\alpha = 1.2$	0.20	7.79	7.71	7.91	94.6
		$\alpha = 0$	−1.05	8.60	8.58	11.60	85.6
		$\alpha = -0.3$	−1.72	8.93	8.91	15.63	71.4
Case B	Proposed	FI	−0.19	8.84	8.91	8.93	94.0
		MSI	−0.06	8.14	8.21	8.15	95.2
		IPW	−0.27	9.22	9.32	9.42	94.8
	NI	FI	−0.24	9.13	9.18	9.29	95.0
		MSI	−0.11	8.34	8.34	8.37	95.0
		IPW	−0.47	9.63	9.59	10.26	92.6
	DR	$\alpha = 1.2$	0.48	7.62	7.52	8.55	90.6
		$\alpha = 0$	0.01	8.08	8.01	8.08	95.4
		$\alpha = -0.3$	−0.42	8.29	8.21	8.85	94.4

SD standard deviation, *SE* standard error, *RMSE* root mean square error, *FI* full imputation, *MSI* mean score imputation, *IPW* inverse probability weighting, *NI* nonignorable, *DR* doubly robust, *AUC* area under ROC curve

report the bias (in percentage of the true AUC), 1000 times the empirical standard deviation (SD) of the estimates, 1000 times the average standard error (SE) estimates, the root mean square error (RMSE) and the 95% confidence interval (CI) coverage.

For both cases A and B, the bias for the proposed method is generally the smallest. The NI method treats the two types of missingness as a whole, and uses one single selection model to describe the verification process. In case A, the bias for NI method is still relatively small compared to the variance. In case B, as the verification process is truly ignorable, the disease model could still be estimated consistently regardless of the misspecified verification model. Therefore, the performance of FI and MSI estimators is good, while the IPW estimator is a bit biased. Although the NI method is not biased seriously, it is less efficient than the proposed method, especially for the IPW estimator. This is because a better understanding of the missingness mechanism adds information to estimating the selection probability. The bias for DR method is small only with approximately correct NI parameter specification ($\alpha = 1.2$ for case A and $\alpha = 0$ for case B), and substantial if the specified parameter is far from the truth. In case B, it is likely that the DR estimator is not very sensitive to α, which explains the good coverage rates even with incorrect α. Although the DR estimator has the smallest variance, it is hard in practice to specify the correct NI parameter.

The SE of all three proposed methods are close to the SD, indicating that the variance estimators capture the true variability. As for the comparison of FI, MSI, and IPW estimators, imputation based estimators (FI and MSI) are more efficient than the IPW estimators, and hence are recommended in practice.

5.5 NACC Data Example

The National Alzheimer's Coordinating Center (NACC) was established in 1999 to facilitate the collaborative research among the 34 past and present Alzheimer's Disease Centers (ADCs) in the USA. We extracted the NACC Minimum Data Set containing over 70,000 patients who made visit to ADCs between January 1984 and November 2005. The mini-mental state examination (MMSE) is a brief 30-point questionnaire test used to screen for cognitive impairment. Our interested scientific question is how well the MMSE score classifies patients with and without AD.

The data set analyzed by Liu and Zhou (2010) consists of 53,063 patients in total, only 11 % of which received gold standard verification. The verification process has two natural steps: in step one, all the alive patients automatically missed the disease status; in step two, a subsample of the dead patients were chosen to undergo the brain autopsy and to verify their AD status. Hence, we denote $V_{1i} = 1$ if a subject was dead, and denote $V_{2i} = 1$ if a dead subject finally received the disease verification. Assume that the first step of missingness is NI and the second step is ignorable. We use the verification model (5.1) and (5.2) and the disease model (5.3), where T is the MMSE test, D is the true AD status, and X are the patient covariates. The covariates that might be associated with the verification or the disease include age at the MMSE test, gender, race, marital status, clinical diagnosis of AD, other disease conditions (i.e., stroke, Parkinson's disease, depression). The proposed method treats the case nonfatality as a source of missingness and models its probability separated from other missingness. As a comparison, the NI method pools two types of missingness together and directly models $Pr(V_{1i}V_{2i} = 1| D_i, T_i, X_i)$.

In Tables 5.2 and 5.3, we compare the NI method and the proposed method in estimating the verification and disease models. For the two-step verification model, the covariate's effect on the first-stage missingness are quite different from that on the second-stage missingness. For example, stroke may increase the chances of death, but does not significantly affect the verification probability for a dead patient; patients with lower MMSE score are more likely to be dead, but among those who died, higher MMSE score is associated with greater probability of verification. Therefore, if we pool the two sources of missingness together and use the one-step NI model instead, the estimated covariate's effect is probably an " average" effect of the two stages. The disease models generally agree with each other for NI and the proposed methods. The comparison of NI estimates and our proposed estimates are shown in Table 5.4. The proposed method gives higher AUC estimates than the NI method. The FI, MSI, and IPW estimators are 0.760 (95 % CI: 0.747, 0.773), 0.759 (95 % CI: 0.745, 0.773), and 0.738 (0.721, 0.755), respectively. Furthermore, Fig. 5.3 shows

Table 5.2 The parameter estimation (log odds ratios) for the verification model using the proposed and NI methods

	Proposed		NI
	Step 1	Step 2	
Intercept	**−2.945 (0.055)**	**−1.465 (0.079)**	**−4.527 (0.089)**
Age (per 10 years increasing)	**0.247 (0.013)**	**−0.174 (0.019)**	**0.086 (0.017)**
Gender (M vs. F)	**0.617 (0.029)**	**0.214 (0.037)**	**0.587 (0.037)**
Race (white vs. others)	**0.802 (0.038)**	**1.350 (0.071)**	**1.696 (0.070)**
Marital status (married vs. others)	**−0.094 (0.027)**	**−0.191 (0.039)**	**−0.195 (0.035)**
Stroke (yes vs. no)	**0.390 (0.034)**	0.033 (0.047)	**0.305 (0.043)**
Parkinson's disease (yes vs. no)	**0.703 (0.051)**	**0.264 (0.064)**	**0.641 (0.058)**
Depression (yes vs. no)	**−0.438 (0.034)**	**0.119 (0.050)**	**−0.202 (0.044)**
Clinical AD (yes vs. no)	**0.195 (0.058)**	**−0.211 (0.039)**	0.079 (0.083)
T: MMSE (per 15 points decreasing)	**0.839 (0.032)**	**−0.444 (0.035)**	**0.203 (0.040)**
D: the gold standard (AD vs non-AD)	**1.016 (0.127)**	—	**0.718 (0.178)**

NI nonignorable, *AD* Alzheimer's disease, *MMSE* mini-mental state examination

Table 5.3 The parameter estimation (log odds ratios) for the disease model using the proposed and NI methods

	Proposed	NI
Intercept	**−1.370 (0.195)**	**−1.101 (0.252)**
Age (per 10 years increasing)	**0.192 (0.033)**	**0.134 (0.034)**
Gender (M vs. F)	**−0.415 (0.074)**	**−0.468 (0.075)**
Race (white vs.others)	0.055 (0.159)	−0.025 (0.175)
Marital status (married vs. others)	0.124 (0.078)	0.129 (0.080)
Stroke (yes vs. no)	−0.042 (0.094)	−0.100 (0.095)
Parkinson's disease (yes vs. no)	**0.265 (0.115)**	0.234 (0.122)
Depression (yes vs. no)	0.063 (0.098)	0.110 (0.099)
Clinical AD (yes vs. no)	**1.891 (0.069)**	**1.881 (0.070)**
T: MMSE (per 15 points decreasing)	**1.063 (0.075)**	**0.784 (0.071)**

NI nonignorable, *AD* Alzheimer's disease, *MMSE* mini-mental state examination

the estimated ROC curve using FI approach under the proposed and the NI method. Under the two-stage verification assumption, the ROC curve is slightly higher than that assuming one-stage verification.

In this example, the proposed selection model does not change the 95 % CI width substantially, but it does change the point estimates of the AUC. Even though the FI and MSI estimators do not directly use the selection probability, these imputation-based estimators could still be affected. This is because the selection and disease probabilities are not distinct in the likelihood function, and we have to specify both

Table 5.4 The AUC estimates using NI method and our proposed method

		AUC	95 % CI
NI	FI	0.735	(0.722, 0.748)
	MSI	0.736	(0.724, 0.747)
	IPW	0.716	(0.698, 0.734)
Proposed	FI	0.760	(0.747, 0.773)
	MSI	0.759	(0.745, 0.773)
	IPW	0.738	(0.721, 0.755)

FI full imputation, *MSI* mean score imputation, *IPW* inverse probability weighting, *NI* nonignorable, *AUC* area under *ROC* curve

models correctly to get the unbiased estimators. The NACC example implies that an unrealistic selection model could obviously lead to biased results. In this data set, about 89 % of the patients missed the AD status, so it does not suffice to use a single selection model to account for all the missing data.

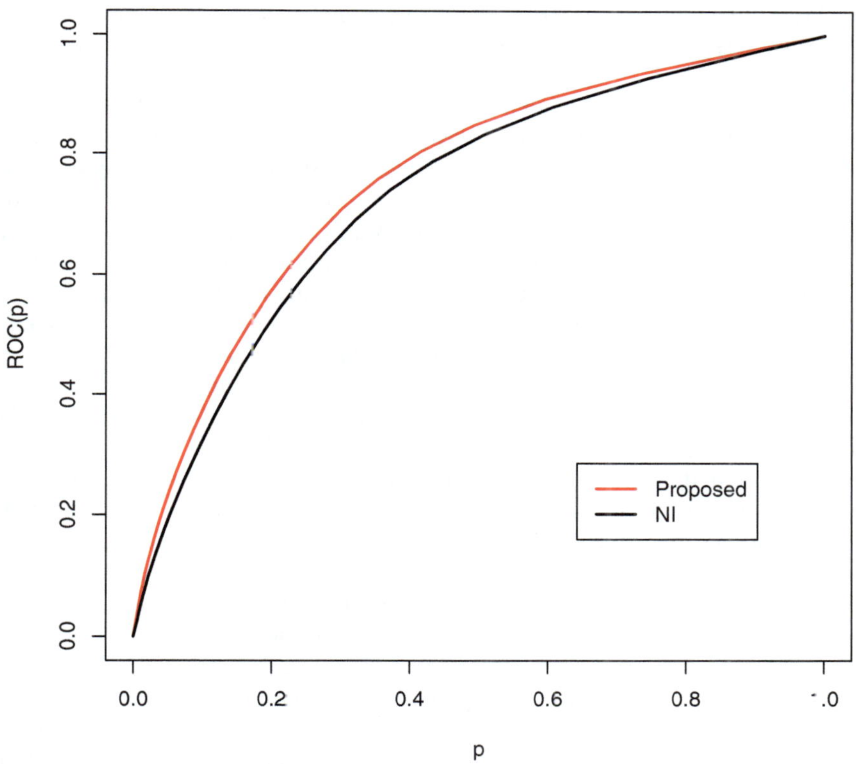

Fig. 5.3 Full imputation (*FI*) estimation of the receiver operating characteristic (*ROC*) curve under the proposed two-stage verification model and the one-stage nonignorable (*NI*) model

5.6 Discussion

In this chapter, we discussed multiple types of missing gold standard in estimating the ROC curve area to extend the results of Liu and Zhou (2010). We assume that different types of ignorable or NI missingness occur sequentially, which are reflected by separate selection models. The overall missingness mechanism might be a mixture of ignorable and NI missingness. The selection and disease probabilities are obtained by maximizing the likelihood. Then the empirical estimators are constructed using imputation or reweighting techniques. The simulation study shows the proposed estimator works well in terms of consistency and CI coverage.

Theoretically, the proposed estimator is generally not robust to model misspecifications, because the likelihood function involves the joint distribution of the disease and verification indicator, and their parameter estimation cannot be separated. That being said, our experience is that mild model misspecification does not create too much bias in the AUC estimators, which is seen in the simulation studies of our previous work (Liu and Zhou 2010). For example, if the true model has a probit link while we specify the logit link, we would expect little bias in the AUC estimators as logit function approximates probit function quite closely. We also found that MSI estimator has slightly better performance than FI and IPW estimators under mild model misspecification. With more severe misspecification, all estimators could have large bias.

As the NI missingness is not nonparametrically testable from the data, we recommended to build up plausible models based on scientific knowledge. In the stages of study design and data collection, careful thoughts about potential missing data are necessary. Then additional information on the reason of missingness can be collected. However, it is quite difficult to gather all the relevant information on the missingness, especially if the missing proportion is high. The missingness may come from quite different sources that could not be explained by a single ignorable or NI selection model. Thus, the heterogeneity of the missingness should be taken into consideration. Stratifying the missingness into several major sources is helpful to remove the heterogeneity, and hence leads to better estimation of the interested parameters. Therefore, the key message of this chapter is that, in practice, if the missingness is known to come from difference sources, it is better to model them separately. When designing new studies, investigators should try their best to collect the information on the reasons of missing data, which could greatly facilitate the model specification. A referee mentioned that machine learning techniques, such as tree-based methods or neural network algorithms are potentially useful to improve the disease and verification models, which is a very interesting extension on the proposed method. However, the difficulty is that, under NI missingness, the disease and verification models need to be estimated jointly, and the model training should be done for both models too, which may be computationally challenging. We leave it as future exploration.

The verification indicator can be also viewed as having more than two categories, indicating different reasons of missingness. Hence, an alternative approach could be directly modeling the verification by a multinomial logistic regression. But the parameters are hard to interpret, and could not explicitly distinguish ignorable versus NI missingness. Our proposed selection models are easy to interpret and implement.

Acknowledgments The authors would like to thank the referees for their insightful comments, which greatly improved the quality of this chapter. This work was supported in part by NIH/NIA grant U01AG016976. Dr. Danping Liu's research is supported by the Intramural Research Program of the National Institute of Health (NIH), *Eunice Kennedy Shriver* National Institute of Child Health and Human Development (NICHD). This chapter does not necessarily represent the findings and conclusions of VA HSR&D. Dr. Xiao-Hua Zhou is presently a core investigator and biostatistics unit director at HSR&D Center of Excellence, Department of Veterans Affairs Puget Sound Health Care System, Seattle, Washington.

References

Alonzo TA, Pepe MS (2005) Assessing accuracy of a continuous screening test in the presence of verification bias. Appl Stat 54:173–190

Baker SG (1995) Evaluating multiple diagnostic tests with partial verification. Biometrics 51: 330–337

Begg CB (1987) Biases in assessment of diagnostic tests. Stat Med 6:411–423

Begg CB, Greenes RA (1983) Assessment of diagnostic tests when disease verification is subject to verification bias. Biometrics 39:207–215

Harel O, Schafer JL (2009) Partial and latent ignorability in missing-data problems. Biometrika 96:37–50

Kosinski AS, Barnhart HX (2003) Accounting for nonignorable verification bias in assessment of diagnostic tests. Biometrics 59:163–171

Liu D, Zhou XH (2010) A model for adjusting for nonignorable verification bias in estimation of ROC curve and its area with likelihood-based approach. Biometrics 66:1119–1128

Liu D, Zhou XH (2011) Semiparametric estimation of the covariate-specific ROC curve in presence of ignorable verification bias. Biometrics 67:906–916

Rodenberg CA, Zhou XH (2000) ROC curve estimation when covariates affect the verification process. Biometrics 56:1256–1262

Rotnitzky A, Faraggi D, Schisterman E (2006) Doubly robust estimation of the area under the receiver-operating characteristic curve in the presence of verification bias. J Am Stat Assoc 101:1276–1288

Zhou XH (1996) A nonparametric ML estimate of an ROC curve area corrected for verification bias. Biometrics 52:310–316

Zhou XH (1998) Comparing correlated areas under the ROC curves of two diagnostic tests in the presence of verification bias. Biometrics 54:349–366

Zhou XH, Castelluccio P (2003) Nonparametric analysis for the ROC areas of two diagnostic tests in the presence of nonignorable verification bias. J Stat Plan Inference 115:193–213

Zhou XH, Castelluccio P (2004) Adjusting for non-ignorable verification bias in clinical studies for Alzheimer's disease. Stat Med 23:221–230

Zhou XH, Rodenberg CA (1998) Estimating an ROC curve in the presence of non-ignorable verification bias. Commun Stat 27:635–657

Chapter 6
Group Sequential Methods for Comparing Correlated Receiver Operating Characteristic Curves

Xuan Ye and Liansheng Larry Tang

Abstract Receiver operating characteristic (ROC) curves are commonly used to measure the performance of diagnostic tests. The ROC curve can be estimated empirically without assuming the distributions of the underlying diagnostic test data. Comparison of the accuracy of two diagnostic tests using ROC curves from the two tests are often conducted using fixed sample designs. However, to address the ethics and efficiency concerns of clinical trial studies, there is a need to employ a group sequential design (GSD) and periodically monitor and analyze the accruing data. In this chapter, we incorporate group sequential methods into the design of comparative diagnostic study with respect to the ROC curves. First, we study the difference between sequential empirical ROC curves on the process level. Then we derive the asymptotic distribution theory for the difference between sequential empirical ROC curves and derive the asymptotic covariance structure for comparative ROC statistics. Relating the difference between empirical ROC curves to the Kiefer process, we also show these results can be used to conduct a GSD using standard software.

6.1 Introduction

Diagnostic testing is important in medical decision making. It provides reliable information about a patient's condition. The health care provider can make plans for managing the patient with the information (Sox et al. 1989) and possibly better understand the disease mechanism through research (McNeil and Adelstein 1976). An early diagnosis can possibly save a patient's life. Diagnostic test accuracy is the ability of the test to discriminate alternative states of health (Zweig and Campbell 1993). A diagnostic test may have binary, ordinal, or continuous results, and the accuracy is measured by comparing the test results to the disease status. For binary results, the accuracy is evaluated using sensitivity and specificity, where sensitivity is the

X. Ye (✉) · L. L. Tang
Department of Statistics, George Mason University, Fairfax, VA 22030, USA
e-mail: xye@masonlive.gmu.edu

L. L. Tang
e-mail: ltang1@gmu.edu

Z. Chen et al. (eds.), *Applied Statistics in Biomedicine and Clinical Trials Design,*
ICSA Book Series in Statistics, DOI 10.1007/978-3-319-12694-4_6

probability of a positive test result given that the patient has the disease, and specificity is the probability of a negative test result given that the patient is non-diseased. For ordinal or continuous results, the receiver operating characteristic (ROC) curve is commonly used. Here, sensitivity and specificity depend on how well the test separates the two groups and which threshold we choose. Given a diagnostic test, we can let the threshold vary from $-\infty$ to ∞, an ROC curve plots all possible pairs of the false positive rate (FPR, i.e., 1-specificity) and the true positive rate (TPR, i.e., sensitivity). Many statistical methods for ROC curves are based on the summary statistic such as the area under the curve (AUC), partial area under the curve, and weighted area under the curve (Zhou et al. 2011). The diagnostic accuracy can be evaluated with a fixed sample design, or a group sequential design GSD. With a fixed sample design, the ROC statistics are estimated after tests are measured on all subjects. And with a GSD, the ROC statistics are estimated at interim analysis points as subjects are accrued. In contrast to its counterpart, the group sequential method allows researchers to terminate the study early, if a candidate diagnostic test is clearly superior or non-inferior to the established diagnostic test under comparison (Jennison and Turnbull 2000). Group sequential method also allows early termination for futility based on conditional estimation of sensitivity and specificity (Pepe et al. 2009). Hence, it addresses the ethical and cost issues in diagnostic trials. Methods have been proposed to apply group sequential methodology to diagnostic test studies (Tang et al. 2008; Tang and Liu 2010; Pepe et al. 2009; Liu et al. 2008; Mazumdar and Liu 2003). The nonparametric sequential methods for the AUC or the weighted AUC (wAUC) statistics in sequentially comparing ROC curves have been introduced, as well as the sample size recalculation. Asymptotic properties of a single sequential empirical ROC curve has been rigorously studied in Koopmeiners and Feng (2011). Understanding the joint asymptotic properties of two sequential empirical ROC curves, as well as the sequential differences of two empirical ROC curves at any FPR, will help us conduct group sequential study on the process level instead of the point level. It is shown in this chapter that they asymptotically follow special Kiefer processes. This implies that for example the sequential differences at different FPRs are also asymptotically jointly normal. Furthermore, the existing results on the summary ROC statistics can be obtained from our findings.

6.2 Method

6.2.1 Group Sequential Method for Comparing ROC Curves

Many diagnostic trials involve the comparison of summary measures of ROC curves. The summary measure of the ROC curve can be in the forms of the AUC, partial AUC, or sensitivity at a given specificity, and they are all special cases of the wAUC (Tang et al. 2008). A fixed sample diagnostic trial can be designed to compare the ROC measures, in which a hypothesis test will be conducted after all sample data are collected. However, to address the cost and ethics issues related to human experimentation, a GSD can be implemented. In a GSD, we conduct interim analyses of accumulating data and the hypothesis is tested at each interim analysis. This method addresses the concerns and is supposed to be more efficient in terms of expected sample sizes since it is possible to end the trial earlier. In a group sequential method, how to control the type I error is important and affects the calculation of the rejection bounds at each interim point. Stopping boundaries proposed by Pocock, O'Brien and Fleming, Kim and Demets (Pocock 1977; O'Brien and Fleming 1979; Kim and Demets 1992) are commonly used to control the overall type I error rate. The Pocock method uses repeated significance tests with constant nominal significance levels. The O'Brien and Fleming method is a test in which the nominal significance levels at each interim analysis increase as the study progresses. In clinical trials, the O'Brien and Fleming's approach is commonly used, as it has wider boundaries initially and narrower ones at later analyses. And the error spending method by Kim and Demets uses a function of the observation information for the type I error spent at each interim analysis, with the maximum of the function being the nominal type I error rate. This approach allows flexibility in deciding the number of interim analyses.

Some research has been done in asymptotic sequential property of a single ROC curve (Koopmeiners and Feng 2011). They derived the asymptotic theory for the sequential empirical ROC curve under the case-control sampling. In this chapter, we study the properties of the difference between two empirical ROC curves and present a method to sequentially compare the empirical curves.

In a comparative diagnostic trial, let $X_{i,D}$ and $X_{i,\bar{D}}$ denote the outcome of the ith diagnostic test for cases and controls, respectively, with $i = 1, 2$. Suppose a larger value is more likely to indicate the disease. The cumulative distribution functions of $X_{i,D}$ and $X_{i,\bar{D}}$ are $F_{i,D}$ and $F_{i,\bar{D}}$ for the case and control populations, respectively. $S_{i,D}$ and $S_{i,\bar{D}}$ are the survival functions for the case and control populations. The sensitivity and specificity are given by $S_{i,D}(c)$ and $F_{i,\bar{D}}(c)$ for a given cutoff value, c. The ROC curve for the ith diagnostic test is defined by

$$ROC_i(t) = S_{i,D}(S_{i,\bar{D}}^{-1}(t)), \qquad t \in [0, 1], \tag{6.1}$$

where $S^{-1}(t) = inf\{x : F(x) \geq (1 - t)\}$. The ROC curve is a plot of sensitivity (TPR) against 1-specificity (FPR), as the threshold value c varies. Assume that there are a total of n_D case subjects and $n_{\bar{D}}$ control subjects in the study. Suppose that we observe $X_{i,D,j} \sim F_{i,D}$, $j = 1, ..., n_D$, representing the measurements of the ith diagnostic test from n_D subjects, and $X_{i,\bar{D},j} \sim F_{i,\bar{D}}$, $j = 1, ..., n_{\bar{D}}$, the measurements of the ith diagnostic test from $n_{\bar{D}}$ subjects, for $i = 1, 2$. Assume that measurements from different subjects are independent, and measurements of tests 1 and 2 within the same subject are possibly correlated. The survival functions, $S_{i,D}$, $S_{i,\bar{D}}$, can be empirically estimated to yield the empirical ROC curve:

$$\widehat{ROC}_i(t) = \hat{S}_{i,D}(\hat{S}_{i,\bar{D}}^{-1}(t)), \qquad i = 1, 2, \tag{6.2}$$

where $\hat{S}_{i,D}(t) = \sum_{j=1}^{n_D} I(X_{i,D,j} > t)/n_D$ and $\hat{S}_{i,\bar{D}}(t) = \sum_{j=1}^{n_{\bar{D}}} I(X_{i,\bar{D},j} > t)/n_{\bar{D}}$. Also, $\hat{S}_{i,\bar{D}}^{-1}(t) = inf\{x : \hat{F}_{i,\bar{D}}(x) \geq (1-t)\}$, where $\hat{F}_{i,\bar{D}}(t) = \sum_{j=1}^{n_{\bar{D}}} I(X_{i,\bar{D},j} \leq t)/n_{\bar{D}}$.

6.2.2 Asymptotic Property

Suppose we have measurements from two diagnostic tests on n_D case subjects and $n_{\bar{D}}$ control subjects, where all subjects are independent. Throughout the chapter, we make the following assumptions:

(A1) $F_{i,D}(x)$ and $F_{i,\bar{D}}(x)$ are continuous distribution functions with continuous densities $f_{i,D}(x)$ and $f_{i,\bar{D}}(x)$, respectively,
(A2) $f_{i,D}(x) > 0$ for $x \in (sup\{x : F_{i,D}(x) = 0\}, inf\{x : F_{i,D}(x) = 1\})$
(A3) $f_{i,\bar{D}}(x) > 0$ for $x \in (sup\{x : F_{i,\bar{D}}(x) = 0\}, inf\{x : F_{i,\bar{D}}(x) = 1\})$
(A4) $\frac{n_D}{n_{\bar{D}}} \to \lambda > 0$ as $n_D \to \infty$ and $n_{\bar{D}} \to \infty$, i.e., the ratio of cases to controls converges to a constant.

Let $\Delta(t) = ROC_1(t) - ROC_2(t)$, $\hat{\Delta}(t) = \widehat{ROC_1}(t) - \widehat{ROC_2}(t)$, and at an interim analysis in a GSD when the proportion of accrued cases among all cases and the proportion of controls among all controls are r_D and $r_{\bar{D}}$, respectively. We define $\hat{\Delta}_{r_D,r_{\bar{D}}}(t) = \widehat{ROC}_{1,r_D,r_{\bar{D}}}(t) - \widehat{ROC}_{2,r_D,r_{\bar{D}}}(t)$. For the sequential empirical $\Delta(t)$ at two different analysis points $(r_D, r_{\bar{D}})$ and $(r'_D, r'_{\bar{D}})$, we let

$$\mathbf{Y} = \begin{pmatrix} n_D^{-1/2}[n_D r_D](\hat{\Delta}_{r_D,r_{\bar{D}}}(t) - \Delta(t)) \\ n_D^{-1/2}[n_D r'_D](\hat{\Delta}_{r'_D,r'_{\bar{D}}}(t) - \Delta(t)) \end{pmatrix},$$

which can be expressed in terms of the empirical $\widehat{ROC}$ and true ROC curves as

$$\begin{pmatrix} 1 & -1 & 0 & 0 \\ 0 & 0 & 1 & -1 \end{pmatrix} \begin{pmatrix} n_D^{-1/2}[n_D r_D](\widehat{ROC}_{1,r_D,r_{\bar{D}}}(t) - ROC_1(t)) \\ n_D^{-1/2}[n_D r_D](\widehat{ROC}_{2,r_D,r_{\bar{D}}}(t) - ROC_2(t)) \\ n_D^{-1/2}[n_D r'_D](\widehat{ROC}_{1,r'_D,r'_{\bar{D}}}(t) - ROC_1(t)) \\ n_D^{-1/2}[n_D r'_D](\widehat{ROC}_{2,r'_D,r'_{\bar{D}}}(t) - ROC_2(t)) \end{pmatrix}.$$

We also let

$$\mathbf{X} = \begin{pmatrix} n_D^{-1/2}[n_D r_D](\widehat{ROC}_{1,r_D,r_{\bar{D}}}(t) - ROC_1(t)) \\ n_D^{-1/2}[n_D r_D](\widehat{ROC}_{2,r_D,r_{\bar{D}}}(t) - ROC_2(t)) \\ n_D^{-1/2}[n_D r'_D](\widehat{ROC}_{1,r'_D,r'_{\bar{D}}}(t) - ROC_1(t)) \\ n_D^{-1/2}[n_D r'_D](\widehat{ROC}_{2,r'_D,r'_{\bar{D}}}(t) - ROC_2(t)) \end{pmatrix}.$$

Assume (A1)–(A4) hold, and let $\frac{f_{i,D}(S^{-1}_{i,\bar{D}}(t))}{f_{i,\bar{D}}(S^{-1}_{i,\bar{D}}(t))}$ be bounded on the interval of [a,b] for some $0 < a < b < 1$. As $n_D \to \infty$ and $n_{\bar{D}} \to \infty$, for any diagnostic test i, $i = 1, 2$,

$$n_D^{-1/2}[n_D r_D](\widehat{ROC}_{i,r_D,r_{\bar{D}}}(t) - ROC_i(t)) \tag{6.3}$$

$$= n_D^{-1/2}[n_D r_D](\hat{S}_{i,D,r_D}(\hat{S}^{-1}_{i,\bar{D},r_{\bar{D}}}(t)) - S_{i,D}(\hat{S}^{-1}_{i,\bar{D},r_{\bar{D}}}(t))) \tag{6.4}$$

$$+ n_D^{-1/2}[n_D r_D](S_{i,D}(\hat{S}^{-1}_{i,\bar{D},r_{\bar{D}}}(t)) - S_{i,D}(S^{-1}_{i,\bar{D}}(t))). \tag{6.5}$$

By applying partial sum process results of vander Vaart and Wellner (1996), we have

$$n_D^{-1/2}[n_D r_D](\hat{S}_{i,D,r_D}(\hat{S}^{-1}_{i,\bar{D},r_{\bar{D}}}(t)) - S_{i,D}(\hat{S}^{-1}_{i,\bar{D},r_{\bar{D}}}(t))) \xrightarrow{d} K_{i,1}(ROC_i(t), r_D), \tag{6.6}$$

and

$$n_{\bar{D}}^{-1/2}[n_{\bar{D}} r_{\bar{D}}](\hat{S}_{i,\bar{D},r_{\bar{D}}}(t) - S_{i,\bar{D}}(t)) \xrightarrow{d} K_{i,2}(S_{i,\bar{D}}(t), r_{\bar{D}}),$$

where $K_{i,1}$ and $K_{j,2}$ are independent Kiefer processes, for $i, j = \{1, 2\}$. A Kiefer process, K(t,r), is a two-parameter zero-mean Gaussian process in t and r with covariance: $Cov(K(t_1, r_1), K(t_2, r_2)) = (t_1 \wedge t_2 - t_1 t_2)(r_1 \wedge r_2)$, where $\wedge$ represents the minimum of two operands. It behaves like a Brownian bridge in t and a Wiener process (Brownian motion) in r. From the equation and the compact differentiability of the inverse function, we have

$$n_D^{-1/2}[n_D r_D](\hat{S}^{-1}_{i,\bar{D},r_{\bar{D}}}(t) - S^{-1}_{i,\bar{D}}(t)) \xrightarrow{d} -\lambda^{1/2}\frac{r_D}{r_{\bar{D}}} \cdot \frac{1}{f_{i,\bar{D}}(S^{-1}_{i,\bar{D}}(t))} K_{i,2}(t, r_{\bar{D}}).$$

Applying the functional delta method,

$$n_D^{-1/2}[n_D r_D](S_{i,D}(\hat{S}^{-1}_{i,\bar{D},r_{\bar{D}}}(t)) - S_{i,D}(S^{-1}_{i,\bar{D}}(t))) \xrightarrow{d} \lambda^{1/2}\frac{r_D}{r_{\bar{D}}} \cdot \frac{f_{i,D}(S^{-1}_{i,\bar{D}}(t))}{f_{i,\bar{D}}(S^{-1}_{i,\bar{D}}(t))} K_{i,2}(t, r_{\bar{D}}). \tag{6.7}$$

Then we rewrite the random vector components as sums of two terms as of Eq. 6.3:

$$\begin{pmatrix} n_D^{-1/2}[n_D r_D](\widehat{ROC}_{1,r_D,r_{\bar{D}}}(t) - ROC_1(t)) \\ n_D^{-1/2}[n_D r_D](\widehat{ROC}_{2,r_D,r_{\bar{D}}}(t) - ROC_2(t)) \\ n_D^{-1/2}[n_D r'_D](\widehat{ROC}_{1,r'_D,r'_{\bar{D}}}(t) - ROC_1(t)) \\ n_D^{-1/2}[n_D r'_D](\widehat{ROC}_{2,r'_D,r'_{\bar{D}}}(t) - ROC_2(t)) \end{pmatrix}$$

$$= \begin{pmatrix} n_D^{-1/2}[n_D r_D](\hat{S}_{1,D,r_D}(\hat{S}^{-1}_{1,\bar{D},r_{\bar{D}}}(t)) - S_{1,D}(\hat{S}^{-1}_{1,\bar{D},r_{\bar{D}}}(t))) \\ n_D^{-1/2}[n_D r_D](\hat{S}_{2,D,r_D}(\hat{S}^{-1}_{2,\bar{D},r_{\bar{D}}}(t)) - S_{2,D}(\hat{S}^{-1}_{2,\bar{D},r_{\bar{D}}}(t))) \\ n_D^{-1/2}[n_D r'_D](\hat{S}_{1,D,r'_D}(\hat{S}^{-1}_{1,\bar{D},r'_{\bar{D}}}(t)) - S_{1,D}(\hat{S}^{-1}_{1,\bar{D},r'_{\bar{D}}}(t))) \\ n_D^{-1/2}[n_D r'_D](\hat{S}_{2,D,r'_D}(\hat{S}^{-1}_{2,\bar{D},r'_{\bar{D}}}(t)) - S_{2,D}(\hat{S}^{-1}_{2,\bar{D},r'_{\bar{D}}}(t))) \end{pmatrix}$$

$$+\begin{pmatrix} n_{\bar{D}}^{-1/2}[n_D r_D](S_{1,D}(\hat{S}^{-1}_{1,\bar{D},r_{\bar{D}}}(t)) - S_{1,D}(S^{-1}_{1,\bar{D}}(t))) \\ n_{\bar{D}}^{-1/2}[n_D r_D](S_{2,D}(\hat{S}^{-1}_{2,\bar{D},r_{\bar{D}}}(t)) - S_{2,D}(S^{-1}_{2,\bar{D}}(t))) \\ n_{\bar{D}}^{-1/2}[n_D r'_D](S_{1,D}(\hat{S}^{-1}_{1,\bar{D},r'_{\bar{D}}}(t)) - S_{1,D}(S^{-1}_{1,\bar{D}}(t))) \\ n_{\bar{D}}^{-1/2}[n_D r'_D](S_{2,D}(\hat{S}^{-1}_{2,\bar{D},r'_{\bar{D}}}(t)) - S_{2,D}(S^{-1}_{2,\bar{D}}(t))) \end{pmatrix},$$

using Eqs. 6.6, 6.7, and Cramér–Wold device (Karr 1993). The summation above converges weakly to

$$\begin{pmatrix} K_{1,1}(ROC_1(t), r_D) \\ K_{2,1}(ROC_2(t), r_D) \\ K_{1,1}(ROC_1(t), r'_D) \\ K_{2,1}(ROC_2(t), r'_D) \end{pmatrix} + \begin{pmatrix} \lambda^{1/2}\frac{r_D}{r_{\bar{D}}}\left(\frac{f_{1,D}(S^{-1}_{1,\bar{D}}(t))}{f_{1,\bar{D}}(S^{-1}_{1,\bar{D}}(t))}\right) K_{1,2}(t, r_{\bar{D}}) \\ \lambda^{1/2}\frac{r_D}{r_{\bar{D}}}\left(\frac{f_{2,D}(S^{-1}_{2,\bar{D}}(t))}{f_{2,\bar{D}}(S^{-1}_{2,\bar{D}}(t))}\right) K_{2,2}(t, r_{\bar{D}}) \\ \lambda^{1/2}\frac{r'_D}{r'_{\bar{D}}}\left(\frac{f_{1,D}(S^{-1}_{1,\bar{D}}(t))}{f_{1,\bar{D}}(S^{-1}_{1,\bar{D}}(t))}\right) K_{1,2}(t, r'_{\bar{D}}) \\ \lambda^{1/2}\frac{r'_D}{r'_{\bar{D}}}\left(\frac{f_{2,D}(S^{-1}_{2,\bar{D}}(t))}{f_{2,\bar{D}}(S^{-1}_{2,\bar{D}}(t))}\right) K_{2,2}(t, r'_{\bar{D}}) \end{pmatrix}$$

uniformly for $t \in [a, b]$, $r_D \in [c, 1]$, and $r_{\bar{D}} \in [d, 1]$ for $0 < c < 1$, $0 < d < 1$. Thus, the random vector **X** is approximately multivariate normal with the covariance matrix given by

$$\Sigma = \begin{pmatrix} a_{11} & a_{12} & a_{13} & a_{14} \\ a_{12} & a_{22} & a_{23} & a_{24} \\ a_{13} & a_{23} & a_{33} & a_{34} \\ a_{14} & a_{24} & a_{34} & a_{44} \end{pmatrix}.$$

See appendix for the derivation of elements a_{ij}.

Hence, the random vector **Y** is approximately normal with the covariance matrix derived approximately in the following:

$$\begin{pmatrix} 1 & -1 & 0 & 0 \\ 0 & 0 & 1 & -1 \end{pmatrix} \Sigma \begin{pmatrix} 1 & 0 \\ -1 & 0 \\ 0 & 1 \\ 0 & -1 \end{pmatrix}$$

$$= \begin{pmatrix} a_{11} + a_{22} - 2a_{12} & a_{13} + a_{24} - 2a_{14} \\ a_{13} + a_{24} - 2a_{14} & a_{33} + a_{44} - 2a_{34} \end{pmatrix}.$$

Without the loss of generality, let $r'_D \geq r_D$ and $r'_{\bar{D}} \geq r_{\bar{D}}$, that is, the proportions $(r'_D, r'_{\bar{D}})$ occur in a later time than $(r_D, r_{\bar{D}})$. Approximately,

$$Cov(\hat{\Delta}_{r_D,r_{\bar{D}}}(t), \hat{\Delta}_{r'_D,r'_{\bar{D}}}(t)) = Cov(\hat{\Delta}_{r_D,r_{\bar{D}}}(t) - \Delta(t), \hat{\Delta}_{r'_D,r'_{\bar{D}}}(t) - \Delta(t))$$

$$= n_D \frac{1}{n_D r_D} \frac{1}{n_D r'_D} (a_{13} + a_{24} - 2a_{14}).$$

And the variance,

$$\begin{aligned} Var(\hat{\Delta}_{r'_D, r'_{\bar{D}}}(t)) &= Var(\hat{\Delta}_{r'_D, r'_{\bar{D}}}(t) - \Delta(t)) \\ &= n_D \frac{1}{n_D r'_D} \frac{1}{n_D r'_D} (a_{33} + a_{44} - 2a_{34}). \end{aligned}$$

Applying the formulas of a_{ij} to the equations above, we have

$$\begin{aligned} & Cov(\hat{\Delta}_{r_D, r_{\bar{D}}}(t), \hat{\Delta}_{r'_D, r'_{\bar{D}}}(t)) = Var(\hat{\Delta}_{r'_D, r'_{\bar{D}}}(t)) \qquad (6.8) \\ = & \frac{1}{n_D r'_D} (ROC_1(t) - ROC_1^2(t)) + \frac{1}{n_{\bar{D}} r'_{\bar{D}}} \left(\frac{f_{1,D}(S_{1,\bar{D}}^{-1}(t))}{f_{1,\bar{D}}(S_{1,\bar{D}}^{-1}(t))} \right)^2 (t - t^2) \\ & + \frac{1}{n_D r'_D} (ROC_2(t) - ROC_2^2(t)) + \frac{1}{n_D r'_D} \left(\frac{f_{2,D}(S_{2,\bar{D}}^{-1}(t))}{f_{2,\bar{D}}(S_{2,\bar{D}}^{-1}(t))} \right)^2 (t - t^2) \\ & - 2 \frac{1}{n_D r'_D} (S_D(S_{1,\bar{D}}^{-1}(t), S_{2,\bar{D}}^{-1}(t)) - ROC_1(t) ROC_2(t)) \\ & - 2 \frac{1}{n_{\bar{D}} r'_{\bar{D}}} \frac{f_{1,D}(S_{1,\bar{D}}^{-1}(t))}{f_{1,\bar{D}}(S_{1,\bar{D}}^{-1}(t))} \frac{f_{2,D}(S_{2,\bar{D}}^{-1}(t))}{f_{2,\bar{D}}(S_{2,\bar{D}}^{-1}(t))} (S_{\bar{D}}(S_{1,\bar{D}}^{-1}(t), S_{2,\bar{D}}^{-1}(t)) - t^2) \end{aligned}$$

for $r'_D \geq r_D$ and $r'_{\bar{D}} \geq r_{\bar{D}}$.

The estimated ROC curves have interesting joint asymptotic properties at the process level as indicated above. We then would be able to analyze ROC curves at different FPRs, say $ROC_1(t_1), ROC_2(t_2)$. And we can do analysis of two ROC curves at multiple points, since they all follow multivariate normal distribution with the variance–covariance stated before.

Furthermore, we can compare multiple points of ROC curves based on weighted average. It can be shown that the sequential weighted average of $\hat{\Delta}(t)$ on several FPRs has asymptotic multivariate normality and its asymptotic covariance matrix can be calculated by $Cov(\sum_{i=1}^{K} \omega_i \hat{\Delta}_{r_D, r_{\bar{D}}}(t_i), \sum_{i=1}^{K} \omega_i \hat{\Delta}_{r'_D, r'_{\bar{D}}}(t_i)) = Var(\sum_{i=1}^{K} \omega_i \hat{\Delta}_{r'_D, r'_{\bar{D}}}(t_i))$, where ω_i is the weight on $\hat{\Delta}_{r_D, r_{\bar{D}}}(t_i)$ with $\sum_{i=1}^{K} \omega_i = 1$. This is due to the fact that $Cov(\hat{\Delta}_{r_D, r_{\bar{D}}}(t_i), \hat{\Delta}_{r'_D, r'_{\bar{D}}}(t_j)) = Cov(\hat{\Delta}_{r'_D, r'_{\bar{D}}}(t_i), \hat{\Delta}_{r'_D, r'_{\bar{D}}}(t_j))$ for $r'_D \geq r_D$ and $r'_{\bar{D}} \geq r_{\bar{D}}$.

6.2.3 Group Sequential Method

To carry out a group sequential test, we analyze the accumulating data in groups rather than after an additional observation as in a fully sequential test or after all data are collected as in a fixed sample test. A GSD is convenient to conduct and provide an opportunity for stopping the trial earlier than planned. It achieves the goals of lower expected sample sizes and shorter average study lengths. GSD methods utilize different strategies of allocating the overall type I error probability.

From the previous theorem, we know that the sequential empirical difference of two ROC curves is also a Gaussian process. The sequential empirical difference at any finite set of analysis points follow a multivariate normal distribution. And the sequential score statistic has an "independent increment" covariance structure (Jennison and Turnbull 2000), which facilitates the sequential comparison of ROC curves and any standard GSD software can be readily applied.

Suppose we are interested in a two-sided test with the hypothesis of H_0 : $ROC_1(t_0) - ROC_2(t_0) = 0$ on a particular FPR t_0, and H_a : $ROC_1(t_0) - ROC_2(t_0) \neq 0$. Let $\Delta(t_0) = ROC_1(t_0) - ROC_2(t_0)$, and $\hat{\Delta}(t_0) = \widehat{ROC_1}(t_0) - \widehat{ROC_2}(t_0)$. Then under H_0, we can do the Z-test with the statistic $Z = \frac{\hat{\Delta}(t_0)}{\sqrt{Var(\hat{\Delta}(t_0))}}$. And for a fixed sample test we reject H_0 if $|Z| > Z_{\alpha/2}$. However, suppose we will do the GSD with a sampling plan of J interim analyses. At the jth analysis, test results are available on the first $n_D r_D^{(j)}$ case subjects and the first $n_{\bar{D}} r_{\bar{D}}^{(j)}$ control subjects, where n_D and $n_{\bar{D}}$ are the maximum case and control sample size, respectively, and $r_D^{(j)}$ and $r_{\bar{D}}^{(j)}$ are the ratios of the case and control subjects accrued so far at jth analysis. Given type I error rate α and power $1 - \beta$ at $\Delta(t_0) = \pm\delta$, the fixed sample size is calculated based on α, β, δ, and $Var(\hat{\Delta}(t_0))$. The maximum sample size for the GSD are proportional to the fixed sample size, and this ratio $R(J, \alpha, \beta)$ depends only on J, α, β and the particular GSD method used.

Consider a GSD plan involving up to J analyses of sample data. At the time of the jth analysis, let $I_j = 1/\sigma^2_{\hat{\Delta}_j(t)}$, $\tau_j = I_j/I_J = \sigma^2_{\hat{\Delta}_J(t)}/\sigma^2_{\hat{\Delta}_j(t)}$. Define $B(\tau_j) = \sqrt{\tau_j I_j}\hat{\Delta}_j(t)$. For $j < k$, $Cov(B(\tau_j), B(\tau_k)) = \tau_j$. This can be proved using the previous finding of Eq. 6.8. Thus, $B(\tau_j)$ behaves asymptotically like a Brownian motion process. Then the standard GSD software like R package gsDesign can be readily applied. Similarly, we can apply the transformation on the sequential weighted average of $\hat{\Delta}(t)$ on several FPRs and come up with the same conclusion. The transformation used is $I_j = 1/Var(\sum_{i=1}^{K} \omega_i \hat{\Delta}_j(t_i))$, $\tau_j = I_j/I_J = Var(\sum_{i=1}^{K} \omega_i \hat{\Delta}_J(t_i))/Var(\sum_{i=1}^{K} \omega_i \hat{\Delta}_j(t_i))$. Define $B(\tau_j) = \sqrt{\tau_j I_j}(\sum_{i=1}^{K} \omega_i \hat{\Delta}_j(t_i))$. Then for $j < k$, again we have $Cov(B(\tau_j), B(\tau_k)) = \tau_j$.

The GSD needs to be specified and the maximum sample sizes need to be determined before conducting the trial. At the first interim analysis, we calculate the Z test statistic based on the empirical estimation of $ROC_1(t_0)$, $ROC_2(t_0)$, and $Var(\hat{\Delta}(t_0))$. We compare the Z statistic to the boundaries of Pocock, O'Brien–Fleming, or error spending method that are calculated to control type I error rate. The boundaries a_j are defined to control the overall type I error rate: $Pr(|Z_j| > a_j \mid \Delta(t_0) = 0)$ for some $j = 1...J$. If this Z statistic falls in the rejection boundaries, we then reject the null hypothesis, and the clinical trial is stopped with null hypothesis rejection and no more subjects will be accrued. Otherwise, we will continue accruing sufficient subjects to be able to proceed to the next analysis point. At the jth analysis, the first

Table 6.1 The values of elements ($\times 10^{-3}$) in observed and theoretical covariance matrix

	Observed covariance matrix				Theoretical covariance matrix			
	$n_D = 200$, $n_{\bar{D}} = 200$							
$\Delta_{0.2,0.3}(0.5)$	3.718	1.850	1.458	0.755	3.720	1.898	1.499	0.782
$\Delta_{0.4,0.5}(0.5)$		1.927	1.490	0.773		1.898	1.499	0.782
$\Delta_{0.5,0.7}(0.5)$			1.529	0.790			1.499	0.782
$\Delta_{1,1}(0.5)$				0.787				0.782

$n_D r_D^{(j)}$ case subjects and the first $n_{\bar{D}} r_{\bar{D}}^{(j)}$ control subjects are used to compute the interim statistic Z_j. We will repeat the process until the last Jth analysis point. At the last analysis, we will either reject the null hypothesis or accept it and stop the clinical trial.

The previous findings and method can also be used to obtain the properties of the sequential wAUC or AUC statistics. Such an extension can be done in comparing summary statistics of two ROC curves through the integration of $\Delta(t)$ from 0 to 1 with regard to any given weight probability measure function. The AUC and pAUC statistic become special cases, as indicated in Tang et al. (2008). More importantly, because of the results in Eq. (6.8), we can compare a wide range of ROC summary measures, including curves at different FPRs or their weighted averages of the ROC curves.

6.3 Simulation Studies

6.3.1 Covariance Matrix

We conduct a simulation study to assess the finite sample properties of the results in Theorem 6.8. Diagnostic test data are drawn from bivariate normal distributions. For a case, the bivariate normal model is $(X_1, X_2)^T \sim N\{(10, 6)^T, \Sigma_1\}$, and for a control, the bivariate normal model is $(Y_1, Y_2)^T \sim N\{(0, 4)^T, \Sigma_2\}$, where

$$\Sigma_1 = \begin{pmatrix} 2 & \rho 2\sqrt{2} \\ \rho 2\sqrt{2} & 4 \end{pmatrix} \quad \text{and} \quad \Sigma_2 = \begin{pmatrix} 1 & \rho \\ \rho & 1 \end{pmatrix}, \quad \text{with } \rho = 0.5 .$$

We conduct 5000 simulation with $n_D = 200, n_{\bar{D}} = 200$, and for the simulated data, we calculate the variance–covariance of the $\Delta(t)$ at various combinations of $r_D, r_{\bar{D}}$ with $t = 0.5$. Here, the ROC curves are estimated with the empirical functions. Then we compare the simulated covariance matrix to the theoretical covariance matrix derived using the results of Theorem 6.8.

6.3.2 Simulated Type I Error Rate in GSDs

To investigate finite sample performance of the GSD procedure, we conduct a simulation study in a two-group sequential test ($J = 2$), and a five-group sequential test ($J = 5$). The null hypothesis of equal ROC(t) is set to be true and the nominal type I error was set to be $\alpha = 0.05$ for two-sided tests. Two set of diagnostic test data are simulated from bivariate normal (binorm) and bivariate lognormal(bilognorm) models. The bivariate normal models is $(X_1, X_2)^T \sim N\{(1, 10)^T, \Sigma_1\}$ for case data. And for control data, the bivariate normal model is $(Y_1, Y_2)^T \sim N\{(0, 8)^T, \Sigma_2\}$, where

$$\Sigma_1 = \begin{pmatrix} 1 & 2\rho \\ 2\rho & 4 \end{pmatrix} \quad \Sigma_2 = \begin{pmatrix} 1 & 2\rho \\ 2\rho & 4 \end{pmatrix} \quad with\ \rho = (0, 0.25, 0.5, 0.75, 0.9).$$

In this case, the ROC curves are identical from the formula of ROC curve under binormal models (Zhou et al. 2011): $ROC(t) = \Phi(a + b\Phi^{-1}(t))$, where $a = (\mu_1 - \mu_0)/\sigma_1$ and $b = \sigma_0/\sigma_1$, (μ_1, σ_1), and (μ_0, σ_0) are the normal parameters in case and control groups. The bivariate lognormal data are generated by taking exponential of the simulated bivariate normal data. Because the ROC curves are invariant to a monotone transformation, the ROC curves under the bivariate lognormal models are also identical. Different numbers of case and control subjects, $n_D, n_{\bar{D}} = (50, 250, 500)$, are considered in our simulation study.

For each simulation setting, 5000 random datasets are generated and the GSD method applied to the simulated data. The Z statistics at each interim analysis point are then calculated based on the empirical ROC difference and estimated variances. The GSD test procedure compares the Z statistics with corresponding test boundaries of design, and the decision of rejection or failing to rejection is obtained for each simulated dataset. We then calculate the overall rejection rates for all simulated datasets. Table 6.3 gives the rejection rates of all different model and sample size combinations with a nominal α level 0.05 under the O'Brien and Fleming's criterion. And Table 6.1 is the results for the Pocock's criterion. As we can see, the simulated type I error rates are close to the nominal rate and tend to be closer as the overall sample sizes increase.

We take the same two identical ROC curves as mentioned above and the null hypothesis of H_0: $\sum_{t=\{0.2,0.5,0.8\}} \Delta(t)/3 = 0$ as an example for the sequential weighted average test. For the simulation with $n_D = 250, n_{\bar{D}} = 250$, and $J = 5$, we get the type I error rates as following. When $\rho = 0$, error $= 0.0526$ for binormal distribution, error $= 0.0768$ for bilognormal distribution. When $\rho = 0.25$, error $= 0.053$ and 0.0694 for binormal and bilognormal distributions, respectively. When $\rho = 0.5$, error $= 0.0514$ and 0.07 for binormal and bilognormal distributions, respectively. When $\rho = 0.75$, error $= 0.0546$ and 0.0654; when $\rho = 0.9$, error $= 0.062$ and 0.0668 for binormal and bilognormal distributions, respectively. More results are shown in Table 6.4.

Table 6.2 Type I error using the O'Brien–Fleming group sequential design (GSD) with $\alpha = 0.05$

			$\rho = 0$		$\rho = 0.25$		$\rho = 0.5$		$\rho = 0.75$		$\rho = 0.9$	
n_D	$n_{\bar{D}}$	t	Binorm	Bilog	Binorm	Bilog	Binorm	Bilog	Binorm	Bilog	Binorm	Bilog
Two-group sequential design ($J = 2$)												
50	50	0.2	0.0694	0.1096	0.0702	0.1030	0.0620	0.0974	0.0598	0.0860	0.0426	0.0580
		0.4	0.0538	0.0898	0.0490	0.0834	0.0436	0.0744	0.0408	0.0680	0.0338	0.0526
		0.5	0.0386	0.0914	0.0414	0.0878	0.0386	0.0874	0.0360	0.0690	0.0260	0.0464
		0.6	0.0384	0.0900	0.0374	0.0794	0.0318	0.0722	0.0252	0.0572	0.0164	0.0356
		0.8	0.0158	0.0362	0.0156	0.0346	0.0124	0.0258	0.0082	0.0180	0.0042	0.0062
250	250	0.2	0.0610	0.0738	0.0572	0.0700	0.0528	0.0642	0.0500	0.0586	0.0554	0.0584
		0.4	0.0436	0.0556	0.0424	0.0560	0.0442	0.0558	0.0472	0.0592	0.0458	0.0562
		0.5	0.0398	0.0696	0.0470	0.0680	0.0462	0.0714	0.0474	0.0718	0.0444	0.0618
		0.6	0.0432	0.0788	0.0408	0.0714	0.0474	0.0778	0.0406	0.0660	0.0402	0.0662
		0.8	0.0352	0.0620	0.0360	0.0590	0.0386	0.0590	0.0302	0.0506	0.0268	0.0390
250	500	0.2	0.0530	0.0604	0.0536	0.0582	0.0524	0.0570	0.0552	0.0542	0.0534	0.0546
		0.4	0.0472	0.0542	0.0536	0.0604	0.0554	0.0592	0.0518	0.0574	0.0474	0.0528
		0.5	0.0510	0.0664	0.0484	0.0604	0.0548	0.0696	0.0488	0.0638	0.0482	0.0588
		0.6	0.01486	0.0644	0.0532	0.0720	0.0488	0.0658	0.0508	0.0670	0.0478	0.0614
		0.8	0.0380	0.0580	0.0388	0.0532	0.0372	0.0528	0.0410	0.0542	0.0360	0.0424
500	500	0.2	0.0544	0.0700	0.0568	0.0704	0.0532	0.066	0.0518	0.0580	0.0542	0.0562
		0.4	0.0514	0.0610	0.0500	0.0562	0.0456	0.0528	0.0466	0.0508	0.0448	0.0458
		0.5	0.0452	0.0608	0.0476	0.0594	0.0532	0.0636	0.0438	0.0578	0.0470	0.0572
		0.6	0.0430	0.0714	0.0484	0.0736	0.0436	0.0668	0.044	0.0608	0.0460	0.0646
		0.8	0.0414	0.0684	0.0418	0.0642	0.0400	0.0616	0.0386	0.0550	0.0384	0.0502

Table 6.2 (continued)

			$\rho = 0$		$\rho = 0.25$		$\rho = 0.5$		$\rho = 0.75$		$\rho = 0.9$	
n_D	$n_{\bar{D}}$	t	Binorm	Bilog	Binorm	Bilog	Binorm	Bilog	Binorm	Bilog	Binorm	Bilog
Five-group sequential design ($J = 5$)												
50	50	0.2	0.0806	0.1394	0.0806	0.1298	0.0716	0.1122	0.0642	0.1026	0.0484	0.0696
		0.4	0.0590	0.0986	0.0500	0.0938	0.0480	0.0842	0.0444	0.0736	0.0338	0.0550
		0.5	0.0426	0.0982	0.0428	0.0942	0.0420	0.0956	0.0360	0.0758	0.0246	0.0444
		0.6	0.0368	0.0980	0.0366	0.0884	0.0320	0.0782	0.0252	0.0568	0.0154	0.0324
		0.8	0.0138	0.0320	0.0134	0.0280	0.0086	0.0208	0.0068	0.0130	0.0030	0.0046
250	250	0.2	0.0664	0.0818	0.0638	0.0790	0.0584	0.0762	0.0570	0.0658	0.0574	0.0642
		0.4	0.0454	0.0612	0.0476	0.0624	0.0454	0.0616	0.0508	0.0636	0.0484	0.0608
		0.5	0.0438	0.0770	0.0484	0.0760	0.0510	0.0790	0.0490	0.0732	0.0442	0.0652
		0.6	0.0468	0.0866	0.0418	0.0766	0.0512	0.0846	0.0434	0.0752	0.0436	0.0688
		0.8	0.0332	0.0634	0.0346	0.0604	0.0382	0.0618	0.0304	0.0484	0.0226	0.0360
250	500	0.2	0.0558	0.0648	0.0560	0.0638	0.0576	0.0620	0.0572	0.0572	0.0542	0.0568
		0.4	0.0486	0.0572	0.0580	0.0638	0.0564	0.0636	0.0548	0.0600	0.0482	0.0550
		0.5	0.0536	0.0712	0.0518	0.0678	0.0566	0.0740	0.0532	0.0674	0.0500	0.0634
		0.6	0.0476	0.0708	0.0518	0.0740	0.0514	0.0718	0.0532	0.0724	0.0498	0.0632
		0.8	0.0390	0.0586	0.0368	0.0576	0.0392	0.0558	0.0400	0.0586	0.0306	0.0456
500	500	0.2	0.0560	0.0770	0.0580	0.0758	0.0556	0.0698	0.0548	0.0644	0.0584	0.0616
		0.4	0.0532	0.0616	0.0512	0.0588	0.0484	0.0552	0.0474	0.0536	0.0450	0.0488
		0.5	0.0470	0.0638	0.0476	0.0630	0.0546	0.0704	0.0462	0.0620	0.0482	0.0620
		0.6	0.0436	0.0736	0.0500	0.0778	0.0462	0.0742	0.0456	0.0670	0.0462	0.0674
		0.8	0.0404	0.0724	0.0428	0.0676	0.0416	0.0670	0.0400	0.0618	0.0386	0.0552

Table 6.3 Type I error using the Pocock GSD with a = 0:05

			$\rho = 0$		$\rho = 0.25$		$\rho = 0.5$		$\rho = 0.75$		$\rho = 0.9$	
n_D	$n_{\bar{D}}$	t	Binorm	Bilog	Binorm	Bilog	Binorm	Bilog	Binorm	Bilog	Binorm	Bilog
Two-group sequential design ($J = 2$)												
50	50	0.2	0.0740	0.1250	0.0740	0.1228	0.0690	0.1174	0.0626	0.0984	0.0412	0.0670
		0.4	0.0536	0.0990	0.0506	0.0966	0.0488	0.0886	0.0378	0.0718	0.0274	0.0456
		0.5	0.0416	0.0954	0.0400	0.0922	0.0382	0.0866	0.0280	0.0666	0.0188	0.0358
		0.6	0.0354	0.0884	0.0312	0.0778	0.0264	0.0656	0.0186	0.0456	0.0088	0.0242
		0.8	0.0114	0.0234	0.0092	0.0204	0.0072	0.0170	0.0038	0.0098	0.0016	0.0032
250	250	0.2	0.0636	0.0812	0.0606	0.0730	0.0588	0.0700	0.0528	0.0656	0.0520	0.0570
		0.4	0.0444	0.0640	0.0484	0.0638	0.0494	0.0668	0.0472	0.0630	0.0446	0.0586
		0.5	0.0434	0.0790	0.0474	0.0770	0.0480	0.0794	0.0416	0.0720	0.0388	0.0654
		0.6	0.0432	0.0896	0.0418	0.0784	0.0420	0.0806	0.0382	0.0682	0.0354	0.0648
		0.8	0.0300	0.0630	0.0306	0.0584	0.0314	0.0590	0.0234	0.0422	0.0160	0.0264
250	500	0.2	0.0574	0.0648	0.0572	0.0668	0.0612	0.0646	0.0590	0.0604	0.0578	0.0532
		0.4	0.0492	0.0592	0.0548	0.0670	0.0542	0.0628	0.0498	0.0582	0.0472	0.0544
		0.5	0.0530	0.0728	0.0540	0.0724	0.0530	0.0718	0.0464	0.0658	0.0504	0.0648
		0.6	0.0494	0.0768	0.0498	0.0762	0.0472	0.0708	0.0484	0.0676	0.0470	0.0628
		0.8	0.0372	0.0554	0.0372	0.0534	0.0358	0.0526	0.0320	0.0480	0.0228	0.0314
500	500	0.2	0.0572	0.0724	0.0598	0.0742	0.0526	0.0660	0.0540	0.0614	0.0586	0.0614
		0.4	0.0538	0.0658	0.0500	0.0596	0.0482	0.0578	0.0462	0.0564	0.0438	0.0486
		0.5	0.0458	0.0630	0.0468	0.0650	0.0508	0.0714	0.0448	0.0616	0.0466	0.0628
		0.6	0.0466	0.0738	0.0476	0.0768	0.0436	0.0706	0.0404	0.0666	0.0452	0.0686
		0.8	0.0400	0.0690	0.0414	0.0688	0.0400	0.0650	0.0356	0.0584	0.0324	0.0506

Table 6.3 (continued)

			$\rho = 0$		$\rho = 0.25$		$\rho = 0.5$		$\rho = 0.75$		$\rho = 0.9$	
n_D	$n_{\bar{D}}$	t	Binorm	Bilog	Binorm	Bilog	Binorm	Bilog	Binorm	Bilog	Binorm	Bilog
Five-group sequential design ($J = 5$)												
50	50	0.2	0.1102	0.1942	0.1016	0.1852	0.0924	0.1634	0.0668	0.1238	0.0444	0.0714
		0.4	0.0660	0.1192	0.0580	0.1106	0.0508	0.0936	0.0346	0.0664	0.0178	0.0342
		0.5	0.0466	0.0974	0.0408	0.0914	0.0378	0.0810	0.0254	0.0562	0.0136	0.0260
		0.6	0.0306	0.0768	0.0296	0.0714	0.0256	0.0594	0.0168	0.0396	0.0050	0.0156
		0.8	0.0064	0.0162	0.0054	0.0130	0.0034	0.0070	0.0024	0.0038	0.0008	0.0014
250	250	0.2	0.0744	0.1028	0.0758	0.1082	0.0674	0.0942	0.0616	0.0886	0.0538	0.0706
		0.4	0.0470	0.0780	0.0534	0.0832	0.0494	0.0784	0.0462	0.0722	0.0376	0.0606
		0.5	0.0476	0.0914	0.0514	0.0910	0.0506	0.0944	0.0436	0.0842	0.0330	0.0640
		0.6	0.0422	0.1032	0.0396	0.0878	0.0416	0.0906	0.0360	0.0730	0.0296	0.0622
		0.8	0.0210	0.0506	0.0248	0.0478	0.0198	0.0462	0.0166	0.0332	0.0086	0.0184
250	500	0.2	0.0688	0.0782	0.0646	0.0774	0.0654	0.0758	0.0628	0.0700	0.0526	0.0558
		0.4	0.0506	0.0656	0.0598	0.0730	0.0520	0.0652	0.0534	0.0684	0.0432	0.0610
		0.5	0.0516	0.0804	0.0504	0.0798	0.0468	0.0768	0.0468	0.0724	0.0396	0.0596
		0.6	0.0504	0.0820	0.0476	0.0782	0.0428	0.0756	0.0460	0.0694	0.0354	0.0578
		0.8	0.0288	0.0508	0.0276	0.0454	0.0248	0.0422	0.0218	0.0362	0.0122	0.0180
500	500	0.2	0.0610	0.0840	0.0626	0.0866	0.0568	0.0796	0.0598	0.0742	0.0536	0.0652
		0.4	0.0522	0.0688	0.0486	0.0722	0.0496	0.0662	0.0488	0.0610	0.0462	0.0592
		0.5	0.0472	0.0780	0.0488	0.0802	0.0470	0.0854	0.0512	0.0738	0.0434	0.0702
		0.6	0.0474	0.0908	0.0490	0.0908	0.0430	0.0852	0.0376	0.0716	0.0398	0.0698
		0.8	0.0328	0.0652	0.0316	0.0640	0.0344	0.0630	0.0272	0.0500	0.0202	0.0372

Table 6.4 Test based on average: Type I error using the O'Brien–Fleming group sequential design (*GSD*) with $\alpha = 0.05$

			$\rho = 0$		$\rho = 0.25$		$\rho = 0.5$		$\rho = 0.75$		$\rho = 0.9$	
n_D	$n_{\bar{D}}$	t	Binorm	Bilog	Binorm	Bilog	Binorm	Bilog	Binorm	Bilog	Binorm	Bilog
Two-group sequential design ($J = 2$)												
50	50	0.2,0.5,0.8	0.0552	0.0974	0.0554	0.0934	0.0552	0.0904	0.0592	0.0892	0.067	0.0864
250	250	0.2,0.5,0.8	0.0512	0.0704	0.0514	0.0658	0.0488	0.0628	0.0502	0.0592	0.0502	0.0534
250	500	0.2,0.5,0.8	0.0528	0.0638	0.0522	0.0626	0.054	0.0622	0.0556	0.0592	0.0582	0.0588
500	500	0.2,0.5,0.8	0.0496	0.068	0.0548	0.067	0.0566	0.0666	0.0542	0.0652	0.0602	0.0694
Five-group sequential design ($J = 5$)												
50	50	0.2,0.5,0.8	0.0602	0.113	0.0584	0.1106	0.064	0.11	0.0742	0.1202	0.103	0.1246
250	250	0.2,0.5,0.8	0.0526	0.0768	0.053	0.0694	0.0514	0.07	0.0546	0.0654	0.062	0.0668
250	500	0.2,0.5,0.8	0.0554	0.0688	0.056	0.0648	0.0592	0.0674	0.061	0.0666	0.0696	0.0684
500	500	0.2,0.5,0.8	0.0528	0.071	0.057	0.0714	0.0562	0.0722	0.0568	0.0674	0.064	0.0802

Table 6.5 Interim test statistics

Interim Z statistic					
FPR	1	2	3	4	5
0.2	1.562	2.174	3.544		
0.4	1.632	2.364	3.386		
0.5	2.202	1.247	2.637		
0.6	1.424	2.019	2.557	2.791	
0.8	1.472	1.692	1.885	2.269	2.218
Boundaries	±4.56	±3.23	±2.63	±2.28	±2.04

FPR false positive rate

6.4 Example

In this section, we illustrate the GSD in a hypothetical lung cancer diagnostic trial. Both computed tomography (CT) and positron emission tomography (PET) can be used for diagnosing the staging of non-small cell lung cancer. The AUC for staging non-small cell lung cancer is between 52 and 85 % for CT and between 81 and 96 % for PET (Lardinois et al. 2003; Silvestri et al. 2003). In our example, we choose the AUCs to be 75 % for CT and 90 % for PET from the reasonable range. Consider testing the null hypothesis of $\Delta(t) = 0$ for $t = \{0.2, 0.4, 0.5, 0.6, 0.8\}$ and correlation between two diagnostic tests' data as $\rho = 0.5$ and are binormally distributed. Our example is a possible case under the alternative hypothesis condition, with $\Delta(t) = \{0.289, 0.182, 0.135, 0.094, 0.032\}$ for $t = \{0.2, 0.4, 0.5, 0.6, 0.8\}$, respectively. In Table 6.5, we show the interim looks of one simulation data with statistics and corresponding boundaries (O'Brien–Fleming) displayed at the bottom.

Suppose $n_D = 250$, $n_{\bar{D}} = 250$, FPR $= 0.5$, and the number of looks is 5. At the first endpoint, with $n_D = 50$, $n_{\bar{D}} = 50$ subjects recruited and tested, the Z statistic is 2.202, which is within the rejection boundaries for the null hypothesis. Thus we fail to reject the null hypothesis, and continue to recruit 50 additional cases and 50 additional controls. The difference between the ROC curves at FPR = 0.5 and its variance can be estimated using the derived formula on the accruing data from the 100 cases and controls. The statistic of 1.247 is calculated and is smaller than the boundary 3.23. Again, we fail to reject the null hypothesis, and continue to recruit another 50 cases and controls. At the third interim analysis with overall 150 cases and controls, we calculate the Z statistic to be 2.637, which is greater than the boundary 2.63. Therefore, we reject the null hypothesis of $\Delta(0.5) = 0$ at this step, and conclude that the two imaging tests are significantly different in their accuracy at the FPR of 0.5.

We also experiment with an example of comparing the average of three ROC points at different FPRs. Suppose FPR $= (0.2, 0.5, 0.8)$ are of interest, and $n_D = 250$, $n_{\bar{D}} = 250$. All other settings remain the same as the previous example. The AUCs are set to be 75 % for CT and 90 % for PET with $\Delta(t) = \{0.289, 0.135, 0.032\}$ for $t = \{0.2, 0.5, 0.8\}$, respectively. The average of the $\Delta(t)$ at the three FPRs is 0.152.

We also reject the null hypothesis, $H_0 : \sum_{t=\{0.2,0.5,0.8\}} (ROC_1(t)/3 - ROC_2(t)/3) = 0$, with the expected sample size to be 111 for either cases or controls.

6.5 Discussion

In this chapter, we have derived asymptotic properties of the sequential differences of two empirical ROC curves at the process level. We then used these results to develop distribution theory for the sequential difference of two empirical ROC curves at an FPR. We also extended the work to the asymptotic properties of the sequential difference of weighted ROC averages at several FPRs. Our approach not only enables us to investigate the difference of two correlated ROC curves but also enables us to investigate the joint behavior of multiple points of two correlated ROC curves' differences and their weighted averages. Based on this, standard GSD software can be readily applied to design group sequential comparative diagnostic tests studies.

Based on the theorems developed, we conducted a simulation study to assess the finite sample properties of the results in Theorem 6.8. The simulation study verified the asymptotic variance–covariance matrix by comparing the theoretical covariance matrix to the observed covariance matrix from the simulated data. We verified that they match each other closely when sample size n is sufficiently large. We also conducted simulation studies, both for one point and for average of multiple points on ROC curves. With α level set to 0.05, the test type I error rate is approximately 0.05 and tend to be closer to the number as we increase the sample sizes.

We further applied the GSD to a lung cancer diagnosis example, and our results clearly illustrate the advantage of sequentially monitoring the comparative diagnostic trial based on our theorem. The example shows that we are able to reject the null hypothesis under the alternative hypothesis with a substantially smaller expected sample size.

In our study, we used empirical cumulative distribution functions and Kernel density estimation to generate an estimate of $\sigma_{\hat{\Delta}(t)}$. Due to the limitation of Kernel density estimation, it will be desirable if we can develop a new nonparametric estimation method for variance without involving density estimation. Currently, we mainly deal with two correlated ROC curves and provide the variance–covariance formula. We will extend the research to more general cases like clustered ROC curves and their differences. We can also apply a similar approach to compare multiple ROC curves.

Appendix

Derivation of the elements a_{ij} in Σ:

$$a_{11} = Var(K_{1,1}(ROC_1(t), r_D)) + Var\left(\lambda^{1/2}\frac{r_D}{r_{\bar{D}}}\left(\frac{f_{1,D}(S_{1,\bar{D}}^{-1}(t))}{f_{1,\bar{D}}(S_{1,\bar{D}}^{-1}(t))}\right)K_{1,2}(t, r_{\bar{D}})\right)$$

$$= r_D(ROC_1(t) - ROC_1^2(t)) + \lambda \frac{r_{\bar{D}}^2}{r_{\bar{D}}} \left(\frac{f_{1,D}(S_{1,\bar{D}}^{-1}(t))}{f_{1,\bar{D}}(S_{1,\bar{D}}^{-1}(t))} \right)^2 (t - t^2),$$

$$\begin{aligned}
a_{12} = {} & Cov\big(n_D^{-1/2}[n_D r_D](\hat{S}_{1,D,r_D}(\hat{S}_{1,\bar{D},r_{\bar{D}}}^{-1}(t)) - S_{1,D}(\hat{S}_{1,\bar{D},r_{\bar{D}}}^{-1}(t))), \\
& n_D^{-1/2}[n_D r_D](\hat{S}_{2,D,r_D}(\hat{S}_{2,\bar{D},r_{\bar{D}}}^{-1}(t)) - S_{2,D}(\hat{S}_{2,\bar{D},r_{\bar{D}}}^{-1}(t)))\big) \\
& + Cov\left(n_D^{-1/2}[n_D r_D](S_{1,D}(\hat{S}_{1,\bar{D},r_{\bar{D}}}^{-1}(t)) - S_{1,D}(S_{1,\bar{D}}^{-1}(t))),\right. \\
& \left. n_D^{-1/2}[n_D r_D](S_{2,D}(\hat{S}_{2,\bar{D},r_{\bar{D}}}^{-1}(t)) - S_{2,D}(S_{2,\bar{D}}^{-1}(t)))\right) \\
= {} & Cov\left(n_D^{-1/2} \sum_{i=1}^{[n_D r_D]} \left(I(X_{1,D,i} > \hat{S}_{1,\bar{D},r_{\bar{D}}}^{-1}(t)) - S_{1,D}(\hat{S}_{1,\bar{D},r_{\bar{D}}}^{-1}(t))\right),\right. \\
& \left. n_D^{-1/2} \sum_{i=1}^{[n_D r_D]} \left(I(X_{2,D,i} > \hat{S}_{2,\bar{D},r_{\bar{D}}}^{-1}(t)) - S_{2,D}(\hat{S}_{2,\bar{D},r_{\bar{D}}}^{-1}(t))\right)\right) \\
& + Cov\left(n_D^{-1/2}[n_D r_D](S_{1,D}(\hat{S}_{1,\bar{D},r_{\bar{D}}}^{-1}(t)) - S_{1,D}(S_{1,\bar{D}}^{-1}(t))),\right. \\
& \left. n_D^{-1/2}[n_D r_D](S_{2,D}(\hat{S}_{2,\bar{D},r_{\bar{D}}}^{-1}(t)) - S_{2,D}(S_{2,\bar{D}}^{-1}(t)))\right) \\
= {} & r_D(S_D(S_{1,\bar{D}}^{-1}(t), S_{2,\bar{D}}^{-1}(t)) - ROC_1(t)ROC_2(t)) \\
& + \lambda \frac{r_{\bar{D}}^2}{r_{\bar{D}}} \frac{f_{1,D}(S_{1,\bar{D}}^{-1}(t))}{f_{1,\bar{D}}(S_{1,\bar{D}}^{-1}(t))} \frac{f_{2,D}(S_{2,\bar{D}}^{-1}(t))}{f_{2,\bar{D}}(S_{2,\bar{D}}^{-1}(t))} (S_{\bar{D}}(S_{1,\bar{D}}^{-1}(t), S_{2,\bar{D}}^{-1}(t)) - t^2).
\end{aligned}$$

The last step is derived by applying the results of sequential empirical process, the compact differentiability of the inverse function and delta method in vander Vaart and Wellner (1996).

$$\begin{aligned}
a_{13} = {} & Cov\left(K_{1,1}(ROC_1(t), r_D), K_{1,1}(ROC_1(t), r'_D)\right) \\
& + Cov\left(\lambda^{1/2} \frac{r_D}{r_{\bar{D}}} \left(\frac{f_{1,D}(S_{1,\bar{D}}^{-1}(t))}{f_{1,\bar{D}}(S_{1,\bar{D}}^{-1}(t))} \right) K_{1,2}(t, r_{\bar{D}}), \lambda^{1/2} \frac{r'_D}{r'_{\bar{D}}} \left(\frac{f_{1,D}(S_{1,\bar{D}}^{-1}(t))}{f_{1,\bar{D}}(S_{1,\bar{D}}^{-1}(t))} \right) K_{1,2}(t, r'_{\bar{D}})\right) \\
= {} & (r_D \wedge r'_D)(ROC_1(t) - ROC_1^2(t)) + (r_{\bar{D}} \wedge r'_{\bar{D}}) \lambda \frac{r_D}{r_{\bar{D}}} \frac{r'_D}{r'_{\bar{D}}} \left(\frac{f_{1,D}(S_{1,\bar{D}}^{-1}(t))}{f_{1,\bar{D}}(S_{1,\bar{D}}^{-1}(t))} \right)^2 (t - t^2).
\end{aligned}$$

$$\begin{aligned}
a_{14} = {} & Cov\big(n_D^{-1/2}[n_D r_D](\hat{S}_{1,D,r_D}(\hat{S}_{1,\bar{D},r_{\bar{D}}}^{-1}(t)) - S_{1,D}(\hat{S}_{1,\bar{D},r_{\bar{D}}}^{-1}(t))), \\
& n_D^{-1/2}[n_D r'_D](\hat{S}_{2,D,r'_D}(\hat{S}_{2,\bar{D},r'_{\bar{D}}}^{-1}(t)) - S_{2,D}(\hat{S}_{2,\bar{D},r'_{\bar{D}}}^{-1}(t)))\big) \\
& + Cov\big(n_D^{-1/2}[n_D r_D](S_{1,D}(\hat{S}_{1,\bar{D},r_{\bar{D}}}^{-1}(t)) - S_{1,D}(S_{1,\bar{D}}^{-1}(t))),
\end{aligned}$$

$$
\begin{aligned}
&n_D^{-1/2}[n_D r'_D](S_{2,D}(\hat{S}^{-1}_{2,\bar{D},r'_{\bar{D}}}(t)) - S_{2,D}(S^{-1}_{2,\bar{D}}(t))))\\
&= (r_D \wedge r'_D)(S_D(S^{-1}_{1,\bar{D}}(t), S^{-1}_{2,\bar{D}}(t)) - ROC_1(t)ROC_2(t))\\
&\quad + (r_{\bar{D}} \wedge r'_{\bar{D}})\lambda \frac{r_D}{r_{\bar{D}}}\frac{r'_D}{r'_{\bar{D}}} \frac{f_{1,D}(S^{-1}_{1,\bar{D}}(t))}{f_{1,\bar{D}}(S^{-1}_{1,\bar{D}}(t))} \frac{f_{2,D}(S^{-1}_{2,\bar{D}}(t))}{f_{2,\bar{D}}(S^{-1}_{2,\bar{D}}(t))}(S_{\bar{D}}(S^{-1}_{1,\bar{D}}(t), S^{-1}_{2,\bar{D}}(t)) - t^2).
\end{aligned}
$$

The last step is again derived by applying the results of sequential empirical process, the compact differentiability of the inverse function and delta method in vander Vaart and Wellner (1996). Similarly, we can get the following elements of the covariance matrix:

$$
\begin{aligned}
a_{22} &= r_D(ROC_2(t) - ROC_2^2(t)) + \lambda \frac{r_D^2}{r_{\bar{D}}} \left(\frac{f_{2,D}(S^{-1}_{2,\bar{D}}(t))}{f_{2,\bar{D}}(S^{-1}_{2,\bar{D}}(t))} \right)^2 (t - t^2),\\
a_{23} &= a_{14},\\
a_{24} &= (r_D \wedge r'_D)(ROC_2(t) - ROC_2^2(t)) + (r_{\bar{D}} \wedge r'_{\bar{D}})\lambda \frac{r_D}{r_{\bar{D}}}\frac{r'_D}{r'_{\bar{D}}} \left(\frac{f_{2,D}(S^{-1}_{2,\bar{D}}(t))}{f_{2,\bar{D}}(S^{-1}_{2,\bar{D}}(t))} \right)^2 (t - t^2),\\
a_{33} &= r'_D(ROC_1(t) - ROC_1^2(t)) + \lambda \frac{r'^2_D}{r'_{\bar{D}}} \left(\frac{f_{1,D}(S^{-1}_{1,\bar{D}}(t))}{f_{1,\bar{D}}(S^{-1}_{1,\bar{D}}(t))} \right)^2 (t - t^2),\\
a_{34} &= r'_D(S_D(S^{-1}_{1,\bar{D}}(t), S^{-1}_{2,\bar{D}}(t)) - ROC_1(t)ROC_2(t))\\
&\quad + \lambda \frac{r'^2_D}{r'_{\bar{D}}} \frac{f_{1,D}(S^{-1}_{1,\bar{D}}(t))}{f_{1,\bar{D}}(S^{-1}_{1,\bar{D}}(t))} \frac{f_{2,D}(S^{-1}_{2,\bar{D}}(t))}{f_{2,\bar{D}}(S^{-1}_{2,\bar{D}}(t))}(S_{\bar{D}}(S^{-1}_{1,\bar{D}}(t), S^{-1}_{2,\bar{D}}(t)) - t^2),\\
a_{44} &= r'_D(ROC_2(t) - ROC_2^2(t)) + \lambda \frac{r'^2_D}{r'_{\bar{D}}} \left(\frac{f_{2,D}(S^{-1}_{2,\bar{D}}(t))}{f_{2,\bar{D}}(S^{-1}_{2,\bar{D}}(t))} \right)^2 (t - t^2).
\end{aligned}
$$

References

Jennison C, Turnbull BW (2000) Group sequential methods with applications to clinical trials. Chapman and Hall, New York

Karr AF (1993) Probability. Springer, New York

Kim K, Demets DL (1992) Sample size determination for group sequential clinical trials with immediate response. Stat Med 11(10):1391–1399

Koopmeiners JS, Feng Z (2011) Asymptotic properties of the sequential empirical ROC, PPV and NPV curves under case-control sampling. Ann Stat 39(6):3234–3261

Lardinois D, Weder W, Hany TF, Kamel EM, Korom S, Seifert B, von Schulthess GK, Steinert HC (2003) Staging of non-small-cell lung cancer with integrated positron-emission tomography and computed tomography. N Engl J Med 348(25):2500–2507

Liu A, Wu C, Schisterman EF (2008) Nonparametric sequential evaluation of diagnostic biomarkers. Stat Med 27(10):1667–1678

Mazumdar M, Liu A (2003) Group sequential design for comparative diagnostic accuracy studies. Stat Med 22(5):727–739

McNeil BJ, Adelstein SJ (1976) Determining the value of diagnostic and screening tests. J Nucl Med 17(6):439–448

Pepe MS, Feng Z, Longton G, Koopmeiners J (2009) Conditional estimation of sensitivity and specificity from a phase 2 biomarker study allowing early termination for futility. Stat Med 28(5):762–779

Pocock SJ (1977) Group sequential methods in the design and analysis of clinical trials. Biometrika 64(2):191–199

O'Brien PC, Fleming TR (1979) A multiple testing procedure for clinical trials. Biometrics 35(3):549–556

Silvestri GA, Tanoue LT, Margolis ML, Barker J, Detterbeck F (2003) The noninvasive staging of non-small cell lung cancerthe guidelines. CHEST J 123(1_suppl):147S –156S

Sox HC, Stern S, Owens D, Abrams HL (1989) Assessment of diagnostic technology in health care: rationale, methods, problems, and directions. National Academies Press, Washington, DC

Tang L, Liu A (2010) Sample size recalculation in sequential diagnostic trials. Biostatistics 11: 151–163

Tang L, Emerson SS, Zhou XH (2008) Nonparametric and semiparametric group sequential methods for comparing accuracy of diagnostic tests. Biometrics 64(4):1137–1145

vander Vaart AW, Wellner J (1996) Weak convergence and empirical processes: with applications to statistics. Springer, New York

Zhou XH, Obuchowski NA, McClish DK (2011) Statistical methods in diagnostic medicine, vol 712. Wiley, Hoboken

Zweig MH, Campbell G (1993) Receiver-operating characteristic (ROC) plot: a fundamental evaluation tool in clinical medicine. Clin Chem 39:561–577

Chapter 7
Nonparametric Covariate Adjustment for the Youden Index

Haochuan Zhou and Gengsheng Qin

Abstract The receiver operating characteristic (ROC) curve has been widely applied to evaluate the accuracy of a diagnostic test. The Youden index (YI) is a popular summary index of the ROC curve. In some diagnostic studies, it is believed that the impact of covariates might influence the accuracy of the diagnostic test. In regards to this consideration, we propose nonparametric estimates for the YI with covariate adjustment for the test results under heteroscedastic regression models. We also investigate the asymptotic properties of the covariate-adjusted YI estimators under normal error and non-normal error model assumptions. Extensive simulation studies are conducted to illustrate the effectiveness and the robustness of the proposed methods. A diabetes data set from a diagnostic study is used to demonstrate the application of the new methods.

7.1 Introduction

Over the past three decades, *Receiver Operating Characteristic* (ROC) curve analysis has drawn attention and gained reputation as a statistical methodology for the evaluation of the discriminating efficiency of medical diagnostic tests. For a diagnostic test with continuous or ordinal outcomes, the ROC curve describes the ability of the test to suitably diagnose for a variety of test cutoff points (Pepe 2003). ROC curves offer a graphical method for statisticians to compare the diagnostic efficiencies of medical tests at various special levels of false positive rates.

Continuous diagnostic test outcomes would be the focus of this research. For a certain disease, let X represent the test result of the control group and Y represent the test result of the case group. Without losing generality, further assume that the larger the test outcome is, the more evidences of abnormality. The sensitivity and the

H. Zhou (✉)
CyberSource, 901 Metro Center Boulevard, M3-5NW Foster City, CA, USA
e-mail: harriszhou@gmail.com

G. Qin
Georgia State University, 30 Pryor Street, Atlanta, GA, USA
e-mail: gqin@gsu.edu

Z. Chen et al. (eds.), *Applied Statistics in Biomedicine and Clinical Trials Design*,
ICSA Book Series in Statistics, DOI 10.1007/978-3-319-12694-4_7

specificity of the test at a given cutoff point of the diagnose are defined as:

$$sensitivity(c) = P(Y \geq c) = 1 - G(c), \quad specificity(c) = P(X \leq c) = F(c),$$

respectively, where G and F are the respective cumulative distributions of the diseased test result X and the non-diseased test result Y. The ROC curve is constructed via plotting $1 - specificity$ versus *sensitivity* for all possible cutoff point c.

The area under the ROC curve (AUC) is a commonly used global index of diagnostic accuracy. With the above assumptions, the AUC would range from 0.5 to 1, where value 0.5 indicates a useless diagnostic test, and value 1 indicates a perfect diagnostic test. Alternatively, Youden (1950) introduced another global index (called the Youden index, YI) for the ROC curve:

$$J = \sup_{c}\{sensitivity(c) + specificity(c) - 1\}. \tag{7.1}$$

The YI is ranged between 0 and 1, where 0 indicates that a test cannot discriminate between non-diseased and diseased groups, and 1 indicates that a test perfectly discriminates between the two groups. The optimal cutoff point is the threshold leading to the maximum summation of *sensitivity* and *specificity* of a diagnostic test. Since the optimal cutpoint may not be unique, let $C = \{c : \sup_c (1 - G(c) + F(c))\}$ represent the collection of all possible optimal cutpoints. For simplicity, we define the optimal cutpoint as follows:

$$c_{o,1} = \inf_{c} C, \quad c_{o,2} = \sup_{c} C.$$

Evidently, $c_{o,1}$ is the unique optimal cutpoint maximizing the sensitivity, and $c_{o,2}$ is the unique optimal cutpoint maximizing the *specificity*. If $c_{o,1} = c_{o,2}$, $c_o \equiv c_{o,1} = c_{o,2}$ is the unique optimal cutpoint. In practice, if the sensitivity is believed to be more important than the specificity, $c_{o,1}$ is suggested as the classifying threshold. In some medical screening applications, $c_{o,2}$ might be preferred under the consideration of controlling false positives. The YI is also frequently used in practice (See Aoki et al. 1997; Grmec and Gasparovic 2001; Demir et al. 2002; Schisterman et al. 2008). For instance, Demir et al. (2002) applied the YI to identify the most reliable indices in distinguishing between thalassemial trait and iron deficiency anemia, and Schisterman et al. (2008) used the YI to analyze a data set on the coronary calcium score, a marker for atherosclerosis. The YI has one advantage over the AUC; by evaluating the YI, one can explore the information of the associated optimal cutoff point. This optimal cutoff point is required in real-world applications because an individual can be classified to be either diseased or healthy by comparing the test value with the optimal cutoff point. The optimal cutoff point has the desirable property of maximizing the overall correct diagnosis rate and therefore minimizing the overall misdiagnosis rate (Kim 2008).

YI is a function of sensitivity and specificity that depends on the unknown diseased and non-diseased population distributions. Under the assumption that the distributions belong to a specific parametric family such as binormal distributions,

Fluss et al. (2005) and Schisterman and Perkins (2007) provided statistical inferences for the YI. Fluss et al. (2005) also suggested some nonparametric methods for the YI and the corresponding cutoff point. Recently, Zhou and Qin (2012) proposed new nonparametric confidence intervals for the YI.

Diagnostic tests often include covariates information, such as patients' age, gender, or race, and such information is known to influence the accuracy of a test. It may be that the definition of testing positive (or negative) should depend on the covariates, or it may be that the accuracy of the test is less than optimal in certain settings (see Pepe 2003). Covariate-adjustment for the summary measures of the ROC curve has thus become necessary in many diagnostic applications. Tosteson and Begg (1988) and Toledano and Gatsonis (1995) used a latent variable ordinal regression to model the distribution of the test results in the diseased and non-diseased populations. Thompson and Zucchini (1989) and Obuchowski (1995) calculated the ROC curve and AUC for a number of distinct combinations of covariates and then applied a general regression model. Pepe (1997, 2000), Dodd and Pepe (2003) proposed a general regression framework and semi-parametric methods to model the dependence of the ROC curve and AUC on the covariates. Zhou et al. (2002) and Pepe (2003) gave a wonderful introduction to why and how to adjust for covariate effects for the ROC curves and a detailed review of the existing methods in estimating a covariate-specific ROC curve.

While the covariate adjustment has been extensively studied for the ROC curve and the AUC in the literature, not much work has been focused on the YI. Faraggi (2003) proposed normal regression models to adjust the AUC and YI for covariates. Schisterman et al. (2006) proposed mixture models for test outcomes with mass at value zero for adjusting the ROC curve and AUC. Yang and Qin (2012) developed empirical likelihood-based inferences for the AUC with covariates. Yao et al. (2010) generalized the approaches of Faraggi (2003) and Schisterman et al. (2006) to construct a covariate-adjusted Mann–Whitney estimator for the AUC. They also mentioned that the methods can be extended to other measures related to ROC curves, but they did not give the details. Since the YI is very important in practice, we believe it is necessary to extend Yao et al.'s work (2010) to inferences on the YI.

This chapter is organized as follows. In Sect. 7.2, we propose covariate-adjusted estimators for the YI under heteroscedastic regression models with normal errors and non-normal errors. In Sect. 7.3, we investigate the asymptotic properties of the estimators. In Sect. 7.4, simulation studies are conducted to evaluate the finite sample performance of the new methods. In Sect. 7.5, a real example is used to illustrate the application of the proposed methods. We give a final remark in Sect. 7.6. The proofs of the main theorems are put in the Appendix.

7.2 Models and Methods

7.2.1 *Heteroscedastic Regression Models for the Test Results*

There are two approaches in the literature to model the relationship between the ROC curve and covariates. The first one is to model the dependence of the ROC curve directly on the covariates. Yao et al. (2010) indicated that this approach loses the connection with the cut-off value and does not allow the prediction of the sensitivity and specificity at a given cutoff conditional on covariates. The second one is to directly model the covariate effects on the test results and obtain the covariate-adjusted ROC curve and its related summary measures through the modeling process. Faraggi (2003) employed the second approach by using a simple linear regression model with normal error. Yao et al. (2010) extended Faraggi's work (2003) by using a nonparametric heteroscedastic regression model. Here we utilize the same models as in Yao et al. (2010). Assume the following nonparametric models for X and Y:

$$X|(Z = z) = \mu_1(z) + \sqrt{\nu_1(z)}\varepsilon_1, \tag{7.2}$$

$$Y|(Z = z) = \mu_2(z) + \sqrt{\nu_2(z)}\varepsilon_2, \tag{7.3}$$

where Z represents the covariate vector, ε_1 and ε_2 are independent standard errors having mean zero and standard deviation one, the range of the variance functions $\nu_1(z)$ and $\nu_2(z)$ is restricted in $\Re^+$ and finite for all $z \in \Re$. In addition, let F_Z and G_Z denote the cumulative distribution functions (c.d.f.) of X and Y at given Z respectively, f_Z and g_Z denote the probability density functions (p.d.f.) of X and Y at given Z, respectively; $F^*(\cdot)$ and $G^*(\cdot)$ denote the c.d.f. of ε_1 and ε_2 respectively; and $f^*(\cdot)$ and $g^*(\cdot)$ denote the p.d.f. of ε_1 and ε_2 respectively. Here, the error distributions F^* and G^* are assumed to be independent of Z. We further assume that for a given covariate value $Z = z$, $P(Y(z) > X(z)) \geq 0.5$, which is equivalent to $\mu_1(z) < \mu_2(z)$ if F^* and G^* are symmetric distributions about 0. This assumption ensures that the value of the YI with given covariate information is between 0 and 1 inclusive.

7.2.2 *Covariate-Adjusted YI Under Normal Error Assumption*

With the covariate Z, both YI and the optimal cutoff point actually are dependent on Z. Let $C(z) = \{c : \sup_c [P(Y \geq c|Z = z)) + P(X \leq c|Z = z) - 1]\}$ represent the collection of possible optimal cutoff points when $Z = z$, $c_{o,1}(z) = \inf_c C(z)$, and $c_{o,2}(z) = \sup_c C(z)$. The YI at given $Z = z$ is

$$\begin{aligned} J(z) &= \sup_c\{P(Y \geq c|Z = z) + P(X \leq c|Z = z) - 1\} \\ &= P(Y \geq c_o(z)|Z = z) + P(X \leq c_o(z)|Z = z) - 1 \\ &= P(X \leq c_o(z)|Z = z) - P(Y \leq c_o(z)|Z = z) \\ &= F_Z(c_o(z)) - G_Z(c_o(z)), \end{aligned} \tag{7.4}$$

where $c_o(z) = c_{o,1}(z)$, or $c_{o,2}(z)$. If the errors ε_1 and ε_2 are assumed to be normally distributed in models (7.2) and (7.3), the YI at $Z = z$ can be expressed as

$$J_N(z) = \Phi\left(\frac{\mu_2(z) - c_o(z)}{\sqrt{\nu_2(z)}}\right) - \Phi\left(\frac{\mu_1(z) - c_o(z)}{\sqrt{\nu_1(z)}}\right), \quad (7.5)$$

where $J_N(z)$ stands for $J(z)$ under normal error. With normality and the assumption that $\mu_2(z) > \mu_1(z)$, $c_o(z)$ has the following closed form:

$$c_o(z) = \frac{\mu_1(z)(b^2 - 1) - a + b\sqrt{a^2 + (b^2 - 1)\nu_1(z)ln(b^2)}}{(b^2 - 1)}, \quad (7.6)$$

where $a = \mu_2(z) - \mu_1(z)$, $b = \sqrt{\nu_2(z)}/\sqrt{\nu_1(z)}$. When $b = 1$, we have

$$c_o(z) = \frac{\mu_1(z) + \mu_2(z)}{2}. \quad (7.7)$$

Under models (7.2–7.3), the mean and variance functions μ_1, μ_2, ν_1, and ν_2 can be consistently estimated via some nonparametric techniques such as the local polynomial regression technique. Let $\widehat{\mu}_1$, $\widehat{\mu}_2$, $\widehat{\nu}_1$, and $\widehat{\nu}_2$ be the local polynomial estimates for μ_1, μ_2, ν_1, and ν_2 by using local polynomial method (see Fan and Gijbels 1996), and $\widehat{c}_o(z)$ be the plug-in estimate of $c_o(z)$. Then the covariate-adjusted estimator for the YI can be defined as follows:

$$\widehat{J}_N(z) = \Phi\left(\frac{\widehat{\mu}_2(z) - \widehat{c}_o(z)}{\sqrt{\widehat{\nu}_2(z)}}\right) - \Phi\left(\frac{\widehat{\mu}_1(z) - \widehat{c}_o(z)}{\sqrt{\widehat{\nu}_1(z)}}\right). \quad (7.8)$$

7.2.3 *Covariate-Adjusted YI Without Normal Error Assumption*

The covariate-adjusted YI in Sect. 7.2.2 is a semi-parametric estimator for the YI based on regression models with normal error distribution assumption for test results. However, this method may be sensitive to departures from the distributional assumption. Therefore, it is necessary to provide a fully nonparametric covariate-adjustment for the YI.

In this section, ε_1 and ε_2 in models (7.2–7.3) are assumed to be distribution free, i.e., both $F^*(\cdot)$ and $G^*(\cdot)$ are unknown distributions. Let $\{(z_{i,x}, x_i) : i = 1 \ldots m\}$ and $\{(z_{j,y}, y_j) : j = 1 \ldots n\}$ be random samples of "non-diseased" subjects and "diseased" subjects from models (7.2–7.3), where $z_{i,x}$ and $z_{j,y}$ are the corresponding observed covariate values in the "non-diseased" and "diseased" samples. Our goal is to estimate $J(z)$ at given z based on these samples.

To estimate $J(z)$ at given z, we have to estimate test values at given $Z = z$ since the mean functions $\mu_i(z)$'s and the variance functions $\nu_i(z)$'s as well as the error distributions $F^*(\cdot)$ and $G^*(\cdot)$ are unknown. Estimating the mean and variance functions can be easily implemented by modern nonparametric methods (e.g., local polynomial method). However, producing a good estimate for the error distribution is a difficult task in nonparametric heteroscedastic regression models. Instead of using the complex estimation of the error distributions, we employ the following procedure which has been applied in Yao et al. (2010):

1. Find nonparametric estimates $\widehat{\mu}_1$, $\widehat{\mu}_2$, $\widehat{\nu}_1$, and $\widehat{\nu}_2$ for μ_1, μ_2, ν_1, and ν_2 by using local polynomial method (see Fan and Gijbels 1996).
2. Find the standardized residuals:

$$\widehat{\varepsilon}_{i,x} = \frac{x_i - \widehat{\mu}_1(z_{i,x})}{\sqrt{\widehat{\nu}_1(z_{i,x})}}, \quad \widehat{\varepsilon}_{j,y} = \frac{y_j - \widehat{\mu}_2(z_{j,y})}{\sqrt{\widehat{\nu}_2(z_{j,y})}}.$$

3. Estimate test values at given $Z = z$ as follows:

$$\widehat{x}_{i,z} = \widehat{\mu}_1(z) + \sqrt{\widehat{\nu}_1(z)}\widehat{\varepsilon}_{i,x}, \quad \widehat{y}_{j,z} = \widehat{\mu}_2(z) + \sqrt{\widehat{\nu}_2(z)}\widehat{\varepsilon}_{j,y}.$$

Then, the nonparametric covariate-adjusted estimator for the YI can be defined as follows:

$$\begin{aligned}\widehat{J}_E(z) &= \sup_c \left[m^{-1}\sum_{i=1}^{m} I(\widehat{x}_{i,z} \le c) - n^{-1}\sum_{j=1}^{n} I(\widehat{y}_{j,z} \le c) \right] \\ &= m^{-1}\sum_{i=1}^{m} I\left(\widehat{x}_{i,z} \le \widehat{c}_{oE}(z)\right) - n^{-1}\sum_{j=1}^{n} I\left(\widehat{y}_{j,z} \le \widehat{c}_{oE}(z)\right)\end{aligned}$$

where $I(\cdot)$ is the indicator function, $\widehat{c}_{oE}(z) = \widehat{c}^{(1)}_{oE}(z)$ or $\widehat{c}^{(2)}_{oE}(z)$ with

$$\widehat{c}^{(1)}_{oE}(z) = \inf_c \left\{ c : \sup_c \left[m^{-1}\sum_{i=1}^{m} I(\widehat{x}_{i,z} \le c) - n^{-1}\sum_{j=1}^{n} I(\widehat{y}_{j,z} \le c) \right] \right\}, \tag{7.9}$$

$$\widehat{c}^{(2)}_{oE}(z) = \sup_c \left\{ c : \sup_c \left[m^{-1}\sum_{i=1}^{m} I(\widehat{x}_{i,z} \le c) - n^{-1}\sum_{j=1}^{n} I(\widehat{y}_{j,z} \le c) \right] \right\}. \tag{7.10}$$

$\widehat{c}^{(i)}_{oE}(z)$'s are empirical estimates for the optimal cutoff point. In practice, $\widehat{c}^{(i)}_{oE}(z)$ can be estimated via numerically searching on a grid of combined samples from X and Y. It is noted that, while $\widehat{c}^{(i)}_{oE}(z)$ lead to the empirical estimate of the YI, $\widehat{c}^{(1)}_{oE}(z)$ maximizes the empirical sensitivity, and $\widehat{c}^{(2)}_{oE}(z)$ maximizes the empirical specificity.

Remark 1. It should be indicated that one advantage of the proposed nonparametric approach is that the estimated covariates-specific YI is invariant to monotone transformation of test results. On the contrary, a parametric procedure forces the covariates to affect the test in a certain scale, and hence the resulting YI is not transformation-free.

Remark 2. In general, the proposed procedure can be used with multi-covariates scenarios. When more than one covariates need to be adjusted, the multivariate smoothing becomes challenging with slower convergence rates and much more intensive computation burden, and it might face the curse of dimensionality problem. However, existing methods for dimension reduction (e.g., additive models) could be a valuable solution in such situation.

7.3 Asymptotic Properties of the Covariate-Adjusted Estimators for the YI

We present the asymptotic properties of the covariate-adjusted estimators for the YI in this section. Firstly, we explore the asymptotic properties of $\widehat{J_N}(z)$ under the normal error assumption. Then we discuss the properties of $\widehat{J_E}(z)$ when there is no specific assumptions for the underlying error distributions.

7.3.1 Asymptotic Properties of $\widehat{J_N}(z)$

Under the normal error assumption, Yao et al. (2010) obtained the asymptotic normality of the covariate-adjusted AUC estimator under models (7.2–7.3) for a given z, and its strong uniform convergence rate. Applying the same arguments, we can derive similar asymptotic properties for $\widehat{J_N}(z)$.

Some notations are presented below for better presenting the asymptotic properties of $\widehat{J_N}(z)$.

$$\zeta_1(z) = E(\varepsilon_1^3|Z = z), \qquad \zeta_2(z) = E(\varepsilon_2^3|Z = z),$$

$$\pi_1(z) = Var(\varepsilon_1^2|Z = z), \qquad \pi_2(z) = Var(\varepsilon_1^2\ Z = z),$$

$$\mathcal{M}_j(\mathcal{K}) = \int \mu^j \mathcal{K}(\mu)d\mu, \text{ for all integer } j \geq 0,$$

$$\mathcal{R}(\mathcal{K}) = \int \mathcal{K}^2(\mu) < \infty, \qquad \mathcal{S}_p = \left(m_{j+l}(\mathcal{K})\right)_{0\leq j,l\leq p}$$

$$\mathcal{K}^*(\mu) = v_1^T \mathcal{S}_p^{-1}(1, \mu, \ldots, \mu^p)^T \mathcal{K}(\mu),$$

$$R(\mathcal{K}^*, \rho) = \int \mathcal{K}^*(\mu)\mathcal{K}^*(\mu/\rho)d\mu, \text{ for any } 0 < \rho < \infty,$$

where $\mathcal{K}(\cdot)$ is a symmetric kernel density function, p is the order of local polynomial methodology. v_k is the $(p + 1) \times 1$ vector with the kth element being 1 and 0 others.

Under some assumptions, for a given z, the local polynomial estimators of the mean and variance functions in models (7.2) and (7.3) are asymptotically normal in distribution, namely,

$$\sqrt{mh_{\mu_1}}\left(\hat{\mu}_1(z) - \mu_1(z), \hat{\nu}_1(z) - \nu_1(z)\right)^\tau \xrightarrow{d} N(\beta_1(z), \Xi_1(z)),$$

$$\sqrt{nh_{\mu_2}}\left(\hat{\mu}_2(z) - \mu_2(z), \hat{\nu}_2(z) - \nu_2(z)\right)^\tau \xrightarrow{d} N(\beta_2(z), \Xi_2(z)),$$

where h_{μ_1} and h_{μ_2} are the bandwidths for estimating μ_1 and μ_2, respectively, and

$$\beta_1(z) = \{\beta_{11}(z), \beta_{12}(z)\}^\tau, \qquad \Xi_1(z) = \xi_{x,ij}(z)_{1\le i,j\le 2},$$

$$\beta_{11} = \frac{\mathcal{M}_{p+1}\mathcal{K}^*}{(p+1)} d_1 \mu_1^{p+1}(z), \qquad \beta_{12} = \frac{\mathcal{M}_{p+1}\mathcal{K}^*}{(p+1)} d_1 \rho_1^{p+1} \nu_1^{p+1}(z),$$

$$\xi_{x,11}(z) = \frac{\mathcal{R}(\mathcal{K}^*)\nu_1(z)}{\theta(z)}, \qquad \xi_{x,22}(z) = \frac{\mathcal{R}(\mathcal{K}^*)\pi_1(z)}{\theta(z)\rho_1},$$

$$\xi_{x,12}(z) = \xi_{x,21}(z) = \frac{\mathcal{R}(\mathcal{K}^*, \rho_1)\zeta_1(z)}{\theta(z)\rho_1}, \qquad d_1 = \lim \left(m h_{\mu_1}^{2p+3}\right)^{1/2}$$

$$\beta_2(z) = \{\beta_{21}(z), \beta_{22}(z)\}^\tau, \qquad \Xi_2(z) = \xi_{y,ij}(z)_{1\le i,j\le 2},$$

$$\beta_{21} = \frac{\mathcal{M}_{p+1}\mathcal{K}^*}{(p+1)} d_2 \mu_2^{p+1}(z), \qquad \beta_{22} = \frac{\mathcal{M}_{p+1}\mathcal{K}^*}{(p+1)} d_2 \rho_2^{p+1} \nu_2^{p+1}(z),$$

$$\xi_{y,11}(z) = \frac{\mathcal{R}(\mathcal{K}^*)\nu_2(z)}{\theta(z)}, \qquad \xi_{y,22}(z) = \frac{\mathcal{R}(\mathcal{K}^*)\pi_2(z)}{\theta(z)\rho_2},$$

$$\xi_{y,12}(z) = \xi_{y,21}(z) = \frac{\mathcal{R}(\mathcal{K}^*, \rho_2)\zeta_2(z)}{\theta(z)\rho_2}, \qquad d_2 = \lim \left(m h_{\mu_2}^{2p+3}\right)^{1/2},$$

$$\rho_i = \lim h_{\nu_i}/h_{\mu_i},\ i = 1, 2, \text{ and } h_{\nu_i} \text{ is the bandwidth for estimating } \nu_i,$$

Based on above asymptotic properties, applying the Cramer–Wald device and Slusky's theorem, we obtain the following theorems for $\widehat{J}_N(z)$.

Theorem 1 *Under assumptions (A1–A5) stated in Appendix, for a given $Z = z$, we have that*

(i) if $\frac{n}{m} \to \infty$, $\sqrt{m h_{\mu,1}}(\hat{J}_N(z) - J_N(z)) \xrightarrow{d} N(M_1(z), V_1(z))$, where

$$M_1(z) = \frac{\partial J_N(z)}{\partial \mu_1(z)}\beta_{11}(z) + \frac{\partial J_N(z)}{\partial \nu_1(z)}\beta_{12}(z),$$

$$V_1(z) = \left(\frac{\partial J_N(z)}{\partial \mu_1(z)}\right)^2 \xi_{x,11}(z) + \left(\frac{\partial J_N(z)}{\partial \nu_1(z)}\right)^2 \xi_{x,22}(z) + \xi_{x,12}(z)\left(\frac{\partial J_N(z)}{\partial \nu_1(z)}\frac{\partial J_N(z)}{\partial \mu_1(z)} + \frac{\partial J_N(z)}{\partial \mu_1(z)}\frac{\partial J_N(z)}{\partial \nu_1(z)}\right).$$

(ii) if $\frac{n}{m} \to 0$, $\sqrt{n h_{\mu,2}}(\hat{J}_N(z) - J_N(z)) \xrightarrow{d} N(M_2(z), V_2(z))$, where

$$M_2(z) = \frac{\partial J_N(z)}{\partial \mu_2(z)}\beta_{21}(z) + \frac{\partial J_N(z)}{\partial \nu_2(z)}\beta_{22}(z),$$

$$V_2(z) = \left(\frac{\partial J_N(z)}{\partial \mu_2(z)}\right)^2 \xi_{y,11}(z) + \left(\frac{\partial J_N(z)}{\partial \nu_2(z)}\right)^2 \xi_{y,22}(z) + \xi_{y,12}(z)\left(\frac{\partial J_N(z)}{\partial \nu_2(z)}\frac{\partial J_N(z)}{\partial \mu_2(z)} + \frac{\partial J_N(z)}{\partial \mu_2(z)}\frac{\partial J_N(z)}{\partial \nu_2(z)}\right),$$

(iii) if $\frac{n}{m} \to \rho$, $0 < \rho < \infty$, $\sqrt{mh_{\mu,1}}(\hat{J}_N(z) - J_N(z)) \xrightarrow{d} N(M_3(z), V_3(z))$, *where*

$$M_3(z) = M_1(z) + \rho^{-\frac{p+1}{2p+3}} M_2(z), \quad V_3(z) = V_1(z) + \rho^{-\frac{2p+2}{2p+3}} V_2(z).$$

The forms of partial derivatives in above equations are given in Appendix.

Theorem 2 *Under assumptions (A1†–A5†) and (A6–A8) stated in Appendix, we have*

$$\sup_{z \in \Re_Z} |\hat{J}_N(z) - J_N(z)| = O(\mathcal{T}_m + \mathcal{W}_n), \tag{7.11}$$

where $\mathcal{T}_m = h_{\mu_1}^{p+1} + \sqrt{log(1/h_{\mu_1})/(mh_{\mu_1})}$, $\mathcal{W}_n = h_{\mu_2}^{p+1} + \sqrt{log(1/h_{\mu_2})/(nh_{\mu_2})}$, h_{μ_i}*'s are bandwidths for estimating* $\mu_i(z)$*'s (i= 1, 2), and* $\Re_Z$ *is the domain of Z.*

7.3.2 Asymptotic Properties of $\widehat{J}_E(z)$

Now, we explore the asymptotic properties of the empirical estimate $\widehat{J}_E(z)$ of $J(z)$ without normality assumption.

Let

$$\varepsilon_{i,x} = \frac{x_i - \mu_1(z_{i,x})}{\sqrt{\nu_1(z_{i,x})}}, \quad \varepsilon_{j,y} = \frac{y_j - \mu_2(z_{j,y})}{\sqrt{\nu_2(z_{j,y})}}.$$

and

$$x_{i,z} = \mu_1(z) + \sqrt{\nu_1(z)}\varepsilon_{i,x}, \quad y_{j,z} = \mu_2(z) + \sqrt{\nu_2(z)}\varepsilon_{j,y}.$$

$$\begin{aligned}\widetilde{J}_E(z) &= \sup_c \left[m^{-1} \sum_{i=1}^{m} I(x_{i,z} \le c) - n^{-1} \sum_{j=1}^{n} I(y_{j,z} \le c) \right] \\ &= m^{-1} \sum_{i=1}^{m} I(x_{i,z} \le \tilde{c}_{oE}(z)) - n^{-1} \sum_{j=1}^{n} I(y_{j,z} \le \tilde{c}_{oE}(z)),\end{aligned}$$

where $\widetilde{c}_{oE}(z) = \widetilde{c}_{oE}^{(1)}(z)$ or $\widetilde{c}_{oE}^{(2)}(z)$, and

$$\widetilde{c}_{oE}^{(1)}(z) = \inf_c \left\{ c : \sup_c \left[m^{-1} \sum_{i=1}^{m} I(x_{i,z} \le c) - n^{-1} \sum_{j=1}^{n} I(y_{j,z} \le c) \right] \right\}, \tag{7.12}$$

$$\widetilde{c}_{oE}^{(2)}(z) = \sup_c \left\{ c : \sup_c \left[m^{-1} \sum_{i=1}^{m} I(x_{i,z} \le c) - n^{-1} \sum_{j=1}^{n} I(y_{j,z} \le c) \right] \right\}. \tag{7.13}$$

$\widetilde{J}_E(z)$ can be treated as a "hypothetical" estimator for $J(z)$ because the mean functions $\mu_i(z)$'s and the variance functions $\nu_i(z)$'s need to be estimated in practice.

If $\mu_i(z)$'s and $\nu_i(z)$'s are known, $\widetilde{J}_E(z)$ is asymptotically an unbiased estimator for $J(z)$.

Theorem 3 *If $n/m \to \rho$ for some $0 < \rho < \infty$, then*

$$E\left[\widetilde{J}_E(z)\right] \longrightarrow J(z), \quad \textit{for a given } z. \tag{7.14}$$

Theorem 4 *Under assumptions (A1†), (A2†), (A4†), (A3*), (A5*), (A6–A8) and (A9) stated in Appendix, if $n/m \to \rho$ for some $0 < \rho < \infty$, then*

$$E\left[\left(\widehat{J}_E(z) - \widetilde{J}_E(z)\right)^2\right] \longrightarrow 0, \quad \textit{for a given } z. \tag{7.15}$$

The asymptotic unbiasness property of $\widehat{J}_E(z)$ can be obtained from Theorem 3 and Theorem 4. But the asymptotic normality of the empirical estimator $\widehat{J}_E(z)$ has eluded us so far. It still is an open research problem.

7.4 Confidence Intervals for the YI and Simulation Study

7.4.1 Confidence Intervals for the Covariate-Adjusted YI

Under the normal error assumption for models (7.2) and (7.3), using the asymptotic distribution of $\widehat{J}_N(z)$, we can construct a normal approximation (NA)-based confidence interval (NA interval) for the YI at given $Z = z$. To avoid plugging in many estimates listed in Theorem 1, we apply the bootstrap method to estimate the bias and variance of the covariate adjusted $\widehat{J}_N(z)$. At given z, resample the original data B times to calculate B bootstrap replications of $\widehat{J}_N(z)$, denoted as $\{\widehat{J}_N^{*b}(z) : b = 1, 2, \ldots, B\}$, then the bias can be estimated by

$$\widehat{M}_3^*(z) = \frac{1}{B}\sum_{b=1}^{B}(\widehat{J}_N^{*b}(z) - \widehat{J}_N(z)),$$

and the variance can be estimated by

$$\widehat{V}_3^*(z) = \frac{1}{B-1}\sum_{b=1}^{B}(\widehat{J}_N^{*b}(z) - \widehat{J}_N(z))^2.$$

Therefore, at given z, we can construct a $(1-\alpha)100\,\%$ NA confidence interval for $J_N(z)$ as:

$$\left(\widehat{J}_N(z) - \widehat{M}_3^*(z) - z_{1-\alpha/2}\sqrt{\widehat{V}_3^*(z)},\ \widehat{J}_N(z) - \widehat{M}_3^*(z) + z_{1-\alpha/2}\sqrt{\widehat{V}_3^*(z)}\right), \tag{7.16}$$

where $z_{1-\alpha/2}$ is the $(1-\alpha/2)$th quantile of the standard normal distribution.

Without the normal error assumption, the confidence interval for the YI at given $Z = z$ should be based on the nonparametric estimate $\widehat{J}_E(z)$. Since the asymptotic distribution of $\widehat{J}_E(z)$ is still unknown, we propose a nonparametric interval for $J(z)$ by using bootstrap method. Let

$$\widehat{J}_{AC}(z) = \frac{\sum_{i=1}^{m} I(\widehat{x}_{i,z} \le \widehat{c}_{oE}(z)) + z_{1-\alpha/2}^2/2}{m + z_{1-\alpha/2}^2} - \frac{\sum_{j=1}^{n} I(\widehat{y}_{j,z} \le \widehat{c}_{oE}(z)) + z_{1-\alpha/2}^2/2}{n + z_{1-\alpha/2}^2}.$$

$\widehat{J}_{AC}(z)$ is inspired by Agresti and Coull's (1998) interval estimate for a binomial proportion which has very good small sample performance. Since $z_{1-\alpha/2}$ is approximately equal to 2 when $\alpha = 0.05$, $\widehat{J}_{AC}(z)$ may be regarded as an adjusted estimate for the difference between two proportions (i.e., $P(X \le c_o(z)|Z = z)$ and $P(Y \le c_o(z)|Z = z)$) by adding two successes and two failures to the pseudo Bernoulli observations. We summarize the bootstrap procedure in the following steps:

(i). Resample of size m, $\widehat{x}_{i,z}^*$'s, with replacement from $\widehat{x}_{i,z}$'s and a resample of size n, $\widehat{y}_{j,z}^*$'s, with replacement from $\widehat{y}_{j,z}$'s.

(ii). Calculate the bootstrap version of $\widehat{J}_{AC}(z)$

$$\widehat{J}_{AC}^*(z) = \frac{\sum_{j=1}^{m} I(\widehat{y}_{j,z}^* \le \widehat{c}_{oE}^*(z)) + z_{1-\alpha/2}^2/2}{m + z_{1-\alpha/2}^2} - \frac{\sum_{i=1}^{n} I(\widehat{x}_{i,z}^* < \widehat{c}_{oE}^*(z)) + z_{1-\alpha/2}^2/2}{n + z_{1-\alpha/2}^2},$$

where $\widehat{c}_{oE}^*(z)$ is the bootstrap version of $\widehat{c}_{oE}(z)$.

(iii). Repeat step (i) and step (ii) B times to obtain the set of bootstrap replications $\{\widehat{J}_{AC}^{*b}(z) : b = 1, 2, \ldots, B\}$ (it is suggested that $B \ge 200$).

Then, the bootstrap variance estimator $V^*(\widehat{J}_{AC}(z))$ is defined as

$$V^*(\widehat{J}_{AC}(z)) = \frac{1}{B-1} \sum_{b=1}^{B} (\widehat{J}_{AC}^{*b}(z) - \bar{J}_{AC}^*(z))^2$$

where $\bar{J}_{AC}^*(z) = \frac{1}{B} \sum_{b=1}^{B} \widehat{J}_{AC}^{*b}(z)$.

Now the new bootstrap (Agresti and Coull normal approximation, ACNA) interval for $J(z)$ is defined as follows:

$$\left(\widehat{J}_{AC}(z) - z_{1-\alpha/2}\sqrt{V^*(\widehat{J}_{AC}(z))},\ \widehat{J}_{AC}(z) + z_{1-\alpha/2}\sqrt{V^*(\widehat{J}_{AC}(z))} \right). \qquad (7.17)$$

7.4.2 Simulation Study

In this section, we conduct simulation study to examine the finite sample performances of the proposed methods for estimating the YI with adjustment for covariates. In the study, we utilize two sets of models to evaluate the efficiency of our methods.

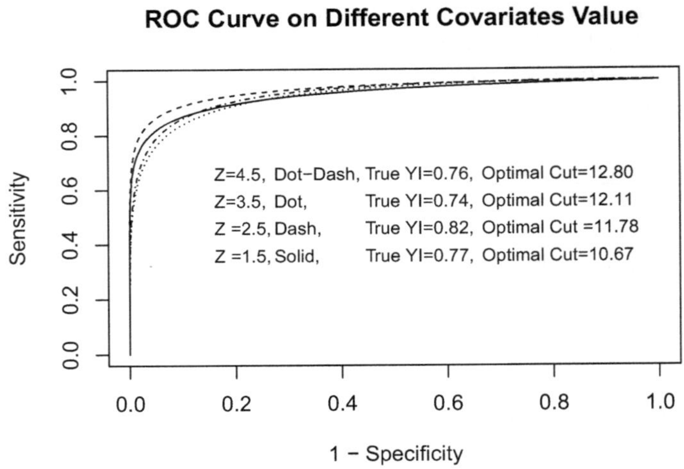

Fig. 7.1 Simulation normal error setting: true receiver operating characteristic (*ROC*) curve, Youden index and optimal cutoff point at different covariate values

In the first situation, we consider the following models for the healthy population and the diseased population:

$$X|Z = 6 + 1.5Z + 1.5\sin(Z) + \sqrt{0.4 + \Phi(2Z - 6)}\varepsilon_1,$$

$$Y|Z = 7.2 + 1.5Z + 1.5\sin(Z) + \sqrt{Z - 0.8} + \sqrt{1.2 + \Phi(2Z - 6)}\varepsilon_2,$$

where both ε_1 and ε_2 follow the standard normal distribution, and Φ is the c.d.f. of standard normal distribution. The simulated observations $\{x_i, z_{i,x}\}$ and $\{y_j, z_{j,y}\}$ for the two populations are generated by drawing Z values from uniform distribution on 1–5 independently, and drawing the errors from $N(0,1)$ independently, where $i = 1, \ldots, m$ and $j = 1, \ldots, n$. We choose the sample sizes to be $n = m = 50$ and $n = m = 100$ to compare performances of the methods at smaller sample size and larger sample size. Figure 7.1 provides an example on how the covariate value impacts the diagnostic accuracy based on the above settings.

In the second situation, we assume the models for the non-diseased and the diseased populations as follows:

$$X|Z = 6 + 1.5Z + 1.5\sin(Z) + \sqrt{0.4 + \Phi(2Z - 6)}\varepsilon_1,$$

$$Y|Z = 8 + 1.5Z + 1.5\sin(Z) + \sqrt{Z - 0.5} + \sqrt{1.5 + \Phi(2Z - 6)}\varepsilon_2,$$

where ε_1, ε_2 follow heavy tail symmetric distribution, namely, the student t-distribution with degree of freedom 4. The purpose of using this setting is to evaluate the performances of the methods when the underlying distributions are missspecified.

Simultaneously selecting the four bandwidths for estimating $J(z)$ here faces the similar issues as in Yao et al. (2010). First, the computational cost is expensive.

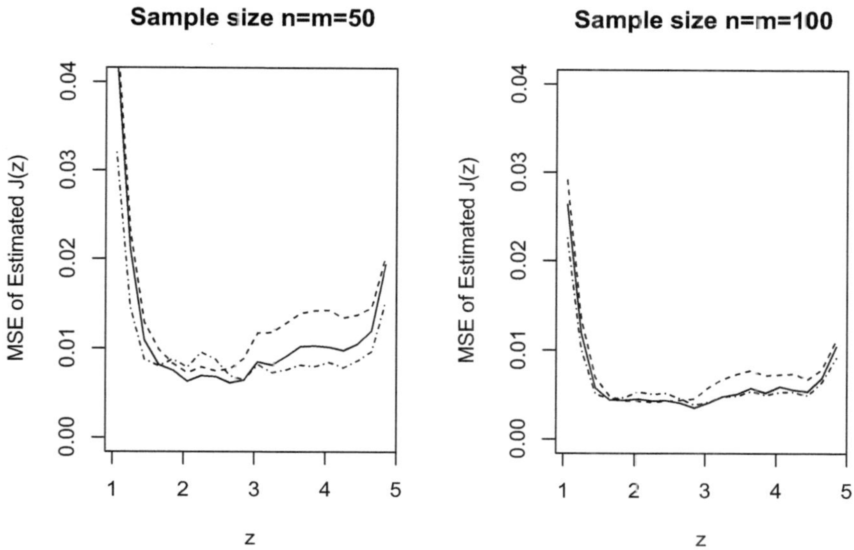

Fig. 7.2 The mean square errors (*MSE*) of the estimators when ε_1 and ε_2 follow the standard normal distribution: *solid line* for $\widehat{J}_N$, *dashed line* for $\widehat{J}_E$, and *dotdash line* for $\widehat{J}_{AC}$

Second, it is too complicated in practice if the criterion for bandwidth selection is based on the asymptotic bias and variance of the estimated YI which involve in complex unknown functions. Lastly, if we apply cross-validation for $J(z)$, there is no observed YI at given $Z = z$. Alternatively, we selected a reasonable path to access the "optimal" bandwidth by the standard leave-one-out cross-validation targeting on minimizing the mean square errors (MSE) of the estimated mean and variance functions. Namely, for given $\{(z_{i,x}, x_i) : i = 1 \ldots m\}$, we select h_{μ_1}, which minimizes $\sum_{i=1}^{m} (x_i - \widehat{\mu}_{1,-i}(z_{i,x}))^2/m$, where $\widehat{\mu}_{1,-i}(z)$ is the local polynomial estimate for $\mu_1(z)$ obtained by leaving $(z_{i,x}, x_i)$ out. Similarly, we can choose h_{μ_2}, h_{ν_1} and h_{ν_2}.

With the generated data, we evaluate the performances of the estimator $\widehat{J}_N(z)$ under normal assumption and the nonparametric estimators $\widehat{J}_E(z)$ and $\widehat{J}_{AC}(z)$ by reporting the MSE at given covariate values. We repeat the simulation for each setting 500 times to calculate MSE at different value of z. From Fig. 7.2, we observe that $\widehat{J}_{AC}(z)$ has the smallest MSE among the three estimators. When sample size increases, the MSE of all estimators decrease as expected, shown in Fig. 7.2 (right). For the second model, which assumed the t-distribution for the errors, the MSE of $\widehat{J}_N(z)$ is significantly larger than those of $\widehat{J}_E(z)$ and $\widehat{J}_{AC}(z)$ (see Fig. 7.3), as expected.

We also examine the 95 % level pointwise NA and ACNA confidence intervals for $J(z)$. The usual bootstrap percentile (BP) confidence interval based on the empirical estimator $\widehat{J}_E(z)$ is also included in the comparisons. In the simulation study, we calculate the average upper bounds and the average lower bounds of these confidence

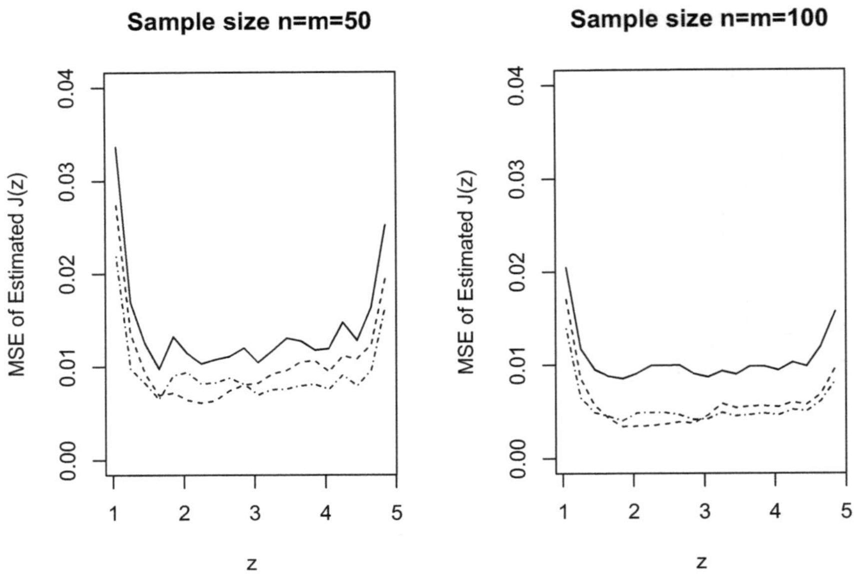

Fig. 7.3 The mean square errors (*MSE*) of the estimators when ε_1 and ε_2 follow t-distribution with degree of freedom 4: *solid line* for $\widehat{J}_N$, *dashed line* for $\widehat{J}_E$, and *dotdash line* for $\widehat{J}_{AC}$

intervals at given z from 500 Monte Carlo runs. In the resampling procedure, we chose $B = 999$ to pursue a better performance. For each Monte Carlo run, we select h_{μ_1}, h_{μ_2}, h_{ν_1}, and h_{ν_2} via leave-one-out cross-validation, and apply the selected bandwidths in the bootstrap procedure.

When the underlying error distribution is normal, from Fig. 7.4, we can see that the ACNA and NA intervals are competitive. The BP pointwise confidence band shows the highest lower band among all three methods, such over estimate of the YI leads to low coverage probability; therefore, its performance is not desired. Overall, the empirical coverage probabilities are lower than the nominal confidence level, specially when z is near the lower and upper bounds of the covariate. When sample size increases, the empirical coverage probabilities of NA and ACNA intervals are closer to the nominal confidence level. When the underlying distribution is a t-distribution, from Fig. 7.5, we observe that ACNA interval performs robustly. Since the underlying distribution is missspecified, the NA interval with the t-distribution error is not competitive to the ACNA interval. Above all, we recommend the ACNA interval in practice.

In another comparative simulation study not reported here, we select the bandwidths as we know the true mean and variance functions. Namely we select h_{μ_1}, which minimizes the true integrated error: $\int [\hat{\mu}_1(z; h_{\mu_1}) - \mu_1(z)]^2 dz$, and choose h_{μ_2}, h_{ν_1}, and h_{ν_2} similarly. Via this approach, we obtained slightly smaller MSE of $\widehat{J}_N(z)$, $\widehat{J}_E(z)$, and $\widehat{J}_{AC}(z)$; also higher empirical pointwise coverage probabilities of $J(z)$, under both simulation settings. Nevertheless, the performance patterns of the

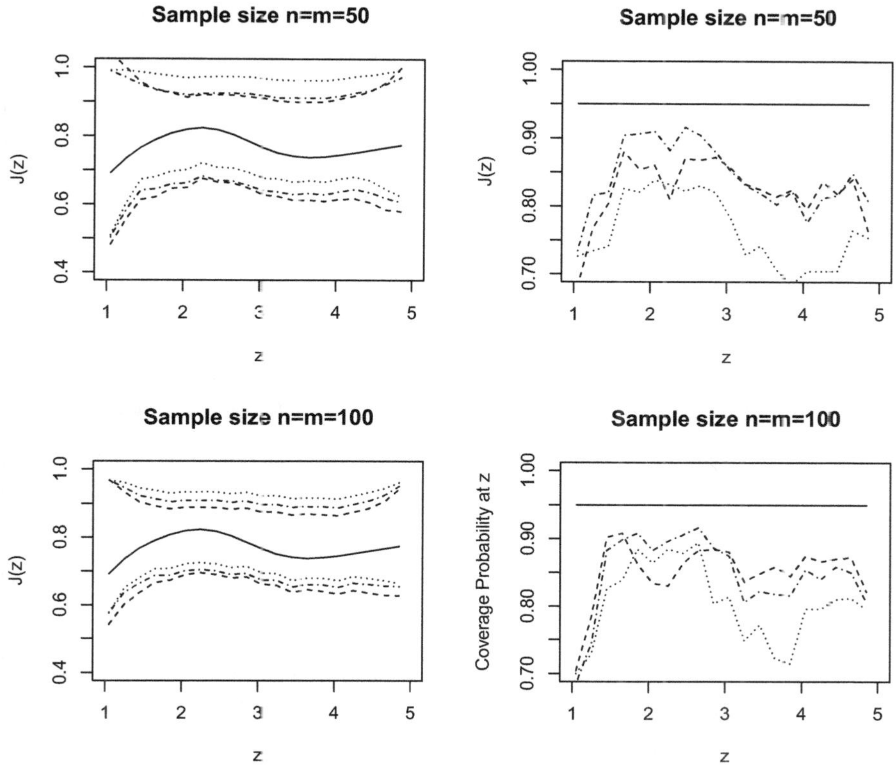

Fig. 7.4 ε_1 and ε_2 follow the standard normal distribution. Left panels: the pointwise confidence bands for $J(z)$: normal approximation (NA) band (*dashed*), bootstrap percentile (BP) band (*dotted*), and Agresti and Coull normal approximation (ACNA) band (*dotdash*). *Solid line* is the curve for the true values of $J(z)$; right panels: the pointwise empirical coverage probability for the proposed confidence intervals, *solid line* is the benchmark, other line types are the same as in left panel

$\widehat{J}_N(z)$, $\widehat{J}_E(z)$, and $\widehat{J}_{AC}(z)$ are similar to the results reported above. Overall, we would like to recommend the ACNA estimate and ACNA interval for the YI in practice.

7.5 Real Application

In this section, we consider the Pima Indians Diabetes Study data set originally discussed by Smith et al. (1988). In the data set, nine variables are recorded: number of times pregnant (V_1), plasma glucose concentration in an oral glucose tolerance test (OGTT; V_2), diastolic blood pressure (mmHg; V_3), triceps skin fold thickness (mm; V_4), 2-h serum insulin (mu U/ml; V_5), body mass index (weight (kg)/(height (m))^2; V$_6$), Diabetes pedigree function (V_7), Age (years) (V_8), Disease Status (0 or

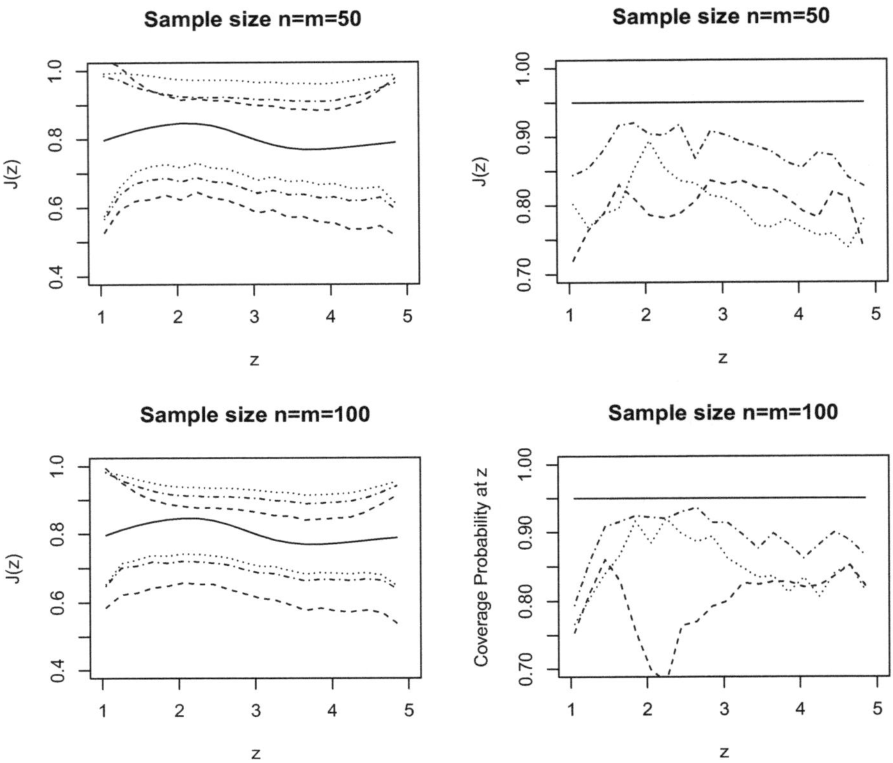

Fig. 7.5 ε_1 and ε_2 follow the t distribution. Left panels: the pointwise confidence bands for $J(z)$: NA band (*dashed*), BP band (*dotted*), and ACNA band (*dotdash*). *Solid line* is the curve for the true values of $J(z)$; right panels: the pointwise empirical coverage probability for the proposed confidence intervals, solid line is the benchmark, other line types are the same as in left panel

1; V_9). There are 268 cases and 500 controls. Two individuals in the case group have OGTT value 0 and three individuals have OGTT value 0. We deleted these five observations in the data analysis. The OGTT is a standard diagnostic test for diabetes. Smith and Thompson (1996) considered the age as a potential covariate that could influence the OGTT results.

First, we consider the situation without covariate adjustment. The OGTT results from case and control groups are not normally distributed based on the Pearson chi-square test for normality (p-value $= 0.001, 0.023$ respectively). The empirical estimate for the YI is $J_E = 0.446$. This estimated YI value indicates that the ability of the OGTT for distinguishing diabetes is mediocre.

Now we consider the effect of age in estimating the YI. The scatter plots of the OGTT results versus age among non-diseased and diseased groups (see Fig. 7.6) do not indicate a strong linear relationship between OGTT and age. It also indicates that the variations in OGTT results over age is non-constant. Consequently, the

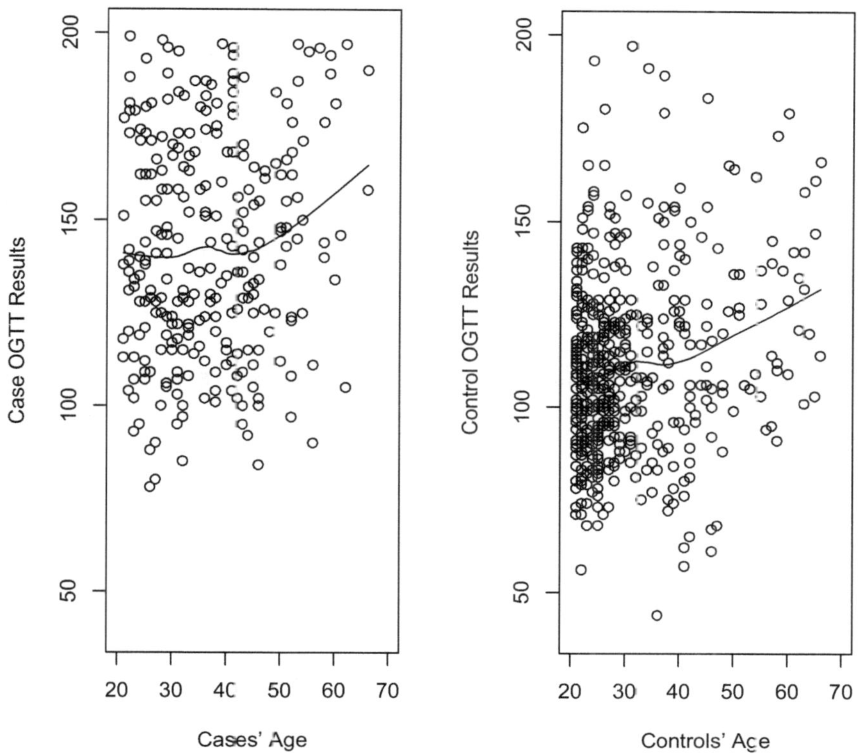

Fig. 7.6 The scatter plot of oral glucose tolerance test (*OGTT*) versus age, *left* for cases, *right* for controls. *Solid lines* are local polynomial estimates for the mean functions

linear regression models employed in Faraggi (2003) cannot be directly applied here. However, the heteroscedastic regression models (7.2) and (7.3) could work for this data set. Figure 7.7. presents the local polynomial regression on the mean and variance functions for both cases and controls, in which, the bandwidth for h_{μ_1}, h_{μ_2} h_{ν_1}, and h_{ν_2} are selected via standard leave-one-out cross validation.

Here, we use the OGTT results of subjects aged between 21 and 66, and produce three covariate-adjusted estimates $\widehat{J_N}(z)$, $\widehat{J_E}(z)$ and $\widehat{J_{AC}}(z)$ for the YI, with 95% pointwise BP band and ACNA band. We also include the YI estimate (denoted as $\widehat{J_L}(z)$) via linear model for comparison. From Fig. 7.8, by heteroscedastic model, it is noticeable that the accuracy of diagnosing diabetes by testing the glucose level in blood varies by age. The diagnostic accuracy of OGTT for younger individuals (age $<$ 30 years) is observed to be more precise than that for individuals aged from 30 years to 35 years. There is a small spike which shows a slightly increasing accuracy for 38-year to 40-year-old individuals, and then the accuracy decreases slowly to about 50 years. When testing individuals are getting older (age $>$ 50 years), the accuracy of OGTT increases, and the confidence bands become wider as age increases. This

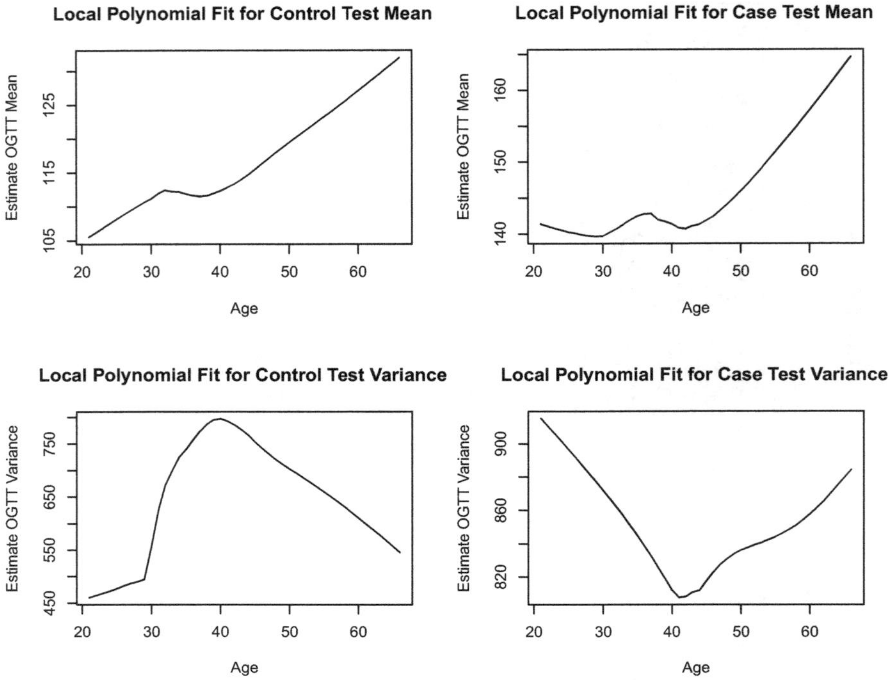

Fig. 7.7 Local polynomial estimates for the mean and variance of oral glucose tolerance test (*OGTT*) results of both case and control

probably is due to the sparseness of observations with age larger than 50. $\widehat{J_L}(z)$ shows an attenuate trend of diagnostic accuracy on OGTT test as varied by age. On the other hand, comparing the estimated age-specific optimal cutoff point to the golden standard (value $=$ 126 mg/dl), the newly proposed method suggests that optimal threshold increases as age increases. This can be interpreted as, for general population, when age increases, the functionality of pancreas decays; therefore, the OGTT test result is expected to be higher since less insulin is secreted from the pancreas. The differences among the three proposed estimates are not obvious. However, we recommend the nonparametric covariate-adjusted estimates for the YI to this data set because it is more flexible and robust than the one with normal error assumption.

7.6 A Final Remark

In this chapter, we have proposed nonparametric covariate-adjusted estimates for the YI. The simulation study conducted here has demonstrated the robustness and

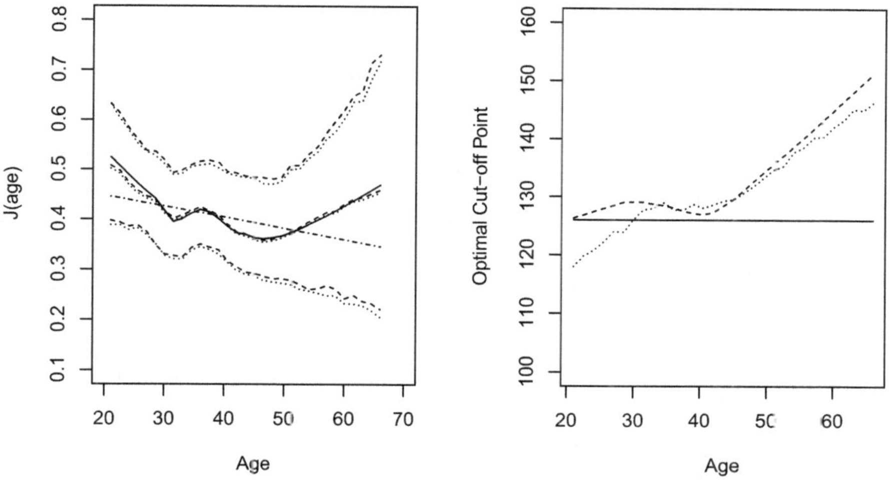

Fig. 7.8 Left panel: Estimates for $J(Age)$: $\widehat{J}_N$ (*solid*), $\widehat{J}_E$ (*dashed*), $\widehat{J}_{AC}$ (*dot*), and $\widehat{J}_L(z)$ (*dotdash*). Pointwise confidence bands for $J(Age)$: BP band (*dashed*), ACNA band (*dot*); right panel: estimate for optimal cutoff: Golden standard (*solid*), estimate under normality error (*dash*), and empirical estimate (*dot*)

effectiveness of the proposed method. Accordingly, we suggest applying the nonparametric approach in real applications. Although some asymptotic properties of the nonparametric covariate-adjusted estimator for the YI have been obtained, its asymptotic distribution is still an open question. While the discussion is limited to the case of the YI in this chapter, the proposed method will be extended to the partial AUC in the future. Global test of covariates effects on the YI is another interesting topic and has not been discussed in literature. Huang and Chen (2008) provided a unified framework for local polynomial regression-based analysis of variance. Their method can be applied to the nonparametric heteroscedastic models for testing global effects of covariates on test outcomes. We will study this topic in the future.

Appendix

Denote the neighborhood of z by $\mathcal{N}(z)$ for given $Z = z$. Following the same arguments in Yao et al. (2010) could lead to the Theorems presented in Sect. 7.3. Here, we first list assumptions applied in Theorems 1–4.

(A1) $\varphi(z)$ is the probability density function of Z. $\varphi(\cdot)$ is continuous in $\mathcal{N}(z)$ and $\varphi(z) > 0$.

(A2) $\nu_1(z) > 0$, $\mu_1^{(p+1)}(\cdot)$, $\nu_1^{(p+1)}(\cdot)$, $\zeta_1(\cdot)$, and $\pi_1(\cdot)$ are continuous in $\mathcal{N}(z)$.

(A3) $h_{\mu_1} \to 0$, $mh_{\mu_1} \to \infty$, $mh_{\mu_1}^{2p+3} \to d_1^2$ for some $d_1 > 0$, $h_{\nu_1}/h_{\mu_1} \to \rho_1$ for some $0 < \rho_1 < \infty$, as $m \to \infty$.

(A4) $\nu_2(z) > 0$, $\mu_2^{(p+1)}(\cdot)$, $\nu_2^{(p+1)}(\cdot)$, $\zeta_2(\cdot)$, and $\pi_2(\cdot)$ are continuous in $\mathcal{N}(z)$.

(A5) $h_{\mu 2} \to 0$, $nh_{\mu 2} \to \infty$, $nh_{\mu 2}^{2p+3} \to d_2^2$ for some $d_2 > 0$, $h_{\nu 2}/h_{\mu 2} \to \rho_2$ for some $0 < \rho_2 < \infty$, as $n \to \infty$.

(A6) $\mathcal{K}^*$ is uniform continuous, absolutely integrable with respect to Lebesgue measure on $\Re$ and of bounded variation, $\mathcal{K}^*(\mu) \to 0$ as $|\mu| \to \infty$, $\int \{|\mu log(|\mu|)|\}^{1/2}|d\mathcal{K}^*(\mu)| < \infty$.

(A7) $E(|X|^s) < \infty$, $\sup_{z \in \Re_Z} \int |x|^s P(Z,X)dy < \infty$ for some $s \geq 2$, where $P(Z,X)$ is the joint density of (Z,X).

(A8) $E(|Y|^s) < \infty$, $\sup_{z \in \Re_Z} \int |y|^s P(Z,Y)dy < \infty$ for some $s \geq 2$, where $P(Z,Y)$ is the joint density of (Z,Y).

The following assumptions are modifications of (A1–A5) which are used in the proof of Theorem 2:

(A1†) $\varphi(\cdot) > 0$ and $\varphi^{(p+1)}(\cdot)$ is bounded and continuous on $\Re_Z$.

(A2†) On the domain $\Re_Z$, $\nu_1(\cdot) > \gamma_1$ for some $\gamma_1 > 0$ and is bounded, $\mu_1(\cdot)$ is bounded, $\mu_1^{(p+1)}(\cdot)$, $\nu_1^{(p+1)}(\cdot)$, $\zeta_1(\cdot)$ and $\pi_1(\cdot)$ are bounded and continuous.

(A3†) $\Xi_m h_{\mu_1}^{\Delta_1} < \infty$ for some $\Delta_1 > 0$, $m^{2\rho_1 - 1}h_{\mu_1} \to \infty$ for some $\rho_1 < 1 - s^{-1}$, where $s > 2$ satisfies (A7).

(A4†) On the domain $\Re_Z$, $\nu_2(\cdot) > \gamma_2$ for some $\gamma_2 > 0$ and is bounded, $\mu_2(\cdot)$ is bounded, $\mu_2^{(p+1)(\cdot)}$, $\nu_2^{(p+1)(\cdot)}$, $\zeta_2(\cdot)$ and $\pi_2(\cdot)$ are bounded and continuous.

(A5†) $\Xi_n h_{\mu 2}^{\Delta_2} < \infty$ for some $\Delta_2 > 0$, $n^{2\rho_2 - 1}h_{\mu_2} \to \infty$ for some $\rho_2 < 1 - s^{-1}$, where $s > 2$ satisfies (A8).

(A^*3) $h_{\mu_1} \to 0$, $m^{\rho_1}h_{\mu_1} \to \infty$ for some $\rho_1 \leq 1 - s^{-1}$, where s satisfies (A7).

(A^*5) $h_{\mu_2} \to 0$, $n^{\rho_2}h_{\mu_2} \to \infty$ for some $\rho_2 \leq 1 - s^{-1}$, where s satisfies (A8).

(A9) $F^*(\cdot)$ and $G^*(\cdot)$ are continuous and monotone increasing on their domains.

Proof of Theorem 1. Theorem 1 directly follows from lemma 1 in Yao et al. (2010) and a simple application of the Cramér-Wald device. The partial derivatives of $J_N(z)$ with respect to the mean and variance functions in Theorem 1 are:

$$\begin{aligned}
\frac{\partial J_N(z)}{\partial \mu_1(z)} &= -\frac{1}{\sqrt{\nu_1(z)}}\phi\left(\frac{c_o(z) - \mu_1(z)}{\sqrt{\nu_1(z)}}\right) \\
&\quad + \frac{\partial c_o(z)}{\partial \mu_1(z)}\left[\frac{1}{\sqrt{\nu_1(z)}}\phi\left(\frac{c_o(z) - \mu_1(z)}{\sqrt{\nu_1(z)}}\right) - \frac{1}{\sqrt{\nu_2(z)}}\phi\left(\frac{\mu_2(z) - c_o(z)}{\sqrt{\nu_2(z)}}\right)\right] \\
\frac{\partial J_N(z)}{\partial \mu_2(z)} &= \frac{1}{\sqrt{\nu_2(z)}}\phi\left(\frac{\mu_2(z) - c_o(z)}{\sqrt{\nu_2(z)}}\right) \\
&\quad + \frac{\partial c_o(z)}{\partial \mu_2(z)}\left[\frac{1}{\sqrt{\nu_1(z)}}\phi\left(\frac{c_o(z) - \mu_1(z)}{\sqrt{\nu_1(z)}}\right) - \frac{1}{\sqrt{\nu_2(z)}}\phi\left(\frac{\mu_2(z) - c_o(z)}{\sqrt{\nu_2(z)}}\right)\right] \\
\frac{\partial J_N(z)}{\partial \nu_1(z)} &= -\frac{1}{2}(c_o(z) - \mu_1(z))\nu_1^{-3/2}\phi\left(\frac{c_o(z) - \mu_1(z)}{\sqrt{\nu_1(z)}}\right) \\
&\quad + \frac{\partial c_o(z)}{\partial \nu_1(z)}\left[\frac{1}{\sqrt{\nu_1(z)}}\phi\left(\frac{c_o(z) - \mu_1(z)}{\sqrt{\nu_1(z)}}\right) - \frac{1}{\sqrt{\nu_2(z)}}\phi\left(\frac{\mu_2(z) - c_o(z)}{\sqrt{\nu_2(z)}}\right)\right] \\
\frac{\partial J_N(z)}{\partial \nu_2(z)} &= -\frac{1}{2}(\mu_2(z) - c_o(z))\nu_2^{-3/2}\phi\left(\frac{\mu_2(z) - c_o(z)}{\sqrt{\nu_2(z)}}\right)
\end{aligned}$$

$$+\frac{\partial c_o(z)}{\partial \nu_2(z)}\left[\frac{1}{\sqrt{\nu_1(z)}}\phi\left(\frac{c_o(z)-\mu_1(z)}{\sqrt{\nu_1(z)}}\right)-\frac{1}{\sqrt{\nu_2(z)}}\phi\left(\frac{\mu_2(z)-c_o(z)}{\sqrt{\nu_2(z)}}\right)\right],$$

and the partial derivatives of $c_o(z)$ with respect to the mean and variance functions are

$$\frac{\partial c_o(z)}{\partial \mu_1(z)}=\frac{b^2 \pm ab(rad)^{-1/2}(-1)}{b^2-1}$$

$$\frac{\partial c_o(z)}{\partial \mu_2(z)}=\frac{-1 \pm ab(rad)^{-1/2}}{b^2-1}$$

$$\frac{\partial c_o(z)}{\partial \nu_1(z)}=-\frac{(\mu_2(z)-\mu_1(z))\nu_2(z)}{(\nu_2(z)-\nu_1(z))^2}\pm$$

$$\left[\frac{\frac{1}{2}\nu_2^{1/2}(z)\nu_1^{-1/2}(z)rad^{1/2}+\frac{1}{2}(\nu_1\nu_2)^{1/2}rad^{-1/2}\left(-ln\frac{\nu_2(z)}{\nu_1(z)}-\frac{\nu_2(z)}{\nu_1(z)}+1\right)(\nu_2(z)-\nu_1(z))}{(\nu_2(z)-\nu_1(z))^2}\right.$$

$$\left.+\frac{(\nu_1(z)\nu_2(z))rad^{1/2}}{(\nu_2(z)-\nu_1(z))^2}\right]$$

$$\frac{\partial c_o(z)}{\partial \nu_2(z)}=\frac{(\mu_2(z)-\mu_1(z))\nu_1(z)}{(\nu_2(z)-\nu_1(z))^2}\pm$$

$$\left[\frac{\frac{1}{2}\nu_1^{1/2}(z)\nu_2^{-1/2}(z)rad^{1/2}+\frac{1}{2}(\nu_1\nu_2)^{1/2}rad^{-1/2}\left(-ln\frac{\nu_2(z)}{\nu_1(z)}+(\nu_2(z)-\nu_1(z)\frac{1}{\nu_2(z)})\right)(\nu_2(z)-\nu_1(z))}{(\nu_2(z)-\nu_1(z))^2}\right.$$

$$\left.+\frac{(\nu_1(z)\nu_2(z))rad^{1/2}}{(\nu_2(z)-\nu_1(z))^2}\right],$$

where $rad=a^2+(b^2-1)\nu_1(z)ln(b^2)$, a and b are defined in Sect. 7.2.2. □

Proof of Theorem 2. Theorem 2 follows from Slusky's theorem and Lemma 2 in Yao et al. (2010).

Proof of Theorem 3. Let

$$J(c;z)=F(X\le c|Z=z)-G(Y\le c|Z=z)\equiv F(c;z)-G(c;z)$$

$$\widetilde{J}_E(c;z)=\widetilde{F}_m(c;z)-\widetilde{G}_n(c;z)$$

where $\widetilde{F}_m(c;z)=\frac{\sum_{i=1}^m I(x_{i,z}\le c)}{m}$, and $\widetilde{G}_n(c;z)=\frac{\sum_{j=1}^n I(y_{j,z}\le c)}{n}$.

By the law of the iterated logarithm (LIL) for empirical process, we have that $\sup_c|\widetilde{F}_m(c;z)-F(c;z)|=O(\sqrt{loglogm/2m})\ a.s.$, and $\sup_c|\widetilde{G}_n(c;z)-G(c;z)|=O(\sqrt{loglogn/2n})\ a.s.$. If $n/m\to\rho$, then

$$\sup_c|\widetilde{J}_E(c;z)-J(c;z)|\le\sup_c|\widetilde{F}_m(c;z)-F(c;z)|+\sup_c|\widetilde{G}_n(c;z)-G(c;z)|$$

$$=O\left(\sqrt{\log\log m/2m}+\sqrt{\log\log n/2n}\right),a.s.$$

which indicates the strong convergence of $\widetilde{J}_E(c;z)$ to $J(c;z)$ uniformly on c for a given z. Consequently, for a given z, $\widetilde{c}_{oE}(z)$ converges to $c_o(z)$ almost surely. Straightforwardly, applying the Lebesgue dominated convergence theorem, $E[\widetilde{J}_E(z)]$ converges to $J(z)$ for a given z. □

Proof of Theorem 4. Let

$$\widehat{J}_E(c;z) = \widehat{F}_m(c;z) - \widehat{G}_n(c;z),$$

where $\widehat{F}_m(c;z) = \frac{\sum_{i=1}^m I(\widehat{x}_{i,z} \leq c)}{m}$, and $\widehat{G}_n(c;z) = \frac{\sum_{j=1}^n I(\widehat{y}_{j,z} \leq c)}{n}$.

First of all we need to show the uniform consistency of $\widehat{J}(c;z)$ on c for a given z. From the strong uniform consistency of $\widehat{\mu}_i(z)$'s and $\widehat{\nu}_i(z)$'s, it follows that for a given z,

$$I(\widehat{x}_{i,z} \leq c) - I(x_{i,z} \leq c) \longrightarrow 0, \ a.s.$$
$$I(\widehat{y}_{i,z} \leq c) - I(y_{i,z} \leq c) \longrightarrow 0, \ a.s.$$

uniformly on c for all i. Therefore, for a given z,

$$\begin{aligned} |\widehat{J}_E(c;z) - \widetilde{J}_E(c;z)| \leq & \left| m^{-1} \sum_{i=1}^m \big(I(\widehat{x}_{i,z} \leq c) - I(x_{i,z} \leq c) \big) \right| \\ & + \left| m^{-1} \sum_{i=1}^m \big(I(\widehat{y}_{i,z} \leq c) - I(y_{i,z} \leq c) \big) \right| \\ & \longrightarrow 0, \ a.s. \end{aligned}$$

uniformly on c. Hence, for given $Z = z$,

$$\sup_c |\widehat{J}_E(c;z) - J(c;z)| \leq \sup_c |\widehat{J}_E(c;z) - \widetilde{J}_E(c;z)| + \sup_c |\widetilde{J}_E(c;z) - J(c;z)| \longrightarrow 0, a.s.$$

Consequently, for a given z, $\widehat{c}_{oE}(z)$ converges to $c_o(z)$ almost surely.

Now define $\widehat{\delta}_{i,z} = \widehat{x}_{i,z} - \widehat{c}_{oE}(z)$, $\delta_{i,z} = x_{i,z} - \widetilde{c}_{oE}(z)$, $\widehat{\omega}_{j,z} = \widehat{y}_{j,z} - \widehat{c}_{oE}(z)$, and $\omega_{j,z} = y_{j,z} - \widetilde{c}_{oE}(z)$. We have

$$\begin{aligned} E[\{\widehat{J}_E(z) - \widetilde{J}_E(z)\}^2] = & E\left[m^{-1} \sum_{i=1}^m \big(I(\widehat{\delta}_{i,z} \leq 0) - I(\delta_{i,z} \leq 0) \big) \right. \\ & \left. - n^{-1} \sum_{j=1}^n \big(I(\widehat{\omega}_{j,z} \leq 0) - I(\omega_{j,z} \leq 0) \big) \right]^2 \\ \leq & \, 2\left[E(T_1^2) + E(T_2^2) \right], \end{aligned}$$

where $T_1 = m^{-1} \sum_{i=1}^m \big(I(\widehat{\delta}_{i,z} \leq 0) - I(\delta_{i,z} \leq 0) \big)$, and $T_2 = n^{-1} \sum_{j=1}^n \big(I(\widehat{\omega}_{j,z} \leq 0) - I(\omega_{j,z} \leq 0) \big)$. Let us explore ET_1^2 first.

$$\begin{aligned} ET_1^2 = & \frac{1}{m^2} E\left[\sum_{i=1}^m \big(I(\widehat{\delta}_{i,z} \leq 0) - I(\delta_{i,z} \leq 0) \big)^2 \right. \\ & + \sum_{i \neq i'} \big(I(\widehat{\delta}_{i,z} \leq 0) I(\widehat{\delta}_{i',z} \leq 0) + I(\delta_{i,z} \leq 0) I(\delta_{i',z} \leq 0) \end{aligned}$$

$$-I(\widehat{\delta}_{i,z} \leq 0)I(\delta_{i',z} \leq 0) - I(\delta_{i,z} \leq 0)I(\widehat{\delta}_{i',z} \leq 0)\Big)\Big]$$

$$\leq \frac{1}{m} + \frac{1}{m^2}\sum_{i \neq i'}\Big[P(\widehat{\delta}_{i,z} \leq 0, \widehat{\delta}_{i',z} \leq 0) + P(\delta_{i,z} \leq 0, \delta_{i',z} \leq 0)$$

$$- P(\widehat{\delta}_{i,z} \leq 0, \delta_{i',z} \leq 0) - P(\delta_{i,z} \leq 0, \widehat{\delta}_{i',z} \leq 0)\Big]$$

By the strong uniform consistency of $\widehat{\mu}_i(z)$'s and $\widehat{\nu}_i(z)$'s and the strong consistency of $\widehat{c}_{oE}(z)$ and $\widetilde{c}_{oE}(z)$, we have that for a given z,

$$\widehat{\delta}_{i,z} \longrightarrow x_{i,z} - c_o(z)\ a.s., \quad \delta_{i,z} \longrightarrow x_{i,z} - c_o(z)\ a.s., \text{ for all } i.$$

So,

$$P(\widehat{\delta}_{i,z} \leq 0, \widehat{\delta}_{i',z} \leq 0) + P(\delta_{i,z} \leq 0, \delta_{i',z} \leq 0) - P(\widehat{\delta}_{i,z} \leq 0, \delta_{i',z} \leq 0) - P(\delta_{i,z} \leq 0, \widehat{\delta}_{i',z} \leq 0) \longrightarrow 0$$

for all $i \neq i'$. Therefore, $ET_1^2 \longrightarrow 0$ as $m \longrightarrow \infty$. Similarly, we can show $ET_2^2 \longrightarrow 0$ as $n \longrightarrow \infty$. Hence, $E\left[\widehat{J}_E(z) - \widetilde{J}_E(z)\right]^2 \longrightarrow 0$. □

References

Agresti A, Coull BA (1998) Approximate is better than 'exact' for interval estimation of binomial proportions. Am Stat 27:119–126

Aoki K, Misumi J, Kimura T, Zhao W, Xie T (1997) Evaluation of cutoff levels for screening of gastric cancer using serum pepsinogen and distributions of levels of serum pepsinogen I, II and of PG I/PG II ratios in a gastric cancer case-control study. J Epidemiol 7:143–151

Demir A, Yarali N, Fisgin T, Duru F, Kara A (2002) Most reliable indices in differentiation between thalassemia trait and iron deficiency anemia. Pediatr Int 44:612–616

Dodd L, Pepe MS (2003) Semiparametric regression for the area under the receiver operating characteristic curve. JASA 98:409–417

Fan J, Gijbels I (1996) Algorithms for computer algebra. Chapman & Hall, London

Faraggi D (2003) Adjusting receiver operating characteristic curves and related indices for covariates. J R Stat Soc Series D 52:179–192

Fluss R, Faraggi D, Reiser B (2005) Estimation of the Youden index and its associated cutoff point. Biom J 47:458–472

Grmec S, Gasparovic V (2001) Comparison of APACHE II, MEES and Glasgow Coma Scale in patients with nontraumatic coma for prediction of mortality. Crit Care 5:19–23

Huang L-S, Chen J (2008) Analysis of variance, coefficient of determination and F-test for local polynomial regression. Ann Statist 5:2025–2550

Kim K (2008) Maximization of the sum of sensitivity and specificity as a diagnostic cutpoint criterion. J Clin Epidemiol 61:517–518

Obuchowski NA (1995) Multireader, multimodality receiver operating characteristic curve studies: hypothesis testing and sample size estimation using an analysis of variance approach with dependent observations. Acad Radiol 1:S22–S29

Pepe MS (1997) A regression modeling framwork for reciever operating characteristics curves in medical diagnostic testing. Biometrika 84:595–608

Pepe MS (1998) Three approaches to regression analysis of reciever operating characteristic curves for continues test results. Biometrics 54:124–135

Pepe MS (2000) An interpretation for the ROC curve and inference using GLM procedures. Biometrika 56:352–359

Pepe MS (2003) The statistical evaluation of medical tests for classification and prediction. Oxford University Press, New York

Schisterman EF, Perkins N (2007) Confidence interval for Youden index and corresponding optimal cut-point. Commun Stat Simul Comput 36:549–563

Schisterman E, Reiser B, Fraaggi D (2006) ROC analysis for markers with mass at zero. Stat Med 23:623–638

Schisterman EF, Faraggi D, Reiser B, Hu J (2008) Youden index and the optimal threshold for markers with mass at zero. Stat Med 27:297–315

Smith PJ, Thompson TJ (1996) Correcting for confounding in analyzing receiver operating characteristic curves. Biom J 38:857–863

Smith JW, Everhart JE, Dickson WC, Knowler WC, Johannes RS (1988) Using the ADAP learning algorithm to forecast the onset of diabetes mellitus. Proc Annu Symp Comput Appl Med Care 9:261–265

Thomas EAC, Myers J (1972) Implications of latency data for threshold and nonthreshold models of signal detection. J Math Psychol 9:253–285

Thompson ML, Zucchini W (1989) On the statistical analysis of ROC curves. Stat Med 8:1277–1290

Toledano A, Gatsonis C (1995) Regression analysis of correlated reciever operating characteristic data. Acad Radiol 2:530–536

Tosteson ANA, Begg CB (1988) A general regression methodology for ROC curve estimation. Med Decis Mak 8:204–215

Yang B, Qin G (2012) Empirical likelihood-based inferences for the area under the ROC curve with covariates. SCI CHINA Math (Science in China Series A) 55:1553–1564

Yao F, Craiu RV, Reiser B (2010) Nonparametric covariate adjustment for receiver operating characteristic curves. Can J Stat 38:27–46

Youden WJ (1950) Index for rating diagnostic tests. Cancer 3:32–35

Zhou H, Qin G (2012) New non-parametric confidence intervals for the Youden index. J Biopharm Stat 22:1244–1257

Chapter 8
Comparative Effectiveness Research Using Meta-Analysis to Evaluate and Summarize Diagnostic Accuracy

Kelly H. Zou, Ching-Ray Yu, Steven A. Willke, Ye Tan and Martin O. Carlsson

Abstract According to the Agency for Healthcare Research and Quality, "comparative effectiveness research is designed to inform health-care decisions by providing evidence on the effectiveness, benefits, and harms of different treatment options. The evidence is generated from research studies that compare drugs, medical devices, tests, surgeries, or ways to deliver health care." Since it is difficult to systematically review each study to generate the best evidence and practice based on the overall diagnostic accuracy, it is useful to conduct a meta-analysis of such studies. Our main aim is to synthesize and to combine studies that yield proportions in a two-sample setting according to a reference standard. Statistical methods for combining sensitivities, specificities, and log diagnostic odds ratios are compared. A summary receiver operating characteristic curve is constructed. Monte Carlo simulation studies are conducted under both homogeneity and heterogeneity assumptions. For illustration purposes, a publically available example in urology is provided.

8.1 Introduction

The Agency for Healthcare Research and Quality (AHRQ) defines that comparative effectiveness research (CER) is "designed to inform health-care decisions by providing evidence on the effectiveness, benefits, and harms of different treatment options," and "the evidence is generated from research studies that compare drugs, medical devices, tests, surgeries, or ways to deliver health care" (see AHRQ 2014).

Meta-analysis is a quantitative method for combining the results of independent studies and for systematically synthesizing summaries and conclusions. The overall results may be used to evaluate therapeutic effectiveness and to plan for new studies. See, e.g., Zou et al. (2004) on the evidence-based medicine and meta-analysis, with a special focus on medical imaging and diagnostic trials. It is typical to use either

K. H. Zou (✉) · C.-R. Yu · Y. Tan · M. O. Carlsson
Pfizer Inc, 235 East 42nd Street Mail Stop: 235/9/1, New York, NY 10017, USA
Tel.: (212) - 733 - 0087
e-mail: Kelly.Zou@pfizer.com

S. A. Willke
The Ohio State University, 281 W. Lane Ave., Columbus, OH 43210, USA

Z. Chen et al. (eds.), *Applied Statistics in Biomedicine and Clinical Trials Design*,
ICSA Book Series in Statistics, DOI 10.1007/978-3-319-12694-4_8

a fixed or a random effects model to conduct a meta-analysis. Appropriate meta-analytic methods help display and visualize the summary measures across individual studies. Such analysis is a critical tool to assess complex information with or without heterogeneity across studies.

According to Cappelleri et al. (2010), in a well-conducted meta-analysis, the following steps are imperative: (1) formulate the study question and establish a protocol; (2) literature search and retrieval; (3) paper selection per protocol; (4) data extraction and quality assessment; (5) analysis and interpretation, weighted average, meta-regression, sensitivity, and subgroup analysis.

In this investigation, we aim to synthesize and to combine outcomes from diagnostic studies based on a reference standard (RS). We also evaluate meta-analytic methods to illustrate and to compare fixed and random effects methods for the following purposes: to display the sensitivities and specificities, to combine the diagnostic odds ratio (DOR) or the log of DOR (LDOR), along with confidence intervals (CI), and to generate a summary receiver operating characteristic (sROC) curve.

A number of seminal papers and textbooks on ROC analysis have been available in the literature (e.g., Metz et al. 1986; Alemayehu and Zou 2012; Swets and Pickett 1982; Zhou et al. 2002; Pepe 2003; Gönen 2007; Krzanowski and Hand 2009; Zou et al. 2011, etc.).

A general tutorial on meta-analysis was published by Normand (1999). In specific applications in combining diagnostic tests, several authors have developed methods and published in the statistical literature (e.g., Walter and Irwig 1988; Moses et al. 1993; Walter et al. 1999; Rutter and Gatsonis 2001; Miller et al. 2009; Dendukuri et al. 2012; Menten et al. 2013). A review article was by Jones and Athanasiou (2009).

This chapter is organized as follows. In Sect. 8.2, we provide notations and assumptions for synthesizing and combining accuracy measures and for generating the sROC curve. Section 8.3 presents a publically available example in urology. In Sect. 8.4, Monte Carlo simulation studies are conducted to compare the meta-analytic methods based on fixed effects versus random effects modeling. Finally, conclusions and discussions are presented in Sect. 8.5.

8.2 Notations, Assumptions, and Summary Measures

We introduce notations and assumptions for combining results from a set of published diagnostic studies. Graphical display, heterogeneity assessment, and meta-analytic methods using univariate and bivariate approaches are described.

Table 8.1 A 2 × 2 table of counts within study k

Binary D_k	Binary RS_k		Marginal count
	0 (Healthy)	1 (Diseased)	
0 (Negative)	TN_k	FN_k	$TN_k + FN_k$
1 (Positive)	FP_k	TP_k	$FP_k + TP_k$
Marginal count	$m_k = TN_k + FP_k$	$n_k = FN_k + TP_k$	$N_k = m_k + n_k$

RS reference standard, *D* diagnosis, *TN* true negative, *FN* false negative, *FP* false positive, *TP* true positive

8.2.1 Notations and Assumptions

A 2 × 2 table of diagnostic accuracy, as shown in Table 8.1, may be formed in each of the kth study ($k = 1, \ldots, K$), first by stratifying the diagnostic results according to the binary reference standard, RS_k (e.g., healthy vs. diseased).

The total sample size N_k (e.g., number of patients) based on binary RS_k and binary diagnosis (D_k) may be decomposed as true positives (TP_k), true negatives (TN_k), false positives (FP_k), and false negatives (FN_k).

8.2.2 Forest Plot and Heterogeneity Assessment

In a forest plot as found in Lewis and Clarke (2001), the results of K individual studies are displayed as squares centered on the point estimate of the result of each study. A horizontal line runs through the square to show each 95 % CI.

The I^2statistic measures the heterogeneity, with low, moderate, and high correspond to the benchmark values, $I^2 = 25$, 50, and 75 %, respectively. This measure is calculated as in Higgins et al. (2003) and is derived as a typical meta-analysis, such that $I^2 = 100\,\% \times (Q - df)/Q$, where Q is Cochran's heterogeneity statistic and df the degrees of freedom.

8.2.3 Univariate Modeling of Sensitivity, Specificity, or LDOR

Furthermore, there are two independent and mutually exclusive groups, stratified by the binary RS_k into x and y samples in a two-sample setting. Traditionally, the x sample represents the healthy subjects, while the y sample represents the diseased subjects.

Within the kth study, for the healthy sample of size m_k among subjects with $RS_k = 0$, the ith subject-level diagnosis ($D_{x,\,k}$) is generated by an independent and identical (*i.i.d.*) distribution, $F(\cdot)$:

$$X_{k,\,i} \sim i.i.d.F\,(x_k),\ i = 1, \ldots, m_k.$$

The specificity for the kth study is

$$Sp_k = TN_k/m_k.$$

Similarly and independently, for the diseased sample of size n_k among subjects whose $RS_k = 1$, the jth subject-level diagnosis ($D_{y,k}$) is generated by an *i.i.d.* distribution $G(\cdot)$:

$$Y_{k,j} \sim i.i.d.G\,(y_k),\, j = 1, \ldots, n_k.$$

The sensitivity for the kth study is

$$Se_k = TP_k/n_k.$$

For subjects pooled between both the x and y groups, the index for all of the observations is given by

$$l = 1,\, \ldots, N_k, where\ N_k = m_k + n_k.$$

Diagnostic reviews start with a set of individual studies presenting estimates of sensitivity and specificity. One intuitive approach is to do separate pooling of sensitivity and specificity using standard methods for proportions. However, sensitivity and specificity are often negatively correlated within studies.

The ratio of the odds of the test being positive if the subject has a disease against the odds of the test being positive if the subject does not have the disease is

$$DOR_k = (TP_k/FN_k)\,/\,(FP_k/TN_k).$$

After a log transformation, the LOR is as given by:

$$LDOR_k = ln\,(DOR_k) = ln\,(TP_k) - ln\,(FN_k) + ln\,(TN_k) - ln\,(FP_k).$$

The standard error (SE) of the estimated $LDOR_k$ is straightforward,

$$[1/\,(TP_k) + 1/\,(FN_k) + 1/\,(TN_k) + 1/\,(FP_k)]^{1/2},$$

along with the associated 95 % CIs constructed accordingly.

Univariate fitting may be conducted using the R function "mada" or "madauni" within the R package named "mada."

To synthesize across all $k = 1, \ldots, K$ studies, both the fixed effects Mantel–Haenszel (MH) found in Robins et al., (1986) and the random effects DerSimonian–Laird (DSL) methods were developed by the authors DerSimonian and Laird (1986).

The sROC curve plots (1–Sp_k, Se_k) across all possible thresholds. One way of constructing an sROC is by assuming that overall $Se = (1\text{-}Sp)^{\theta}$, where θ is an accuracy parameter within a Lehman family for fitting (see, e.g., Holling et al., 2012).

8.2.4 Bivariate Joint Modeling of Sensitivity and Specificity

Although it appears to be intuitive and straightforward to analyze sensitivity and specificity separately, it is more appropriate to assume that sensitivity and specificity values are negatively correlated due to the different thresholds (i.e., cutoff points) used across different studies.

A possible cause for this negative correlation between sensitivity and specificity is that studies may have used different thresholds to define positive and negative test results. In some cases, this may have been done explicitly due to studies using different cutoff points to classify a continuous biochemical measurement as either positive or negative. In other situations, there may have been implicit variations in thresholds between studies due to differences in observers, laboratories, or equipment. Unlike other sources of variation, a difference in threshold leads to a particular pattern between sensitivity and specificity.

Therefore, it is more appropriate to employ bivariate joint modeling of sensitivity and specificity. See recent developments by Reitsma et al. (2005), which, according to Harbord et al. (2007), is equivalent to the hierarchical sROC (HSROC) analysis proposed by Rutter and Gatsonis (2001).

For model fitting in SAS, see Macaskill (2004) and Reitsma et al. (2005). For model fitting in *R*, a linear mixed model with known variances is available under the "reitsma" function within the R package "mada." Variance components may be estimated using fixed, restricted maximum likelihood (REML, as the default) or maximum likelihood (ML) methods.

Furthermore, meta-regression based on other transformation methods beyond logit may be conducted, as in Doebler et al. (2012). Additional relevant publications are by Arends et al. (2008), Trikalinos et al. (2012), Dehabreh et al. (2012), Trikalinos et al. (2013), and Leeflang et al. (2013). The sROC curves may be formed based on the above bivariate or multivariate models, accordingly.

8.3 An Illustrative Example in Urology

We illustrate our methods on a publically available example on computed tomography (CT) scans of urolithiasis, published by Niemann et al. (2008). Prospective and retrospective studies from 1995 to 2007 are based on comprehensive literature searches via PubMed, Medline, and Cochrane Library.

Low-dose CT scan (with < 3 mSv dose applied for the entire CT examination) is the diagnostic test for the detection of urolithiasis, i.e., a stone located in the ureter. There are a total of $K=7$ studies, and each study provides the counts of urolithiasis from low-dose CT to determine urolithiasis. See Table 8.2 for extracted study-level data from these studies.

The R packages "rmeta" developed by Lumley (2012) and "mada" developed by Doebler (2013) are used to conduct all analyses described below and to generate tables and figures.

Table 8.2 Classifications in each of the seven studies on low-dose CT to detect urolithiasis

Study (k)	#Healthy (m_k)	TN_k	FP_k	#Diseased (n_k)	TP_k	FN_k	Sp_k	Se_k	DOR_k	$LDOR_k$
1	23	22	1	37	36	1	0.957	0.973	792.000	6.675
2	29	28	1	80	77	3	0.966	0.962	718.667	6.577
3	62	61	1	147	142	5	0.984	0.966	1732.400	7.457
4	14	12	2	102	96	6	0.857	0.941	96.000	4.564
5	40	38	2	102	99	3	0.950	0.971	627.000	6.441
6	24	23	1	101	98	3	0.958	0.970	751.333	6.622
7	142	133	9	158	154	4	0.937	0.975	568.944	6.344

TN true negative, *FP* false positive, *TP* true positive, *FN* false Negative, *Sp* specificity, *Se* sensitivity, *DOR* diagnostic odds ratio, *LDOR* log diagnostic odds ratio, *CT* computed tomography

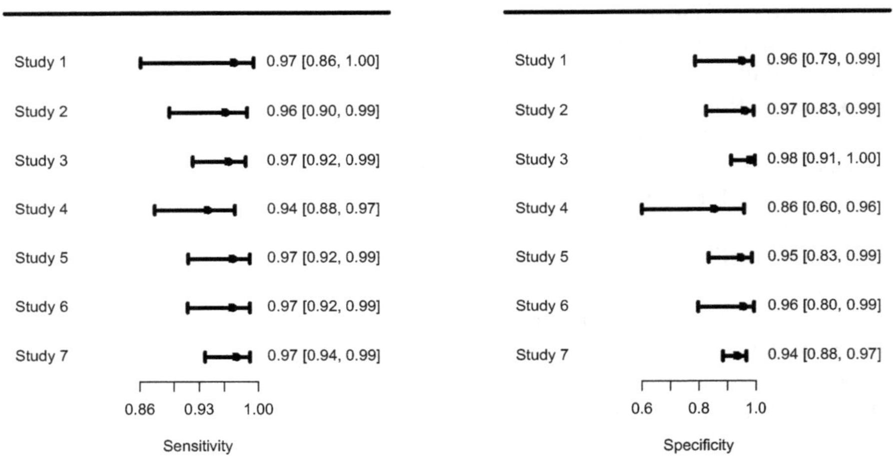

Fig. 8.1 A forest plot of the specificity and sensitivity measures

The estimated correlation of sensitivities and false positive rates is -0.778, with a 95 % CI of (-0.965, -0.061). Because of such a wide CI, both univariate and bivariate analyses are conducted for the purpose of comparisons.

The heterogeneity across studies is assessed, and the corresponding $I^2 \approx 0$, which is low across all studies. In Figs. 8.1 and 8.2, the forest plots of Sp_k, Se_k, and $LDOR_k$ are displayed. Table 8.3 compares results based on the fixed effects (MH) and random effects (DSL) models.

Figure 8.3 demonstrates the sROC curve, where the full area under the curve (AUC) under the sROC curve is 0.991. In comparison, by using bivariate modeling (see Reitsma, 2005), which is equivalent to the HSROC approach (see Rutter and Gatsonis, 2001), the estimated AUCs under the sROC curves are 0.922 via REML and 0.932 via ML estimation methods.

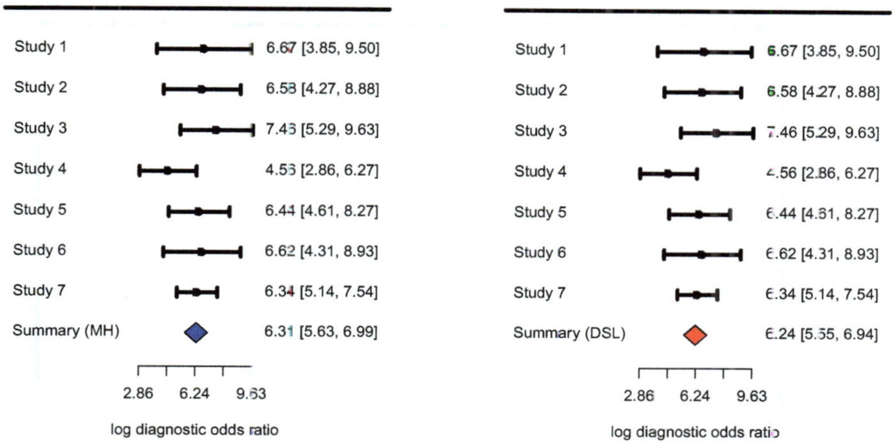

Fig. 8.2 Forest plot of log diagnostic odds ratios via the fixed effects and random effects models using two methods. The combination methods used are as follows: panel 2a (left), fixed effects (MH = Mantel–Haenszel); panel 2b (right), random effects (*DSL* = DerSimonian–Laird)

Table 8.3 Combined results based on seven studies on low-dose CT to detect urolithiasis by the fixed effects and random effects models

Meta-analytic method	Combined *LDOR*	95 % CI of the LDOR
Fixed effects (MH)	6.312	(5.629, 6.995)
Random effects (DSL)	6.244	(5.545, 6.942)

LDOR log diagnostic odds ratio, *CI* confidence interval, *MH* Mantel–Haenszel, *DSL* DerSimonian–Laird, *CT* computed tomography

8.4 Monte Carlo Simulations

In each setting, we assume either homogeneity or heterogeneity across $K = 10$ studies. The true accuracy is predetermined to compare fixed (MH) and random (DSL) effects methods. Variations in terms of the underlying sensitivity and specificity are considered using realistic and extreme scenarios.

We generate $k = 1, \ldots, K$ ($K = 10$) sets of study-level data with either small or large sample sizes, $m_k = n_k = \{25, 50\}$, with a total sample size of $N_k = \{50, 100\}$. To investigate the performances, either homogeneity or heterogeneity is assumed across all studies.

For simplicity, specificity and sensitivity have independent binomial distributions, where

$$X_k \sim Binomial(m_k, Sp_k),$$

with $Sp_k = \{0.5, 0.7, 0.9\}$ for the health subjects, and

$$Y_k \sim Binomial(m_k, Se_k),$$

with $Se_k = \{0.5, 0.7, 0.9\}$ for the diseased subjects.

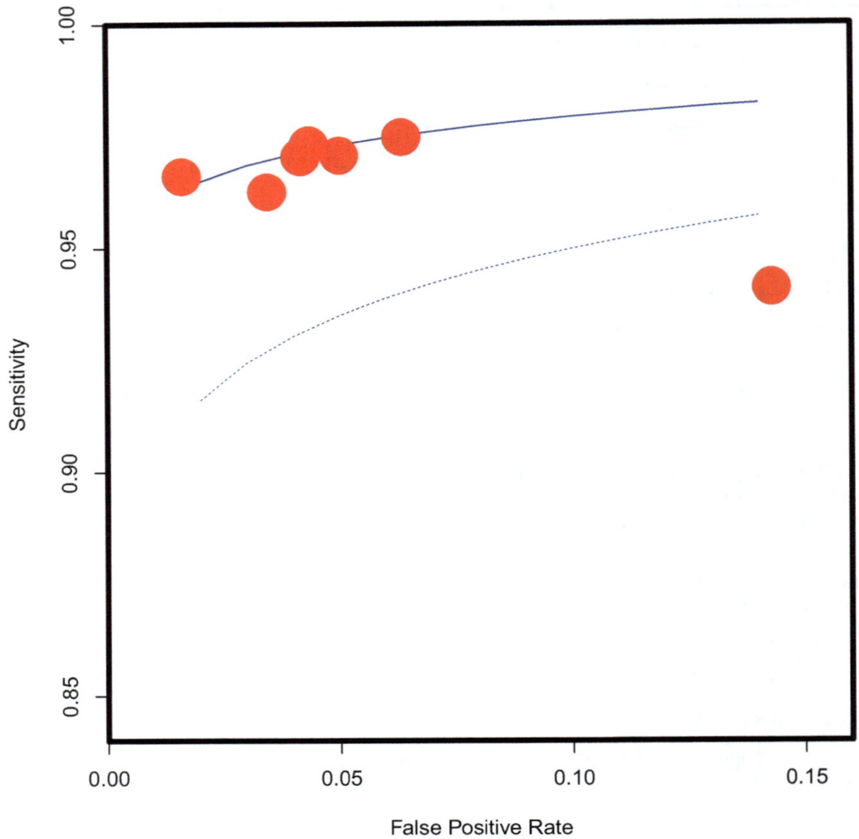

Fig. 8.3 The summary of ROC curve in a restricted ROC space. ROC receiver operating characteristic

With $MC = 10{,}000$ replicates for each scenario, Tables 8.4 and 8.5 show the mean bias, mean squared errors (MSE), and coverage probability (with 95 % as the nominal level) for small and large study sample sizes, respectively.

We have found that the random effects model tends to yield higher coverage with comparable MSE. Nevertheless, the choice of method may depend on heterogeneity across all studies and the correlation between sensitivities and specificities due to the different thresholds used across studies.

8.5 Conclusions and Discussions

According to principles of evidence-based medicine in Sackett et al. (1996), we must strive to achieve "the conscientious, explicit, and judicious use of current best evidence in making decisions about the care of individual patients." The CER must be applied appropriately and correctly. For example, as Normand (1999) has

Table 8.4 Monte Carlo simulation results for $k = 1, \ldots, K = 10$ studies with 10,000 replicates at the 95 % nominal coverage level when sample sizes are small, $N_k = m_k + n_k = 25 + 25 = 50$

Study variability	Underlying accuracy			Fixed effects (MH) method[a]			Random effects (DSL) method[a]			
	Sp_k	Se_k	$LDOR_k$	Mean bias	MSE	Coverage probability (%)	Mean I^2 (%)	Mean bias	MSE	Coverage probability (%)
Homogeneity across all studies $\forall k = 1, \ldots, 10$	0.5	0.5	0	0.0006	0.032	91.1	0	0.0006	0.033	96.3
	0.5	0.7	0.8473	−0.0048	0.036	92.0	0	−0.0047	0.036	96.4
	0.5	0.9	2.1972	0.1683	0.086	87.5	0	0.1366	0.066	94.3
	0.7	0.7	1.6946	−0.0102	0.038	93.2	0	−0.0159	0.038	96.6
	0.7	0.9	3.0445	0.1841	0.102	86.5	0	0.1281	0.070	94.4
	0.9	0.9	4.3944	0.4240	0.273	71.2	0	0.2464	0.131	89.9
Heterogeneity with partial Homogeneity $k = 1, \ldots, 5$ and $k = 6, \ldots, 10$	0.5 0.7	0.5 0.7	0 1.6946	0.1621	0.057	80.3	49.0	0.1600	0.057	89.4
	0.7 0.9	0.7 0.9	1.6946 4.3944	0.2337	0.101	77.3	76.3	0.2288	0.097	84.8

Sp specificity, *Se* sensitivity, *LDOR* log diagnostic odds ratio, *MH* Mantel–Haenszel, *DSL* DerSimonian–Laird
[a]LDOR as the outcome of interest

Table 8.5 Monte Carlo simulation results for $k = 1, \ldots, K = 10$ studies with 10,000 replicates at the 95 % nominal coverage level when sample sizes are large, $N_k = m_k + n_k = 50 + 50 = 100$

Study variability	Underlying accuracy			Fixed effects (MH) method[a]			Random effects (DSL) method[a]			
	Sp_k	Se_k	$LDOR_k$	Mean bias	MSE	Coverage probability (%)	Mean I^2 (%)	Mean bias	MSE	Coverage probability (%)
Homogeneity across all studies $\forall k = 1, \ldots, 10$	0.5	0.5	0	0.0009	0.016	91.4	0	0.0009	0.016	96.4
	0.5	0.7	0.8473	−0.0031	0.018	92.2	0	−0.0043	0.018	96.1
	0.5	0.9	2.1972	−0.0002	0.031	93.8	0	0.0265	0.290	96.6
	0.7	0.7	1.6946	−0.0063	0.019	93.4	0	−0.0113	0.019	96.7
	0.7	0.9	3.0445	−0.0020	0.033	94.0	0	0.0104	0.031	96.9
	0.9	0.9	4.3944	0.0106	0.050	93.8	0	−0.0056	0.045	96.9
Heterogeneity with partial homogeneity $k = 1, \ldots, 5$ and $k = 6, \ldots, 10$	0.5 0.7	0.5 0.7	0 1.6946	−0.0030	0.016	92.6	24.8	−0.0048	0.016	96.4
	0.7 0.9	0.7 0.9	1.6946 4.3944	−0.0100	0.024	94.7	58.8	−0.0154	0.024	97.1

Sp specificity, *Se* sensitivity, *LDOR* log diagnostic odds ratio, *MH* Mantel–Haenszel, *DSL* DerSimonian–Laird
[a]LDOR as the outcome of interest

suggested, systematically combining complex information across individual studies, the overall results have greater power than that of an analysis conducted study by study. If several studies have conflicting conclusions, a meta-analysis can better identify those associated with an overall effect (e.g., an accurate diagnosis for a beneficial treatment).

In this research, we have compared the synthesis methods to display and combine individual diagnostic accuracy (e.g., *Sp* and *Se*), *LDOR*, and to use both univariate and bivariate approach to model sensitivity and specificity, as well as to generate a single sROC curve. We have illustrated these methods on an example in urology. We have also compared the performances of the fixed and the random effects models by Monte Carlo simulations. We have only shed some light on the performances of fixed effects versus random effects models, as well as the impact of underlying parameters and sample sizes.

Further research is needed to examine issues arising from the prevalence of the disease, systematic publication biases, and various combinations of *Sp* and *Se* values. For example, since sensitivity and specificity measures tend to be negatively correlated, a bivariate approach should be considered, rather than a marginal univariate analysis.

It is worth emphasizing that several other best practices such as using a checklist under the Standards for Reporting of Diagnostic Accuracy Studies (2008), in short, "STARD" and in Bossuyt et al. (2003), towards complete and accurate reporting of studies of diagnostic accuracy may be conscientiously applied when conducting a meta-analysis of diagnostic studies. A quality assessment tool for diagnostic accuracy studies (QUADAS), by Whiting et al. (2003; 2004; 2011) and the University of Bristol (2014), may also be utilized.

Acknowledgments This chapter is dedicated to and in memory of Professor Charles E. Metz of the University of Chicago, Professor Harry S. Wieand of the University of Pittsburgh, Professor Donald D. Dorfman of the University of Iowa, Dr. Robert F. Wagner of the Food and Drug Administration, and Professor W. J. Hall of the University of Rochester, who have made substantial contributions to the field of receiver operating characteristic analysis.

The views in this chapter may not necessarily reflect those of Pfizer Inc. where four authors (K.H.Z.; C.-R.Y; Y.T; M.O.C.) are employed or the Ohio State University where the remaining author (S.A.W.) is enrolled. The authors are grateful for the constructive comments from a number of colleagues. No editorial support was provided.

References

Agency for Healthcare Research and Quality (2014) What is comparative effectiveness research. http://effectivehealthcare.ahrq.gov/index.cfm/what-is-comparative-effectiveness-research1. Accessed 15 January 2014

Alemayehu D, Zou KH (2012) Applications of ROC analysis in medical research: recent developments and future directions. Acad Radiol 19:1457–1464

Arends LR, Hamza TH, van Houwelingen JC, Heijenbrok-Kal MH, Hunink MG, Stijnen T (2008) Bivariate random effects meta-analysis of ROC curves. Med Decis Making 28:621–638

Bossuyt PM, Reitsma JB, Bruns DE et al (2003) Towards complete and accurate reporting of studies of diagnostic accuracy: the STARD initiative. BMJ 326:41–44

Cappelleri JC, Ioannidis JPA, Lau J (2010) Meta-analysis of therapeutic trials. In: Chow S-C (ed) Encyclopedia of biopharmaceutical statistics, 3rd edn. Informa Health Care/CRC, London, pp 768–779

Dendukuri N, Schiller I, Joseph L et al (2012) Bayesian meta-analysis of the accuracy of a test for tuberculous pleuritis in the absence of a gold standard reference. Biometrics 68:1285–1293

DerSimonian R, Laird N (1986) Meta-analysis in clinical trials. Control Clin Trials 7:177–188

Doebler P (2013) Meta-analysis of diagnostic accuracy (mada). http://cran.r-project.org/web/packages/mada/mada.pdf. Accessed 15 January, 2014

Gönen M (2007) Analyzing receiver operating characteristic curves with SAS®. SAS Institute Inc: Cary

Harbord RM, Deeks JJ, Egger M, Whiting P, Sterne JA (2007) A unification of models for meta-analysis of diagnostic accuracy studies. Erratum Biostat. 2008;9:779

Higgins JP, Thompson SG, Deeks JJ et al (2003) Measuring inconsistency in meta-analyses. BMJ 327:557–560

Holling H, Böhning W, Böhning D (2012) Meta-analysis of diagnostic studies based upon SROC-curves: a mixed mode approach using the Lehmann family. Statistical Modelling 12:347–375

Jones CM, Athanasiou T (2009) Diagnostic accuracy meta-analysis: review of an important tool in radiological research and decision making. Br J Radiol 82:441–446

Krzanowski WJ, Hand DJ (2009) ROC curves for continuous data. Chapman & Hall/CRC, Boca Raton

Leeflang MM, Deeks JJ, Takwoingi Y, Macaskill P (2013) Cochrane diagnostic test accuracy reviews. Syst Rev 2:82

Lewis S, Clarke M (2001) Forest plots: trying to see the wood and the trees. BMJ 322:1479–1480

Lumley T (2012) Meta-analysis (rmeta). http://cran.r-project.org/web/packages/rmeta/rmeta.pdf. Accessed 15 January, 2014

Macaskill P (2004) Empirical Bayes estimates generated in a hierarchical summary ROC analysis agreed closely with those of a full Bayesian analysis. J Clin Epidemiol 57:925–932

Menten J, Boelaert M, Lesaffre E (2013) Bayesian meta-analysis of diagnostic tests allowing for imperfect reference standards. Stat Med 32:5398–5413

Metz CE (1986) ROC methodology in radiologic imaging. Invest Radiol 21:720–733

Miller SW, Sinha D, Slate EH et al (2009) Bayesian adaptation of the summary ROC curve method for meta-analysis of diagnostic test performance. J Data Sci 7:349–364

Moses LE, Shapiro D, Littenberg B (1993) Combining independent studies of a diagnostic test into a summary ROC curve: data-analytic approaches and some additional considerations. Stat Med 12:1293–1316

Niemann T, Kollmann T, Bongartz G (2008) Diagnostic performance of low-dose CT for the detection of urolithiasis: a meta-analysis. AJR Am J Roentgenol 191:396–401

Normand S (1999) Meta-analysis: formulating, evaluating, combining, and reporting. Stat Med 18:321–359

Pepe MS (2003) The statistical evaluation of medical tests for classification and prediction. Oxford University, Oxford

Reitsma JB, Glas AS, Rutjes AW, Scholten RJ, Bossuyt PM, Zwinderman AH (2005) Bivariate analysis of sensitivity and specificity produces informative summary measures in diagnostic reviews. J Clin Epidemiol 58:982–990

Robins J, Greenland S, Breslow NE (1986) A general estimator for the variance of the Mantel-Haenszel odds ratio. Am J Epidemiol 124:719–723

Rutter CM, Gatsonis CA (2001) A hierarchical regression approach to meta-analysis of diagnostic test accuracy evaluations. Stat Med 20:2865–2884

Sackett DL, Rosenberg WM, Gray JA et al (1996) Evidence based medicine: what it is and what it isn't. BMJ 312:71–72

Standards for the Reporting of Diagnostic Accuracy Studies (2008) STARD checklist. http://www.stard-statement.org. Accessed 15 January, 2014

Swets JA, Pickett RM (1982) Evaluation of diagnostic systems: methods from signal detection theory. Academic, New York

Trikalinos TA, Kulasingam S, Lawrence WF (2012) Chapter 10: deciding whether to complement a systematic review of medical tests with decision modeling. J Gen Intern Med 27(Suppl 1):S76–S82

Trikalinos TA, Hoaglin DC, Schmid CH (2013) Empirical and simulation-based comparison of univariate and multivariate meta-analysis for binary outcomes. Rockville, MD: Agency for Healthcare Research and Quality, US

University of Bristol (2014). A quality assessment tool for diagnostic accuracy studies. http://www.bris.ac.uk/quadas. Accessed 15 January, 2014

Walter SD, Irwig LM (1988) Estimation of test error rates, disease prevalence and relative risk from misclassified data: a review. J Clin Epidemiol 41:923–937

Walter SD, Irwig L, Glasziou PP (1999) Meta-analysis of diagnostic tests with imperfect reference standards. J Clin Epidemiol 52:943–951

Whiting P, Rutjes AW, Reitsma JB et al (2003) The development of QUADAS: a tool for the quality assessment of studies of diagnostic accuracy included in systematic reviews. BMC Med Res Methodol 3:25

Whiting P, Rutjes AW, Dinnes J et al. (2004) Development and validation of methods for assessing the quality of diagnostic accuracy studies. Health Technol Assess 8:iii, 1–234

Whiting PF, Rutjes AW, Westwood ME et al (2011) QUADAS-2: a revised tool for the quality assessment of diagnostic accuracy studies. Ann Intern Med 155:529–536

Zhou XH, Obuchowski NA, McClish DK (2002) Statistical methods in diagnostic medicine. Wiley, New York

Zou KH, Fielding JR, Ondategui-Parra S (2004) What is evidence-based medicine? Acad Radiol 11:127–133

Zou KH, Liu A, Bandos AI et al (2011) Statistical evaluation of diagnostic performance: topics in ROC Analysis. Chapman & Hall/CRC, Boca Raton

Part III
Innovative Clinical Trial Designs and Analysis

Chapter 9
Some Characteristics of the Varying-Stage Adaptive Phase II/III Clinical Trial Design

Gaohong Dong

Abstract Conventionally, adaptive phase II/III clinical trials are carried out with a strict two-stage design. Dong (Stat Med 33(8):1272–1287) recently proposed a varying-stage adaptive phase II/III clinical trial design, in which the number of further investigational stages is determined based upon data accumulated to the interim analysis. In this design, following the first stage, an intermediate stage can be adaptively added to obtain more data, so that a more informative decision could be made. This design considers two plausible study endpoints with one of them initially designated as the primary endpoint. Based on the interim results, another endpoint can be switched as the primary endpoint. Dong (Stat Med 33(8):1272–1287) has showed relations of design parameters (e.g., thresholds and percent of alpha allocated in the two-stage setting) as well as the trial design properties under the alternative hypotheses for both plausible endpoints. Here, we explore characteristics of the design when the alternative hypothesis for only one of the two endpoints is true, and the treatment effect for another endpoint is null (an extremely worst case) or lower than what was anticipated per trial design. The simulations show that the statistical power of the varying-stage adaptive phase II/III clinical trial design (Dong, Stat Med 33(8):1272–1287) is less sensitive to a low realized treatment effect.

9.1 Introduction

Different from conventional separate phase II and phase III clinical trials, a seamless phase II/III trial design addresses study objectives of phase II and phase III within a single trial. This uninterrupted adaptive design has advantages of combining conventional phase II and phase III operationally and inferentially into a single study (e.g., Bretz et al. 2006; Gallo et al. 2006; Jennison and Turnbull 2006), particularly to (1) accelerate drug development process by reducing "white space" between the two clinical trial phases, (2) gain statistical efficiency by using first-stage data on the patients treated with the new therapy with the dose selected for the second stage, thus

G. Dong (✉)
Biometrics & Statistical Sciences, Novartis Pharmaceuticals Corporation,
One Health Plaza, East Hanover, NJ 07936, USA
e-mail: gaohong.dong@novartis.com

Z. Chen et al. (eds.), *Applied Statistics in Biomedicine and Clinical Trials Design*,
ICSA Book Series in Statistics, DOI 10.1007/978-3-319-12694-4_9

reduce the sample size needed for the second stage, and (3) get long-term safety data earlier since the patients in stage I are followed longer as compared to conventional phase II study. Adaptive phase II/III clinical trial designs have been extensively studied (e.g., Bauer and Köhne 1994; Cui et al. 1999; Müller and Schäfer 2001; Todd and Stallard 2005; Bischoff and Miller 2009; Bretz et al. 2009). More recently, in 2010, the US Food and Drug Administration (FDA) released the draft guidance of adaptive design clinical trials for drugs and biologics (FDA 2010).

Frequently, there are situations in which researchers are in dilemma to make "go or no-go" decision and/or to select "best" dose arm(s), since interim data from the first stage may not provide sufficient data for their decision making. In this case, it is challenging to follow a strict two-stage plan. Therefore, we proposed a varying-stage adaptive phase II/III clinical trial design, in which we consider whether there is a need to have an intermediate stage to obtain more data, so that a more informative decision could be made regarding whether the trial can be advanced to the final confirmatory stage (Dong 2014). In our proposed design, two study endpoints are considered plausible. The endpoint 1 is initially designated as the primary study endpoint. The endpoint 2 can be switched as the primary study endpoint if the endpoint 1 does not seem sensitive to show treatment effect, whereas the endpoint 2 appears a better measure of clinical benefit for the study.

Dong (2014) has showed relations of design parameters (e.g., thresholds and percent of alpha allocated in the two-stage setting) as well as the trial design properties under the alternative hypotheses for both plausible endpoints. Here, we explore characteristics of the design when the alternative hypothesis for only one of the two endpoints is true, and the treatment effect for another endpoint is null or low compared to what was anticipated per the trial design. In Sect. 2, we briefly introduce the varying-stage adaptive phase II/III clinical trial design as presented in Dong (2014), then show some characteristics of this design in Sect. 3. In Sect. 4, we summarize the findings of this chapter and discuss some future research with the varying-stage adaptive phase II/III clinical trial design.

9.2 Varying-Stage Adaptive Phase II/III Clinical Trial Design

Consider a clinical trial that is initially planned with two study endpoints, up to three stages, K dose arms of the study treatment and one control arm. Let $D = \{1, 2, \ldots, K\}$ be the full index set of dose arms of the study treatment, and θ_{ik} be the parameter of interest with respect to the ith endpoint for the kth dose arm ($k = 0$ for the control arm). The elementary null hypothesis for the comparison between the kth dose arm of the study treatment and the control arm is:

$$\mathrm{H}_{0ik} : \theta_{ik} = \theta_{i0}, \text{vs } \mathrm{H}_{1ik} : \theta_{ik} > \theta_{i0}, \text{ where, } i = 1, 2 \text{ for endpoint; } k \in D \quad (9.1)$$

The global null hypothesis with respect to the ith endpoint is

$$H_{0i} : \bigcap_{k \in D} H_{0ik} = H_{0i1} \bigcap H_{0i2} \bigcap \cdots \bigcap H_{0iK}, \text{ where } i = 1,2 \text{ for endpoint} \quad (9.2)$$

Let p_{ijk} be the p-value of the elementary null hypothesis (H_{0ik}) testing for the difference between the kth dose arm ($k \in D$) and the control arm with respect to the ith endpoint ($i = 1, 2$) at the jth stage ($j = 1, 2, 3$), and p_{ij} be the p-value of the global null hypothesis (H_{0i}) testing at the jth stage with respect to the ith endpoint. The p-values p_{ijk} and p_{ij} are based on the data from the jth stage only. Let $\alpha_i^{(j)}$ be the prespecified threshold parameter for the ith endpoint at the jth stage.

9.2.1 Initial Learning Stage (Phase II)

Figure 9.1 shows the flow chart of the varying-stage adaptive phase II/III clinical trial design. The initial stage is considered as a learning stage (phase II). Following this stage, the first interim analysis is performed. As shown in Fig. 9.1a, if $p_{11} < \alpha_1^{(1)}$, the endpoint 1 is kept as the primary study endpoint as initially planned. Following this, inefficacious/harmful dose arm(s) will be dropped and sample size adjustment for the final stage will be performed (path A_1). If $p_{11} \geq \alpha_1^{(1)}$ and $p_{21} < \alpha_2^{(1)}$, then the endpoint 2 will be chosen as the primary study endpoint. With respect to the new primary study endpoint (endpoint 2), inefficacious/harmful dose arm(s) will be dropped, and sample size adjustment will be performed for the next stage (path A_2). Otherwise, the primary endpoint cannot be decided based on the current interim data. Therefore, two further study stages need to be planned: one is intermediate stage; another one is confirmatory stage (path A_3). The intermediate stage is considered as an extension of phase II, from which more data will be obtained, so that more informative decisions can be made.

9.2.2 Intermediate Stage (Extended Phase II)

The second interim analysis is conducted following the intermediate stage. For this interim analysis, a combination test is performed to incorporate data obtained from the initial stage and the intermediate stage. The combined p-values are based on a combination function $C(p_{i1}, p_{i2})$, where p_{i1} and p_{i2} are p-values from the two disjoint stages—initial stage and intermediate stage, respectively, for the ith endpoint ($i = 1, 2$). We use Fisher's product combination method (Fisher 1932; Bauer and Köhne 1994) to combine p-values. Hence $C(p_{i1}, p_{i2}) = p_{i1} p_{i2}$. One should note that Fisher's p-value combination method requires the independence of the two p-values. As the two disjoint stages comprise two separate cohorts of patients (or two independent samples in another word), the p-values p_{i1} and p_{i2} are independent and fulfill the independence requirement of Fisher's p-value combination method.

Corresponding to the combined overall p-value $C(p_{11}, p_{12}) < \alpha_1^{(2)}$, or $C(p_{11}, p_{12}) \geq \alpha_1^{(2)}$ and $C(p_{21}, p_{22}) < \alpha_2^{(2)}$, similar design flows (path B_1 and path B_2, respectively) to the first interim analysis can be followed to switch primary

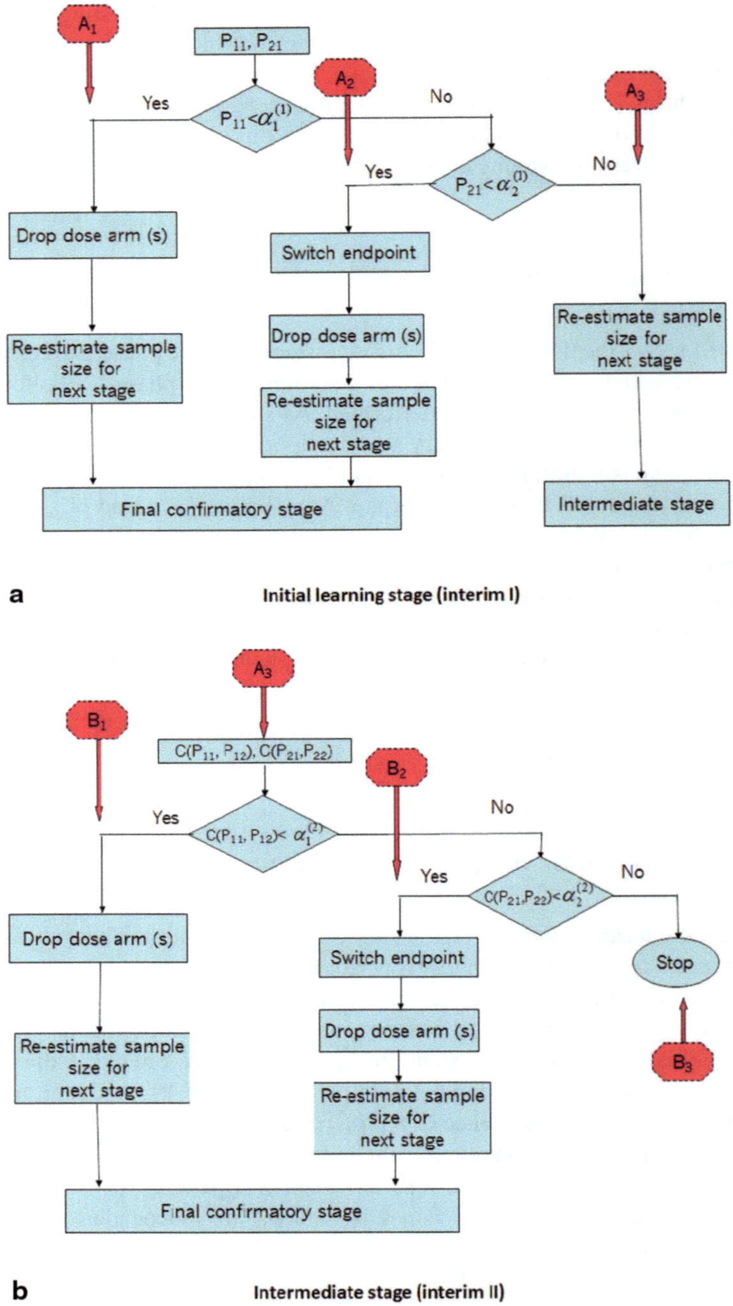

Fig. 9.1 Flow chart of the varying-stage adaptive phase II/III clinical trial design

study endpoint, drop inefficacious/harmful dose arm(s), and perform sample adjustment for the final confirmatory stage. Otherwise, the trial will be stopped for futility (path B_3).

9.2.3 Final Confirmatory Stage (Phase III)

The final stage is considered as a confirmatory phase III stage. Following the completion of the final stage, the final analysis will be performed. Similar to the second interim analysis, the final analysis incorporates data from previous stage(s) via a combination test. The statistical significance will be demonstrated by comparing the combined p-value against a critical value with respect to the primary study endpoint.

The parameters $\alpha_1^{(1)}$ and λ play important roles in the varying-stage adaptive phase II/III clinical trial design. These parameters can be determined based on the feasibility of sample size, statistical power, and anticipated alpha allocation. The parameter λ mainly impacts alpha allocation and thus the expected sample size. The threshold probability $\alpha_1^{(1)}$ mainly contributes to the chance to have a trial follow A_1 path. In the current setting, we select the most effective dose(s) (with the smallest p-value(s) or combine p-value(s)) from the early stage(s) for the final stage. See Dong (2014) for details on the prespecified threshold parameters $\alpha_1^{(1)}$, $\alpha_2^{(1)}$, $\alpha_1^{(2)}$, and $\alpha_2^{(2)}$; multiplicity; and sample size re-estimation.

9.2.4 Combined p-Values and Critical Values for the Final Analysis

For a phase II/III clinical trial, based on interim results, usually one or two doses of the study treatment are chosen for the final confirmatory stage. However, without loss of generality, let S be the index set of the dose arms chosen for the final confirmatory stage, $S \subseteq D$. Following the closed testing procedure (Marcus et al. 1976), to reject the elementary null hypothesis H_{0is} for the dose arm s, $s \in S$ and $i = 1, 2$ for study endpoint, all intersection null hypotheses $H_{0i,J}$: $\bigcap_{k\in J} H_{0ik} (s \in J \subseteq D = \{1,2,\ldots, K\})$ including the dose arms dropped from an interim analysis have to be rejected as long as these intersection null hypotheses contain H_{0is}.

Let D_1 be a closed set for the first stage, such that $s \in D_1$. For a three-stage setting, the same D_1 applies to the second stage as there are no dose arm changes from interim I. For the final stage, since some dose arms would have been dropped, the set D_1 is reduced to S_1 and the intersection null hypothesis H_{0i,D_1}: $\bigcap_{k\in D_1} H_{0ik}$ is reduced to H_{0i,S_1}: $\bigcap_{k\in S_1} H_{0ik}$, such that $s \in S_1 \subseteq D_1 \subseteq D = \{1,2,\ldots, K\}$. Let p_{i1,D_1} and p_{i2,S_1} be p-values corresponding to H_{0i,D_1} and H_{0i,S_1} for a two-stage setting, and p_{i1,D_1}, p_{i2,D_1}, and p_{i3,S_1} be corresponding p-values for a three-stage setting. To reject the null hypothesis H_{0is} for the selected dose arm s with respect to the ith endpoint, the combined p-values and corresponding critical values for the final analysis are

Table 9.1 Combined p-values and critical values for the final analysis to reject H_{0is} for the selected dose arm s

Trial path	Final analysis	
	Combined p-value, for any S_1 and D_1 such that $s \in S_1 \subseteq D_1 \subseteq D$ and $s \in S_1 \subseteq S \subseteq D$	Critical value
A_1	$p_{11,D_1} p_{12,S_1}$	$\alpha_1^{(1)} c_{\alpha^*}$
A_2	$p_{21,D_1} p_{22,S_1}$	$\alpha_2^{(1)} c_{\alpha^*}$
A_3B_1	$p_{11,D_1} p_{12,D_1} p_{13,S_1}$	$\alpha_1^{(2)} c_{\alpha^*}$
A_3B_2	$p_{21,D_1} p_{22,D_1} p_{23,S_1}$	$\alpha_2^{(2)} c_{\alpha^*}$

listed in Table 9.1, where $c_{\alpha^*} = \exp\left(-0.5\chi^2_{\alpha^*,4}\right)$ and $\chi^2_{\alpha^*,4}$ is the $(1-\alpha^*)$ quantile of the χ^2 distribution with four degrees of freedom. For α^*, see the next section; for the distributions of conditional p-values and combined p-values, see Dong (2014).

9.2.5 *Type I Error Rate and Alpha Allocation*

To achieve family-wise type I error controlled at α level, the final analysis is performed at the significance level of α^*. Following a closed testing procedure (Marcus et al. 1976), to reject the null hypothesis H_{0is} for the selected dose arm s, all intersection null hypotheses containing H_{0is} have to be rejected at the significance level α^*. Following Dong (2014), the type I error rate for the two-stage setting is as follows:

$$\mathrm{ER_{II}} = \alpha^* \left[\alpha_1{}^{(1)} + \left(1 - \alpha_1{}^{(1)}\right)\alpha_2{}^{(1)}\right] = \lambda\alpha \tag{9.3}$$

where λ is the percent of alpha allocated for the two-stage setting. The type I error rate for the three-stage setting is

$$\begin{aligned}\mathrm{ER_{III}} &= \alpha^* \left\{-\alpha_1^{(2)}\left(1-\alpha_2^{(1)}\right)\ln\left(\alpha_1^{(1)}\right) - \alpha_2^{(2)}\ln\left(\alpha_2^{(1)}\right)\left[1-\alpha_1^{(1)} + \alpha_1^{(2)}\ln\left(\alpha_1^{(1)}\right)\right]\right\} \\ &= (1-\lambda)\,\alpha \end{aligned} \tag{9.4}$$

To control the overall Type I error rate at α, we require that α^* satisfies

$$\mathrm{ER} = \mathrm{ER_{II}} + \mathrm{ER_{III}} \le \alpha \tag{9.5}$$

9.3 Characteristics of the Varying-Stage Adaptive Phase II/III Clinical Trial Design

For the varying-stage adaptive phase II/III clinical trial design, Dong (2014) has showed statistical power, probabilities of trial paths, and expected sample size (EN) under the alternative hypotheses for both plausible endpoints. Here, we explore

Table 9.2 Distribution of the two endpoints for simulations

Study endpoint	Distribution			
	Control	Dose 1	Dose 2	Dose 3
1	$N(40, 20^2)$	$N(45, 20^2)$	$N(47, 20^2)$	$N(49, 20^2)$
2	$N(10, 15^2)$	$N(14, 15^2)$	$N(15, 15^2)$	$N(17, 15^2)$

characteristics of the design when the alternative hypothesis for only one of the two endpoints is true, and the treatment effect for another endpoint is null or lower than what was anticipated per trial design. Same as Dong (2014), we control the family-wise type I error rate at the level of $\alpha = 0.05$ (two-sided), apply 80 % conditional power to re-estimate the sample size for the final stage, and assume the two endpoints are normally distributed (Table 9.2). Following Bretz et al. (2009), we use a closed Dunnett test procedure. For simplicity and simulation purpose, we set the sample size for the first stage $n_1 = 35$/arm, which could detect the maximal assumed treatment effect $\tau = 0.45$ for the dose arm 3 at the significance level of $\alpha_1 = 0.20$ with the power = 70% approximately. We set the sample size for the intermediate stage in the same way as the initial stage, but considered the data from the first two stages.

9.3.1 *Simulation Under the Alternative Hypothesis for the Endpoint 1*

Tables 9.3 and 9.4 present the simulation results under the alternative hypothesis for the endpoint 1 and the null hypothesis for the endpoint 2. Given λ, as $\alpha_1^{(1)}$ increases, the condition for the trial to follow the trial path A_1 is relaxed; therefore, the probability of the path A_1 and the power for the path A_1 increase. With a relaxed condition to the path A_1, an increased sample size is needed to obtain a stronger evidence in path A_1. Consequently, the trial has a higher overall statistical power, which results in a decreased probability of trial early stop due to futility (path A_3B_3). As $\alpha_1^{(1)}$ increases, there is not much change in the power for the path A_3B_1 and the probability of the trial following the path A_3B_1.

Given $\alpha_1^{(1)}$, as λ increases, there is not much change in the power and probability of the trial path A_1. However, as more alpha is allocated to the two-stage setting (with an increased λ), sample size is reduced and overall statistical power is decreased. Consequently, the probability of trial early stop due to futility (path A_3B_3) increases.

The total power for the endpoint 2 (paths A_2 and A_3B_2), which is the type I error rate under the null hypothesis H_{02} for the endpoint 2, is less than 0.015. Therefore, type I error rate under H_{02} is well controlled at the nominal level of $\alpha = 0.05$.

Table 9.3 Simulated power under the alternative hypothesis for the endpoint 1

λ	$\alpha_1^{(1)}$	Trial path				Total power
		A_1	A_2	A_3B_1	A_3B_2	
50 %	0.05	0.3802	0.0065	0.3198	0.0035	0.7100
	0.06	0.4129	0.0069	0.3075	0.0023	0.7296
	0.07	0.4291	0.0057	0.3065	0.0013	0.7426
	0.08	0.4441	0.0061	0.3051	0.0024	0.7577
	0.09	0.4714	0.006	0.2972	0.0024	0.7770
	0.10	0.4941	0.0053	0.2890	0.0013	0.7897
60 %	0.05	0.3815	0.0083	0.2792	0.0029	0.6719
	0.06	0.4080	0.0078	0.2929	0.0027	0.7114
	0.07	0.4202	0.0076	0.2798	0.0024	0.7100
	0.08	0.4539	0.0084	0.2711	0.0024	0.7358
	0.09	0.4688	0.0076	0.2635	0.0013	0.7412
	0.10	0.4711	0.0066	0.2722	0.0024	0.7523
70 %	0.05	0.3873	0.0101	0.2417	0.0022	0.6413
	0.06	0.4164	0.0096	0.2348	0.0028	0.6636
	0.07	0.4289	0.0092	0.2457	0.0013	0.6851
	0.08	0.4522	0.0100	0.2404	0.0023	0.7049
	0.09	0.4676	0.0097	0.2291	0.0022	0.7086
	0.10	0.4711	0.0085	0.2380	0.0018	0.7194

9.3.2 *Simulation Under the Alternative Hypothesis for the Endpoint 2*

The simulated statistical power, sample size, and trial path probability under the alternative hypothesis for the endpoint 2 and the null hypothesis for the endpoint 1 are provided in Tables 9.5 and 9.6. The simulation results are very similar to those under the alternative hypothesis for the endpoint 1, but for the parameters related to the endpoint 2 instead.

9.3.3 *Comparison to the Simulation Results Under the Alternative Hypotheses for Both Endpoints*

In general, these simulation results under an alternative hypothesis for either endpoint are consistent with those under the hypotheses for both endpoints as reported in Dong (2014). For example, given λ, as $\alpha_1^{(1)}$ increases, the probability and statistical power of the two-stage setting as well as the overall power increase. Since

Table 9.4 Simulated probability and sample size for each trial path under the alternative hypothesis for the end point 1

λ	$\alpha_1^{(1)}$	Trial path										EN
		A_1		A_2		A_3B_1		A_3B_2		A_3B_3		
		Prob	n	Prob	n	Prob	n	Prob	n	Prob	n	
50 %	0.05	0.4169	78	0.0281	101	0.3478	116	0.0106	147	0.1966	84	93.8
	0.06	0.4539	83	0.0337	109	0.3340	123	0.0110	159	0.1674	84	98.2
	0.07	0.4723	88	0.0362	115	0.3348	126	0.0129	166	0.1438	84	102.1
	0.08	0.4844	93	0.0416	123	0.3345	129	0.0141	168	0.1254	84	106.2
	0.09	0.5142	98	0.0431	127	0.3216	131	0.0145	173	0.1066	84	109.5
	0.10	0.5422	100	0.0452	134	0.3146	135	0.0113	181	0.0867	84	112.1
60 %	0.05	0.4195	71	0.0295	91	0.3021	112	0.0094	139	0.2395	84	87.7
	0.06	0.4487	80	0.0338	103	0.3187	120	0.0108	151	0.1880	84	95.0
	0.07	0.4628	81	0.0373	108	0.3042	121	0.0102	155	0.1855	84	95.5
	0.08	0.4949	85	0.0397	113	0.2959	125	0.0106	163	0.1589	84	98.6
	0.09	0.5147	89	0.0428	118	0.2896	129	0.0104	173	0.1425	84	102.0
	0.10	0.5233	94	0.0472	124	0.2972	132	0.0111	167	0.1212	84	106.3
70 %	0.05	0.4236	65	0.0292	82	0.2621	110	0.0070	131	0.2781	84	83.0
	0.06	0.4578	71	0.0314	92	0.2553	114	0.0076	137	0.2479	84	86.4
	0.07	0.4681	75	0.0364	98	0.2680	118	0.0066	147	0.2209	84	89.8
	0.08	0.4952	80	0.0399	106	0.2615	123	0.0079	147	0.1955	84	93.6
	0.09	0.5159	84	0.0429	110	0.2497	125	0.0076	155	0.1839	84	95.9
	0.10	0.5184	86	0.0461	111	0.2598	125	0.0090	160	0.1667	84	97.6

a priori of the simulations is to re-estimate the sample size for the final stage based on 80 % conditional power, and the two endpoints are assumed independent and equally plausible with similar treatment effect, the sample sizes for the three scenarios under the alternative hypothesis (hypotheses): (a) for the endpoint 1, (b) for the endpoint 2, and (c) for both endpoints are very similar for each pair of parameters λ and $\alpha_1^{(1)}$. As expected, when the treatment effect for an endpoint is lower than what was anticipated per trial design, the overall statistical power becomes lower. For example, when $\lambda = 70\%$ and $\alpha_1^{(1)} = 0.1$, power $= 0.7194$, 0.6864, and 0.8869 for the three scenarios, respectively. One should note that the scenarios (a) and (b) may be extremely worst cases as one endpoint is assumed as expected but a null treatment effect is assumed for another endpoint. When the treatment effect is 80 % of the anticipated effect in another endpoint, the power is 0.8025 and 0.8308 for the first two scenarios, respectively (Table 9.7), which are not too far to the power of 0.8869 under the alternative hypotheses for both endpoints. As a reference but not a head-to-head comparison, for a single-stage trial designed with a similar primary endpoint to those described in Table 9.2 and with two-sided $\alpha = 0.05$ and power $= 90\,\%$, statistical power can

Table 9.5 Simulated power under the alternative hypothesis for the endpoint 2

λ	$\alpha_1^{(1)}$	Trial path				Total power
		A_1	A_2	A_3B_1	A_3B_2	
50 %	0.05	0.0125	0.3764	0.0080	0.3072	0.7041
	0.06	0.0141	0.4003	0.0070	0.2873	0.7087
	0.07	0.0136	0.4147	0.0061	0.2904	0.7248
	0.08	0.0126	0.4313	0.0078	0.2802	0.7319
	0.09	0.0123	0.4417	0.0081	0.2643	0.7264
	0.10	0.0127	0.4433	0.0083	0.2667	0.7310
60 %	0.05	0.0155	0.3763	0.0068	0.2782	0.6768
	0.06	0.0140	0.4010	0.0054	0.2845	0.7049
	0.07	0.0138	0.4123	0.0039	0.2703	0.7003
	0.08	0.0165	0.4312	0.0054	0.2581	0.7112
	0.09	0.0157	0.4439	0.0046	0.2471	0.7113
	0.10	0.0169	0.4509	0.0039	0.2394	0.7111
70 %	0.05	0.0186	0.3777	0.0036	0.2452	0.6451
	0.06	0.0164	0.4073	0.0047	0.2314	0.6598
	0.07	0.0188	0.4238	0.004	0.2309	0.6775
	0.08	0.0170	0.4267	0.0040	0.2224	0.6701
	0.09	0.0182	0.4460	0.049	0.2185	0.6876
	0.10	0.0180	0.4435	0.0042	0.2207	0.6864

be reduced to 73 % if treatment effect is reduced to 80 %; and statistical power can be reduced to 5 % if treatment effect is down to null. Therefore, the simulations show that the statistical power of the varying-stage adaptive phase II/III clinical trial design (Dong 2014) is less sensitive to a low realized treatment effect compared to the anticipated treatment effect per trial design. This finding is due to an advantage of the varying-stage adaptive phase II/III clinical trial design with two plausible study endpoints.

9.4 Discussion

In the varying-stage adaptive phase II/III clinical trial design (Dong 2014), following the first stage, an intermediate stage can be adaptively added to obtain more data, so that a more informative decision could be made regarding whether the trial can be advanced to the final confirmatory stage. Therefore, this design is a two-stage setting or three-stage setting depending on whether there is an intermediate stage added as an extended learning stage between the initial learning stage (phase II) and the confirmatory stage (phase III). This design considers two plausible study endpoints with

Table 9.6 Simulated probability and sample size for each trial path under the alternative hypothesis for the end point 2

λ	$\alpha_1^{(1)}$	Trial path										EN
		A1		A2		A3B1		A3B2		A3B3		
		Prob	n	Prob	n	Prob	n	Prob	n	Prob	n	
50 %	0.05	0.0529	111	0.4115	77	0.0288	149	0.3307	115	0.1761	84	94.6
	0.06	0.0617	108	0.4367	83	0.0372	157	0.3094	122	0.1550	84	99.6
	0.07	0.0694	115	0.4512	86	0.0376	164	0.3107	125	0.1311	84	102.8
	0.08	0.0793	123	0.4629	91	0.0426	172	0.2995	129	0.1157	84	107.6
	0.09	0.0882	127	0.4807	96	0.0491	177	0.2848	131	0.0972	84	111.5
	0.10	0.0978	132	0.4798	98	0.0494	179	0.2858	132	0.0872	84	113.8
60 %	0.05	0.0479	89	0.4101	70	0.0222	140	0.3006	112	0.2192	84	88.2
	0.06	0.0568	103	0.4362	78	0.0258	155	0.3043	118	0.1769	84	94.6
	0.07	0.0687	106	0.4472	81	0.0235	158	0.2909	121	0.1697	84	96.7
	0.08	0.0814	113	0.4673	84	0.0268	161	0.2783	125	0.1462	84	99.8
	0.09	0.0886	119	0.4846	88	0.0320	169	0.2656	129	0.1292	84	103.7
	0.10	0.1048	121	0.4870	92	0.0330	176	0.2601	129	0.1151	84	106.5
70 %	0.05	0.0480	83	0.4084	64	0.0117	132	0.2640	109	0.2679	84	82.9
	0.06	0.0584	92	0.4423	70	0.0140	139	0.2500	115	0.2353	84	86.8
	0.07	0.0713	98	0.4606	74	0.0159	148	0.2484	119	0.2038	84	90.1
	0.08	0.0808	105	0.4658	79	0.0179	156	0.2396	122	0.1959	84	93.8
	0.09	0.0918	110	0.4815	82	0.0201	157	0.2351	124	0.1715	84	96.3
	0.10	0.1046	114	0.4840	86	0.0228	166	0.2379	127	0.1507	84	100.2

Table 9.7 Powers when only 80 % of anticipated treatment effect for an endpoint (λ = 70 % and $\alpha_1^{(1)} = 0.1$)

Scenario	Under alternative hypothesis for endpoint 1		Under alternative hypothesis for endpoint 2		Under alternative hypotheses for both endpoints
	No (0 %) treatment effect for endpoint 2	80 % treatment effect for endpoint 2	No (0 %) treatment effect for endpoint 1	80 % treatment effect for endpoint 1	
Total power	0.7194	0.8025	0.6864	0.8308	0.8869

one of them initially designated as the primary endpoint, and controls family-wise type I error rate in a strong sense. This chapter additionally explores characteristics of the design when the alternative hypothesis for only one of the two endpoints is true, and the treatment effect for another endpoint is null (an extremely worst case) or lower than what was anticipated per trial design. Since two plausible endpoints are considered in the varying-stage adaptive phase II/III clinical trial design, as shown in our simulations, the statistical power of the design is less sensitive to a low realized treatment effect compared to the anticipated treatment effect per the trial design. As also discussed in Dong (2014), the parameters λ and $\alpha_1^{(1)}$ have a great impact to the design. The parameter λ mainly impacts alpha allocation and thus expected sample size, and the threshold probability $\alpha_1^{(1)}$ mainly contributes to the chance to have a trial follow A_1 path.

For the simulations presented in this chapter, we assume that the two endpoints are independent. When the two endpoints are correlated, there is a power loss at a certain degree (Dong 2014). Other areas that can be improved in the future were discussed in Dong (2014), of which it is worth noting that the dose arm(s) with smallest p-value(s) or combined p-value(s) is(are) selected for the final stage in the current form of the proposed design.

Point estimate and confidence interval have been proposed and studied more for two-stage designs. For some two-stage designs (e.g., one with O'Brien Fleming boundary), the regular confidence interval without adjusting for interim looks may still provide good information for the medical researchers and reviewers for proper decision making. However, as of today, a satisfactory method to construct point estimate and confidence interval for phase II/III clinical trials has not been established, which is mainly due to: (a) Some methods have a good bias reduction for point estimate, but their variance are unfortunately substantially increased (Kimani et al. 2013); (b) some methods are only developed for point estimate or confidence interval, but not for both. Recently, Bowden and Glimm (2008) and Bretz et al. (2009) discussed uniformly minimum variance conditional unbiased estimate (UMVCUE); Carreras and Brannath (2013) developed a new method of shrinkage estimator; Kimani et al. (2013) published a uniformly minimum variance unbiased estimator by considering futility stopping; and Bowden and Glimm (2014) proposed point estimate for a K:L:1 three-stage setting phase II/III design. We are currently evaluating what point estimators are suitable for the varying-stage adaptive phase II/III clinical trial design. In addition, a reviewer and an editor pointed out that the proposed design is quite complex with the adaptive features. We have simplified this design to consider one study endpoint only, as in many therapeutic areas, the primary study endpoint is well established. This simplified design will be reported in a future paper.

Acknowledgement The author would like to sincerely thank Dr. Weichung Joe Shih, Dr. Dirk Moore, Dr. Hui Quan, and Dr. Stephen Marcella for their advices, sincerely thank Dr. Aiyi Liu for his invitation for the 2013 ICSA and ISBS Joint Statistical Conference, sincerely thank an anonymous reviewer and the editor Dr. Yi Tsong for their helpful comments, and thank the editors for their invitation of this chapter.

References

Bauer P, Köhne K (1994) Evaluation of experiments with adaptive interim analyses. Biometrics 50(4):1029–41

Bischoff W, Miller F (2009) A seamless phase II/III design with sample-size re-estimation. J Biopharm Stat 19(4):595–609

Bowden J, Glimm E (2008) Unbiased estimation of selected treatment means in two-stage trials. Biom J 50(4):515–527

Bowden J, Glimm E (2014) Conditionally unbiased and near unbiased estimation of the selected treatment mean for multistage drop-the-losers trials. Biom J 56(2):332–349

Bretz F, Schmidli H, Koenig F, Racine A, Maurer W (2006) Confirmatory seamless phase II/III clinical trials with hypotheses selection at interim: general concepts (with discussion). Biom J 48:623–634

Bretz F, Koenig F, Brannath W, Glimm E, Posch M (2009) Adaptive designs for confirmatory clinical trials. Stat Med 28(8):1181–1217

Carreras M, Brannath W (2013) Shrinkage estimation in two-stage adaptive designs with midtrial treatment selection. Stat Med 32(10):1677–1690

Cui L, Hung HMJ, Wang SJ (1999) Modification of sample size in group sequential clinical trials. Biometrics 55:853–857

Dong G (2014) A varying-stage adaptive phase II/III clinical trial design. Stat Med 33(8):1272–1287

Fisher RA (1932). Statistical methods for research workers, 4th edn. Oliver & Boyd, London

Food and Drug Administration (2010) Adaptive design clinical trials for drugs and biologics (draft FDA guidance). http://www.fda.gov/downloads/Drugs/GuidanceComplianceRegulatoryInformation/Guidances/UCM201790.pdf. Accessed 14 Feb 2014

Gallo P, Chuang-Stein C, Dragalin V, Gaydos B, Krams M, Pinheiro J (2006) Adaptive designs in clinical drug development—an executive summary of the PhRMA working group. J Biopharm Stat 16(3):275–283

Jennison C, Turnbull BW (2006) Confirmatory seamless phase II/III clinical trials with hypotheses selection at interim: opportunities and limitations. Biom J 48:650–655

Kimani PK, Todd S, Stallard N (2013) Conditionally unbiased estimation in phase II/III clinical trials with early stopping for futility. Stat Med 32(17):2893–2910

Marcus R, Peritz E, Gabriel K (1976) On closed testing procedures with special reference to ordered analysis of variance. Biometrika 63(3):655–660

Müller HH, Schäfer H (2001) Adaptive group sequential designs for clinical trials: combining the advantages of adaptive and of classical group sequential approaches. Biometrics 57:886–891

Todd S, Stallard N (2005) A new clinical trial design combining phase 2 and 3: sequential designs with treatment selection and a change of endpoint. Drug Inf J 39:109–118

Chapter 10
Collective Evidence in Drug Evaluation

Qian H. Li

Disclaimer: The views presented in this chapter are the author's own views.

Abstract Multiple doses, endpoints, and tests are used in several clinical studies to establish drug efficacy. Statistical evaluation relies heavily on multiplicity adjustments within one study to control the type I error rate. The use of multiplicity adjustment procedures (MAPs) sometimes leads to conclusions that may not seem logical. As drug efficacy evaluation involves aspects such as assessing efficacy, selecting optimal doses, and labeling claims, incorporating all the aspects under the umbrella of controlling type I error may not be an optimum strategy. Alternatively, a practical approach that uses collective evidence is proposed to evaluate multiple studies, doses, endpoints, and tests. Instead of controlling the type I error, specific types of errors are controlled, such as the error of wrongly approving an ineffective drug and the error of labeling false information. With the collective evidence approach, the need of MAPs in individual studies is debated when multiple studies are available.

10.1 Introduction

Drug efficacy evaluation usually is based on evidence from multiple clinical studies that assess multiple doses using multiple endpoints and tests. The multiplicity issues arising from the clinical studies are classic problems in drug evaluation and have been heavily studied by the regulatory agencies, pharmaceutical and biotech industries, and research institutes (Chuang-Stein et al. [3]; Committee for Proprietary Medical Products (CPMP) by EMEA [4]; Pocock [16]; Proschan and Waclawiw [17]; Shih and Quan [18]). The majority of statistical methods, such as the closed testing procedure

Q. H. Li (✉)
National Institute of Health, National Center for Complementary and Alternative Medicine,
Democracy Blvd., Suite 401, Bethesda, MD 20892-5475, USA
Tel.: 301-594-8018 6707
e-mail: Qian.li@nih.gov

Z. Chen et al. (eds.), *Applied Statistics in Biomedicine and Clinical Trials Design*,
ICSA Book Series in Statistics, DOI 10.1007/978-3-319-12694-4_10

(Marcus et al. [12]), Bonferroni correction, and Hochberg procedure (Hochberg [7]), referred to as multiplicity adjustment procedures (MAPs), have been developed based on the logic that multiplicity, such as multiple doses, endpoints, or tests, increases the chance of detecting a statistically significant result from an ineffective drug. Commonly used analogies of the multiplicity issues have been situations such as betting on a horse race or buying lottery tickets, where increasing the number of horses that one bets on, or the number of tickets that one purchases, would increase chances of winning.

These horse race and lottery analogies have, at times, misled the understanding of multiplicity issues in drug evaluation and disguised rudimentary differences between drug evaluation and such games of chance. In a race, the determination of the winning horse does not depend upon the distance between the winner and the losing horses. That is, the relative speeds of the losing horses do not matter. However, in drug evaluation, the efficacy determination of the drug depends upon the collective performance of individual doses, endpoints, and studies. If only one dose shows a statistically significant treatment effect while none of the other doses show any trend of efficacy, the evidence is less convincing for an efficacious drug than the case where multiple doses show trend of efficacy. Therefore, multiplicity in drug evaluation may not necessarily increase the chance to claim that an ineffective drug is efficacious when information is evaluated collectively.

In this chapter, a practical approach to evaluate evidence collectively is proposed. This method controls the specific types of errors encountered in drug evaluation, such as the error rate of wrongly approving an ineffective drug and the error rate of labeling false information. Moreover, it controls the consistency of evidence. Sect. 10.2 discusses the problems of applying MAPs. Section 10.3 presents the concept of the collective evidence and describes the practical approach. Section 10.4 covers the application of collective evidence in cases of multiple studies, doses, endpoints (including co-primary endpoints and secondary endpoints) and tests. Two cases are discussed in Sect. 10.5 to illustrate the use of collective evidence in understanding the effect of drugs. Throughout this chapter, one-sided p values and one-sided statistical significant levels are used unless otherwise specified.

10.2 Problems of Applying MAPs

Prespecification is vital in the protocol development to ensure careful planning in study design, experiment procedures, endpoint selection, and statistical analysis plans, etc. However, it can be problematic to prespecify decision rules, which are MAPs, in the individual study protocols. The intention of the prespecified decision rule is to reduce the chance of claiming success, yet the selection of the decision rules appears somewhat arbitrary. The same study results may reach different conclusions depending upon the choice of the decision rules. For instance, p values 0.040 and 0.012 were observed for high and low doses, respectively, in a study. If the closed testing procedure using high dose to protect low dose was prespecified, the results

Table 10.1 *P* values of two studies with two doses in each study

	1-sided *p* values	
	High dose	Low dose
Study 1	0.028	0.015
Study 2	0.025	0.013

would not pass the decision rule and would yield an inconclusive conclusion. However, if either the Hochberg procedure or Bonferroni correction was prespecified, the low dose would be considered to be efficacious. Clearly, these distinct conclusions are the result of the prespecified decision rules, which are inflexible and, to a certain extent, arbitrary.

Another problem is that the MAPs may overvalue the isolated effect. To illustrate this, consider a study with three parallel doses and a control arm. If both high and medium doses yielded *p* values of 0.500 and the low dose yielded 0.001, both the Hochberg and Bonferroni procedures would conclude that the low dose was efficacious, despite the fact that there was no sign of efficacy in the other doses. Unless other information supported that this drug had narrow therapeutic window, the evidence would not be considered convincing. Whereas if three doses from high to low yielded *p* values of 0.028, 0.025, and 0.015, respectively, some MAPs would consider such evidence inconclusive. Thus, only looking at the performance of the individual doses rather than the totality evidence may not lead to useful conclusions.

The problem can be more confusing when data from more than one study are available. In fact, two phase 3 studies have been the requirement by the US Food and Drug Administration (FDA) for the purpose of establishing substantial evidence (US FDA [19]; US FDA [20]). Suppose that two phase 3 studies were conducted to support a claim. Also, suppose that two doses, high and low, were included in both studies and a closed testing procedure using high dose to protect low dose was placed in each study. The *p* values of the two doses from both studies were listed in Table 10.1. Following the closed testing procedure, study 1 would be concluded as a "failed" study since it failed to pass the closed testing procedure, whereas study 2 would be considered a successful study. However, the fundamental question of the efficacy of the drug has not been answered.

The application of the MAPs is to protect the type I error. However, the meaning of the type I error is not clear since it covers different types of errors that may occur in various aspects and stages of drug evaluation. Errors can occur when deciding if a drug works, selecting the optimal doses, and labeling drug information with selective endpoints, etc. When deciding if a drug is efficacious, it is necessary to control the error rate of wrongly approving an ineffective drug. When selecting the optimal doses, it is necessary to reduce the error rate of selecting suboptimal doses. When labeling drugs, it is necessary to limit the error rate of providing false information. These different types of errors play different roles in the drug evaluation process and may not necessarily be controlled simultaneously. It is easy to understand that the error of selecting suboptimal doses, or the error of false labeling information would not occur if the drug is concluded to be ineffective. On the other hand, the error made in efficacy decisions should not be impacted by the decision of selecting the optimal doses and the decision of drug labeling. Therefore, it may be less confusing to differentiate the types of errors in drug evaluation and control the different types of error rates separately.

10.3 Concept of Collective Evidence

10.3.1 The Two Types of Logic

In preparation for discussing the alternative approach proposed, two types of logic are considered. Mathematically, the "OR" logic is the union of all events and represented as $E_1 \cup E_2 \cup \ldots \cup E_K$; the "AND" logic is the intersection of all events and formulated as $E_1 \cap E_2 \cap \ldots \cap E_K$, where E_k, $k = 1, 2, \ldots, K$, are events. The K events can be the number of bets that is put down in a horse race for example, or K doses, K endpoints, or K individual studies in drug evaluation. The "OR" logic is the basis for most of the MAPs where success is claimed if one event out of the K events is true. On the contrary, the success definition with the "AND" logic requires that all events are true. The main feature of the collective evidence approach is to include the "AND" logic.

A discussion of Fig. 10.1 illustrates the concept of collective evidence. In Fig. 10.1, the blue area represents the rejection region of Bonferroni correction to control the error rate at the level of 0.025 for two independent p values p_1 and p_2. The Bonferroni correction can be written as $P(p_1 \leq 0.0125 \cup p_2 \leq 0.0125) < 0.025$ or can be written as $P(p_{(1)} \leq 0.0125 \cap p_{(2)} \leq 1.000) < 0.025$ where $p_{(1)}$ and $p_{(2)}$ are ordered p values of p_1 and p_2. Notice that the Bonferroni correction is rewritten using the AND logic, although it can be simplified to $P(p_{(1)} \leq 0.0125) < 0.025$ as the event of a p value less than 1 is always true. Using γ_1, γ_2 to denote the p value cut points for the ordered p values, respectively, the decision rule for the Bonferroni correction can be written as $(\gamma_1, \gamma_2) = (0.0125, 1.000)$. This rejection region allows the success claim if one of the p values is 0.0125 or less. It is important to understand that the Bonferroni correction is not the only way of controlling the error rate at the level of 0.025. The green area represents another rejection region that controls error rate at the level of 0.025, that is, $P(p_{(1)} \leq 0.025 \cup p_{(2)} \leq 0.5125) \leq 0.025$. The decision rule is $(\gamma_1, \gamma_2) = (0.025, 0.5125)$. This green rejection region supports the success claim if the smaller p value is less than or equal to 0.025 and the larger p value is less than 0.5125. The orange area represents yet another rejection region that controls the same error rate with decision rule $(\gamma_1, \gamma_2) = (0.050, 0.275)$. This decision rule covers the rejection region that allows the smaller p value to be 0.050 or less and the larger one has to be 0.275 or less. Notice that both the orange and green rejection regions use the AND logic.

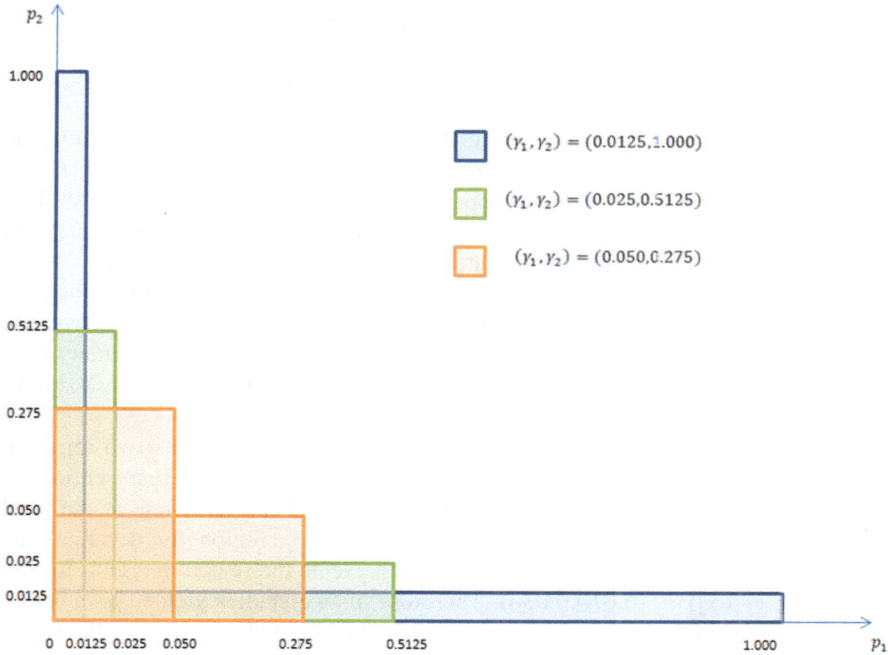

Fig. 10.1 Rejection regions that control the error at the level of 0.025 under different decision rules

10.3.2 The Formulation of the Collective Evidence Approach

The concept of collective evidence was originally proposed by Li and Huque (Li and Huque [10]) for the purpose of evaluating multiple studies and was extended to the evaluation of co-primary endpoints by Li (Li [9]). The concept of collective evidence approach can be described as follows:

1. Similar to a single hypothesis testing scenario, individual null and alternative hypotheses, H_{0k} and H_{Ak}, are used to test each individual event E_k and the test yields p value $p_k, k = 1, 2, \ldots, K$. Null represents no effect, while the alternative is the complement. The K p values are ranked as $p_{(1)} \leq p_{(2)} \leq \ldots \leq p_{(K)}$.
2. Next is to formulate the overall hypothesis to test if a drug works. An overall null hypothesis represents the case that all the individual null hypotheses H_{0k}, $k = 1, 2, \ldots, K$, are true, i.e., an ineffective drug. The corresponding alternative is that at least one of the individual alternatives is true. The overall null and corresponding alternative are denoted as $H_0^{1/K}$ and $H_A^{1/K}$, respectively, and formulated as

$$H_0^{1/K} : \bigcap_{k=1}^{K} H_{0k} \text{ versus } H_A^{1/K} : \bigcup_{k=1}^{K} H_{Ak}$$

The error of wrongly rejecting the overall null is defined as

$$P_{H_0^{1/K}}(p_{(1)} \le \gamma_1 \cap p_{(2)} \le \gamma_2 \cap \ldots \cap p_{(K)} \le \gamma_K),$$

where $\gamma_1 \le \gamma_2 \le \ldots \le \gamma_K$ is a set of the decision rule. The error rate is controlled at the level of $\alpha(H_0^{1/K})$ under $H_0^{1/K}$. When the events are independent studies, $\alpha(H_0^{1/K})$ represents the error rate of wrongly approving an ineffective drug. For two studies, the error rate $\alpha(H_0^{1/2})$ is usually controlled at the level of $0.025^2 = 0.000625$ (Li and Huque [10]). This level of error rate arises from the requirement of two statistically significant studies as the substantial evidence for drug approval. When the events are correlated endpoints within one study, $\alpha(H_0^{1/K})$ represents the error rate of wrongly claiming an ineffective drug to be efficacious. For two co-primary endpoints in one study, the error rate $\alpha(H_0^{1/2})$ is controlled at the level of 0.025 (Li [9]).

To further illustrate the point discussed here, Fig. 10.2 presents two rejection regions for two independent studies in the coordinates p_1 and p_2, representing results of the two studies. Both rejection regions control the error rate at the level of 0.000625. The orange area represents the rejection region for decision rule $(\gamma_1, \gamma_2) = (0.025, 0.025)$ and the green area represents the rejection region for decision rule $(\gamma_1, \gamma_2) = (0.010, 0.036)$. Therefore, if two studies yielded p values of (0.010,0.030), this could be considered as convincing evidence for an efficacious drug.

3. In addition, another set of overall hypotheses is formulated to test if all events present efficacy—a reflection of consistency among all events. The overall alternative requires that all events show efficacy. The overall null is therefore that at least one event does not have efficacy. The overall null and alternative are denoted as $H_0^{K/K}$ and $H_A^{K/K}$, respectively, and formulated as

$$H_0^{K/K} : \bigcup_{k=1}^{K} H_{0k} \text{ versus } H_A^{K/K} : \bigcap_{k=1}^{K} H_{Ak}$$

The level of the error should be controlled at the level of $\alpha(H_0^{K/K})$ under the overall null hypothesis $H_0^{K/K}$. It has been shown (Li [9]) that the error rate $\alpha(H_0^{K/K})$ of rejecting the null is

$$P_{H_0^{K/K}}(p_{(1)} \le \gamma_1 \cap p_{(2)} \le \gamma_2 \cap \ldots \cap p_{(K)} \le \gamma_K) \le \gamma_K,$$

where γ_K is the largest p value cut point of the decision rule $\gamma_1 \le \gamma_2 \le \ldots \le \gamma_K$. For the decision rule $(\gamma_1, \gamma_2) = (0.010, 0.036)$ presented in Fig. 10.2, $\alpha(H_0^{2/2})$ is controlled at the level of 0.036 while $\alpha(H_0^{1/2})$ is controlled at the level of 0.000625.

4. It is important to emphasize that $\alpha(H_0^{K/K})$ has different meaning from $\alpha(H_0^{1/K})$. Take multiple studies as an example, where the error rate of wrongly approving

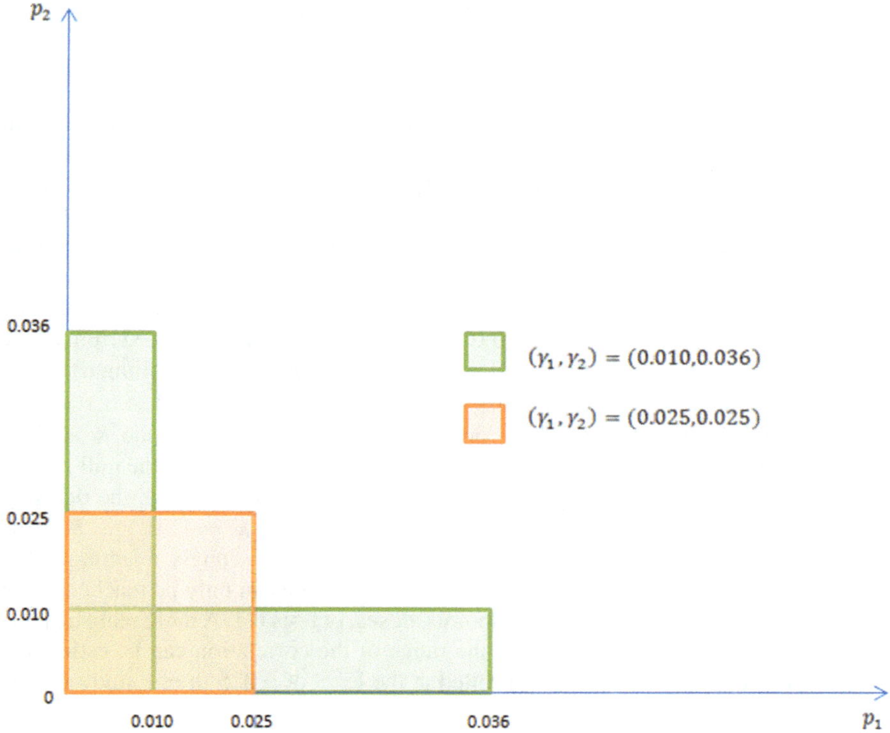

Fig. 10.2 Rejection regions that control the error rate at the level of 0.000625 for two independent studies

an ineffective drug is controlled at the level of $\alpha(H_0^{1/K})$. The error rate of accepting the hypothesis that all studies present consistent evidence when it is false is controlled at the level of $\alpha(H_0^{K/K})$. It makes common sense that $\alpha(H_0^{1/K})$ should be more stringent in comparison to $(H_0^{K/K})$, as the error of approving an ineffective drug is more serious than the error of claiming consistent evidence when in fact that efficacy is not consistently presented among studies. For two studies, $\alpha(H_0^{1/2})$ is controlled at the level of *0.000625*, while $\alpha(H_0^{2/2})$ is controlled at the level of *0.025* for a decision rule *(0.025, 0.025)*. For two co-primary endpoints, $\alpha(H_0^{1/2})$ is controlled at the level of *0.025*, while $\alpha(H_0^{2/2})$ can be controlled at the level of *0.030* for a decision rule *(0.023, 0.030)*.

The calculation of the decision rules has been described in detail in papers by Li and Huque (Li and Huque [10]) and Li (Li [9]) and various sets of decision rules can be calculated. The original approach of collective evidence requires that the decision rule be prespecified. Since prespecifying a decision rule can be arbitrary and can cause trouble, a practical approach is proposed to reduce the burden of the prespecifying decision rule.

10.3.3 The Practical Approaches to Evaluate Evidence Collectively

To reduce the burden of selecting and prespecifying decision rules, the practical approach uses only one set of decision rules for each K. The following set of decision rules can be considered for independent studies: $(\gamma_1, \gamma_2) = (0.025,\ 0.025)$, $(\gamma_1, \gamma_2,\ \gamma_3) = (0.025,\ 0.025,\ 0.100)$, and $(\gamma_1, \gamma_2,\ \gamma_3,\ \gamma_4) = (0.025,\ 0.025,\ 0.100,\ 0.150)$ for $K=2,\ 3,$ and $4,$ respectively. The ideal evidence for $K=2$ is to have two studies demonstrate statistical significance at the same level of 0.025, therefore, the decision rule $(\gamma_1, \gamma_2) = (0.025,\ 0.025)$ should be considered for $K=2$. The decision rule $(\gamma_1, \gamma_2,\ \gamma_3) = (0.025,\ 0.025,\ 0.100)$ for $K=3$ is developed from $K=2$ by adding $\gamma_3 = 0.100$. The choice of γ_3 is primarily driven by controlling $\alpha(H_0^{3/3})$, the error rate of wrongly rejecting the overall null $H_0^{3/3}$, at the level of 0.100. The decision rule for $K=4$ is similarly derived. Note that, the larger the K is, it is reasonable to accept higher levels of error rates of wrongly rejecting the null $H_0^{K/K}$.

In cases of co-primary endpoints, doses, or tests within one study, the decision rules that are recommended are formed with $\gamma_k = 0.025,\ k = 1,\ 2, \ldots,\ K$. This choice will conservatively control the error rate $\alpha(H_0^{1/K})$, wrongly rejecting $H_0^{1/K}$ in one study, at the level of 0.025. This level of error rate can only be reached when correlation among the co-primary endpoints, doses, or tests is 1. A more realistic level of error rate can be calculated when the range of the correlation can be estimated. The error rate $\alpha(H_0^{K/K})$ is also controlled at the level of 0.025 in one study for the recommended decision rule.

If the p values of the study results satisfy the decision rules, all error rates are adequately controlled. However, it may not be reasonable to require all study results to satisfy the decision rules for drug approval. For example, if the p values of two studies are *(0.020, 0.028)*, this may be considered as convincing evidence for an effective drug. It is therefore necessary to establish the standard of convincing evidence. To address this, two quantities are proposed, one to measure the worst inflation and the other for consistency.

The worst inflation is the maximum possible error that could be observed and is defined in (10.1) below. It is the probability of observing the kth p value $p_{(k)}$ that equals to $\max(\gamma_k, pv_{(k)})$ or less, where $pv_{(k)},\ k = 1,\ 2,\ \ldots,\ K$, are the ordered observed p values. The relative inflation is calculated using formula (10.2).

$$Max.\ Inflated\ error = P\left(\bigcap_{k=1}^{K} p_{(k)} \le \max\left(\gamma_k, pv_{(k)}\right)\right) \quad (10.1)$$

$$\%\ of\ Inflation = \frac{P\left(\bigcap_{k=1}^{K} p_{(k)} \le \max(\gamma_k, pv_{(k)})\right) - P\left(\bigcap_{k=1}^{K} p_{(k)} \le \gamma_k\right)}{P\left(\bigcap_{k=1}^{K} p_{(k)} \le \gamma_k\right)} \quad (10.2)$$

For example, if the observed p values of two independent studies are *(0.020, 0.028)*, the inflation is

Table 10.2 Examples of max. inflation and consistency using decision rule (0.025, 0 025)

Observed p values	Max. inflated error (%)	Consistency
0.020, 0.026	0.000675 (8.0 %)	17.0 %
0.021, 0.026	0.000675 (8.0 %)	14.1 %
0.026, 0.026	0.000676 (8.2 %)	0.0 %
0.027, 0.027	0.000729 (16.6 %)	0.0 %
0.025, 0.028	0.000775 (24.0 %)	8.4 %
0.020, 0.030	0.000875 (40.0 %)	28.3 %
0.030, 0.030	0.000900 (44.0 %)	0.0 %
0.010, 0.036	0.001175 (88.0 %)	73.5 %
0.025, 0.036	0.001175 (88.0 %)	31.1 %
0.030, 0.036	0.001160 (101.6 %)	17.0 %

$$Max.\ Inflated\ error = P\left(p_{(1)} \le 0.025 \cap p_{(2)} \le 0.028\right) = 0.000775$$

$$\%\ of\ Inflation =$$

$$\frac{P\left(p_{(1)} \le 0.025 \cap p_{(2)} \le 0.028\right) - P\left(p_{(1)} \le 0.025 \cap p_{(2)} \le 0.025\right)}{P\left(p_{(1)} \le 0.025 \cap p_{(2)} \le 0.025\right)} = 24\%.$$

The consistency is another measure that helps assess the variation of the observed results against the decision rule ($\gamma_1, \gamma_2, \ldots, \gamma_K$). There can be several ways of assessing the consistency. The measure introduced here is the sample variance of the relative ratio of the ordered observed p value $pv_{(k)}$ versus the corresponding component of decision rule γ_k, for $k = 1, 2, \ldots, K$. The ratios are considered as the normalized observed p values by the components of the decision rule. The calculation can be written as (10.3):

$$Consistency = \sqrt{\frac{1}{K-1}\sum_{k=1}^{K}\left(\frac{pv_{(k)}}{\gamma_k} - \frac{1}{K}\sum_{k=1}^{K}\frac{pv_{(k)}}{\gamma_k}\right)^2} \tag{10.3}$$

For the same example above, the consistency is calculated as:

$$Consistency = \sqrt{\left(\frac{0.028}{0.025} - 0.96\right)^2 + \left(\frac{0.020}{0.025} - 0.96\right)^2} = 22.6\%.$$

Table 10.2 lists the calculation of the inflation and consistency of some observed p values for the case of two independent studies using decision rule (0.025, 0.025).

The collective evidence approach uses one set of predetermined criteria which control the desired level of error rates. To make the decision flexible and evidence based, the evidence obtained from the study calculated as the maximum inflation and consistency are also taken into consideration. An inflation of 24 % with less than 22.6 % consistency for two studies (p values are 0.020, 0.028) may be considered as convincing evidence. However, the approval decision should be determined in conjunction with the disease indication, drug safety profiles, and availability of other drugs for the same indication in the market. Other factors such as the selection of outcome measures and the similarity of study design among the studies included for evaluation may also be factored in for the decision making.

10.4 Collective Evidence in Drug Evaluation

As discussed earlier, it can be helpful to divide the error into different types, i.e., the error of wrongly approving an ineffective drug, the error of wrongly choosing the optimal doses, and the error of false labeling drug information. The first logical step in drug evaluation is to evaluate if a drug is efficacious by controlling the error rate of wrongly approving an ineffective drug. Once it is concluded that the drug is efficacious and reasonably safe, the next step is to identify the optimal doses. Selection of optimal drug doses is not discussed, as it involves evaluating the risk–benefit ratio and possibly pharmacokinetic information which is beyond the scope of this chapter. The discussion of the multiple doses is focused on the efficacy evaluation here. The next step is the labeling decision by controlling the error rate of labeling false information. The error rates are discussed in this section for cases of multiple studies, doses, endpoints, and tests.

10.4.1 Multiple Studies

The total evidence from multiple studies can be obtained by conducting a meta-analyses or using the collective evidence approach. For either approach, the first step is to decide which studies are to be included in the evaluation, since diversely designed studies may not always be informative when evaluating evidence collectively. The studies should be selected based on the study population, design, and the conduct of the studies, rather than the results of studies. It is also important to select studies based on a well-defined patient population. Study design factors, such as blinding, treatment duration, endpoints, and usage of concomitant medications, are important considerations as well. The conduct of the studies, such as the time period and condition of implementation, can be crucial too. For example, studies of seasonal allergic rhinitis may need to be conducted during allergy seasons when high levels of pollen are apparent in the air. If heavy rain occurs, the participants may not be exposed to sufficient allergen to develop allergic reactions. Inadequate exposure could be a legitimate reason to exclude the study, whereas, certain design differences may not be a valid reason to exclude studies. For instance, study endpoints may be evaluated differently among studies in allergic conjunctivitis studies. The redness of the eyes can be evaluated either by study subjects themselves or by practitioners. This may not be a valid reason to exclude studies even though it can be argued that the self evaluation may inherit larger variability than that from the practitioners. To obtain an unambiguous analysis, a good practice is to develop an integrative analysis plan to prespecify criteria for study selection.

The following step is to select a statistical method to evaluate the evidence collectively. Patient-level meta-analyses to poll studies have been popular approaches and are desirable if the number of studies is large and all studies are similarly designed. The collective evidence approach can be desirable in situations when it is important to understand the individual study results and consistency among them; also when differences in study design prohibit study pooling and cause difficulties in interpretation for meta-analyses.

The collective evidence approach for independent studies is relatively easy to use and interpret. To illustrate, take another hypothetical example of a set of *p* values from three independent studies. The evaluation could be simple if the results satisfy the decision rule for $K = 3$, $(\gamma_1, \gamma_2, \gamma_3) = (0.025, 0.025, 0.100)$. The error rate should be controlled at the level of 0.000156 based on $P(\bigcap_{k=1}^{3} p_{(k)} \leq \gamma_k) = 6\gamma_1\gamma_2\gamma_3 - 3\gamma_3\gamma_1^2 - 3\gamma_2^2\gamma_1 + \gamma_1^3$. If the observed *p* values were *0.001, 0.020*, and *0.120*, it would be necessary to calculate the inflation and consistency using Formulas (10.2) and (10.3). The % inflation and consistency is 24.0 and 58.9 %, respectively. Suppose that the results were obtained from three studies used to support allergic conjunctivitis and redness was the primary endpoint. Further, assume that the endpoint was assessed by the patients in the study yielding the *p* value of 0.120 and the other two were assessed by physicians. If patients were less trained, the reporting variability could be larger than the clinician reported outcomes. Hence, the level of inflation and consistency could be considered reasonable for recommending approval. Even if the endpoints were assessed consistently in all three studies, such results might reflect a possible situation that the drug worked for certain patients that were included in the studies, perhaps not consistently. Depending upon the consistency level and the observed maximum *p* value, it might be useful to further investigate who were more likely to benefit from the drug and who were not.

10.4.2 Multiple Doses to Support Efficacy Evaluation

The evaluation of multiple doses may serve two different purposes: the efficacy evaluation and the selection of the optimal doses. Discussion in this chapter is focused on the efficacy evaluation only.

A typical multiple dose study design includes parallel arms of several doses and placebo where MAPs are traditionally applied. As a result of the stringent significance levels by controlling the type I error, the sample sizes for each arm need to be increased. The application of MAPs could limit the enthusiasm and feasibility to include multiple doses, which are imperative for better understanding of the efficacy as well as dose–response relationship.

It could be suggested that the MAPs for multiple doses in individual studies do not appear to be useful in either efficacy evaluation or the identification of the optimal doses. The fact that all doses show the trend of efficacy is strong evidence against an

Table 10.3 Illustration of strategies of evaluating two doses in two studies using the practical collective evidence approach

	p values		Strategy 1		Strategy 2	
Study	High dose	Low dose	Trend test	Inflate error for studies	Inflated error for dose	Inflated error for studies
1	0.028	0.015	0.023	0.000625 (0 %)	0.028	0.000775 (24 %)
2	0.024	0.013	0.021		0.025	

ineffective drug. It can be even stronger evidence if a reasonable dose–response relationship is demonstrated consistently in multiple studies. Some believe that MAPs are necessary for identifying the effective doses. The counter argument could be made that if a drug is efficacious, many of the dose levels should be efficacious. Whether the dose levels can reach statistical significance is a matter of sample size and treatment difference. Instead of identifying the efficacious doses by the significance, a helpful strategy is to determine the optimal doses, which should be based on the risk–benefit profiles, effect sizes, and other information. If p values play any roles in the identification of the optimal doses, the rank of the p values is usually sufficient. It is unnecessary to use any adjusted p values because the rank of either adjusted or unadjusted p values is the same.

An exception to keep in mind is that certain drugs may have a narrow therapeutic window where many doses may not support the efficacy. In those cases, the understanding of the dose–response relationship is more important than adjusting p values. The efficacy can then be established by a consistent dose–response relationship in multiple studies.

Evaluation of multiple doses should depend upon the study design. For a typical phase III study, two or three doses that are likely to be the optimal doses are selected based on information from early phase studies. It is expected that all doses would demonstrate efficacy to a certain degree. Two strategies are discussed to evaluate multiple doses collectively. The first one is to use directional tests to establish the efficacy by modeling the dose–response trend. This requires a good understanding of the true dose–response which could be obtained from early phases of clinical studies. Guidance on the directional tests, also referred to as the trend tests, is discussed by Li and Lagakos (Li and Lagakos [11]). When multiple studies are available, the trend tests should be first performed within individual studies. Then the p values obtained from the trend tests should be evaluated using the practical collective evidence approach. The second strategy is to evaluate the multiple doses within the individual studies first by using the practical collective evidence approach, then to evaluate the evidence across studies. The two strategies are illustrated in the following hypothetical example, using two studies with two doses in each study. The p values of high and low doses of the two studies as well as the results of the two strategies are listed in Table 10.3.

- To illustrate strategy 1, assume from early phase studies that decreased trend was observed as the dose increased. The pseudo-dose indicators were coded as

2 for the low dose and 1 for the high dose. The p values of the trend tests were hypothetical values, 0.023 and 0.021 for studies 1 and 2, respectively. The results satisfied the two-study decision rule $(\gamma_1, \gamma_2) = (0.025, 0.025)$.

- To illustrate strategy 2, the worst inflated error for multiple doses for each study was calculated first. The decision rule used for two doses was $(\gamma_1, \gamma_2) = (0.025, 0.025)$. The worst inflated error due to two doses for study 1 was 0.028, a result by assuming the worst possible correlation between two doses (a very conservative approach). Similarly, the worst inflation for study 2 was 0.025. The worst inflation for two studies was then calculated as 0.000775 with 24 % inflation. The consistency was 8.4 %. If the correlation between two doses was known or can be estimated, the inflated error could be calculated relatively accurately and should be smaller than that presented in Table 10.3. It can be concluded that the evidence of efficacy is convincing.

If MAPs are applied to this example, depending upon the choice of the procedure, it is likely that results in study 1 are considered inconclusive. The statistical decision rules across studies are unavailable.

Strategy 1 should also be considered when many doses are included in a single study, such as phase II dose ranging studies. Strategy 1 should be particularly useful for drugs with narrow therapeutic windows where a nonlinear dose–response trend could be specified.

10.4.3 Multiple Endpoints

Diseases are multifaceted entities where one endpoint is usually insufficient to describe a certain aspect of a disease or reflect disease changes. Therefore, multiple endpoints are used in clinical studies. Endpoints are chosen based on the study objectives, usually the indications for drugs. For example, a drug approved for chronic obstruction pulmonary disease (COPD) can have indications as a bronchodilator, to reduce exacerbation, or to prolong survival. Each indication is evaluated by a set of prespecified endpoints. The endpoints are usually organized as the primary, secondary, and exploratory endpoints in the study protocols. The primary endpoints are defined by the medical communities, including the FDA, and are crucial for the approval of drug indications. The selection of the secondary endpoints is relatively flexible and may depend upon the secondary objectives or features relevant to the primary endpoints and a particular drug. The exploratory endpoints may be less relevant to the indication and often are included in the study for other purposes.

In efficacy evaluations, the primary endpoints must demonstrate clinically and statistically significant benefits in order for the indication to gain approval. The secondary endpoints should be supportive of the primary endpoints by showing trend of treatment benefit. Clearly, the primary and secondary endpoints play different roles and have different expectations in efficacy evaluation. The natural hierarchical order among the different types of endpoints implies that the secondary endpoints would not contribute any additional error in the efficacy evaluation for a specific indication. Hence, no MAPs are needed because of the hierarchical structure of the different types of endpoints for evaluating a specific indication.

In the labeling process, the primary endpoints of the approved indication are always described in the label. What is less clear is the selection of the secondary endpoints. Again, because of the natural hierarchical order, MAPs are not needed for the different types of endpoints in labeling process. However, MAPs may be considered for the multiple secondary endpoints in labeling. This is discussed in detail in a later section.

10.4.4 Co-Primary Endpoints

Often more than one primary endpoint is used to evaluate a disease condition. European Medicines Agency (EMEA) (Committee for Proprietary Medical Products (CPMP) by EMEA [4]) requires all co-primary endpoints to be statistically significant at the level of one-sided 0.025. The limitation of this approach is that as more co-primary endpoints are used, it becomes more difficult to show all endpoints statistically significant. The ordinary least squares (OLS) and generalized least squares (GLS) tests proposed by O'Brien (O'Brien [15]) consider consolidating all co-primary endpoints into one test. Another practice is to develop one composite primary endpoint by combining all co-primary endpoints. The problems of the composite endpoints are widely discussed in the literature (Kip et al. [8]; Montori et al. [13]). The main problem of the O'Brien's OLS and GLS tests as well as the composite endpoints is that they may disguise the heterogeneity in treatment responses among the co-primary endpoints.

The approach of collective evidence is similar to EMEA's approach which emphasizes the understanding of individual performance of all co-primary endpoints. The collective evidence approach simply recognizes the room of flexibility when controlling the error rate of wrongly rejecting the null hypotheses. When there are multiple studies, similar to the case of multiple doses, the collective evidence of the co-primary endpoints is to first calculate the maximum inflated error within each study. Using the maximum inflated error of the individual studies, the maximum inflated error for all studies is then calculated as well as the consistency index. Again, a hypothetical example is used to illustrate the application in a scenario of two studies using two co-primary endpoints. The p values as well as the results of applying the practical collective evidence approach are listed in Table 10.4.

10.4.5 Secondary Endpoints

This section focuses on the discussion of controlling the error rate of labeling false information due to multiple secondary endpoints. Often, the statistically significant

Table 10.4 Illustration of evaluating two co-primary endpoints using the practical collective evidence approach

Study	Primary 1	Primary 2	Inflated error of co-primary endpoints at the level of 0.025	Inflated error of two studies at the level of 0.000625
1	0.023	0.030	0.030	0.000875 (40 %)
2	0.018	0.025	0.025	

secondary endpoints are labeled. With such practice, the more endpoints that are evaluated, the higher chance to show statistical significance. For this reason, it may be necessary to use MAPs to control the error rate of labeling false information, however, not within individual studies when multiple studies are available.

Without loss of generality, the case of two studies is illustrated. Suppose that both studies evaluate Endpoints A and B. Let A_1 and A_2 represent the results of Endpoint A from study 1 and study 2, respectively, and B_1 and B_2 for Endpoint B from study 1 and study 2, respectively. If a MAP is used in the individual studies, the logic should be written as

$$(A_1 \cup B_1) \cap (A_2 \cup B_2) = A_1A_2 \cup A_1B_2 \cup A_2B_1 \cup B_1B_2$$

The logic controls the error rate for four possible outcomes A_1A_2, A_1B_2, A_2B_1, and B_1B_2 that have the potential to become statistically significant or positive, when they are in fact false. With a close look of the four possible outcomes, it is only possible to claim A_1A_2 or B_1B_2, as they represent the situations where the same endpoint is significant in both studies. The outcomes A_1B_2 and A_2B_1 would never be considered in the label in reality as they represent the cases that endpoint A is significant in one study as well as B is significant in the other. Thus, it is unnecessary to control the error that would never be committed.

Alternatively, if each endpoint is first evaluated across studies collectively, the only possible outcomes are A_1A_2 or B_1B_2. Then it makes sense to apply MAPs to control error due to the two possible outcomes to make claim. For instance, if the error rate of labeling false information should be controlled at the level of 0.025 and there are ten secondary endpoints, applying the Bonferrion correction, each endpoint should be controlled at $\alpha(H_0^{1/K}) = 0.0025$ for K studies. Notice that it is not recommended that the level of error rate for the secondary endpoints be as stringent as the error rate of wrongly approving an ineffective drug. The mistake of wrongly approving an ineffective drug is a more serious matter than that of labeling a false endpoint. In practice, p values that are significant at level of 0.025 consistently across studies are labeled, which is more stringent than necessary. Hence, the adjustment with MAPs may not be necessary unless the number of secondary endpoints is in the scale of hundreds and more.

Often, it is useful to order the secondary endpoints based on the clinical importance in the integrative statistical analysis plan. This is equivalent to using the closed testing procedure on the secondary endpoints. So, the clinically more relevant endpoints are labeled if there is consistently convincing evidence across studies.

It can be further debated whether only placing the significant secondary endpoints in drug labels is an efficient way of communicating drug information. For clinically important secondary endpoints, the statistically insignificant results may be as important to share as the significant ones with patients and practitioners. Insignificant results may inform practitioners that the drug has not shown convincing evidence on certain clinically important secondary endpoints.

10.4.6 Multiple Tests

In this chapter, multiple tests are referred to as performing multiple analyses on the same endpoint and using the same set of data, which is different from the multiple tests for different endpoints, such as gene analyses. Multiple tests are commonly used in clinical studies and usually structured as the primary analysis and secondary analyses (or sensitivity analyses). The primary endpoints are often analyzed using multiple methods, usually with the prespecified primary analysis in an intent-to-treat (ITT) population and several secondary analyses. The multiple tests are used to ensure a good understanding of the treatment benefit from the primary analysis and relatively consistent evidence across all tests.

It is important that all the primary and secondary analyses should be valid and reasonable analyses. Valid analyses are unbiased under null. Reasonable analyses are those that the power under alternative is not seriously distorted and the treatment benefit is not overly underestimated or exaggerated. For example, baseline-carry-forward is sometimes used in missing data imputation and a valid analysis under null. However, this approach may not be a reasonable analysis as it could be overly conservative and the test result would be biased towards null if the treatment is to prevent disease from deterioration. In other scenarios, the approach could exaggerate the treatment difference if the disease symptoms can be improved over time without treatment. The worst-case-carry-forward approach is another valid test under null; however, it is not considered reasonable, as it could overly exaggerate the treatment differences under alternatives in certain scenarios. Another valid test is the test for proportions. It may not be a reasonable test when there are differential dropouts between treatment arms, perhaps due to toxicities.

It may not be equitable that the primary analysis is the most powerful analysis or the only important analysis in making conclusion. This is particularly true when handling missing outcome data. Often missing outcome data are missing-not-at-random and there is not one imputation approach that is better than others. The good practice is to prespecify one imputation method for the primary analysis. Multiple methods, served as sensitivity analyses, are used to confirm that the result of the primary analysis does not deviate from other imputation methods too much and that the impact of the missing data is small. In addition, the totality of evidence obtained from multiple tests may enhance the understanding of treatment difference. For example, the family of weighted log-rank tests and the proportional hazard model are all similarly structured (Harrington and Fleming [6]) and are valid tests under null, but can be sensitive to different types of treatment differences revealed in the data. The commonly used log-rank test, the unweighted test, is more sensitive to differences manifested later than the Wilcoxin log-rank test which is more sensitive to differences exhibited earlier. The discussion here is not to undermine the importance of prespecifying the primary analysis. Prespecifying one primary analysis is particularly important when reporting the results in publications and drug labels. The rule of thumb is to report the primary analysis, rather than by picking the best results among all analyses, while all analysis results should be taken into consideration for decision making and interpretation.

It can also be argued that multiple tests may not necessarily inflate the type I error rate, given that all tests are reasonable and valid. A valid test has a 0.025 chance to reach statistical significance under null. The chance for the majority of the tests to show statistical significance together cannot be larger than 0.025 under null. Following the principle of collective evidence, it would not be convincing evidence if only one test shows a significant result, while other analyses lack statistical significance. Conversely, the evidence would be considered convincing if the majority of the tests reveal statistically significant (or close to) results.

10.5 Case Studies

10.5.1 Case 1: The Primary Endpoint Failed

All relevant information discussed in this case can be found in the FDA advisory briefing package (US [21]). Spiriva Handihaler (tiotropium) was first approved for maintenance treatment of COPD based on forced exploratory volume in 1 second (FEV_1). In 2009, the sponsor submitted the results of a study titled understanding the potential long-term impacts on function with tiotropium (UPLIFT) seeking several usage indications, among them, COPD exacerbation. UPLIFT was a randomized, double-blinded, and placebo-controlled multicenter study. A total of 5993 COPD patients were randomly assigned to tiotropium or placebo in a 1:1 ratio, 2987 to tiotropium and 3006 to placebo. The patients were treated over a 4-year period. Another 6-month study that was conducted in approximately 2000 COPD veterans (VA) was also available. The exacerbation results of the two studies are summarized in Table 10.5. As can be seen from Table 10.5, the primary endpoint for exacerbation, the time from randomization to the first exacerbation episode, was statistically significant in both studies. The average risk reduction over time in both studies was about 15 % in tiotropium in comparison to placebo. All the secondary endpoints listed in Table 10.5 were statistically significant at the two-sided level of 0.050. Despite the statistically significant results shown in two studies, the approval of the exacerbation indication was debated among FDA's statistical reviewers and in the advisory committee meeting.

Table 10.5 Summary of exacerbation results in the UPLIFT and VA studies

	UPLIFT			VA study		
	Tio $N=2986$	Placebo $N=3006$	Ratio (p val)	Tio $N=914$	Placebo $N=915$	Ratio (p val)
Median time (month)	16.7	12.5	0.86 (<0.001)	–	–	0.83 (0.034)
Total # of events	6691	7183	–	376	446	–
Rate (#/p-y)	0.73	0.85	0.86 (<0.001)	0.71	0.88	0.81 (0.037)
# of exacerbation days/p-y	12.1	13.6	0.89 (0.001)	10.0	12.6	0.79 (0.056)

The complication was that the primary endpoint of the UPLIFT study was the rates of decline in FEV_1. UPLIFT failed to show any difference in rates of decline in FEV_1. Exacerbation was a secondary endpoint in the UPLIFT study. Furthermore, the study prespecified a closed testing procedure requiring that the primary endpoints show statistically significant treatment differences before testing the secondary endpoints.

Following the prespecified decision rule, it was argued that because the primary endpoint failed, the secondary endpoints should no longer be tested for the reason of protecting type I error. Consequently, there was no sufficient evidence for the exacerbation indication.

An opposing view stated that overly emphasizing the prespecified statistical decision rules could be problematic, and the fact that multiple studies were available could have reduced the need to use the decision rule. The prespecified decision rule was not necessarily scientifically valid as it was based on the expectation to the study, which was a hypothesis to be tested. The gambling nature of the prespecified decision rule made the selection appear to be arbitrary. In UPLIFT, the study allowed patients to take any COPD treatments available in the market. The expectation of tiotropium slowing down the deterioration of pulmonary function at the design stage may no longer be valid over the course of the study as COPD treatments evolved over time. Furthermore, when multiple studies were available, the error rate of wrongly approving an indication could be tightly protected.

The advisory committee voted to approve the exacerbation indication. This case exemplified the arbitrary nature of the prespecified decision rules. If the Bonferroni procedure was prespecified, no one would question the efficacy on exacerbation for the exact same study results. The lesson learned is that the evidence-based drug evaluation should not rely on the prespecified decision rule, particularly when multiple studies are available. The collective evidence approach can be useful in post hoc evaluation. In this case, when applying the practical approach proposed in this chapter, as both the UPLIFT and VA studies were statistically significant at the 2-sided level of 0.050, there was no error inflation with the decision rule $(\gamma_1, \gamma_2) = (0.025, 0.025)$.

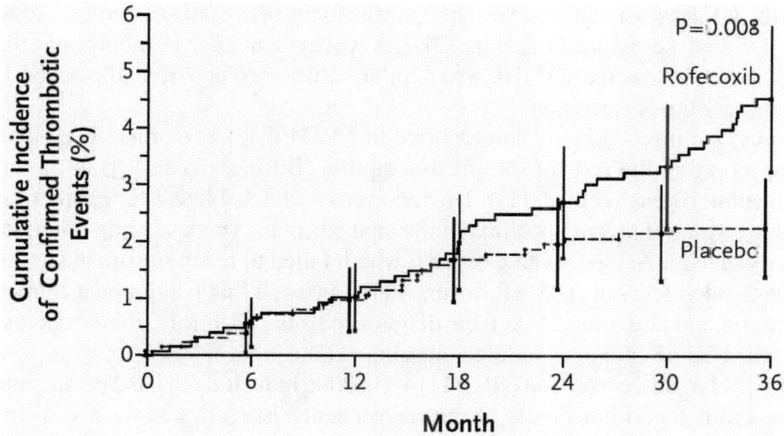

Fig. 10.3 Cumulative CV events curves observed in APPROVe

The error rate of wrongly approving an ineffective drug was indeed tightly protected at the level of 0.000625. The fact that all secondary endpoints were highly significant in both studies further supported the efficacy of tiotropium for treating exacerbation.

10.5.2 Case 2: Dispute on Vioxx (rofecoxib) Cardiovascular Risk

Rofecoxib is a COX-2 agent that was first approved by the FDA in 1999 and withdrawn from market in 2004 due to cardiovascular risk findings in the adenomatous polyp prevention on Vioxx (APPROVe) study (Bresalier et al. [1]). The APPROVe study was a randomized, double-blinded, parallel-grouped, and placebo-controlled study to evaluate the occurrence of neoplastic polyps in patients with a history of colorectal adenomas. Eligible patients were randomized to rofecoxib 25 mg daily or placebo in a 1:1 ratio; 1287 receiving rofecoxib 25 mg and 1299 receiving placebo. At a planed interim analysis, 46 patients developed at least 1 confirmed thrombotic event over 3059 patient-year in the rofecoxib group, and 26 events over 3327 patient-year in the placebo group. The hazard ratio was 1.92 (p value = 0.008) and the cardiovascular risk (CV) risk in rofecoxib was statistically significantly greater compared with placebo. The cumulative incidence curves of the confirmed thrombotic events of the two groups were shown in Fig. 10.3 (Bresalier et al. [1]).

The APPROVe results were published in 2005 in the *New England Journal of Medicine* (NEJM) (Bresalier et al. [1]). In the paper, it was stated that a test of the proportional-hazard (PH) assumption, evaluating the interaction between the treatment and a time logarithm, was specified in the statistical analysis plan for analyzing the cardiovascular risk. Based on this test, the p value of the interaction was statistically significant (two-sided p value = 0.010). It was therefore concluded that the CV risk between the two groups was not proportional over time. Additional post hoc analyses indicated that the CV risk was evident after 18 months of rofecoxib treatment, whereas the CV risk was similar between rofecoxib and placebo for the first 18 months of treatment.

Later, the investigation team reported to NEJM that an error had been identified when reporting the test for the PH assumption (Business Wire [2]) in the original publication (Bresalier et al. [1]). The reported result used linear time rather than the time logarithm that was specified in the analysis plan. The test using the time logarithm yielded a 2-sided p value of 0.07, which failed to reach statistical significance at the 2-sided level of 0.05. However, Merck insisted that using linear time was an appropriate analysis based on their diagnostic tests. Therefore, their conclusion of CV risk after 18 months would be unchanged (Business Wire [2]).

NEJM issued a correction (NEJM [14]) in 2006 indicating that the prespecified test using a time logarithm should be the correct analysis. As this analysis did not reach statistical significance, the PH assumption was not rejected. Therefore, a conclusion about the CV risk of rofecoxib should not be made for treatment after 18 months.

An important lesson learned from this case is the interpretation of multiple tests of the PH assumption. Both tests, using linear time or logarithm of time, are valid and reasonable tests. The prespecified test is not necessarily the best test. On the other hand, it is a good statistical practice to report data using the prespecified test. In disputing the PH assumption, although the test using a time logarithm does not reach statistical significance at the two-sided level of 0.05, a p value of 0.07 was considered marginally significant. Adding the evidence from the test using linear time, which was statistically significant, the totality of evidence demonstrated that the CV risk ratio was not constant over time. However, the fact that risk ratio was not constant over time did not infer the absence of the CV risk in the first 18 months of the rofecoxib treatment. The interaction tests simply could not answer if rofecoxib caused harm in the first 18 months of treatment.

It is important to reemphasize that the collective evidence approach is not to abandon the prespecification and planning. On the contrast, careful planning and designing experiments, prespecifying the experiment procedures, hierarchy of endpoints, the primary analyses, and all other secondary or sensitivity analyses, as well as safety measures and evaluation are imperative for achieving scientific rigor. However, throughout the discussion of the chapter, prespecifying a decision rule in a study appears to add more confusion in drug evaluation.

10.6 Remarks

Drug evaluation is a complex process that involves multidisciplines including medical, drug safety, statistical, clinical pharmacology, chemistry, and preclinical reviews. The decision is based on collective evidence from all disciplines, a different level of synthesizing evidence collectively. Still, drug efficacy is the key element, as none of the other evaluations would be necessary if a drug was ineffective. This explains why there have been significant efforts to develop statistical methodologies to define systematic approaches to control the error of wrongly approving an ineffective drug. The collective evidence approach is an effort to enrich and improve the systematic approaches.

The collective evidence approach reintroduces the "AND" logic which has been overlooked in drug evaluation. With this foundation, the approach takes all available evidence in decision making, controls various errors occurring in drug evaluation, balances the need for consistency among evidence, and allows reasonable variation. The proposed practical approach may reduce the burden of arbitrarily selecting prespecified decision rules in the individual study protocols. It is noteworthy that this approach does not relax the standard of drug approval; rather it provides an alternative way of evaluating evidence with proven scientific rigor.

Rigidly using the collective evidence approach can also be problematic. As discussed earlier, drugs having narrow therapeutic windows may not have multiple doses supporting the efficacy. However, the collective evidence approach can be applied to examine if a consistent dose–response relationship is exhibited in multiple studies. The application of the collective evidence approach may need special care in drug safety evaluation as well. The safety evaluation usually takes a less conservative approach. On one hand, the risk signal that occurred in one study or one dose can be valuable information for practitioners and patients. On the other hand, a trend of risks consistently occurring in multiple studies, albeit statistically insignificant, can raise serious concerns.

This discussion does not cover the multiplicity issues occurring in subgroup analyses, multiregion studies, and interim analyses. The problems noted in such situations may not all be simple multiplicity problems. Nevertheless, the principles of the collective evidence approach can be applied in evaluating evidence when these multiplicity issues occur.

For future research in the area of collective evidence, utility function can be an alternative approach to summarizing evidence collectively. Eriksen and Keller (Eriksen and Keller [5]) proposed a quantitative way of combining evidence from clinical efficacy and safety data to preclinical safety data of drugs using utility function. This idea can be extended to combine multiple endpoints, multiple doses, and multiple studies. More research needs to be done to further develop this approach.

Acknowledgment The author would like to thank a referee's thoughtful comments and constructive suggestions.

References

Bresalier RS, Sandler RS, Quan H (2005) Cardiovascular events associated with rofecoxib in a colorectal adenoma chemoprevention trial. NEJM 352(11):1092–102

Business Wire (2006) Merck corrects description of a statistical method used in APPROVe study—study results unchanged. http://www.businesswire.com/news/home/20060-

530005860/en/Merck-Corrects-Description-Statistical-Method-APPROVe-Study. Accessed 30 May 2006
Chuang-Stein C, Stryszak P, Dmitrienko A et al. (2007) Challenge of multiple co-primary endpoints: a new approach. Stat Med 26:1181–1192
Committee for Proprietary Medical Products (CPMP) by EMEA (2001) Points to consider on multiplicity issues in clinical trials. Biometrical J 43:1039–1048
Eriksen S, Keller R (1993) A multi-attribute-utility-function approach to aeighing the risks and benefits of pharmaceutical agent. Med Decis Mak 13:188–125
Harrington DP, Fleming TR (1982) A class of rank test procedures for censored survival data. Biometrika 69:133–143
Hochberg Y (1988) A sharper Bonferroni procedure for multiple tests of significance. Biometrika 75:800–802
Kip KE, Hollabaugh K, Marroquin OC et al. (2008) The problem with composite end points in cardiovascular studies. J Am Coll Cardiol 51(7):701–707
Li QH (2009) Evaluating co-primary endpoints collectively in clinical trials. Biometrical J 51(1):137–145
Li QH, Huque MF (2003) A decision rule for evaluating several independent clinical trials collectively. J Biopharm Stat 13:621–628
Li QH, Lagakos SW (2006) On the Relationship between directional and omnibus statistical tests. Scand J Stat 33:239–246
Marcus R, Peritz E, Gabriel KR (1976) On closed testing procedures with special reference to ordered analysis of variance. Biometrika 63:655–660
Montori VM, Permanyer-Miralda G, Ferreira-González I et al. (2005) Validity of composite end points in clinical trials. BMJ 330:594–596
NEJM (2006) Correction on cardiovascular events associated with rofecoxib in a colorectal adenoma chemoprevention trial. NEJM 355:221
O'Brien PC (1984) Procedures for comparing samples with multiple endpoints. Biometrics 40:1079–1087
Pocock SJ (1997) Clinical trials with multiple outcomes: a statistical perspective on their design, analysis, and interpretation. Control Clin Trials 18(6):530–545
Proschan MA, Waclawiw MA (2000) Practical guidelines for multiplicity adjustment in clinical trials. Control Clin Trials 2:527–539
Shih WJ, Quan H (1999) Planning and analysis of repeated measures at key time-points in clinical trials sponsored by pharmaceutical companies. Stat Med 18:961–973
US FDA (1995) Statement regarding the demonstration of effectiveness of human drug products and devices. Fed Regist 60:39180–39181 (Docket No. 9500230) Accessed 1 Aug 1995
US FDA (1998) Guidance for industry providing clinical evidence of effectiveness for human drug and biological products. http://www.fda.gov/downloads/Drugs/.../Guidances/ucm078749.pdf. Accessed May 1998
US FDA (2009) Pulmonary-allergy drugs advisory committee package. http://www.fda.gov/downloads/advisorycommittees/committeesmeetingmaterials/drugs/pulmonary-allergydrugs-advisorycommittee/ucm190463.pdf Briefing package. Accessed 19 Nov 2009

Chapter 11
Applications of Probability of Study Success in Clinical Drug Development

Ming-Dauh Wang

Abstract The dominant approach to sample size determination for a clinical trial in regulatory review-driven pharmaceutical research has long been by assuming fixed values of parameters under competing hypotheses, i.e., null versus alternative representing futility and desired efficaciousness of a tested drug. A sample size is then determined to ensure sufficient statistical power for differentiating between the null and alternative hypotheses, while controlling the probability of wrongly rejecting the null. This approach bears the criticism of ignoring the variability inherent with the unknown parameters. To improve sample size determination, accounting for variability of parameters has recently been gaining application in pharmaceutical-conducted clinical trials. The common intent of this increased interest is to better predict the probability of a successful trial, which is often termed probability of study success (PrSS) or probability of success (POS). We discuss the important role that PrSS can play in clinical trial design and decision making throughout medical product development. A few examples are given for illustration.

11.1 Introduction

The dominant approach to sample size determination (SSD) for a clinical trial in regulatory review-driven pharmaceutical research has long been by assuming fixed values of parameters under the competing hypotheses. Although the approach is straightforward, and in many cases a formula can be readily applied for a quick sample size calculation, it bears the criticism of oversimplifying assumptions by overlooking the inherent uncertainty of the assumptions. This would inevitably bias, either over or under, the sample size needed for providing the expected power for achieving the study goal. Along with other statistical measures to improve efficiency of drug development (O'Neill 2006), this long-recognized issue has now emerged as a topic for a serious consideration.

M.-D. Wang (✉)
Eli Lilly and Company, Indianapolis, USA
e-mail: wang_ming-dauh@lilly.com

Z. Chen et al. (eds.), *Applied Statistics in Biomedicine and Clinical Trials Design*,
ICSA Book Series in Statistics, DOI 10.1007/978-3-319-12694-4_11

As alternatives to the conventional approach, methods that incorporate variability of parameters in SSD are gaining popularity in pharmaceutical research. A natural approach to consideration of parameter variability in SSD is incorporating it through a Bayesian framework, which in the clinical trial setting has been recently termed probability of study success (PrSS) (Wang et al. 2013), probability of success (POS) (Chuang-Stein 2006), or assurance (O'Hagan et al. 2005; Bobbs and Carlin 2008). Although its use in drug development, especially in registration studies, has only happened recently (Wang et al. 2013; Chuang-Stein 2006), Bayesian SSD has been a topic of research for decades (Raiffa and Schlaifer 1961; Spiegelhalter and Freedman 1986; Adcock 1988; Weiss 1997; Wang and Gelfand 2002). The growing application of PrSS in the pharmaceutical industry is also encouraged by the increasing openness of regulators toward the use of Bayesian methods in pharmaceutical research (Price and LaVange 2014). Despite the fact that Bayesian analysis for confirmatory trials intended for drug approval is still controversial, Bayesian SSD for designing confirmatory trials has been found acceptable. Moreover, information-based Bayesian SSD for exploratory trials not intended for registration tends to foster efficiency in preregistration drug development.

Bayesian SSD or PrSS is considered in this chapter for the case of hypothesis testing. The Bayesian perspective of the sample size of a trial is in the probability that the trial is predicted to achieve the intended hypothesis with the given sample size, not conditional on fixed parameter values, but based on prior-based Bayesian inference. For a registration trial that uses a frequentist test of hypothesis for analysis of the primary endpoint, the interest is in the predictive probability of the trial giving a statistically significant test result. Thus, it is a Bayesian–frequentist mixed prediction, which can also be applied to designing exploratory trials in lieu of a conventional frequentist sample size calculation. Alternatively, a purely Bayesian approach to SSD employs Bayesian inference also in the final analysis. An inferential framework of Bayesian SSD is developed in Sect. 11.2. The Bayesian approaches are illustrated with some clinical trial applications in Sect. 11.3. Concluding remarks are given in Sect. 11.4.

11.2 Bayesian Inference of PrSS

11.2.1 Hypothesis Testing as the Objective of a Clinical Trial

Consider a clinical trial that is conducted to test the effect of an experimental drug (treatment 1) on an endpoint of interest in comparison with another treatment (treatment 2), with the measurement of the endpoint denoted by X_i for treatment $i, i = 1, 2$. The distribution of X_i is assumed to be defined by parameter $\theta_i, i = 1, 2$, where both X_i and θ_i could be multidimensional. Suppose the trial is designed to test a null hypothesis $H_0 : \mathcal{M}(\theta_1, \theta_2) \in R$ against the alternative $H_a : \mathcal{M}(\theta_1, \theta_2) \in R^c$, where $\mathcal{M}$ is a metric that measures the distance between θ_1 and θ_2, R is a subspace in the Euclidean space, and R^c is the complement of R in the space. With n_i patients enrolled

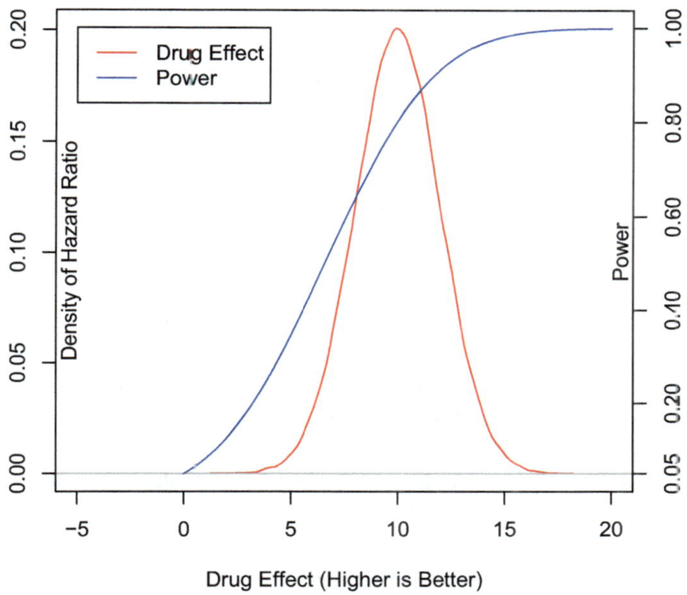

Fig. 11.1 Illustration of probability of study success (PrSS)

to receive treatment i, let $X_i = \{X_{i1}, \ldots, X_{in_i}\}, i = 1, 2$ be data observed at the end of the study. For ease of presentation denote $X = \{X_i, i = 1, 2\}$, $\theta = \{\theta_i, i = 1, 2\}$, and $\boldsymbol{n} = \{n_i, i = 1, 2\}$.

Suppose a test statistic $T(X)$ is prespecified in the statistical analysis plan for the test statistic to test H_a against H_0 at the end of the trial, given α as the level of type 1 error rate typical of regulatory requirement. Usually, fixed values of θ under H_0 and H_a are assumed for sample size calculation without consideration of their variability. For example, the difference $\Delta = \theta_1 - \theta_2$ (assumed univariate) is often of interest, and $H_0 : \Delta = \Delta_0$ is tested again $H_a : \Delta = \Delta_a$. A conventional method of SSD would calculate the $\boldsymbol{n}$ that gives at least a probability of $1 - \beta$ (or power) for exhibiting $T(X) > t_\alpha$ under H_a, where t_α is the $100(1-\alpha)$th percentile of T under H_0. To note, Δ_0 is often a pre-set value agreed upon by the sponsor and the regulatory agency, and Δ_a is commonly chosen as representing the clinically desired value. The power thus calculated is highly dependent on the assumed value of Δ_a. Figure 11.1 illustrates the dependence.

11.2.2 Prediction of PrSS for Determination of Sample Size

Instead of assuming fixed values, a distribution (red curve in Fig. 11.1) that reflects up-to-date knowledge of θ can be assumed. Then the mean of the power (blue curve in Fig. 11.1) over the distribution is more representative of what the trial can offer, which is the PrSS. Using the more general notation, let the prior distribution of θ be denoted as $\pi(\theta)$. At the time of designing a trial, the data X is yet unobserved, which is predicted given the prior $\pi(\theta)$ and the assumed density $f(x|\theta)$. That is, the predictive density of X is derived by

$$\tilde{f}(x) \propto \int f(x|\theta)\pi(\theta)d\theta.$$

Then the PrSS is defined as

$$PrSS = \int I\{T_0(x) > t_\alpha|x\}\tilde{f}(x)dx, \quad (11.1)$$

where T_0 is the statistical test under H_0, and I is the indication function. The sample size is then selected to ensure PrSS is greater than a minimum accepted threshold γ.

By considering uncertainty of assumptions, the PrSS is typically lower than the power that would result from a conventional power calculation for a given sample size. It indicates that conventional SSD tends to over-estimate the power of a trial, and the PrSS approach would better reflect the ability of a trial in achieving the intended objective. Notwithstanding the downward adjustment by PrSS, our recommendation is to keep the same standards for the PrSS approach as would be for a conventional calculation, e.g., $\gamma = 0.9$ for a registration trial and $\gamma = 0.7$ for a phase 2 trial.

The PrSS concept has been earlier proposed and applied to conducting interim analysis of an ongoing trial (Spiegelhalter et al. 2004; Dmitrienko and Wang 2006; Wang 2007), which is called the "predictive power" approach, as an alternative to the "conditional power" approach (Posch and Hunsberger 1995). Application of the methodology to clinical trial design could be seen as a special case of its use for interim analysis, as no interim data are available for update and the prediction of needed sample size is purely based on pre-study prior knowledge. This frequentist and Bayesian mixed approach is more appropriate for registration-oriented clinical trials because frequentist analysis for the primary endpoint is usually required. As long as control of type 1 error is shown to be adequately maintained and measures for guarding patient safety are well addressed, this approach for determining the sample size for a registration trial is not opposed by regulatory agencies (Wang et al. 2013).

Though a frequentist test and its resulting p value are still generally required for judging the success of a trial intended for regulatory approval, for preregistration drug development, p values are often not conducive to decision making. An alternative is to also conduct Bayesian analysis at the end of the study that would provide a statement about θ in terms of probability, which is easier to use in deciding on subsequent steps for the drug in development. In our notation, this posterior probability is $Pr(\theta \in H_a|X)$, which is the updated probability of the alternative hypothesis at the end of the trial and would indicate success of the trial if it is higher than another pre-specified threshold $\eta > 0$. Upon observing $X = x$ at the end of the trial, $Pr(\theta \in H_a|X)$ is realized as

$$Pr(\theta \in H_a|x) = \int I\{\theta \in H_a\}g(\theta|x)d\theta,$$

where

$$g(\theta|x) \propto f(x|\theta)\pi^*(\theta)$$

if another prior $\pi^*(\theta)$ is used for the final analysis. Then SSD is made by the calculation of PrSS expressed by

$$PrSS = \int I\{Pr(\theta \in H_a|x) > \eta\}\tilde{f}(x)dx, \quad (11.2)$$

so as to meet the preselected threshold probability γ. For differentiation $\pi(\theta)$ used for pre-study design is called the design prior and $\pi^*(\theta)$ assigned for final analysis is called the analysis prior (Brutti et al. 2008). Different opinions are held for whether the two priors should be assumed different. We recommend that for a registration trial the sponsor utilizes the most objective knowledge about θ to form the prior at the design stage. Meanwhile, to avoid concern about too much subjectivity, a non-informative prior is suggested for the analysis.

Returning to the previous comment on the downward adjusting property of PrSS by the predictive power approach in comparison with conventionally calculated power, the statement still holds true if the analysis prior is non-informative. However, more informative and optimistic priors for analysis could swing PrSS upward.

Although analytical formulas may be derived for simple cases, PrSS can generally be approximated by simulation. For the predictive power approach in (11.1), the algorithm for a given sample size $\boldsymbol{n}$ is:

1. Simulate a value of θ from $\pi(\theta)$.
2. Conditioned on the value of θ, simulate $\boldsymbol{n}$ observations from $f(x|\theta)$.
3. Given the observations, examine if $T_0(x) > t_\alpha$ as a success.
4. Repeat the above steps many times; the proportion of successes is an estimate of PrSS.

For the fully Bayesian approach in (11.2), the simulation procedure would be

1. Simulate a value θ from the design prior $\pi(\theta)$.
2. Conditioned on the value of θ, simulate $\boldsymbol{n}$ observations from $f(x|\theta)$.
3. Given the observations and the analysis prior $\pi^*(\theta)$, calculate the posterior probability $Pr(\theta \in H_\text{a}|x)$ and examine if it is greater than η as a success.
4. Repeat the above steps many times; the proportion of successes is an estimate of PrSS.

The number of simulations needed in step 4 of the simulation procedures would depend on the complexity of sampling from the distribution of the test statistic $T_0(X)$ in the predictive power approach or computing $Pr(\theta \in H_\text{a}|x)$ in the fully Bayesian approach. In particular, Markov chain Monte Carlo (MCMC) is often applied in the latter case, and thus it requires convergence check to ensure well-performed calculation of PrSS.

11.3 Applications

In this section, several examples of PrSS are presented.

11.3.1 Example 1

One phase 2 study was designed to compare a few doses of an experimental drug with placebo as the primary objective. As a secondary objective, it also included a marketed comparator arm for comparison with placebo as a benchmark. The primary endpoint was the change in a vital sign from baseline to 6 weeks. The conventional approach was used for calculating the sample size needed for comparing the drug with placebo at a 2-sided 0.1 significance level, which resulted in a group sample size of 29 for the experimental drug doses and placebo to give a power of 0.8. At the same time, we applied PrSS to determine the sample size needed for the comparator group, by utilizing study results of the comparator available in the literature. Of a similar idea, there is a recent promotion for borrowing historical data to enrich controls in clinical trials (Neuenschwander et al. 2010 ; Viele et al. 2014).

The endpoint was assumed normally distributed as $N(\mu_1, \sigma_1^2)$ for the comparator and $N(\mu_2, \sigma_2^2)$ for placebo, and the tested hypotheses were $H_0 : \mu_1 - \mu_2 \leq 0$ against $H_a : \mu_1 - \mu_2 > 0$. We employed the fully Bayesian approach defined in (11.2) to calculate the PrSS. For the design prior $\pi(\theta)$, normal-gamma priors were applied for the comparator and placebo as

$$\frac{1}{\sigma_i^2} = \tau \sim Gamma(\nu, \beta), E(\tau) = \nu\beta$$

$$\mu_i|\tau \sim N\left(\mu_{i0}, \frac{1}{n_{i0}\tau}\right),$$

where n_{i0}'s can be viewed as prior numbers of subjects contributing to the PrSS calculation. The actual values used in the PrSS calculation were $n_{10} = n_{20} = 10$, $\mu_{10} = 6$, $\mu_{20} = 0$, $\nu = 9$, and $\beta = 1/(9 \times 81)$. A more stringent 0.9 was chosen for the posterior probability threshold η. In this application, the analysis prior $\pi^*(\theta)$ was assigned the same as the design prior $\pi(\theta)$. PrSS was calculated based on 10,000 simulated trials for a range of sample sizes. The curve of PrSS versus sample size is graphed in Fig. 11.2.

To attain a PrSS of 0.8 for the comparison of the comparator with placebo, a sample size of 15 for the comparator was selected, while the sample size for placebo was maintained at 29 as determined by the frequent calculation for its comparison with the experimental drug doses. Still given 29 for placebo, a conventional calculation would yield 16 for the comparator at the 1-sided 0.1 significance level as corresponding to $\eta = 0.9$. Although there was almost no difference in the determined sample size made by using the PrSS approach in this case, variability in the parameters had been appropriately considered. A more appreciable reduction in sample size would result

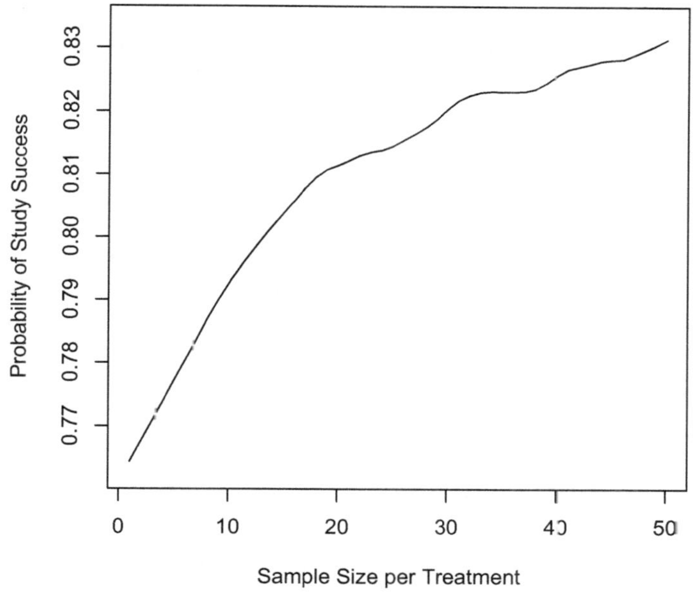

Fig. 11.2 Probability of study success

from application of a stronger analysis prior. In addition, the specified Bayesian analysis at the end of the trial was intended for providing a summary in terms of posterior probability to better facilitate decision making.

Regarding the choice of the analysis prior being the same as the design prior, we adopted the more prevalent practice in the earlier Bayesian SSD literature (Adcock 1988; Raiffa and Schlaifer 1961). This was a phase 2 study not intended for supporting label application, but to inform the company's decision on whether or not to move forward to investing on phase 3 registration trial phase. Thus, the use of informative prior in this application of PrSS received no regulatory concern.

11.3.2 Example 2

Another phase 2 trial was to compare three doses of a drug with placebo on an efficacy endpoint, and simultaneously to compare with a marketed agent on a safety endpoint. Both endpoint were changes from baseline in the corresponding efficacy and safety measures. In other words, the objective was to show that at least one of the tested drug doses was not only more efficacious than placebo but also not worse than the active comparator in terms of the known safety concern.

Denote the efficacy and safety responses at dose level $d (d = 0$ for placebo) as $Y^E(d)$ and $Y^S(d)$, which have $\mu^E(d)$ and $\mu^S(d)$ as their means, respectively. For the active comparator, the safety response was assumed to be $N(\mu_C, \sigma_C^2)$. Then the specific hypotheses were:

$$H_a : \{\mu^E(d) - \mu^E(0) > 8\} \text{ and } \{\mu^S(d) - \mu_C < 0\} \text{ for at least one } d > 0,$$
$$H_0 : \text{Otherwise.}$$

For this case, existing data suggested that both the efficacy and safety effects are dose dependent, showing improved efficacy response and worse safety response with increasing dose. Thus, we assumed the following *E*max-model based dose response curves for $Y^E(d)$ and $Y^S(d)$:

$$Y_E(d) \sim \frac{Emax^E \times d}{ED50^E + d} + e^E = \mu^E(d) + e^E$$
$$Y_S(d) \sim \frac{Emax^S \times d}{ED50^S + d} + e^S = \mu^S(d) + e^S,$$

where $Emax^E$ and $Emax^S$ are maximum achievable efficacy and safety effect sizes at the infinite dose, $ED50^E$ and$ED50^S$ are the doses at which half sizes of $Emax^E$ and $Emax^S$ are achieved, respectively, and $e^E \sim N(0, \sigma_E^2)$ and $e^S \sim N(0, \sigma_S^2)$ are normally distributed random errors. Also, according to existing data, $Y^E(d)$ and $Y^S(d)$ are negatively correlated, with the correlation coefficient denoted by ρ, which was assumed fixed at -0.3 in this example, but can be assumed random as well.

With the available in-house and literature data, the design prior $\pi(\theta)$ was assigned as:

$$Emax^E \sim N(-16, 4^2),\ log(ED50^E) \sim N(2.08, 0.5^2),\ \sigma_E^2 = 7.5^2$$
$$Emax^S \sim N(0.6, 0.15^2),\ log(ED50^S) \sim N(3.6, 0.9^2),\ \sigma_S^2 = 0.3^2$$
$$\mu_C \sim N(0.3, 0.1^2),\ \sigma_C^2 = 0.3^2.$$

Variances of the random errors σ_E^2, σ_S^2, σ_C^2 were assumed fixed, which could also be relaxed to be random. Despite the use of informative priors for the design of the trial, the study team felt the final analysis should be fully driven by the trial data instead of the prior information. Therefore, the analysis prior $\pi^*(\theta)$ was assumed fairly non-informative:

$$Emax^E \sim N(0, 100^2),\ log(ED50^E) \sim N(0, 100^2),\ \sigma_E^2 \sim IGamma(0.5, 0.0005)$$
$$Emax^S \sim N(0, 100^2),\ log(ED50^S) \sim N(0, 100^2),\ \sigma_S^2 \sim IGamma(0.5, 0.0005)$$
$$\mu_C \sim N(0, 100^2),\ \sigma_C^2 \sim IGamma(0.5, 0.0005).$$

Following the simulation procedure for the fully Bayesian approach with $\eta = 0.5$, PrSS was calculated for different scenarios, each based on 1000 simulated trials. Given the richer information on the safety endpoint of the active comparator, the

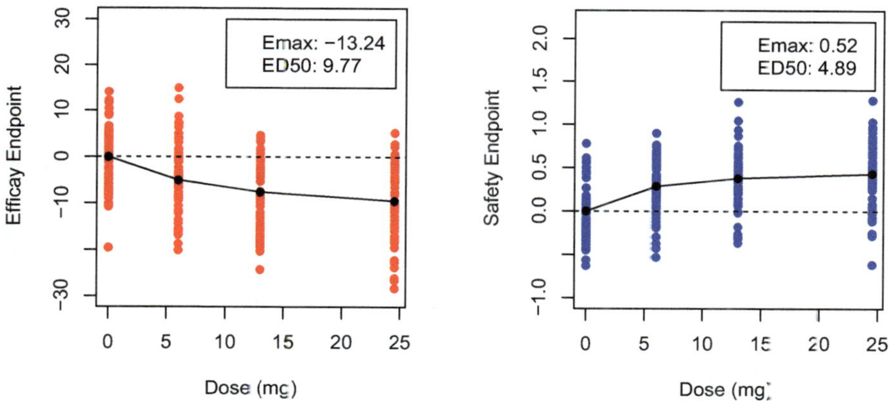

Fig. 11.3 Outcome of a simulated trial

Table 11.1 Probability of study success (PrSS)

Posterior probability	Group sample size[a]				
threshold η	30	40	50	60	70
0.5	0.67	0.68	0.69	0.71	0.73
0.6	0.62	0.66	0.67	0.69	0.70
0.7	0.58	0.60	0.61	0.62	0.64
0.8	0.55	0.57	0.59	0.61	0.62

[a] Half the size for the active comparator

sample size for the active comparator was set as half that of the other groups. One simulated trial is shown in Fig. 11.3, where nonlinear least squares fits for the efficacy and safety endpoint are presented. The simulation results are summarize in Table 11.1. For this trial, the expectation was to have a PrSS greater than 0.70, so it was decided to enroll and complete 60 patients for each of placebo and the tested drug doses and 30 patients for the active comparator.

On the selection of $\eta = 0.5$, there was discussion of its appropriate level among the study team. A consensus was reached that a lower hurdle as $\eta = 0.5$ be adopted to avoid terminating a potential effective drug with a high probability in early phase drug development. One alternative was to lower the superiority cutoff for efficacy in H_a, e.g., from 8 to 6, and allow for an $\eta > 0.5$. Nevertheless, targeting 8 had its clinical significance and thus was not compromised for other considerations.

11.3.3 Example 3

This example concerns an ongoing phase 3 major adverse cardiovascular events (MACE) registration trial. One dose of a drug is being tested against placebo on top of background therapies to show a hazard reduction in a composite of cardiovascular events, such as cardiovascular death, stroke, etc. The trial was designed by the

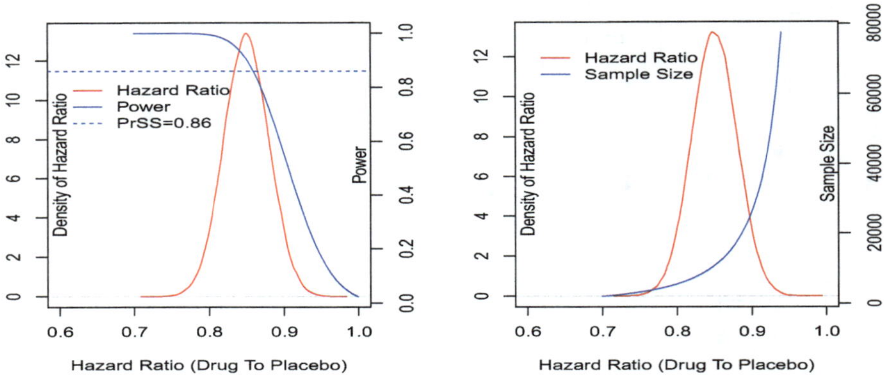

Fig. 11.4 Probability of study success (*PrSS*) and sample size of a major adverse cardiovascular events (MACE) trial

conventional frequentist approach, but is being monitored using a Bayesian approach for event and enrollment prediction in a blinded manner. In the middle of the trial, a Bayesian analysis was conducted to reassess the number of subjects needed to be enrolled. This reassessment of power was based on published information of the correlation between reduction in the MACE event rate and decrease in a particular biomarker.

A 13.75% of patients receiving placebo was estimated to experience a MACE event during exposure to study treatment. At the end of the trial, a log-rank test will be performed to see if the log hazard ratio of the drug to placebo is significantly less than 0, with a 2-side significance level of 0.05. Along with other assumptions, the initial power calculation determined $11,000$ patients were to be enrolled to the trial with a $1:1$ ratio between the drug and placebo.

The predictive power version of PrSS in (11.1) was applied to reassess the study power. Given the biomarker data from a previous phase 2 study of the drug and publications of certain similar MACE trials, it was estimated that at the tested dose of the drug the relative risk reduction would be normally distributed as $N(0.85, 0.03)$, which was employed as the design prior. With $10,000$ simulated trials, simulation results are summarized in Fig. 11.4. The left panel of Fig. 11.4 shows the power curve as a function of the hazard ratio given the elicited distribution, where the blue dotted line indicates PrSS $= 0.86$. This suggested the need of an increased sample size should a PrSS $= 0.9$ be desired. From another perspective, if a power of 0.9 is expected, the right panel of Fig. 11.4 depicts the needed sample size given an assumed hazard ratio.

11.4 Discussion

The information-based PrSS approach to SSD in drug development was described in this chapter, where variability of parameters is considered in power assessment as opposed to the fixed-value approach conventionally employed. We laid out two PrSS inferential paradigms, the predictive power and fully Bayesian approaches. The former is a more widely accepted option for registration trials under current regulatory view of a successful trial, while the latter is preferred for preregistration trials for more effective facilitation of early drug development. A few examples were given for illustration of PrSS implemented using the two paradigms.

We suggest prior elicitation, particularly for the design prior, for the application of PrSS be conducted in a most objective manner possible. At the same time, extra caution needs to be exercised as it has been shown that early-phase drug effect tends to be biased upward (Wang et al. 2006; Kirby et al. 2012; Chuang-Stein et al. 2010). Thus, appropriate adjustment of prior knowledge against inflation of effect size is a wise measure. Though PrSS has been our present focus, a more comprehensive perspective concerning overall correct (true negative or positive) or wrong decision (false negative or positive) has been promoted (Wang et al. 2006). Furthermore, the PrSS approach herein considered can be extended to trials with an adaptive design nature, such as seamless phase 2/3 trials (Inoue et al. 2002) or those allowing mid-course sample size reestimation (Wang 2007).

Increasing application of Bayesian statistics in regulatory approval-driven clinical trials was long foretold (Geisser 1992), which has come true in the area of medical devices (Campbell 2011). There is no reason not to believe that Bayesian methods, such as PrSS, applied in registration trials for drugs and biologics should only continue to gain ground for improvement of drug development efficiency.

Acknowledgments The author thanks Paul Berg, Grace Li, and Karen Price of Eli Lilly and Company and the two anonymous referees for their helpful reviews and valuable comments that resulted in the improved quality of the chapter.

References

Adcock CJ (1988) A Bayesian approach to calculating sample sizes. The Stat 37:433–439

Bobbs BP, Carlin BP (2008) Practical Bayesian design and analysis for drug and device clinical trials. J Biopharm Stat 18:54–80

Brutti P, De Santis F, Gubbiotti S (2008) Robust Bayesian sample size determination in clinical trials. Stat Med 27:2290–2306

Campbell G (2011) Bayesian statistics in medical devices: innovation sparked by the FDA. J Biopharm Stat 21:871–887

Chuang-Stein C (2006) Sample size and the probability of a successful trial. Pharm Stat 5:305–309

Chuang-Stein C, Kirby S, French J, Kowalski K, Marshall S, Smith MK, Bycott P, Beltangady M (2010) A quantitative approach for making go/no-go decisions in drug development. Drug Inf J 45:187–202

Dmitrienko A, Wang M-D (2006) Bayesian predictive approach to interim monitoring in clinical trials. Stat Med 25:2178–2195

Geisser S (1992). On the curtailment of sampling. Can J Stat 20:297–309

Inoue LYT, Thall PF, Berry DA (2002) Seamlessly expanding a randomized phase II trial to phase III. Biometrics 58:823–831

Kirby S, Burke J, Chuang-Stein C, Sin C (2012) Discounting phase 2 results when planning phase 3 clinical trials. Pharm Stat 11:378–385

Neuenschwander B, Capkun-Niggli G, Branson M, Spiegelhalter DJ (2010) Summarizing historical information on controls. Clin Trials 7:5–18

O'Hagan A, Steven JW, Campbell MJ (2005) Assurance in clinical trial design. Pharm Stat 4: 187–201

O'Neill RT (2006) FDA's critical path initiative: a perspective on contributions of Biostatistics. Biom J 48:559–564

Posch M, Hunsberger SA (1995) Designed extension of studies based on conditional power. Biometrics 51:1315–1324

Price K, LaVange L (2014) Bayesian methods in medical product development and regulatory reviews. Pharm Res 13:1–2

Raiffa H, Schlaifer R (1961). Applied statistical decision theory. Cambridge University Press, Cambridge

Spiegelhalter DJ, Freedman LS (1986) A predictive approach to selecting the size of a clinical trial, based on subjective clinical opinion. Stat Med 5:1–13

Spiegelhalter DJ, Abrams KR, Myles JP (2004) Bayesian approach to clinical trials and health-care evaluation. Wiley, Chichester

Viele K, Berry S, Neuenschwander B, Amzal B, Chen F, Enas N, Hobbs B, Ibrahim JG, Kinnersley N, Lindborg S, Micallef S, Roychoudhury S, Thompson L (2014) Use of historical control data for assessing treatment effects in clinical trials. Pharm Stat 13:41–54

Wang M-D (2007) Sample size reestimation by Bayesian prediction. Biom J 49:365–377

Wang F, Gelfand AE (2002) A simulation-based approach to Bayesian sample size determination for performance under a given model and for separating models. Stat Sci 17:193–208

Wang S-J, Hung HMJ, O'Neill RT (2006) Adapting the sample size planning of phase III trial based on phase II data. Pharm Stat 5:85–97

Wang Y, Fu H, Kulkarni P, Kaiser C (2013) Evaluating and utilizing probability of study success in clinical development. Clin Trials 10:407–413

Weiss R (1997) Bayesian sample size calculation for hypothesis testing. The Stat 46:185–191

Chapter 12
Treatment Effect Estimation in Adaptive Clinical Trials: A Review

Ying Yang and Huyuan Yang

Abstract Adaptive design has been increasingly widely discussed and accepted in the community of clinical trials. Currently, statisticians and clinicians are focusing more on the hypothesis testing of the adaptive clinical trials. Since adaptive design allows adaptation or modification to some aspects of clinical trials in the middle course of the trial, it is still not clear whether and how treatment effect estimation may be affected at the end of study as this research area has not been widely explored. In this chapter, we would like to discuss the impact of adaptation on the treatment effect estimation and compare some adjustment techniques in the adaptive trials based on simulation results.

12.1 Introduction

Adaptive design has received a great deal of attention. According to Food and Drug Administration (FDA) guidance (2010), *an adaptive design clinical study* is defined as a study that includes a prospectively planned opportunity for modification of one or more specified aspects of the study design and hypotheses based on analysis of data (usually interim data) from subjects in the study. The range of possible study design modifications that can be planned in the prospectively written protocol is broad, for example, randomization procedure, study eligibility criteria, total sample size of the study, primary endpoint, etc. It is well known that bias from analyses can be introduced when there are choices made based on unblinded analyses of data. An adaptive design approach that can adjust the study sample size to avoid both an underpowered study (because of an overly optimistic parameter estimate such as low variance or large treatment-effect size) and an excessively large study (because of an overly conservative estimate of variance or effect size) might increase the study efficiency and the ability to achieve the study goal.

Y. Yang (✉)
Food and Drug Administration Center for Devices and Radiological Health,
20993 Silver Spring, MD, USA,
e-mail: ying.yang@fda.hhs.gov

H. Yang
Takeda Pharmaceuticals International Co., 35 Landsdowne Street, 02139 Cambridge, MA, USA

Z. Chen et al. (eds.), *Applied Statistics in Biomedicine and Clinical Trials Design*,
ICSA Book Series in Statistics, DOI 10.1007/978-3-319-12694-4_12

There are two issues related to adaptive design methods. One is the potential type I error inflation due to the adaption process in design, analysis, or conduct flaws. The other is the positive study results that are difficult to interpret irrespective of having control of type I error. The size of the potential bias and the possible solutions to eliminate the bias are not yet well understood. Adjustments that appropriately control the type I error rate are not directed at controlling the bias that has been introduced into the effect estimate. Because there is limited experience with the less well-understood adaptive design methods, the size of this bias and the conditions that may influence the size are not yet generally well understood.

Bauer and Einfalt (2006) conducted a literature review and found that sample size reestimation is most commonly used in practice. Most researches focus on how to control type I error. However, how the data from multiple stages (before adaption and after adaption) are combined to estimate the treatment effect and how the estimation bias due to adaption process is eliminated are not well understood. In this chapter, we will focus on this issue.

Sample size reestimation has two types. One is based on nuisance parameter without breaking the treatment codes. It has little effect on standard statistical inference. The other type is based on the observed estimate of treatment effect, which may inflate the type I error rate of the traditional test statistic, compromise the statistical power, and bias the sample mean estimate of parameter and its confidence interval in the trial end. In this chapter, we will investigate how big the bias is and what adjustment or adaptation is available to perform valid statistical inference if the observed treatment effect at the interim time of the trial is used to increase sample size to test a smaller worthwhile effect size.

12.2 Confidence Interval and Point Estimation

An important issue besides hypothesis testing is the estimation of treatment effect upon completion of the study. Subjects are equally assigned to the new treatment or the control. Assume that the observations are normally distributed with means μ_e and μ_c respectively for the two arms and a common variance σ^2. Let $\delta = \mu_e - \mu_c$ be the true treatment difference. Consider the following two-sided hypotheses:

H_0: $\delta = 0$ vs. H_a: $\delta \neq 0$.

Let n_0 be the originally planned sample size per arm. Without loss of generality, we assume that only one interim analysis is performed when $n_1 (n_1 < n_0)$ subjects in each arm have completed the study (called first stage). Denote $t_1 = n_1/\, n_0$ as the information time. A new sample size $N = n_1 + K$ per arm, where $K \geq 0$, is calculated based on the first n_1 observations.

At the end of the study, the usual maximum likelihood estimates of δ based on all the data is the natural estimate of δ.

$$\hat{\delta} = \frac{n_1}{N}\hat{\delta}_1 + \frac{K}{N}\hat{\delta}_2$$

where $\hat{\delta}_1$ and $\hat{\delta}_2$ are estimators of δ based on data before and after interim analysis, respectively. In other words, $\hat{\delta}$ is a weighted linear combination of $\hat{\delta}_1$ and $\hat{\delta}_2$, with weighs depending on n_1 and K. If the study is stopped at the time of interim analysis for futility or significant efficacy, we may have $K = 0$ and $\hat{\delta} = \hat{\delta}_1$. Since $E(\hat{\delta}_2|\hat{\delta}_1) = \delta$, $E(\hat{\delta}|\hat{\delta}_1) = \frac{n_1}{N}\hat{\delta}_1 + \frac{K}{N}\delta$

and we have

$$E(\hat{\delta}) = E(E(\hat{\delta}|\hat{\delta}_1)) = \delta + E\left\{\frac{n_1}{N}(\hat{\delta}_1 - \delta)\right\}$$

Obviously, the maximum likelihood estimate is biased. The second term is the bias and we denote this by $b(\delta)$.

Proschan et al. (2003) used Bayesian ideas to combine prior information with the first-stage data to determine the final sample size. But the analysis of the final data does not require specification of prior distribution. To combine the data from the two stages, they proposed a weighted estimate similar to $\hat{\delta}$ with weight inversely proportional to standard deviation of each stage. They further modified the estimate by using the pooled variance based on all data from each arm. Finally, the final estimate and confidence interval for δ are written as

$$\hat{\delta}_P = \frac{\sqrt{t_1 n_1}\hat{\delta}_1 + \sqrt{(1-t_1)K}\hat{\delta}_2}{\sqrt{t_1 n_1} + \sqrt{(1-t_1)K}}$$

and

$$\left(\hat{\delta}_P - \frac{\sqrt{2}z_{\alpha/2}s}{\sqrt{t_1 n_1} + \sqrt{(1-t_1)K}}, \hat{\delta}_P + \frac{\sqrt{2}z_{\alpha/2}s}{\sqrt{t_1 n_1} + \sqrt{(1-t_1)K}}\right)$$

respectively, where s^2 is the pooled variance based on all N observations per arm.

Lawrence et al. (2003) constructed point estimation and a confidence interval based on an adaptive test statistic, which is a generalization form of Cui et al. (1999). Let $t^* = N/n_0$ denote the information time based on the new total sample size. The point estimate is written as

$$\hat{\delta}_L = \frac{t_1\hat{\delta}_1 + \sqrt{(1-t_1)}\sqrt{t^* - t_1}\hat{\delta}_2}{t_1 + \sqrt{(1-t_1)}\sqrt{t^* - t_1}}$$

The upper and lower limits of the confidence intervals are

$$\frac{t_1\hat{\delta}_1 + \sqrt{(1-t_1)}\sqrt{t^* - t_1}\hat{\delta}_2 \pm z_{\alpha/2}\lambda^{-1}}{t_1 + \sqrt{(1-t_1)}\sqrt{t^* - t_1}}$$

where $\lambda^{-1} = \sqrt{\frac{2\sigma^2}{n_0}}$ is the drift parameter.

If we replace $t_1 = n_1/n_0$ and $t^* = N/n_0$ in the formulas calculating $\hat{\delta}_P$ and $\hat{\delta}_L$, we find

$$\hat{\delta}_P = \frac{\sqrt{\frac{n_1}{n_0}n_1}\hat{\delta}_1 + \sqrt{(1-\frac{n_1}{n_0})(K-n_1)}\hat{\delta}_2}{\sqrt{\frac{n_1}{n_0}n_1} + \sqrt{(1-\frac{n_1}{n_0})(K-n_1)}} = \frac{n_1\hat{\delta}_1 + \sqrt{(n_0-n_1)(N-n_1)}\hat{\delta}_2}{n_1 + \sqrt{(n_0-n_1)(N-n_1)}}$$

and

$$\hat{\delta}_L = \frac{\frac{n_1}{n_0}\hat{\delta}_1 + \sqrt{(1-\frac{n_1}{n_0})(\frac{N}{n_0}-\frac{n_1}{n_0})}\hat{\delta}_2}{\frac{n_1}{n_0} + \sqrt{(1-\frac{n_1}{n_0})(\frac{N}{n_0}-\frac{n_1}{n_0})}} = \frac{n_1\hat{\delta}_1 + \sqrt{(n_0-n_1)(N-n_1)}\hat{\delta}_2}{n_1 + \sqrt{(n_0-n_1)(N-n_1)}}$$

Therefore, $\hat{\delta}_P$ and $\hat{\delta}_L$ are the same. So are the confidence intervals.

Both $\hat{\delta}_P$ and $\hat{\delta}_L$ give conservative estimate of treatment effect. They do not require a sample size adjustment rule to be prespecified in advance. The important feature of both estimators is that the final sample size is restricted to be at least as large as originally planned. In other words, early stopping for either futility or benefit is not allowed.

12.3 Numerical Computation and Simulation Results

In this section, we will further understand the bias of the estimators discussed in the above section: the usual maximum likelihood estimate (MLE), Lawrence estimator (LHE), and Proschan estimator (PLH). A simulation study is performed to compare their biases and the actual coverage probability of confidence intervals. In this simulation, we set the intended type 1 error rate $\alpha = 0.05$, intended type-2 error rate $\beta = 0.1$, the assumed true treatment effect $\delta_0 = 0.4$, and the standard deviation $\sigma = 1$ under a fixed study design; 132 subjects per arm are required to reject the null.

The total sample size is reestimated after observing the treatment improvement with a sample of n_1 according to the following rule:

- If $\hat{\delta}_1 \leq 0$ or $\hat{\delta}_1 > 0.4,\ N = n_0$
- If $0 < \hat{\delta}_1 \leq 0.4,\ N = n_0 \times (\delta_0/\hat{\delta}_1)^2$

Due to limited resources, the final sample size for each arm cannot go beyond the maximum number of patients being allowed. The maximum number of patients per arm is set at 300 in the simulation.

First, we simulate the case of an interim look which is performed after 43 subjects are observed in each group with the true difference $\delta = 0, 0.1, 0.2, 0.3$, and 0.4. The mean additional sample size, coverage probability, 95 % confidence interval, mean bias, and mean square error are presented in Table 12.1 based on 20,000 replicated samples. Results show that the coverage probability of the confidence interval is very close to 95 % in each of the scenarios assessed. Both Lawrence et al. and Proschan et al. estimators have smaller bias than MLE.

Second, we simulate the cases for various timing of the interim analyses, with 20,000 replicated samples. Results (not shown here) also show that the biases of all estimators are close to zero. Mean square errors (MSE) of the estimators are summarized in Table 12.2. It is noticed that the maximum likelihood estimate does not behave very badly. It fluctuates depending on the true difference. When the initial guess is closer to the truth, MSE of MLE is almost same as that obtained by Lawrence et al. and Proschan et al. methods.

Table 12.1 Mean additional sample size, coverage probability, 95 % confidence interval, mean bias, and mean square error

True difference	Mean additional sample size	Coverage		Bias		Mean square error	
		MLE	LHE/PHL	MLE	LHE/PLH	MLE	LHE/PHL
0	73	0.9457	0.9488	−0.0104	−0.0056	0.0119	0.0119
0.1	88	0.9416	0.9485	−0.0053	−0.0028	0.0120	0.0117
0.2	90	0.9436	0.9499	0.0028	0.0018	0.0120	0.0116
0.3	77	0.9449	0.9492	0.0087	0.0048	0.0120	0.0117
0.4	55	0.9493	0.9492	0.0113	0.0062	0.0121	0.0121

Table 12.2 Mean square errors of $\hat{\delta}$

Time of interim look	True δ	MLE	LHE/PHL
$t_1 = 0.25$	0.1	0.0124	0.0121
	0.2	0.0124	0.0121
	0.3	0.0123	0.0120
	0.4	0.0126	0.0126
$t_1 = 0.5$	0.1	0.0123	0.0119
	0.2	0.0123	0.0117
	0.3	0.0120	0.0117
	0.4	0.0120	0.0122
$t_1 = 0.75$	0.1	0.0124	0.0120
	0.2	0.0126	0.0120
	0.3	0.0121	0.0120
	0.4	0.0112	0.0119

12.4 Discussion

Sample size determination is an essential part of clinical trial design. An adaptive procedure allows the study to be extended based on the observed data so that a significant result may be obtained on the basis of additional data which may otherwise end with an inconclusive result. However, the final sample size in a clinical trial with an adaptive procedure is a random variable due to its dependence on the interim data. The usual maximum likelihood estimate of treatment effect is biased and the confidence interval based on the normal distribution is not valid.

In this chapter, we show that Lawrence et al. (2003) and Proschan et al. (2003) provide the same treatment effect and confidence interval. Although estimates using both methods are biased, confidence interval has correct coverage probability. The coverage probability of adaptive confidence interval is very close to 0.95 for each scenario.

Simulation studies also show that the maximum likelihood estimate does not behave very badly. However, the maximum likelihood estimate and its confidence interval are not encouraged in the analysis of adaptive clinical trials because confidence intervals that use normal distribution are not valid.

Although it is not covered here, it will be more desirable to further explore the estimation of treatment effect in adaptive designs with early stopping rules. For example, Denne (2000) proposed a bias-adjusted estimate when sample size is reestimated using Proschan and Hunsberger (1995) method. However, Denne's bias-adjusted estimate depends on the exact strategy choosing K. Confidence intervals were not discussed in Denne's paper. Rosenberger and Hu (1999) proposed nonparametric bootstrap confidence intervals in the adaptive design that can modify allocation probability to favor the treatment performing better during the study. Since the final sample size is a random variable and the distribution of conventional test statistic is no longer normal, developing a nonparametric confidence interval would be an interesting topic of research.

References

Bauer P, Einfalt J (2006) Application of adaptive designs—a review. Biom J 48:493–506

Cui L, Hung HMJ, Wang SJ (1999) Modification of sample size in group sequential clinical trials. Biometrics 55:853–857

Denne JS (2000) Estimation following extension of a study on the basis of conditional power. J Biopharm Stat 10(2):131–144

FDA CDER, CBER (Feb 2010) Guidance for industry, adaptive design clinical trials for drugs and biologics

Lawrence J, Hung HMJ (2003) Estimation and confidence intervals after adjusting the maximum information. Biom J 45:143–152

Proschan MA, Hunsberger SA (1995) Designed extension of studies based on conditional power. Biometrics 51:1315–1324

Proschan MA, Liu Q, Hunsberger S (2003) Practical midcourse sample size modification in clinical trials. Control Clin Trials 24:4–15

Rosenberger W, Hu F (1999) Bootstrap methods for adaptive designs. Stat Med 18:1757–1767

Chapter 13
Inferiority Index, Margin Functions, and Hybrid Designs for Noninferiority Trials with Binary Outcomes

George Y. H. Chi

Abstract In the design of noninferiority (NI) trials with binary outcomes, two basic problems are invariably present. The first problem pertains to the appropriateness of a fixed margin. The two-step fixed margin approach recommended in the Food and Drug Administration (FDA) guidance to industry on NI trials (US FDA, Guidance to industry: non-inferiority clinical trials, 2010) relies on the availability of relevant historical data and expert clinical knowledge and experience to provide the assurance that the derived fixed margin is appropriate. Nonetheless, it still needs an objective measure for assessing its stringency. The FDA approach has its merit in that the fixed margin is determined empirically using the best control response rate and control effect estimates and the best clinical judgment. This feature should be retained in a new design. However, once this fixed margin has been determined, one is faced with the second problem of what appropriate margin to use when the control rate from the NI trial differs from the estimated control response rate. This question was raised by the FDA Anti-infective Division at the November 2011 Anti-infective Advisory Committee meeting. A hybrid design for NI trials with binary outcomes is proposed here that integrates the FDA's fixed margin approach with a variable margin by applying the theory of inferiority index developed for Bernoulli distributions. The inferiority index is an objective measure of the relative stringency of a margin, and it can be used to define a special margin function that retains the empirical nature of the fixed margin but also allows the margin to vary.

13.1 Introduction

In the late 1980s, Food and Drug Administration's (FDA's) Anti-infective Division received submissions that include many active control studies. The Division was wrestling with the difficult issue of how to set the noninferiority (NI) margin. Its efforts resulted in the 1992 FDA Anti-infective Points-to-Consider Guidance (US FDA 1992) which reflects the Division's best thinking at the time. The guidance recognized that the nature of the problem lies in the fact that the margin is depended upon

---

G. Y. H. Chi (✉)
Janssen R&D, LLC, Raritan, NJ 08869, USA
e-mail: gchi@its.jnj.com

Z. Chen et al. (eds.), *Applied Statistics in Biomedicine and Clinical Trials Design*,
ICSA Book Series in Statistics, DOI 10.1007/978-3-319-12694-4_13

the true control response rate which is generally unknown. Therefore, the guidance provided the following margin function to be used for guiding the selection of the NI margin for the rate difference (RD) measure $\delta_{RD} = p_T - p_C$, where p_T and p_C are the response rates for treatment and control, respectively, in a parallel randomized active control trial. The margin function is actually a step function defined to take the value of -0.20, for $p_C \leq 0.80$, the value of -0.15, for $0.80 < p_C \leq 0.90$, and the value of -0.10, for $p_C > 0.90$. However, since the control response rate p_C is not known ahead of time, it is estimated from the NI trial data. The margin function is then applied retrospectively using the estimate $\hat{p}_C$ obtained from the NI trial. Various authors, including Weng and Liu (1994), Bristol (1996), Röhmel (1998, 2001), and Senn (2000) had discussed problems associated with the discontinuous nature of this function and the retrospective nature of its application. Röhmel and Senn also proposed different continuous margin functions. Munk, Skipka and Stratmann (2005) and Zhang (2006) considered NI hypotheses with variable margins that are defined by general margin functions with some regularity properties. However, the concept of a margin function did not receive its due attention from the regulatory authority, probably due to a lack of justification for the choice of margin function and a lack of an accompanied methodology.

In the FDA Guidance to Industry on NI Trials (US FDA 2010), a two-step fixed margin approach is recommended. In this approach, an estimate of the control response rate p_C and an estimate of the control effect (CE) are obtained first from available and relevant historical data. Then from the knowledge and experience of clinical experts, a fraction of the CE estimate is determined as the fixed margin which represents the amount of CE loss that can be tolerated or deemed clinically irrelevant. This two-step fixed margin approach is empirically based and reflects the best clinical judgment as to the degree of stringency required. This is the current practice for most NI trials. However, this two-step fixed margin approach cannot address the question as to what would be the appropriate margin to use in the event the true control response rate p_C from the current NI trial appears to differ from the empirically based estimate of the control response rate p_C. Indeed, at the November 2011 FDA Anti-Infective Advisory Committee meeting discussing the design of hospital-acquired and ventilation-associated bacterial pneumonia (HABP/VABP) NI trials, the FDA Anti-Infective Division posed the following questions among others to the Committee. First, is the fixed margin derived using the two-step procedure for the HABP/VABP trials appropriate? Second, what margin should one use in the event the control response rate p_C from the NI trial appears to deviate from the empirically based estimate? However, the Committee did not provide an answer to this question.

In this chapter, a hybrid NI design for the RD measure that is defined by a special linear margin is presented to address the above two questions raised by the FDA Anti-Infective Division. In Sect. 13.2, the convergence theorem for the test statistic associated with a general fixed margin NI hypothesis is established for the RD measure. This test statistic is more efficient than the classical Wald test and comparable to the likelihood ratio test because it captures the heterogeneity of variance at the boundary of the inferiority null hypothesis. This convergence theorem is used later to establish the convergence theorem for the test statistic associated with hybrid NI hypothesis. In Sect. 13.3, it is shown that there is an index function linking the standard inferiority index under the normal distributions to the RD measure and the control response rate. Upon setting the index at a specific value in its inverse function, one derives a margin function with a degree of stringency specified by that index. This margin function also accommodates the potential heterogeneity of variance through the variance ratio. Then, in Sect. 13.4, through an application of the index and margin function in tandem, it is shown how one can integrate a given fixed margin into a linear margin that can be used to define a variable margin NI hypothesis which will be termed a hybrid NI hypothesis. This hybrid design has the explicit degree of stringency as measured by the index function at the empirically determined fixed margin and control response rate. In addition, it can accommodate the adjustment of the margin in the event the control response rate from the NI trial deviates somewhat from the empirically based estimate of the control response rate. This hybrid design therefore can address both questions posed by the FDA Anti-Infective Division discussed earlier and is consistent with the spirit stated in the Investigational New Drug (IND) Application Format and Content (US FDA 2013) which mentions among other things that "a protocol for a phase 2 or 3 investigation should be designed in such a way that, if the sponsor anticipates that some deviation from the study design may become necessary as the investigation progresses, alternatives or contingencies to provide for such deviation are built into the protocols at the outset." The performance of the test statistic associated with the hybrid NI hypothesis is investigated and its results discussed, and an application to the design of HABP/VABP trials is given. The chapter concludes with a discussion.

13.2 The Scaled Relative Difference Measure and the Relative Difference Measure

In this section, the scaled rate difference (SRD) measure for Bernoulli distributions is first introduced and the related convergence theorem for the test statistic associated with its fixed margin NI hypothesis is proved. The corresponding convergence theorem for the test statistic associated with the fixed margin NI hypothesis for the RD is then deduced. The reason the scaled difference measure is important is because it takes into account potential differences in the variance through the variance ratio. This property is then passed to the RD measure through its relationship with the SRD measure. The reason this is important is because under Bernoulli distributions, at the boundary of the inferiority null, the variances are different since the treatment and control have different response rates. Furthermore, the slope of the variance function of Bernoulli distributions changes dramatically outside the range of (0.30, 0.70) as the response rate approaches 0 or 1 (Chi and Koch 2012). This property is then also captured in the hybrid design for the RD measure.

13.2.1 The Scaled Relative Difference Measure

The scaled rate difference (SRD) measure plays an interesting and important role in the development of the hybrid design which will become evident later. Consider an active control trial with a treatment T, a control C and a clinical outcome X of interest. Assume that the smaller the value of X, the worse is the outcome. Let X_T and X_C denote outcomes on subjects treated with T and C, and $F_{X_T}(t)$ and $F_{X_C}(t)$ denote their distributions with means μ_T and μ_C and variances σ_T^2 and σ_C^2 respectively.

Let $\delta_{SRD} = \frac{\mu_T - \mu_C}{\sigma_C}$ denote the SRD measure and $\delta_{SRD,\,o}$ denote a fixed NI margin for δ_{SRD}. The adjective "relative" is used to emphasize the fact that the measure is defined relative to the control C. However, for simplicity, it may henceforth simply be referred to as the scaled difference measure. Then, an NI hypothesis for the scaled difference measure δ_{SRD} defined by the margin $\delta_{SRD,\,o}$ is given by Eq. 13.1.

$$H_{SRD,\,o}: \delta_{SRD} \le \delta_{SRD,\,o} \quad \text{vs} \quad .H_{SRD,a}: \delta_{SRD} > \delta_{SRD,\,o}. \tag{13.1}$$

Now, if furthermore, the distribution F_{X_T} and F_{X_C} have finite third and fourth central moments denoted, respectively, by $\mu_T^{(3)}$ and $\mu_C^{(3)}$, and $\mu_T^{(4)}$ and $\mu_C^{(4)}$, then Li and Chi (2011) proved Theorem 1.

For simplicity, it suffices for the purpose of this chapter to assume that the variance ratio $\sigma^2 = \frac{\sigma_T^2}{\sigma_C^2}$ is known and $\sigma^2 = \sigma_o^2$ for some fixed number σ_o^2. In the general setting where the variance ratio $\sigma^2 = \frac{\sigma_T^2}{\sigma_C^2}$ is not known, the forthcoming discussion can be similarly developed with an appropriate adjustment to the asymptotic variance given in Eq. 13.2 resulting in a correspondingly larger variance. This general case will be discussed elsewhere.

Theorem 1 Assuming that the variance ratio $\sigma^2 = \frac{\sigma_T^2}{\sigma_C^2}$ is known and $\sigma^2 = \sigma_o^2$ for some fixed number σ_o^2. Then at the boundary of the inferiority null hypothesis in Eq. 13.1, the test statistic defined by $\hat{T}_{SRD} = \sqrt{n}(\hat{\delta}_{SRD} - \delta_{SRD,\,o})$ converges asymptotically to a normal distribution $N(0, \Sigma^2_{SRD,\,o})$, where the asymptotic variance $\Sigma^2_{SRD,\,o}$ is given by Eq. 13.2,

$$\Sigma^2_{SRD,\,o} = \left(1+\sigma_o^2\right) + \frac{\delta^2_{SRD,\,o}}{16}\left[\frac{\mu_T^{(4)} - \sigma_T^4}{\sigma_T^4} + \frac{\mu_C^{(4)} - \sigma_C^4}{\sigma_C^4}\right] - \frac{\delta_{SRD,\,o}}{2}\left[\frac{\mu_T^{(3)}}{\sigma_C\sigma_T^2} + \frac{\mu_C^{(3)}}{\sigma_C^3}\right]. \tag{13.2}$$

The following two corollaries follow directly from Theorem 1.

Corollary 1 *When $X_T \sim N\left(\mu_T, \sigma_T^2\right)$ and $X_C \sim N\left(\mu_C, \sigma_C^2\right)$ are normally distributed, then assuming that the variance ratio $\sigma^2 = \frac{\sigma_T^2}{\sigma_C^2}$ is known and $\sigma^2 = \sigma_o^2$ for some fixed number σ_o^2 then at the boundary of the inferiority null hypothesis in Eq. 13.1, the test statistic $\hat{T}_{SRD} = \sqrt{n}(\hat{\delta}_{SRD} - \delta_{SRD,\,o})$ converges asymptotically to* *a normal distribution* $N(0, \Sigma^2_{SRD,o})$ *where the asymptotic variance* $\Sigma^2_{SRD,o}$ *is given by Eq. 13.3,*

$$\Sigma^2_{SRD,o} = \left(1+\sigma_o^2\right) + \frac{\delta^2_{SRD,o}}{4}. \tag{13.3}$$

Proof The proof follows from Theorem 1 by noting that for normal distributions, their third central moments are $\mu_T^{(3)} = 0$ and $\mu_C^{(3)} = 0$ and their fourth central moments are $\mu_T^{(4)} = 3\sigma_T^4$ and $\mu_C^{(4)} = 3\sigma_C^4$ respectively. ■

Corollary 2 *When* $X_T \sim Bernoulli(p_T)$ *and* $X_C \sim Bernoulli(p_C)$ *are Bernoulli distributed, assuming that the variance ratio* $\sigma^2 = \frac{\sigma_T^2}{\sigma_C^2}$ *is known and* $\sigma^2 = \sigma_o^2$ *for some fixed number* σ_o^2 *then at the boundary of the inferiority null hypothesis in Eq. 13.1, the test statistic* $\hat{T}_{SRD} = \sqrt{n}(\hat{\delta}_{SRD} - \delta_{SRD,o})$ *converges asymptotically to a normal distribution* $N(0, \Sigma^2_{SRD,o})$ *where the asymptotic variance* $\Sigma^2_{SRD,o}$ *is given by Eq. 13.4,*

$$\Sigma^2_{SRD,o} = \left(1+\sigma_o^2\right)\left[1 + \frac{\delta^2_{SRD,o}}{16\sigma_C^2\sigma_o^2}\right] + \frac{\delta^2_{SRD,o}}{2}. \tag{13.4}$$

Proof The proof follows from Theorem 1 by noting that for the Bernoulli distributions, their third central moments $\mu_T^{(3)} = p_T(1-p_T)(1-2p_T)$ and $\mu_C^{(3)} = p_C(1-p_C)(1-2p_C)$, and their fourth central moments $\mu_T^{(4)} = p_T(1-p_T)(1-2p_T)^2 + \sigma_T^4$ and $\mu_C^{(4)} = p_C(1-p_C)(1-2p_C)^2 + \sigma_C^4$, respectively. ■

Now for obvious reason, under Bernoulli distributions, the scaled difference measure δ_{SRD} will be called the SRD measure. The importance of the SRD measure under normal distributions or the SRD measure under the Bernoulli distributions is that by definition, it accommodates for potential differences between the variance of the treatment and the variance of the control through their variance ratio. Hence, it is the natural parameter to consider if one cannot assume homogeneity of variance. This property is captured in the asymptotic variance of their test statistics associated with the fixed margin NI hypothesis in Eq. 13.1. In the next section, it will be shown how this property can be transferred to the RD measure under the Bernoulli distributions, which is a measure that is more commonly used in practice. Analogous derivation can be done for all other binary effect measures as discussed in Chi and Koch (2012), but will not be discussed here.

13.2.2 The Rate Difference Measure

The rate difference (RD) measure $\delta_{RD} = \mu_T - \mu_C$ under normal distributions has been discussed in Chi (2012) within the context of the Behrens–Fisher problem under the NI hypothesis. It will be further dealt with elsewhere in the context of design of bioequivalence study for highly variable drugs. For the purpose of this chapter, the focus is on the RD measure $\delta_{RD} = p_T - p_C$ under the Bernoulli distributions.

Under the Bernoulli distributions, the relationship between the SRD measure δ_{SRD} and the RD measure δ_{RD} is given by Eq. 13.5,

$$\delta_{RD} = f_{RD}(\delta_{SRD}, p_C) = \sigma_C \delta_{SRD} = \sqrt{p_C(1 - p_C)}\, \delta_{SRD}. \tag{13.5}$$

Let $\delta_{SRD,\,o}$ be a fixed NI margin for δ_{SRD} associated with a given control response rate $p_{C,o}$ Then, Eq. 13.5 indicates that

$$\delta_{RD,o} = \sqrt{p_{C,o}(1 - p_{C,o})}\, \delta_{SRD,\,o} \tag{13.6}$$

is the corresponding NI margin for the RD measure δ_{RD} at the same control response rate $p_{C,o}$.

Let the NI hypothesis for the RD measure δ_{RD} corresponding to the NI hypothesis in Eq. 13.1 for the SRD measure δ_{SRD} be defined by

$$H_{RD,o}\colon \delta_{RD} \le \delta_{RD,o} \quad \text{vs} \quad H_{RD,a}\colon \delta_{RD} > \delta_{RD,o}. \tag{13.7}$$

Then, using the test statistic $\hat{T}_{SRD} = \sqrt{n}(\hat{\delta}_{SRD} - \delta_{SRD,\,o})$ in Corollary 2 for the SRD measure as the pivoting statistic, one can derive Theorem 2 for the RD measure δ_{RD}.

Theorem 2 When $X_T \sim Bernoulli(p_T)$ and $X_C \sim Bernoulli(p_C)$ are Bernoulli distributed, assuming that the variance ratio $\sigma^2 = \frac{\sigma_T^2}{\sigma_C^2}$ is known and $\sigma^2 = \sigma_o^2$ for some fixed number σ_o^2 then at the boundary of the inferiority null hypothesis in Eq. 13.7, the test statistic defined by $\hat{T}_{RD} = \sqrt{n}(\hat{\delta}_{RD} - \delta_{RD,o})$ asymptotically converges to a normal distribution $N(0,\ \Sigma^2_{RD,o})$, where the asymptotic variance $\Sigma^2_{RD,o}$ is given by Eq. 13.8,

$$\Sigma^2_{RD,o} = \left[\left(\sigma^2_{C,o} + \sigma^2_{T,o}\right)\left(1 + \frac{\delta^2_{RD,o}}{16\sigma^2_{C,o}\sigma^2_{T,o}}\right) + \frac{\delta^2_{RD,o}}{2}\right] - \left[\left(1 - 2p_{C,o}\right)\delta_{RD,o}\right], \tag{13.8}$$

where $\sigma^2_{C,o} = p_{C,o}(1 - p_{C,o})$ and $\sigma^2_{T,o} = \sigma^2_{C,o}\sigma^2_o$.

Proof The result follows from an application of the Taylor theorem to the function $\delta_{RD} = f_{RD}(\sigma_C,\ \delta_{SRD})$ given by Eq. 13.5 and the test statistic $\widehat{T}_{SRD}$ of Corollary 2, and calculating the product term. ■

It is of interest to point out that the asymptotic variance of $\widehat{T}_{RD}$ takes into consideration the variance differences through the relationship between δ_{RD} and δ_{SRD} as given by Eq. 13.7 to arrive at Theorem 2. Equation 13.8 shows that the asymptotic variance adjusts for the rate of change of the variance function for the Bernoulli distribution at $p_{C,o}$, since $(1 - 2p_{C,o}) = \frac{\mathrm{d}}{\mathrm{d}p_C}\, p_C(1 - p_C)|_{p_C = p_{C,o}}$. This is important because as discussed in Chi and Koch (2012), the variance of the Bernoulli distribution decreases to 0 as response rate approaches 1 and the rate of change in the variance function of Bernoulli distributions begins to accelerate when the response rate exceeds 0.7 and dramatically so as the response rate approaches 1 (or 0). As shown in Chi and Koch (2012), Theorem 2 for the test statistic $\hat{T}_{RD}$ is already an improvement over the corresponding classical Wald test for control response rate in the range (0.5, 1). This improvement is quite substantial for control response rate p_C that approaches 1 due to the fact that the difference in the variance at the boundary of the inferiority null has been taken into account in the test statistic $\hat{T}_{RD}$. As just noted, this difference in variance at the boundary of the inferiority null needs to be accounted for since the rate of change of the variance function of the Bernoulli distribution changes dramatically as the control response rate p_C approaches 1. One can show that this improvement is a result of the fact that the inequality $\left[\left(\sigma^2_{C,o} + \sigma^2_{T,o}\right)\frac{\delta^2_{RD,o}}{16\sigma^2_{C,o}\sigma^2_{T,o}} + \frac{\delta^2_{RD,o}}{2}\right] < \left[\left(1 - 2p_{C,o}\right)\delta_{RD,o}\right]$ holds for $0.5 < p_{C,o} < 1$ at the boundary of the inferiority null. In addition, within this range of (0.5, 1), the performance of the test statistic $\hat{T}_{RD}$ is comparable to the likelihood ratio test as shown in Chi and Koch (2012).

Remark 1 It should be pointed out that similar results can be established for other binary effect measures, including odds ratio, log odds ratio, relative risk and relative risk reduction by utilizing the corresponding relationship between the SRD measure δ_{SRD}, and each of these binary effect measures analogous to that given by Eq. 13.5 between δ_{SRD} and δ_{RD}. Details of these derivations may be found in Chi and Koch (2012). They are outside the scope of this chapter and is not discussed further here.

In the above derivation thus far, the fixed margins $\delta_{SRD,\,o}$ or $\delta_{RD,o}$ are assumed to have been given and are associated with a given assumed control response rate $p_{C,o}$. For example, $\delta_{SRD,\,o}$ or $\delta_{RD,o}$ could have been determined through the FDA's two-step fixed margin approach (US FDA 2010). But the fixed margins $\delta_{SRD,\,o}$ and $\delta_{RD,o}$ are generally not given by an explicit margin function of the control response rate. The desire to have such a function is apparent in the 1992 FDA Anti-Infective Guidance (US FDA 1992), where it was suggested that a step function, as mentioned earlier, linking the control response rate p_C to the RD measure δ_{RD} should be used, albeit it was retrospectively implemented. Since then, other continuous margin functions have been proposed by various authors as discussed in Chi and Koch (2012). Can an explicit margin function be derived between δ_{RD} and p_C in a natural way that has all the desired properties? The answer is yes, and it is shown in Sect. 13.3 that the SRD measure δ_{SRD} again plays a critical role in establishing such an explicit margin function through its relationship to the inferiority index and the control response rate. Then, in Sect. 13.4, it is shown how to use the empirically derived fixed margin $\delta_{RD,o}$ and control response rate $p_{C,o}$ to define a special margin functions for δ_{RD} with an empirically based degree of stringency. This special margin function for δ_{RD} is then used to integrate the given empirically derived fixed margin into a linear margin called the hybrid margin.

13.3 The Inferiority Index and Margin Function

The definition of an inferiority index between two distributions was defined in Li and Chi (2011) as follows. Again consider an active control trial with a treatment T, a control C, and a clinical outcome X of interest. Assume that the smaller the value of X, the worse is the outcome. Let X_T and X_C denote outcomes on subjects treated with T and C, and $F_{X_T}(t)$ and $F_{X_C}(t)$ denote their cumulative distributions, respectively.

Definition The *inferiority index of the distribution* F_{X_T} *relative to the distribution* F_{X_C} is the quantity

$$\rho = \rho(F_{X_T}, F_{X_C}) = Sup_{-\infty<t<\infty}\,[F_{X_T}(t) - F_{X_C}(t)]. \tag{13.9}$$

The inferiority index $\rho(F_{X_T}, F_{X_C})$ measures the one-sided maximum separation between the distributions F_{X_T} and F_{X_C} and represents the excess proportion of subjects under treatment T compared to that under treatment C that responded prior to some point t^* at which the maximum separation occurs. Since $0 \leq \rho < 1$ is a probability, it can be viewed as an index measuring the *degree of inferiority* of F_{X_r} relative to F_{X_C}. The inferiority index defined in Eq. 13.9 is simply the one-sided distributional analogue of the Kolmogorov–Smirnov statistics. It reflects the distributional differences resulting from various moment differences between the two distributions. For other related distributional concepts, one may refer to the discussion in Li and Chi (2011). An important and useful property of $\rho(F_{X_T}, F_{X_C})$ is that it is *invariant* under parallel location and scale transformations, i.e., if a and $b > 0$ are constants, then $\rho\left(F_{\frac{X_T-a}{b}}, F_{\frac{X_C-a}{b}}\right) = \rho(F_{X_T}, F_{X_C})$.

13.3.1 The Standard Index and Margin Functions Under Normal Distributions

First consider the inferiority index under normal distributions. Let $X_T \sim N(\mu_T, \sigma_T^2)$ and $X_C \sim N(\mu_C, \sigma_C^2)$ be normally distributed with μ_T, μ_C and σ_T^2, σ_C^2 denoting the respective means and variances of their distributions F_{X_T} and F_{X_C}. Let $X_T^* = (X_T - \mu_C)/\sigma_C$ and $X_C^* = (X_C - \mu_C)/\sigma_C$ denote the parallel location and scale transformation of X_T and X_C relative to X_C, respectively. Then, $X_T^* \sim N(\delta_{SRD}, \sigma^2)$ and $X_C^* \sim N(0,1)$, where $\delta_{SRD} = (\mu_T - \mu_C)/\sigma_C$ is the scaled difference measure and $\sigma^2 = \sigma_T^2/\sigma_C^2$ is their variance ratio. It then follows from the invariance property that

$$\rho = \rho(F_{X_T}, F_{X_C}) = \rho(F_{X_T^*}, F_{X_C^*}) = Sup_{-\infty<t<\infty}\,[\Phi((t - \delta_{SRD})/\sigma) - \Phi(t)], \tag{13.10}$$

where Φ denotes the standard normal distribution. In light of Eq. 13.10, the inferiority index between two normal distributions will be called the *standard inferiority index* and denoted by $\rho_S = \rho(F_{X_T}, F_{X_C})$ for short. From Eq. 13.10, one can see that ρ_S is linked naturally to the scaled difference measure δ_{SRD} and the variance ratio σ^2 by the function $g_S(\delta_{SRD}, \sigma)$ as defined by Eq. 13.11.

$$\rho_S = g_S(\delta_{SRD}, \sigma) = \begin{cases} [2\Phi(-\delta_{SRD}/2) - 1], & -\infty < \delta_{SRD} \le 0, \text{if } \sigma^2 = 1 \\ \Phi((t^* - \delta_{SRD})/\sigma) - \Phi(t^*), & -\infty < \delta_{SRD} \le 0, \text{if } \sigma^2 \neq 1 \end{cases}, \tag{13.11}$$

where $t^* = \frac{-\delta_{SRD}\,\sigma^{-2} - \sqrt{\delta_{SRD}^2\,\sigma^{-2} + (1-\sigma^{-2})\,\log\sigma^2}}{(\sigma^{-2}-1)}$ denote the point at which the supremum in Eq. 13.10 is attained. The function $\rho_S = g_S(\delta_{SRD}, \sigma)$ is called *the standard inferiority index function,* or simply the *standard index function* for short. For any value $\delta_{SRD,\,o}$ of the scaled difference measure δ_{SRD} and any value σ_o^2 of the variance ratio σ^2, the standard inferiority index function $g_S(\delta_{SRD,\,o}, \sigma_o)$ assigns an inferiority index value $\rho_{S,o}$ indicating the degree of stringency of $\delta_{SRD,\,o}$ at the given variance ratio σ_o^2.

Conversely, for a specified level of the standard inferiority index $\rho_S = \rho_{S,o}$, there is a *standard margin function* $\delta_{SRD}(\sigma\,|\,\rho_{S,o})$, which is defined by Eq. 13.12.

$$\delta_{SRD}(\sigma\,|\,\rho_{S,o}) = \begin{cases} -2\Phi^{-1}\left(\frac{\rho_{S,o}+1}{2}\right) < 0, & \text{for } \sigma = 1, \quad 0 \le \rho_{S,o} < 1 \\ g_S^{-1}(\rho_{S,o}, \sigma), & \sigma \in (\sigma_1(\rho_{S,o}), \sigma_2(\rho_{S,o}))\ \&\ \sigma \neq 1, \quad 0 \le \rho_{S,o} < 1 \end{cases}. \tag{13.12}$$

For a given inferiority index value of $\rho_{S,o}$, the interval $(\sigma_1(\rho_{S,o}), \sigma_2(\rho_{S,o}))$ in Eq. 13.12 is determined by setting $\delta_{SRD} = 0$ under the second alternative in Eq. 13.11 when $\sigma^2 \neq 1$ as shown by Eq. 13.13.

$$\begin{aligned} \rho_s &= \Phi\left(\frac{t_{max}\,(0, \sigma\,(\rho_s))}{\sigma}\right) - \Phi(t_{max}\,(0, \sigma\,(\rho_s)) \\ &= \Phi(-\sqrt{(1-\sigma^{-2})\log\sigma^2}/(1-\sigma^{-2})\sigma) - \Phi(-\sqrt{(1-\sigma^{-2})\log\sigma^2}/(1-\sigma^{-2})). \end{aligned} \tag{13.13}$$

In Eq. 13.12, when the variance ratio $\sigma = 1$, the margin function $\delta_{SRD}(\sigma\,|\,\rho_{S,o})$ is given by $-2\Phi^{-1}\left(\frac{\rho_{S,o}+1}{2}\right)$, which is derived from the first alternative in Eq. 13.11. For variance ratio $\sigma \in (\sigma_1(\rho_{S,o}), \sigma_2(\rho_{S,o}))$ and $\sigma \neq 1$, the inverse function $g_S^{-1}(\rho_{S,o}, \sigma)$ is solved implicitly from the second alternative in Eq. 13.11.

For a specified value of the inferiority index $\rho_S = \rho_{S,o}$, the standard margin function $\delta_{SRD}(\sigma\,|\,\rho_{S,o})$ in Eq. 13.12 has the same degree of stringency given by $\rho_{S,o}$ throughout the interval $(\sigma_1(\rho_{S,o}), \sigma_2(\rho_{S,o}))$. Then, for any given variance ratio σ_o^2, the margin function defines a fixed margin $\delta_{SRD,\,o} = \delta_{SRD}(\sigma_o\,|\,\rho_{S,o})$ that can be used to define a fixed margin NI hypothesis for δ_{SRD} as given in Eq. 13.14 with the degree of stringency $\rho_{S,o}$.

$$\begin{aligned} H_{SRD,\,o}&: \delta_{SRD} \le \delta_{SRD,\,o} = \delta_{SRD}(\sigma_o\,|\,\rho_{S,o}) \quad \text{vs.} \\ H_{SRD,a}&: \delta_{SRD} > \delta_{SRD,\,o}(\sigma) = \delta_{SRD}(\sigma_o\,|\,\rho_{S,o}). \end{aligned} \tag{13.14}$$

Therefore, if the fixed NI margin $\delta_{SRD,\,o} = \delta_{SRD}(\sigma_o | \rho_{S,o})$ happens to be derived from the margin function defined by Eq. 13.12 at a specified standard inferiority index level $\rho_{S,o}$ and a given variance ratio σ_o^2, then Corollary 1 would be applicable and the NI hypothesis in Eq. 13.14 may be rejected at the $\alpha = 0.025$ level of significance if the test statistic $\widehat{T}_{SRD,\,o} = \sqrt{n}\,(\widehat{\delta}_{SRD} - \delta_{SRD}(p_{C,o} | \rho_{S,\,o}))/\Sigma_{SRD,\,o} > 1.96$.

13.3.2 The Standard Index and Margin Functions Under the Bernoulli Distributions

Now let $X_T \sim Bernoulli\,(p_T)$ and $X_C \sim Bernoulli\,(p_C)$ be two independent Bernoulli random variables with distributions $F_{X_T}(t) = 1 - p_T$, at $t = 0$ and $= p_T$, at $t = 1$, and $F_{X_C}(t) = 1 - p_C$, at $t = 0$ and $= p_C$, at $t = 1$. Assuming $p_T < p_C$, then from the definition of the inferiority index given in Eq. 13.9, it follows that $\rho(F_{X_T}, F_{X_C}) = [F_{X_T}(0) - F_{X_C}(0)] = -(p_T - p_C) = -\delta_{RD}$. Thus, based on the definition given by Eq. 13.9, the inferiority index between two Bernoulli distributions is simply equal to the negative of the RD measure δ_{RD} and is not a function of the variance ratio σ^2. What this implies is that the index $\rho(F_{X_T}, F_{X_C}) = -\delta_{RD}$ cannot account for any potential difference in the variance between the treatment and control. This is important because as discussed in Chi and Koch (2012), for Bernoulli distributions, the slope of the variance function changes dramatically outside the range (0.3, 0.7) when the response rate moves towards 1 (or 0). This is the precise reason why one needs to adjust the margin for the RD measure by σ_C if one wants to be able to define a margin function that properly accounts for the anticipated differences in the rate of change of σ_T and σ_C at the boundary of the inferiority null hypothesis. This is especially relevant when the control response rate is outside the range of (0.30, 0.70). This is consistent with the intuition that as the control response rate p_C moves closer to 1 (or 0), then the NI margin should become tighter and tighter. Therefore, the inferiority index as defined in Eq. 13.9 would not be useful under Bernoulli distributions and a different strategy is needed. The alternative strategy is to use the standard index function ρ_S given in Eq. 13.11 under the normal distributions for the Bernoulli distributions. This strategy is possible on account of Theorem 3.

13.3.2.1 Linking the Standard Inferiority Index to the Scaled Rate Difference Measure δ_{SRD}

Theorem 3: Let $\{X_{T,i}\}_{i=1}^{n}$ and $\{X_{C,i}\}_{i=1}^{n}$ be two independent random Bernoulli samples, where $X_{T,i} \sim Bernoulli\,(\,p_T)$ and $X_{C,j} \sim Bernoulli\,(\,p_C)$. Let $\widehat{p}_T = \sum_{i=1}^{n} X_{T,i}/n$ and $\widehat{p}_C = \sum_{j=1}^{n} X_{C,j}/n$ denote the sample means of X_T and X_C, respectively, and $\widehat{p}^*_{T,n} = \sqrt{n}[(\widehat{p}_T - p_C)/\sigma_C]$ and $\widehat{p}^*_{C,n} = \sqrt{n}[(\widehat{p}_C - p_C)/\sigma_C]$ denote their parallel location and scale transforms. Let $\rho_n = \rho(F_{\widehat{p}^*_{T,n}}, F_{\widehat{p}^*_{C,n}})$ denote the inferiority index between the distributions of the two transformed statistics. Then,

$$\lim_{n\to\infty} \rho(F_{\widehat{p}^*_{T,n}}, F_{\widehat{p}^*_{C,n}}) = \rho_S(\Phi(\delta_{SRD}, \sigma^2), \Phi) \tag{13.15}$$

where $\rho_S(\Phi(\delta_{SRD}, \sigma^2), \Phi)$ is the standard inferiority index between the cumulative normal distribution $\Phi(\delta_{SRD}, \sigma^2)$ and the standard normal distribution Φ, where $\delta_{SRD} = (p_T - p_C)/\sigma_C$ with $\sigma_C = \sqrt{p_C(1-p_C)}$ and $\sigma^2 = \sigma_T^2/\sigma_C^2$ with $\sigma_T = \sqrt{p_T(1-p_T)}$.

Proof: It follows from the central limit theorem that $\widehat{p}_T \sim N(p_T, \sigma_T^2/n)$ and $\widehat{p}_C \sim N(p_C, \sigma_C^2/n)$, where $\sigma_T^2 = p_T(1-p_T)$ and $\sigma_C^2 = p_C(1-p_C)$. Then, one has $\widehat{p}^*_{T,n} = \sqrt{n}[(\widehat{p}_T - p_C)/\sigma_C] \sim N(\delta_{SRD}, \sigma^2)$ and $\widehat{p}^*_{C,n} = \sqrt{n}[(\widehat{p}_C - p_C)/\sigma_C] \sim N(0, 1)$, where $\delta_{SRD} = (p_T - p_C)/\sigma_C$ and $\sigma^2 = \sigma_T^2/\sigma_C^2$. Then, Eq. 13.15 follows from the definition of inferiority index, its invariance property under parallel location and scale transformation and an application of the Berry–Esseen theorem (Berry 1941, Esseen 1942) on the uniform convergence of the central limit theorem. Details are omitted. ■

Then, from Eqs. 13.11 and 13.15, one has

$$\rho_S = \rho_S(\Phi(\delta_{SRD}, \sigma^2), \Phi) = g_S(\delta_{SRD}, \sigma). \tag{13.16}$$

Therefore, Theorem 3 and Eq. 13.16 show that the SRD measure $\delta_{SRD} = (p_T - p_C)/\sigma_C$ and the variance ratio $\sigma^2 = \sigma_T^2/\sigma_C^2$ under the Bernoulli distributions are asymptotically linked to the standard inferiority index ρ_S by the standard index function g_S. Now, by substituting the functional relationship between p_T, p_C, and δ_{SRD} as given by $\pi_T(p_C, \delta_{SRD})$ in Eq. 13.17,

$$p_T = \pi_T(p_C, \delta_{SRD}) = p_C + \sigma_C\delta_{SRD} = p_C + \sqrt{p_C(1-p_C)}\,\delta_{SRD}, \tag{13.17}$$

into the variance ratio $\sigma^2 = p_T(1-p_T)/p_C(1-p_C)$ in Eq. 13.16, one derives the index function g^*_{SRD},

$$\begin{aligned}\rho_S &= g^*_{SRD}(\delta_{SRD}, p_C)\\ &= g_S\left(\delta_{SRD}, \sqrt{\frac{\pi_T(p_C, \delta_{SRD})(1-\pi_T(p_C, \delta_{SRD}))}{p_C(1-p_C)}}\right), \text{ for } \delta_{SRD} < 0 \text{ and } 0 < p_C < 1.\end{aligned} \tag{13.18}$$

Equation 13.18 shows that the standard inferiority index ρ_S is now asymptotically linked to SRD measure δ_{SRD} and the control response rate p_C by the function g^*_{SRD} which is defined through the composition of the standard index function g_S and the variance ratio as a function of δ_{SRD} and p_C given by $\sigma^2 = \gamma(\delta_{SRD}, p_C) = \frac{\pi_T(p_C, \delta_{SRD})(1-\pi_T(p_C, \delta_{SRD}))}{p_C(1-p_C)}$, where π_T is defined in Eq. 13.17. The key point here is that the index function g^*_{SRD} has now incorporated the variance ratio σ^2 into its relationship, even though it now appears to be only a function of δ_{SRD} and p_C. This index function g^*_{SRD} then allows one to use the standard inferiority index ρ_S as an objective measure for assessing the degree of stringency for any value of the SRD measure $\delta_{SRD} = \delta_{SRD,\,o}$ at any control response rate $p_C = p_{C,o}$. Conversely, upon setting the standard inferiority index ρ_S at a specific level $\rho_{S,o}$ in its inverse function g^{*-1}_{SRD}, which is derived from the inverse function g^{-1}_S through Eq. 13.18, one derives a margin function $\delta_{SRD}\,(p_C|\rho_{S,\,o})$ for the SRD measure δ_{SRD} as given by Eq. 13.19,

$$\delta_{SRD}\,(p_C|\rho_{S,\,o}) = g^{*-1}_{SRD}(\rho_{S,\,o}, p_C). \tag{13.19}$$

This specific indexed margin function corresponds to a level curve of the surface of the index function g^*_{SRD} given in Eq. 13.18 by setting the index level $\rho_S = \rho_{S,\,o}$. Thus, in a given application, if the control response rate p_C is thought to be equal to $p_{C,o}$, then Eq. 13.20

$$\delta_{SRD,\,o} = \delta_{SRD}(p_{C,o}|\rho_{S,\,o}) = g^{*-1}_{SRD}(\rho_{S,\,o}, p_{C,o}) \tag{13.20}$$

defines a fixed margin at the control response rate $p_{C,o}$ with the degree of stringency $\rho_{S,\,o}$. With this fixed margin $\delta_{SRD,\,o}$, the NI hypothesis for δ_{SRD} can then be stated as

$$H_{SRD,\,o}:\ \delta_{SRD} \le \delta_{SRD,\,o} = \delta_{SRD}(p_{C,o}|\rho_{S,\,o}) \quad \text{vs.}$$
$$H_{SRD,a}:\ \delta_{SRD} > \delta_{SRD,\,o} = \delta_{SRD}(p_{C,o}|\rho_{S,\,o}) \tag{13.21}$$

and Corollary 2 would be applicable. It shows that the test statistic $\widehat{T}_{SRD,\,o}$ at the boundary of the inferiority null of Eq. 13.21 for the SRD measure δ_{SRD} converges asymptotically to a normal distribution. The inferiority null hypothesis in Eq. 13.21 may be rejected at the $\alpha = 0.025$ significance level if the test statistic $\widehat{T}_{SRD,\,o} = \sqrt{n}\,(\widehat{\delta}_{SRD} - \delta_{SRD}(p_{C,o}|\rho_{S,\,o}))/\Sigma_{SRD,\,o} > 1.96$.

13.3.2.2 Linking the Standard Inferiority Index to the Rate Difference Measure δ_{RD}

The relationship between δ_{SRD} and δ_{RD} is given by $\delta_{SRD} = f_{RD}(\delta_{RD}, p_C) = \delta_{RD}/\sigma_C$. Upon substituting this relationship into Eq. 13.18, one obtains the index function g^*_{RD} given in Eq. 13.22,

$$\rho_S = g^*_{RD}(\delta_{RD},\ p_C) = g^*_{SRD}(f_{RD}(\delta_{RD}, p_C),\ p_C), \quad \text{for } 0 < p_C < 1, \tag{13.22}$$

which links the standard inferiority index ρ_S to δ_{RD} and p_C. From Eq. 13.22, one can derive the margin function given by Eq. 13.23 that links ρ_S and p_C to δ_{RD} given by

$$\delta_{RD} = g^{*-1}_{RD}(\rho_S, p_C), \text{ for } 0 < \rho_S < 1 \text{ and } 0 < p_C < 1. \tag{13.23}$$

Analogous to the case for the SRD measure δ_{SRD}, one can use the index function g^*_{RD} defined by Eq. 13.22 to assess the degree of stringency of any value of the RD measure $\delta_{RD} = \delta_{RD,o}$ at any given control response rate $p_C = p_{C,o}$. Similarly, by setting the standard index $\rho_S = \rho_{S,o}$ in Eq. 13.23, one can define a specific indexed margin function for δ_{RD} given by Eq. 13.24

$$\delta_{RD}(p_C|\rho_{S,o}) = g^{*-1}_{RD}(\rho_S, o, p_C), \text{ for } 0 < p_C < 1 \tag{13.24}$$

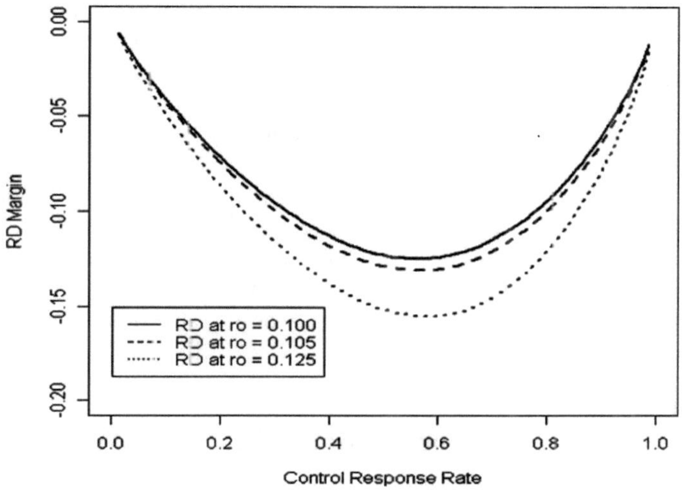

Fig. 13.1 Margin functions $\delta_{RD}(p_C|\rho_S)$ for inferiority index ρ_S =0.10, 0.105, and 0.125. *RD* rate difference

with a degree of stringency given by $\rho_{S,o}$. Now, for a given $p_C = p_{C,o}$, the indexed margin function Eq. 13.24 defines a fixed margin $\delta_{RD,o} = \delta_{RD}(p_{C,o}|\rho_{S,o}) = g_{RD}^{*-1}(\rho_{S,o}, p_{C,o})$ for the RD measure δ_{RD}. Note that the fixed margin $\delta_{RD,o}$ has now been adjusted for σ_C via δ_{SRD} through f_{RD} in Eq. 13.22. One can then use this fixed margin $\delta_{RD,o}$ to define a NI hypothesis relative to δ_{RD} with the degree of stringency $\rho_{S,o}$ as given by Eq. 13.25,

$$\begin{aligned} H_{RD,o} &: \delta_{RD} \leq \delta_{RD,o} = \delta_{RD}(p_{C,o}|\rho_{S,o}) \quad \text{vs.} \\ H_{RD,a} &: \delta_{RD} > \delta_{RD,o} = \delta_{RD}(p_{C,o}|\rho_{S,o}). \end{aligned} \tag{13.25}$$

Theorem 2 shows that the test statistic $\widehat{T}_{RD,o}$ at the boundary of the inferiority null of Eq. 13.25 for the RD measure δ_{RD} converges asymptotically to a normal distribution. The inferiority null hypothesis in Eq. 13.25 may be rejected at the $\alpha = 0.025$ significance level if the test statistic $\widehat{T}_{RD,o} = \sqrt{n}\,(\widehat{\delta}_{RD} - \delta_{RD}(p_{C,o}|\rho_{S,o}))/\Sigma_{RD,o} > 1.96$.

It is of interest to note that the inverse function defined by Eq. 13.23 defines a family of margin functions given by Eq. 13.26

$$\{\delta_{RD}(p_C|\rho_S) = g_{RD}^{*-1}(\rho_S, p_C), \quad \text{for } 0 < \rho_S < 1 \text{ and } 0 < p_C < 1\} \tag{13.26}$$

as illustrated in Fig. 13.1.

By setting the standard index ρ_S equal to a specific value $\rho_{S,o}$, then $\delta_{RD}(p_C|\rho_{S,o})$ defines an indexed margin function with a stringency level of $\rho_{S,o}$ for δ_{RD} as a function of the control response rate p_C. This entire margin function $\delta_{RD}(p_C|\rho_{S,o})$ will have the same degree of stringency $\rho_{S,o}$ at every control response rate p_C, for $0 < p_C < 1$. Furthermore, at the given index level $\rho_{S,o}$, the margin function $\delta_{SRD}(p_C|\rho_{S,o})$ defined by Eq. 13.19 and the margin function $\delta_{RD}(p_C|\rho_{S,o})$

defined by Eq. 13.24 are equally stringent with the same degree of stringency $\rho_{S,o}$. At a given control response rate $p_{C,o}$, these margin functions define equally stringent NI hypotheses as given by Eqs. 13.21 and 13.25. However, the performance of the test statistics $\hat{T}_{SRD,\,o}$ and $\hat{T}_{RD,o}$ for their respective NI hypotheses, Eqs. 13.21 and 13.25, may differ. Similar derivations can be done for other binary effect measures by using their corresponding functional relationship with the SRD measure δ_{SRD} or the RD measure δ_{RD} to arrive at equally stringent margin functions for these binary effect measures. These equally stringent margin functions can then be used to define equally stringent NI hypotheses. The relative performance of the test statistics for these equally stringent NI hypotheses can then be investigated. One may refer to Chi and Koch (2012) for a discussion of such an investigation comparing the RD measure and the log odds ratio measure.

13.4 A Hybrid Design for the Rate Difference Measure

It has been shown in Sect. 13.2 how to improve the efficiency of the test statistic for testing the fixed margin NI hypothesis in Eq. 13.7 by incorporating the information on the variance ratio at the boundary of the inferiority null of Eq. 13.7 into its asymptotic variance. In Sect. 13.3, an index function g^*_{RD} has been derived in Eq. 13.22 that links the RD measure δ_{RD} and control response rate p_C to the standard inferiority index ρ_S. Furthermore, its inverse function g^{*-1}_{RD} in Eq. 13.23 links the standard inferiority index ρ_S and control response rate p_C to the RD measure δ_{RD} so that by setting the standard inferiority index ρ_S at a specified level $\rho_{S,o}$, the inverse function then defines a margin function $\delta_{RD}(p_C|\rho_{S,o})$ given by Eq. 13.24 which has the degree of stringency $\rho_{S,o}$.

In this section, these results are combined to produce a hybrid design for NI trials with binary outcomes intended to address the question of how to set a margin and what margin to use in the event the true control response rate appears to deviate from the assumed control response rate.

13.4.1 An Empirically Based Margin Function for the Rate Difference Measure

How to set the NI margin is a problem that has been around for quite a while. The FDA's proposed two-step empirically based fixed margin approach is really a very good approach. However, it needs to be supplemented by an objective measure of the degree of stringency of the empirically derived fixed margin, and in addition, the fixed margin design needs to be modified to be able to accommodate variability in the margin in the event the true control response rate actually deviates from the assumed rate. It is the purpose of this section to show how the index function g^*_{RD} defined by Eq. 13.22 and the margin function g^{*-1}_{RD} defined by Eq. 13.23 can be used in tandem to address both issues in a hybrid design that preserves the empirical nature of FDA's fixed margin approach.

Now consider the problem of designing an NI trial with binary outcomes using the RD measure δ_{RD}. Assume that relevant historical studies involving the active control and placebo are available. Using the FDA's two-step fixed margin approach described above, one can derive an estimate $p_{C,o}$ for the control response rate p_C and a conservative estimate of the CE. Furthermore, with input from clinical experts, an NI margin $\delta_{RD,o}$ is derived which represents the maximum amount of loss of the CE that can be tolerated.

Then, from the pair of empirically based estimates $(\delta_{RD,o}, p_{C,o})$, one can derive the degree of stringency of the margin $\delta_{RD,o}$ at $p_{C,o}$ from the index function g^*_{RD} defined by Eq. 13.22, which is given by

$$\rho_{S,o} = g^*_{RD}(\delta_{RD,o}, p_{C,o}). \tag{13.27}$$

Now, the index $\rho_{S,o}$ given by Eq. 13.27 is *empirically based* because it is derived from the empirically based estimates $(\delta_{RD,o}, p_{C,o})$ through the index function g^*_{RD} as defined by Eq. 13.27.

Using this empirically based index $\rho_{S,o}$, one can define an empirically based margin function through the inverse function g^{*-1}_{RD} given by Eq. 13.24, or Eq. 13.28,

$$\delta_{RD}(p_C|\rho_{S,o}) = g^{*-1}_{RD}(\rho_{S,o}, p_C), \text{ for } 0 < p_C < 1. \tag{13.28}$$

It is obvious that when this margin function is evaluated at the estimate $p_{C,o}$, it should yield the empirically based margin $\delta_{RD,o}$, i.e., one has

$$\delta_{RD}(p_{C,o}|\rho_{S,o}) = \delta_{RD,o}. \tag{13.29}$$

Thus, from the empirically based pair of estimates $(\delta_{RD,o}, p_{C,o})$, one is able to derive the corresponding empirically based standard inferiority index $\rho_{S,o}$ through the index function g^*_{RD} as given by Eq. 13.27. Then, using empirically based index $\rho_{S,o}$, one can define an empirically based margin function $\delta_{RD}(p_C|\rho_{S,o})$ given by Eq. 13.28 that has the degree of stringency given by $\rho_{S,o}$. Thus, out of the family of possible margin functions defined by Eq. 13.26, one identifies a special indexed margin function $\delta_{RD}(p_C|\rho_{S,o})$ that is based on the empirically based pair of estimates $(\delta_{RD,o}, p_{C,o})$.

Hence, it has now been shown that from the empirically based pair of estimates $\delta_{RD}(p_C|\rho_{S,o})$, one can derive its *implicit* degree of stringency $\rho_{S,o}$ through the index function $g^*_{RD}(\delta_{RD}, p_C)$ given by Eq. 13.22. In actual practice, based on the degree of stringency $\rho_{S,o}$, one may opt to further tighten or relax the empirically derived fixed margin $\delta_{RD,o}$ as deemed appropriate. Now assume that such adjustment has been done if needed. Then, one can simply define the NI hypothesis in Eq. 13.25 using this empirically based margin $\delta_{RD,o}$ and test the inferiority null hypothesis using Theorem 2. This approach without the link to the standard index function ρ_S is essentially what has routinely been done. But as noted earlier, the FDA Anti-Infective Division has posed the question as to what margin to use in the event the control response rate from the current NI trial appears to deviate from the estimated control response rate $p_{C,o}$? Obviously, by simply defining an NI hypothesis (Eq. 13.25) based on an empirically derived fixed margin, one will not be able to address this question. So, further work is needed and is discussed in the next section.

13.4.2 A Hybrid Design with a Linear Margin

Now consider the NI hypothesis in Eq. 13.30

$$H_{RD,o}: \delta_{RD} \le \delta_{RD}(p_C|\rho_{S,o}) \quad \text{vs} \quad H_{RD,a}: \delta_{RD} > \delta_{RD}(p_C|\rho_{S,o}), 0 < p_C < 1. \tag{13.30}$$

Unlike the NI hypotheses in Eq. 13.25, the NI hypothesis in Eq. 13.30 is actually defined by a margin function, and not by a fixed margin. But it is not just any margin function. It is a natural and empirically derived margin function with the empirically determined degree of stringency $\rho_{S,o}$. In Zhang (2006), the author starts off with a given margin function and develops his method for a general variable margin. In Sect. 13.4.1, a natural and special indexed margin function is derived with the empirically determined degree of stringency. In this section, this empirically based margin function will be used to integrate the fixed margin into a linear margin for the hybrid design to be proposed.

Figure 13.1 displays the graphs of margin function $\delta_{RD}(p_C|\rho_S)$ at three selected degrees of stringency. From these graphs, one can see that the power for testing the NI hypothesis in Eq. 13.30 will be low if the true control response rate p_C is considerably larger (or smaller) than the empirically based estimate $p_{C,o}$ because the margin is getting tighter as p_C approaches 1 (or 0).

Since the index function g^*_{RD} is continuously differentiable, it follows from the implicit function theorem that the margin function $\delta_{RD}(p_C|\rho_{S,o})$ given by Eq. 13.28 is continuously differentiable and its derivative is given by

$$\frac{\partial \delta_{RD}(p_C|\rho_{S,o})}{\partial p_C} = \frac{\partial g^{*-1}_{RD}(\rho_{S,o}, p_C)}{\partial p_C} = -\frac{\frac{\partial g^*_{RD}}{\partial p_C}}{\frac{\partial g^*_{RD}}{\partial \delta_{RD}}}. \tag{13.31}$$

Now consider the first-order Taylor approximation of the margin function $\partial\delta_{RD}(p_C|\rho_{S,o})$ expanded around the point $p_{C,o}$ given in Eq. 13.32 as illustrated by Fig. 13.2:

$$\begin{aligned} L(p_C|\rho_{S,o}, p_{C,o}) &= g^{*-1}_{RD}(\rho_{S,o}, p_C)|_{p_C=p_{C,o}} + \frac{\partial g^{*-1}_{RD}(\rho_{S,o}, p_C)}{\partial p_C}|_{p_C=p_{C,o}}(p_C - p_{C,o}) \\ &= \delta_{RD}(p_{C,o}|\rho_{S,o}) + \frac{\partial g^{*-1}_{RD}(\rho_{S,o}, p_{C,o})}{\partial p_C}(p_C - p_{C,o}) = \delta_{RD,o} \\ &\quad + \frac{\partial g^{*-1}_{RD}(\rho_{S,o}, p_{C,o})}{\partial p_C}(p_C - p_{C,o}). \end{aligned} \tag{13.32}$$

The expression in the linear approximation $L(p_C|\rho_{S,o}, p_{C,o})$ in Eq. 13.32 is equal to the fixed margin $\delta_{RD,o}$ plus the linear term $\frac{\partial g^{*-1}_{RD}(\rho_{S,o}, p_{C,o})}{\partial p_C}(p_C - p_{C,o})$. If the true control response rate p_C from the NI trial turns out to be equal to $p_{C,o}$, then $L(p_{C,o}|\rho_{S,o}, p_{C,o}) = \delta_{RD,o}$. But if p_C deviates from $p_{C,o}$, then the margin is equal to the given fixed margin $L(p_C|\rho_{S,o}, p_{C,o}) = \delta_{RD,o}$ plus the deviation term

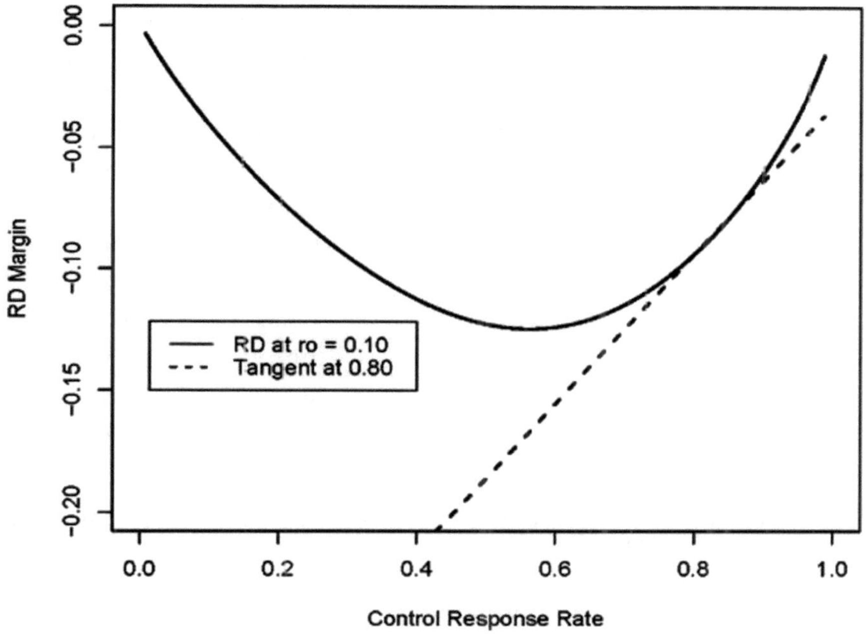

Fig. 13.2 First-order Taylor approximation to the margin function $\delta_{RD}(p_C|\rho_{S,o} = 0.10)$ at $p_{C,o} = 0.80$. RD rate difference

$\frac{\partial g^{*-1}_{RD}(\rho_{S,o},p_{C,o})}{\partial p_C}(p_C - p_{C,c})$, which represents a first-order adjustment to the margin $\delta_{RD,o}$ for the deviation.

The linear margin $L(p_C|\rho_{S,o}, p_{C,o})$ is called a hybrid margin because it *explicitly integrates* the given empirically derived pair $(\delta_{RD,o}, p_{C,o})$ based on FDA's two-step fixed margin approach with a variable term $\frac{\partial g^{*-1}_{RD}(\rho_{S,o},p_{C,o})}{\partial p_C}(p_C - p_{C,o})$ that can accommodate the possibility that the true control response rate p_C may deviate somewhat from the best empirically based estimate of the control response rate $p_{C,o}$.

Now a natural question to ask is how stringent is the linear margin $L(p_C|\rho_{S,o}, p_{C,o})$? The empirically based margin function $\delta_{RD}(p_C|\rho_{S,o})$ has the stringency $\rho_{S,o}$, so the linear margin function $L(p_C|\rho_{S,o}, p_{C,o})$ cannot be at this same stringency level except at $p_C = p_{C,o}$. But the important point to note is that this linear margin has approximately the same degree of stringency $\rho_{S,o}$ as the margin function $\delta_{RD}(p_C|\rho_{S,o})$ in a certain interval around $p_{C,o}$. For example, with $(\delta_{RD,o}, p_{C,o}) = (-0.10, 0.80)$, this interval is approximately (0.75, 0.90) as shown in Table 13.1.

Therefore, now one may consider the following hybrid NI hypothesis as approximately equivalent to the NI hypothesis in Eq. 13.30 within a certain interval of p_C:

$$\begin{aligned} &H_{RD,o} : \delta_{RD} \leq L(p_C|\rho_{S,o}, p_{C,o}) \quad \text{vs} \\ &H_{RD,a} : \delta_{RD} > L(p_C|\rho_{S,o}, p_{C,o}), p_{o,L} < p_C < p_{o,R}. \end{aligned} \tag{13.33}$$

Table 13.1 Comparing the margin functions $\delta_{RD}(p_C|\rho_{S,o})$ and $L(p_C|\rho_{S,o}, p_{C,o})$ with Taylor expansion at $p_{C,o} = 0.80$

True control	Margin function	
Response ate p_C	$\delta_{RD}(p_C\|\rho_{S,o})$	$L(p_C\|\rho_{S,o}, p_{C,o})$
0.50	– 0.1228	– 0.1859
0.55	– 0.1246	– 0.1706
0.60	– 0.1239	– 0.1553
0.65	– 0.1207	– 0.1399
0.70	– 0.1146	– 0.1246
0.75	– 0.1058	– 0.1093
0.80	– 0.0939	– 0.0939
0.85	– 0.0789	– 0.0767
0.90	– 0.0601	– 0.0614
0.95	– 0.0360	– 0.0460

The hybrid NI hypothesis (Eq. 13.32) can be equivalently written as the NI hypothesis in Eq. 13.33,

$$\begin{aligned} H_{RD,o} &: \delta_{RD} - L(p_C|\rho_{S,o}, p_{C,o}) \le 0 \quad \text{vs} \\ H_{RD,a} &: \delta_{RD} - L(p_C|\rho_{S,o}, p_{C,o}) > 0,\, p_{o,L} < p_C < p_{o,R}. \end{aligned} \tag{13.34}$$

13.4.3 The Test Statistic for the Hybrid Design NI Hypothesis

Now consider a binary outcome trial and let $\{X_{T,i}\}_{i=1}^{n}$ and $\{X_{C,i}\}_{i=1}^{n}$ be two independent random Bernoulli samples, where $X_{T,i} \sim Bernoulli(p_T)$ and $X_{C,j} \sim Bernoulli(p_C)$. Let $\hat{p}_T = \sum_{i=1}^{n} X_{T,i}/n$ and $\hat{p}_C = \sum_{j=1}^{n} X_{C,j}/n$ denote the sample means of X_T and X_C, respectively.

Consider the statistic

$$\hat{\Delta}_{RD} = [\hat{\delta}_{RD} - L(\hat{p}_C|\rho_{S,o}, p_{C,o})]. \tag{13.35}$$

Then,

$$E(\hat{\Delta}_{RD}) = E[\hat{\delta}_{RD} - L(\hat{p}_C|\rho_{S,o}, p_{C,o})] = \delta_{RD} - L(p_C|\rho_{S,o}, p_{C,o}).$$

Let

$$\hat{\Delta}_{RD,o} = [\hat{\Delta}_{RD} - E(\hat{\Delta}_{RD}|H_o)]. \tag{13.36}$$

The asymptotic normality of the test statistic $\hat{\Delta}_{RD,o}$ at the inferiority null of the hybrid NI hypothesis (Eq. 13.33 or Eq. 13.34) is established in Theorem 4.

Theorem 4 The statistic $\sqrt{n}\hat{\Delta}_{RD,o}$ is asymptotically normal $N(o, \sum(p_C|H_o))$ at the boundary of the inferiority null of Eq. 13.33 or Eq. 13.34, where

$$\sum{}^2(p_C|H_o) = \sum{}^2_{RD,o}(p_C|H_o) + \left[2\left(\frac{\partial g^{*-1}_{RD}(\rho_{S,o}, p_{C,o})}{\partial p_C}\right) + \left(\frac{\partial g^{*-1}_{RD}(\rho_{S,o}, p_{C,o})}{\partial p_C}\right)^2\right] p_C(1-p_C), \tag{13.37}$$

and

$$\Sigma^2_{RD,o}(p_{C,o}|H_o) = \left[\left(\sigma^2_{C,o} + \sigma^2_{T,o}\right)\left(1 + \frac{\delta^2_{RD,o}}{16\sigma^2_{C,o}\sigma^2_{T,o}}\right) + \frac{\delta^2_{RD,o}}{2}\right] - \left[\left(1-2p_{C,o}\right)\delta_{RD,o}\right]$$

is the variance of the statistic under the fixed margin NI hypothesis (Eq. 13.25) with the fixed margin $\delta_{RD,o} = \delta_{RD}(p_{C,o}|\rho_{S,o})$, $\sigma^2_o = \frac{\sigma^2_{T,o}}{\sigma^2_{C,o}}$, where $\sigma^2_{C,o} = p_{C,o}(1-p_{C,o})$, $\sigma^2_{T,o} = p_{T,o}(1-p_{T,o})$, and $p_{T,o} = p_{C,o} + \delta_{RD,o}$.

Proof The proof follows from the central limit theorem and a derivation of the asymptotic variance of

$$\sqrt{n}\widehat{\Delta}_{RD,o} = \sqrt{n}\left[\widehat{\delta}_{RD} - \delta_{RD}\left(p_{C,o}|\rho_{S,o}\right)\right] - \left[\frac{\partial g^{*-1}_{RD}(\rho_{S,o}, p_{C,o})}{\partial p_C}\left(\widehat{p}_C - p_C\right) + \frac{\partial g^{*-1}_{RD}\left(\rho_{S,o}, p_{C,o}\right)}{\partial p_C}\left(p_C - p_{C,o}\right)\right]$$

by applying Eq. 13.8 of Theorem 2. ■

Hence, the hybrid test statistic,

$$\widehat{T}^{HB}_{RD,o} = \frac{\sqrt{n}\,\widehat{\Delta}_{RD,\,o}}{\sqrt{\Sigma(p_C|H_o)}} \sim N(0,1), \tag{13.38}$$

where the unknown true p_C may be substituted by the sample proportion $\widehat{p}_C$. The hybrid inferiority hypothesis in Eq. 13.33 or Eq. 13.34 may be rejected at the $\alpha = 0.025$ significance level if $\widehat{T}^{HB}_{RD,o} = \sqrt{n}\frac{[\widehat{\delta}_{RD} - \mathcal{L}(\widehat{p}_C|\rho_{S,o}, p_{C,o})]}{\Sigma(\widehat{p}_C|H_o)} > 1.96$.

13.4.4 The Performance of the Hybrid Test Statistic $\widehat{T}^{HB}_{RD,o}$

It should be pointed out that the focus of the hybrid NI design is still on the fixed margin $\delta_o = \delta_{RD}(p_{C,o}|\rho_{S,o})$ at the assumed control response rate $p_C = p_{C,o}$, even though one has added the flexibility in the event the true control response rate p_C may deviate somewhat from $p_{C,o}$. Therefore, it would be of interest to investigate the performance of the test $\widehat{T}^{HB}_{RD,o}$ at $p_{C,o}$.

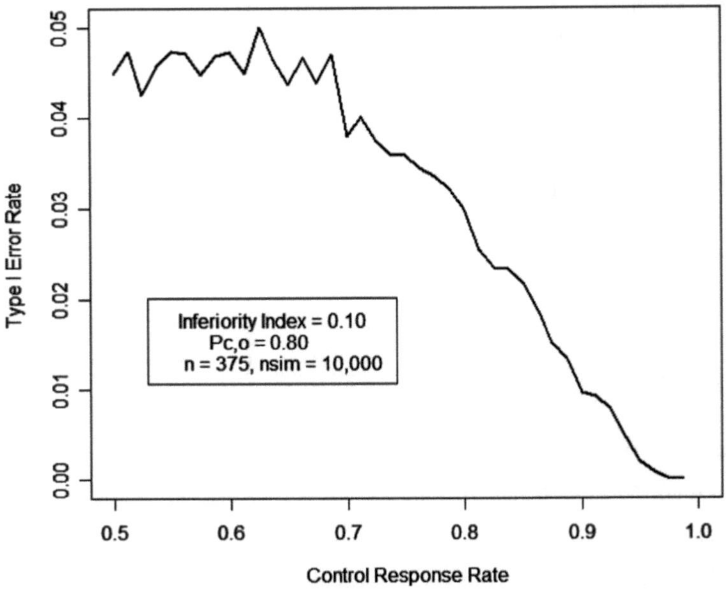

Fig. 13.3 Simulated overall type I error rate for hybrid design with the linear margin $\mathcal{L}(p_C|\rho_{S,o}, p_{C,o})$, where $\rho_{S,o} = 0.10$, $P_{c,o} = 0.80$, and $\alpha = 0.025$

13.4.4.1 Simulation of the Type I Error Rate

The type I error rate of $\widehat{T}_{RD,o}^{HB}$ is given by

$$\alpha(p_C) = 1 - \Phi\left(\frac{\sqrt{n}\widehat{\Delta}_{RD,o}}{\sqrt{\Sigma\,(p_C|H_o)}}\right). \tag{13.39}$$

Figure 13.3 displays the simulated type I error rate as a function of the true control response rate p_C. It shows that at the one-sided nominal significance level of 0.025, the type I error rate will be somewhat inflated when the true control response rate $p_C \leq p_{C,o}$. This should be expected because the true p_C is unknown and is being estimated by $\widehat{p}_C$. Furthermore, for $p_C < p_{C,o}$, the margin becomes more liberal, whereas for $p_C > p_{C,o}$, the margin becomes tighter. Therefore, by using a piecewise linear margin as discussed in Remark 3 should improve the type I error control substantially for $p_C < p_{C,o}$.

In light of the type I error rate inflation when $p_C = p_{C,o}$, one may wish to control this by lowering the significance level α. Table 13.2 and Fig. 13.4 show that if the overall significance level is lowered to approximately $\alpha = 0.020$, then the simulated type I error rate when $p_C = p_{C,o}$ is roughly controlled at 0.025.

However, instead of lowering the significance level $\alpha = 0.025$ to 0.020, it might be more preferable to consider replacing the linear margin $\mathcal{L}(p_C|\rho_{S,o}, p_{C,o})$ by a piecewise linear margin constructed by joining together two or more (if necessary) linear

Table 13.2 Simulated unadjusted and adjusted type I error rates for hybrid design with Taylor expansion at the point $p_{C,o} = 0.80$

True control	Significance level	
Response rate p_C	0.025	0.020
0.50	0.0448	0.0398
0.55	0.0473	0.0383
0.60	0.0472	0.0415
0.65	0.0436	0.0370
0.70	0.0378	0.0376
0.75	0.0358	0.0302
0.80	0.0298	0.0248
0.85	0.0217	0.0167
0.90	0.0096	0.0082
0.95	0.0020	0.0011

margins $\mathcal{L}(p_C|\rho_{S,o}, p_{C,o,1})$ and $\mathcal{L}(p_C|\rho_{S,o}, p_{C,o,2})$ at their point of intersection. For example, by piecing together $\mathcal{L}(p_C|\rho_{S,o}, p_{C,o,1})$ with $p_{C,o,1} = 0.65$ and $\mathcal{L}(p_C|\rho_{S,o}, p_{C,o})$ with $p_{C,o} = 0.80$ would improve substantially the approximation by the linear margin $\mathcal{L}(p_C|\rho_{S,o}, p_{C,o})$ alone as illustrated in Fig. 13.5. This would further improve the type I error control for $p_C < p_{C,o}$.

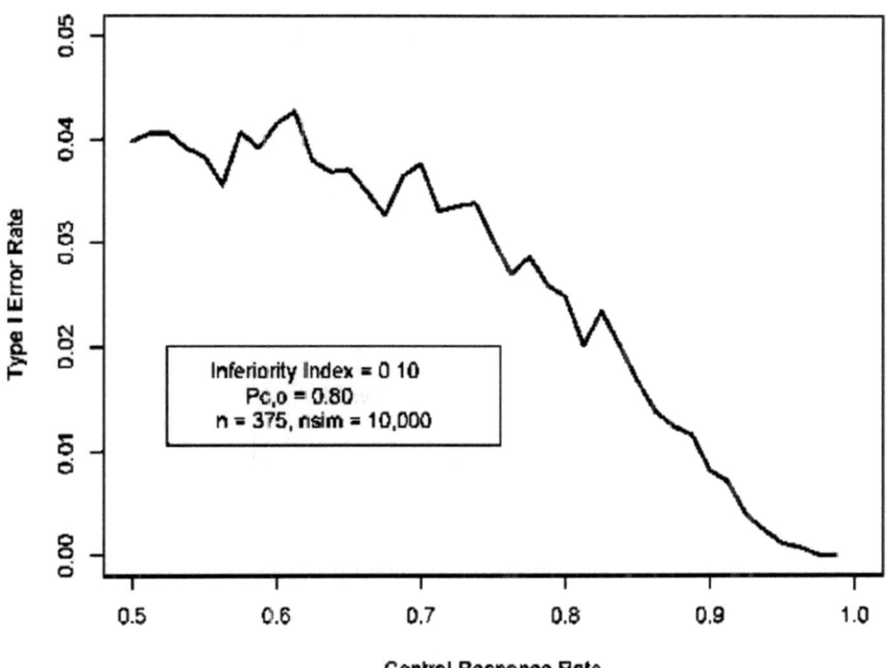

Fig. 13.4 Simulated overall type I error rate for hybrid design with the linear margin $\mathcal{L}(p_C|\rho_{S,o}, p_{C,o})$, where $\rho_{S,o} = 0.10$, $P_{c,o} = 0.80$, and $\alpha = 0.020$

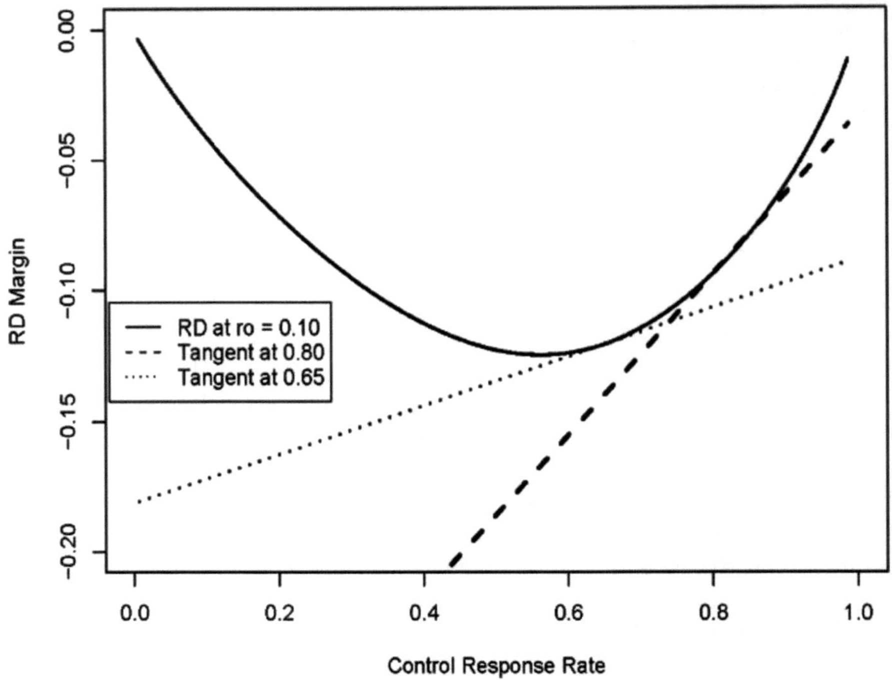

Fig. 13.5 Constructing piecewise linear margin for hybrid design with linear margin $\mathcal{L}(p_C|\rho_{S,o}, p_{C,o})$ expanded around $p_{C,o} = 0.65$ and 0.80. RD rate difference

13.4.4.2 Power Function

To derive the power function for the test statistic $\widehat{T}_{RD,o}$, one notes that under the specific alternative hypothesis $H_{sa}: \delta_{RD}(p_C) \equiv 0$, it follows from Eq. 13.35 that

$$E(\widehat{\Delta}_{RD}|H_{sa}) = E[\widehat{\delta}_{RD} - \mathcal{L}(\widehat{p}_C|\rho_{S,o}, p_{C,o})|H_{sa}] = -\mathcal{L}(p_C|\rho_{S,o}, p_{C,o}). \quad (13.40)$$

Now, let

$$\begin{aligned}\widehat{\Delta}_{RD,a} &= \widehat{\Delta}_{RD} - E\left(\widehat{\Delta}_{RD}|H_{sa}\right) = \widehat{\Delta}_{RD} + \mathcal{L}\left(p_C|\rho_{S,o}, p_{C,o}\right)\\ &= \left[\widehat{\delta}_{RD} - \frac{\partial g_{RD}^{*-1}(\rho_{S,o}, p_{C,o})}{\partial p_C}(\widehat{p}_C - p_C)\right].\end{aligned} \quad (13.41)$$

Then, it follows that under the specific alternative $H_{sa}: \delta_{RD}(p_C) \equiv 0$, $\sqrt{n}\,\widehat{\Delta}_{RD,a} \sim N(0, \Sigma(p_C|H_{sa}))$, where the asymptotic variance $\Sigma(p_C|H_{sa})$ is given by

$$\Sigma(p_C|H_{sa}) = \left[2 + 2\left(\frac{\partial g_{RD}^{*-1}(\rho_{S,o}, p_{C,o})}{\partial p_C}\right) + \left(\frac{\partial g_{RD}^{*-1}(\rho_{S,o}, p_{C,o})}{\partial p_C}\right)^2\right] p_C(1 - p_C). \quad (13.42)$$

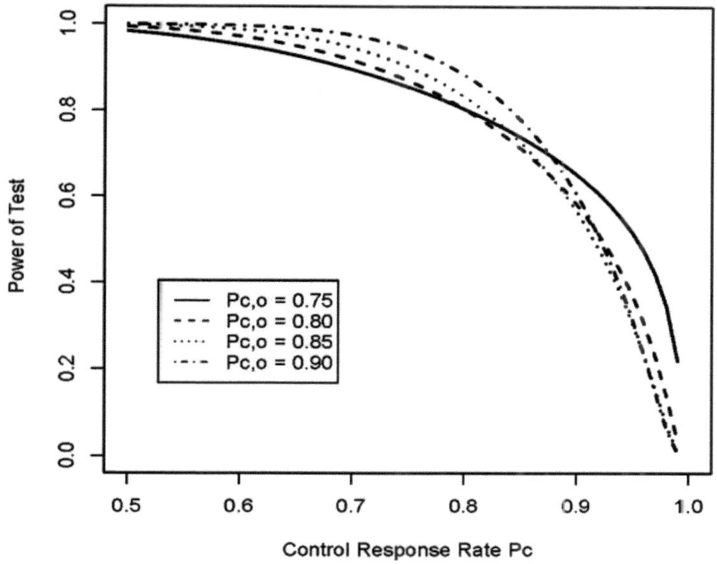

Fig. 13.6 Power functions for hybrid design with linear margin $\mathcal{L}(p_C|\rho_{S,o}, p_{C,o})$ at expansion points $p_{C,o} = 0.75, 0.80, 0.85$, and 0.90 and $n = 386$, $\alpha = 0.025$

Thus,

$$\widehat{T}^{HB}_{RD,sa} = \frac{\sqrt{n}\,\widehat{\Delta}_{RD,\,a}}{\sqrt{\Sigma(p_C|H_{sa})}} \sim N(0,1). \tag{13.43}$$

Now, from Eqs. 13.32 and 13.41, one has

$$\widehat{T}^{HB}_{RD,o} = \widehat{T}^{HB}_{RD,sa}\frac{\sqrt{\Sigma(p_C|H_{sa})}}{\sqrt{\Sigma(p_C|H_o)}} - \frac{\sqrt{n}[\mathcal{L}(p_C|\rho_{S,o}, p_{C,o})]}{\sqrt{\Sigma(p_C|H_o)}}. \tag{13.44}$$

Therefore, it follows that the power function is given by,

$$1-\beta = 1 - \Phi\left(\frac{1.96\sqrt{\Sigma\,(p_C|H_o)} + \sqrt{n}\mathcal{L}(p_C|\rho_{S,o}, p_{C,o})}{\sqrt{\Sigma\,(p_C|H_{sa})}}\right). \tag{13.45}$$

Now for the power function plot in Fig. 13.6, $n = 386$ was selected because it corresponds to an 80 % power for the hybrid design with a linear margin $\mathcal{L}(p_C\ \rho_{S,o}, p_{C,o})$, where $\rho_{S,o} = 0.10$ and $p_{C,o} = 0.80$. Similarly, for Fig. 13.7, $n = 516$ corresponds to a 90 % power for the hybrid design with a linear margin $\mathcal{L}(p_C|\rho_{S,o}, p_{C,o})$, where $\rho_{S,o} = 0.10$ and $p_{C,o} = 0.80$. Both power plots in Figs. 13.6 and 13.7 show that the power drops off quickly when $p_C > p_{C,o}$ due to the dramatic change in variance as $p_C \rightarrow 1$. The deflation in type I error rate for $p_C > p_{C,o}$ might be a desirable feature since it raises a natural barrier to prevent ejection of the inferiority null of Eq. 13.33 or 13.34 when the true control response rate p_C is much greater than the assumed control response rate $p_{C,o}$.

The powers for selected true control response rate p_C in the plots in Figs. 13.6 and 13.7 are given in Table 13.3.

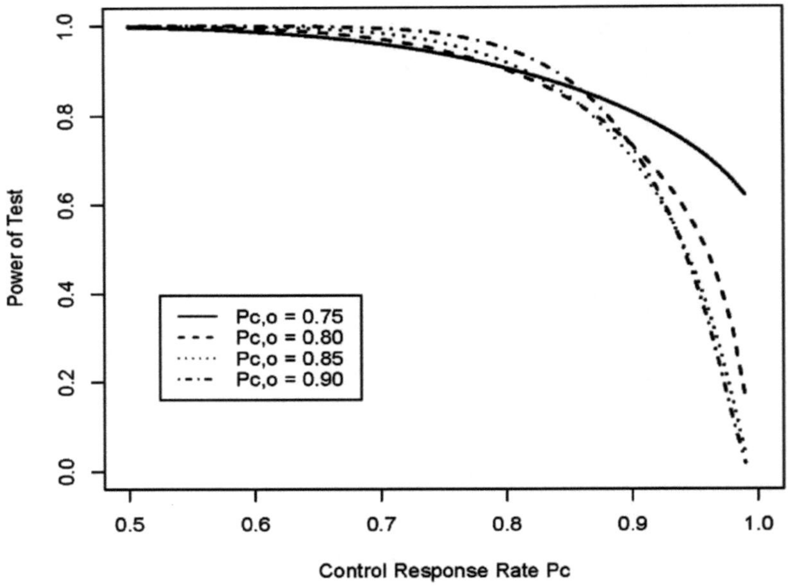

Fig. 13.7 Power functions for hybrid design with linear margin $\mathcal{L}(p_C|p_{S,o}, p_{C,o})$ at expansion points $p_{C,o} = 0.75$, 0.80, 0.85, and 0.90 and $n = 516$, $\alpha = 0.025$

Table 13.3 Pointwise power across p_C at a significance level of $\alpha = 0.025$ and different expansion point $p_{C,o}$

		Expansion point $p_{C,o}$			
Sample size for hybrid design p_C	p_C	0.75	0.80	0.85	0.90
375	0.70	0.895	0.917	0.946	0.975
(80 % Power for $p_{C,o} = 0.80$)	0.75	0.855	0.869	0.902	0.943
	0.80	0.803	0.803	0.832	0.883
	0.85	0.738	0.712	0.725	0.779
	0.90	0.651	0.581	0.564	0.604
	0.95	0.515	0.369	0.305	0.312
500	0.70	0.959	0.969	0.983	0.994
(90 % Power for $p_{C,o} = 0.80$)	0.75	0.936	0.943	0.961	0.981
	0.80	0.905	0.901	0.918	0.949
	0.85	0.863	0.836	0.840	0.877
	0.90	0.807	0.733	0.703	0.729
	0.95	0.726	0.549	0.446	0.428

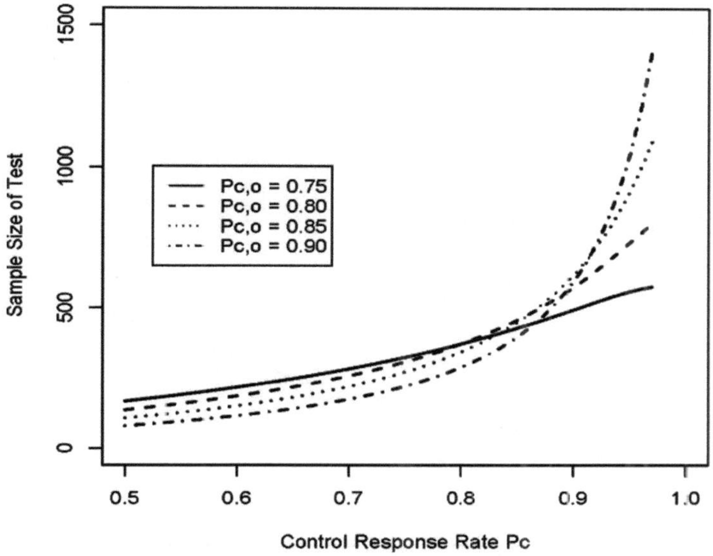

Fig. 13.8 Plots of sample size per group at $\alpha = 0.025$ and 80 % power for hybrid design with linear margin $\mathcal{L}(p_C|\rho_{S,o}, p_{C,o})$ at $\rho_{S,o} = 0.10$ and expansion points $p_{C,o} = 0.75$, 0.80, 0.85, and 0.90

13.4.4.3 Sample Size Calculation

From Eq. 13.44, the sample size formula is derived by setting

$$-z_{1-\beta} = \frac{1.96\sqrt{\Sigma(p_C|H_o)} + \sqrt{n}\,\mathcal{L}(p_C|\rho_{S,o}, p_{C,o})}{\sqrt{\Sigma(p_C|H_{sa})}}.$$

Solving for n, one obtains,

$$n = \frac{\left(1.96\sqrt{\Sigma(p_C|H_o)} + z_{1-\beta}\sqrt{\Sigma(p_C|H_{sa})}\right)^2}{\mathcal{L}^2(p_C|\rho_{S,o}, p_{C,o})}. \quad (13.46)$$

Figures 13.8 and 13.9 display the sample size plots for the hybrid design with linear margin $\mathcal{L}(p_C|\rho_{S,o}, p_{C,o})$ at the expansion points $p_{C,o} = 0.75$, 0.80, 0.85, and 0.90 (Table 13.4).

As discussed in Sect. 13.4.3.1, if one also wishes to control the type I error rate at $p_C = p_{C,o}$ at $\alpha = 0.025$, then one needs to increase the sample size accordingly. Table 13.5 shows the sample size needed for such adjustment.

13.4.5 An Application to the Design of HABP/VABP Trials

The FDA Anti-infective Advisory Committee convened in November 2011 to discuss issues related to the design of NI trials for HABP and VABP [US FDA (2011)]. In

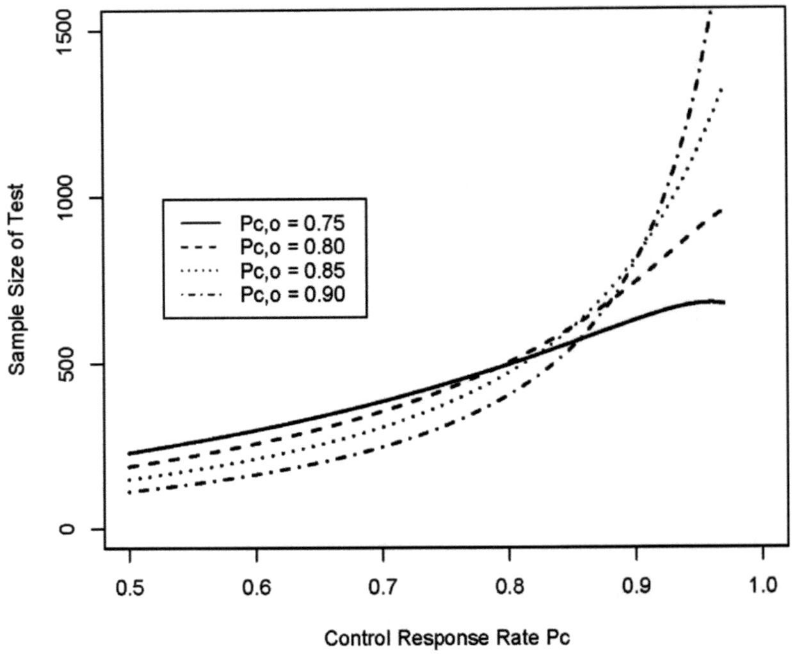

Fig. 13.9 Plots of sample size per group at $\alpha = 0.025$ and 90 % power for hybrid design with linear margin $\mathcal{L}(p_C | \rho_{S,o}, p_{C,o})$ at $\rho_{S,o} = 0.10$ and expansion points $p_{C,o} = 0.75$, 0.80, 0.85, and 0.90

Table 13.4 Selected sample size per group at $\alpha = 0.025$ for hybrid design with linear margin $\mathcal{L}(p_C | \rho_{S,o}, p_{C,o})$ at $\rho_{S,o} = 0.10$ and expansion points $p_{C,o} = 0.75$, 0.80, 0.85, and 0.90

	Power	
Taylor expansion point $P_{C,o}$	80 %	90 %
0.75	323	435
0.80	386	516
0.85	450	605
0.90	593	798

Table 13.5 Unadjusted and adjusted sample size per group for hybrid design with Taylor expansion at the point $p_{C,o} = 0.80$

	Significance level	
Power	0.025	0.020
0.80	386	400
0.90	516	529

the briefing book provided to the Committee members, FDA presented the following data based on two historical placebo-controlled studies and five recent active control studies (Table 13.6).

The estimated control survival rate is equal to 80 %. An estimate of the CE is given by CE = [(0.52 − 0.23) − 0.09] = 0.20, which is obtained by taking the difference

Table 13.6 Estimated mortality rates and 95 % confidence intervals

	Mortality rate	95 % CI
Placebo	62 %	(52 %, 71 %)
Control	20 %	(18 %, 23 %)

Table 13.7 Sample size calculated by FDA for the rate difference measure δ_{RD}

Power	HABP	VABP
80 %	834	714
90 %	1114	894

HABP hospital-acquired bacterial pneumonia, *VABP* ventilation-associated bacterial pneumonia

between a conservative estimate of the mortality rate under placebo (52 %) and a conservative estimate of the mortality rate under control (23 %) and then subtract 9 % to account for factors that may impact on the underlying assumptions of constancy and assay sensitivity. The proposed NI margin was then set at $\delta_{RD,\,o} = -\text{CE} \times \frac{1}{2} = -0.20 \times \frac{1}{2} = -0.10$, where the fraction of one half is based on clinical judgment regarding the size of the margin. FDA posed to the Committee several questions, including the following: What margin should one use in the event the control survival rate from the NI trial appears to deviate from the estimated control survival rate of 80 %?

For the RD measure δ_{RD}, FDA calculated the sample sizes required for 80 and 90 % power at a significance level of 0.025 after an adjustment of 60 %/70 % microbiologic evaluability rate for HABP/VABP trials, respectively, as given in Table 13.7.

Thus, with the given fixed margin of $\delta_{RD,o} = -0.10$ at an estimated survival rate of $p_{C,o} = 0.80$ (equivalent to a 20 % mortality rate), the degree of stringency for the empirically derived pair $(\delta_{RD,o},\ p_{C,o}) = (-0.10, 0.80)$ can be assessed using the standard index function in Eq. 13.22 and is equal to $\rho_{S,o} = g^*_{RD}(\delta_{RD,o}, p_{C,o}) = g^*_{RD}(-0.10,\ 0.80) = 0.1057$. Now, for simplicity of discussion, consider rounding it to an index level of $\rho_{S,c} = 0.10$ instead of the actual index level of 0.1057, since type I error simulations, power plots, and sample size calculations presented previously used the index level of 0.10. This is equivalent to considering a margin of $\delta_{RD,o} = -0.0939$ instead of the margin of $\delta_{RD,o} = -0.10$, at $p_{C,o} = 0.80$. Now upon setting the inferiority index level to $\rho_{S,o} = 0.10$ in the margin function given by Eq. 13.24, one obtains the special indexed margin function $\delta_{RD}(p_C|0.10) = g^{*-1}_{RD}(0.10,\ p_C)$ with the degree of stringency specified by $\rho_{S,o} = 0.10$. After applying the Taylor expansion around the point $p_{C,o} = 0.80$, one finds the linear margin function is equal to

$$\begin{aligned} \mathcal{L}(p_C|\rho_{S,o},\ p_{C,o}) &= \mathcal{L}(p_C|0.10,\ 0.80) = \delta_{RD}(p_C|0.10) \\ &\quad + \frac{\partial g^{*-1}_{RD}}{\partial p_C}(0.10,\ 0.80)(p_C - 0.80) \\ &= -0.0939 + 0.3066\,(p_C - 0.80). \end{aligned}$$

The hybrid NI hypothesis is then defined by

$$H_o: \ \delta_{RD} - [-0.0939 + 0.3066\,(p_C - 0.80)] \leq 0$$

$$vs.$$

$$H_a: \ \delta_{RD} - [-0.0939 + 0.3066\,(p_C - 0.80)] > 0. \tag{13.47}$$

Based on the hybrid design that has just been discussed in Sect. 13.4, to test the hybrid NI hypothesis (Eq. 13.47) at the expansion point $p_{C,o} = 0.80$ with a significance level of $\alpha = 0.025$ and a power of 80 %, a sample size of $n = 386$ subjects per group would be needed (see Table 13.3, Table 13.4 or Table 13.5). Now the sample size per group needed for an HABP/VABP trial is given by 643/551, reflecting an adjustment for a 60 %/70 % microbiologic evaluability rate, or for a total sample size of 1286/1102. On the other hand, for the fixed margin NI hypothesis, the sample size per group is $n = 283$. After adjusting for 60 %/70 % microbiologic evaluability rate, this gives rise to a sample size per group of 472/404 or a total sample size of 944/809 for HABP/VABP trials (see Chi and Koch 2012), reflecting a 36.2 %/36.4 % increase.

Thus, one can see that at a significance level of $\alpha = 0.025$ and a power of 80 %, the flexibility realized in a hybrid NI design with a linear margin $\mathcal{L}(p_C | \rho_{S,o}, p_{C,o})$ derived at the empirically based inferiority index value of $\rho_{S,o} = 0.10$ and the expansion point $p_{C,o} = 0.80$, which is the estimated control response rate, is gained at the cost of about a 36 % increase in the size over that required for a corresponding fixed margin NI design.

Now the hybrid design with its NI hypothesis given by Eq. 13.33 or 13.34 has a linear margin $\mathcal{L}(p_C | \rho_{S,o}, p_{C,o})$ that allows the true control response rate p_C to deviate somewhat from the assumed control response rate of 0.80 at the design stage. If the true control response rate $p_C > 0.80$, then from the type I error simulations, one knows that the probability of rejecting the null of Eq. 13.33 or Eq. 13.34 is low and very low when $p_C > 0.90$. However, with the given sample size, the test still has about 60 % power in rejecting the margin given by $\mathcal{L}(0.90|0.10,\ 0.80) = -0.0614$ at $p_C = 0.90$, which is very comparable to the margin $\delta_{RD}(0.90|\rho_{S,o}) = g_{RD}^{*-1}(0.10,\ 0.90) = -0.0601$ based on the margin function in Eq. 13.24 as shown in Table 13.1. The power of the test also decreases rapidly as p_C moves away from 0.80 towards 1. However, if the true $p_C < 0.80$, then there is inflation in the type I error rate despite the adjustment. Without adjustment by lowering the nominal significance level from $\alpha = 0.025$, one may consider a better alternative discussed earlier by constructing a piecewise linear margin by joining another linear margin $\mathcal{L}(p_C | \rho_{S,o}, p_{C,1})$ derived from first-order Taylor expansion of the same indexed margin function $\delta_{RD}(p_C | \rho_{S,o})$ at another point $p_{C,1}$, where $0.50 < p_{C,1} < p_{C,o}$, with the original linear margin $\mathcal{L}(p_C | \rho_{S,o}, p_{C,o})$. Phillips (2003) has actually constructed piecewise linear margin based on consensus opinions of clinical experts. It is not linked to any index function and is unrelated to the piecewise linear margin as discussed in this chapter. The theoretical properties of an NI design with a piecewise linear margin has been investigated by Zhang (2006) for the likelihood ratio test. The method developed there may be applicable to the hybrid design with a piecewise linear margin. It should be of practical interest to investigate this matter further for the RD measure along the line as suggested in Sect. 13.5.

13.5 Summary Discussion

At the November 2011 FDA Anti-Infective Advisory Committee (US FDA 2011) meeting discussing the design of HABP or VABP trials, the agency posed several questions to the Committee. This chapter attempts to address two of the questions. The first question concerns the appropriateness of the empirically derived fixed margin associated with an estimated control response rate using FDA's two-step procedure. The second question pertains to what margin one should use when the expected control response rate p_C from the NI trial appears to deviate from the estimated control response rate $p_{C,o}$. Should one use the same margin or a different margin? If one is to use a different margin, then what should that margin be? Is there a prospective strategy that one can use to address this problem?

The hybrid NI hypothesis proposed in this chapter is defined by a special linear margin, $\mathcal{L}(p_C|\rho_{S,o}, p_{C,o})$, which is the first-order Taylor expansion of a specific indexed margin function around the estimated control response rate $p_{C,o}$. The specific indexed margin function is defined as follows. First, derive the index value $\rho_{S,o} = g^*_{RD}(\delta_{RD,o}, p_{C,o})$ from the index function given in Eq. 13.22 at the empirically derived pair $(\delta_{RD,o}, p_{C,o})$. Therefore, $\rho_{S,o}$ is an empirically derived inferiority index value. Next, set the index ρ_S in the margin function $\delta_{RD} = g^{*-1}_{RD}(\rho_S,\ p_C)$ given in Eq. 13.23 equal to this empirically derived index value $\rho_{S,o}$ which defines the specific margin function $\delta_{RD}(p_C|\rho_{S,o}) = g^{*-1}_{RD}(\rho_{S,o},\ p_C)$ given by Eq. 13.24. Now define the linear margin given by $\mathcal{L}(p_C|\rho_{S,o}, p_{C,o}) = \delta_{RD}(p_{C,o}|\rho_{S,o}) + \frac{\partial g^{*-1}_{RD}(\rho_{S,o},p_C)}{\partial p_C}(p_C - p_{C,o})$ as the first-order Taylor approximation to the margin function $\delta_{RD}(p_C|\rho_{S,o})$ expanded around $p_C = p_{C,o}$. Clearly, $\mathcal{L}(p_{C,o}|\rho_{S,o}, p_{C,o}) = \delta_{RD}(p_{C,o}|\rho_{S,o}) = \delta_{RD,o}$ when $p_C = p_{C,o}$. Thus, if the true control response rate $p_C = p_{C,o}$, then the hybrid margin reduces to the given fixed margin, but if the true control response rate $p_C \neq p_{C,o}$, then the hybrid margin adjusts the given fixed margin $\delta_{RD}(p_{C,o}|\rho_{S,o}) = \delta_{RD,o}$ by the quantity $\frac{\partial g^{*-1}_{RD}(\rho_{S,o},p_C)}{\partial p_C}(p_C - p_{C,o})$. Hence, the linear margin integrates the empirically derived pair $\delta_{RD,o},\ p_{C,o})$ with a variable component that adjusts for the deviation $(p_C - p_{C,o})$. Thus, the NI hypothesis defined by such a linear margin is called a hybrid design. Such a hybrid design conveys the stringency of the margin through the empirically derived index value $\rho_{S,o}$ and at the same time also has the flexibility to adjust for the margin in the event the control response rate from the trial deviates from the estimated control response rate $p_{C,o}$. Of course, this flexibility of a hybrid design is gained at the cost of a 33 % increase in sample size compared to that required for a fixed margin design for the example considered.

The linear margin $\mathcal{L}(p_C|\rho_{S,o}, p_{C,o})$ tends to be more liberal if the true control response rate is in the range of $0.50 < p_C < p_{C,o}$. For example, with $(\delta_{RD,o}, p_{C,o}) = (-0.10,\ 0.80)$, the linear margin closely approximates the margin function $\delta_{RD}(p_C|\rho_{S,o})$ only for p_C over the range (0.75, 0.90). One may try to minimize this type I error rate inflation by lowering the overall significance level. But this approach would be too drastic and still would not fully resolve the problem. An alternative strategy is to construct a piecewise linear margin by joining two linear margins $\mathcal{L}(p_C|\rho_{S,o}, p_{C,1})$ and $\mathcal{L}(p_C|\rho_{S,o}, p_{C,o})$ at their point of intersection, where $0.50 < p_{C,1} < p_{C,o}$ along the line of Phillips (2003) and Zhang (2006) who demonstrated the asymptotic convergence of the likelihood ratio test statistic for the NI hypothesis defined by a piecewise linear margin. However, an even better strategy is to define a spline function that joins the two linear margins by smoothing out the corner where they intersect [Reinsch (1967), Byrne and Chi (1972), De Boor (2001)]. Such a spline margin would have the regularity property required for the estimate as well as for the asymptotic convergence of the test statistic associated with such hybrid NI hypothesis. The idea of a hybrid design with an empirically determined spline margin based on the special indexed margin function $\delta_{RD}(p_C|\rho_{S,o})$ deserves further investigation because it can provide margins closely matching those from the margin function $\delta_{RD}(p_C|\rho_{S,o})$ throughout the interval (0.50, 1) and has sufficient regularity properties required for the convergence theorem to hold. All of these hybrid designs are of special appeal because they integrate the FDA's two-step fixed margin approach with the flexibility of a variable margin and their associated test statistics have reasonable performance characteristics by taking advantage of the improvement made by the convergence theorem (Theorem 2) under fixed margin for the RD measure. However, these positive attributes come with a 36 % increase in sample size over those required under a fixed margin NI hypothesis.

Looking beyond binary outcome trials, some of the ideas used in this chapter can be extended to normal distributions to provide a natural framework for handling problems involving heterogeneity of variance, such as in establishing bioequivalence of highly variable drugs. Unlike the case under Bernoulli distributions, where for a given index value, the margin is simply a function of the control response rate p_C, under normal distributions, for a given index value, the margin would be a function of the variance of the control σ_C and the variance ratio σ^2 when not assumed to be known.

Post Note: In this chapter, the author has corrected an error that appeared in the original paper by Li and Chi (2011). Specifically, in Eq. 13.7 on page 293 of the Li and Chi (2011) paper, the number "4" appearing in the denominator of the third term should be replaced by the number "2" as shown in Eq. 13.2 in the present chapter. This correction has no impact under normal distributions. But under Bernoulli distributions, the impact of this correction is to increase the variance S in Corollary 2 of Li and Chi (2011) on page 298 by an amount $\frac{\delta^2(\rho,\sigma)}{1+\sigma^2}$ and thus the variance there should be $S = \left\{1 + \frac{\delta^2(\rho,\sigma)}{16\sigma_C^2\sigma^2}\right\} + \frac{\delta^2(\rho,\sigma)}{1+\sigma^2}$. It should also be pointed out that at the end of this same corollary, the variance estimate $\widehat{\sigma}_C^2$ is missing by a factor of ½ and it should be given by $\widehat{\sigma}_C^2 = \frac{1}{2}\left[\frac{\widehat{p}_T(1-\widehat{p}_T)}{\sigma^2} + \widehat{p}_C(1-\widehat{p}_C)\right]$.

This same error also appears in Chi and Koch (2012). Specifically, at the end of Theorem 2 of Chi and Koch (2012), the variance $\Sigma_{SRD,\,o}^2$ should be given by $\Sigma_{SRD,\,o}^2 = \left(1+\sigma_o^2\right)\left(1 + \frac{\delta_{SRD,\,o}^2}{16\sigma_C^2\sigma_o^2}\right) + \frac{\delta_{SRD,\,o}^2}{2}$ as given in Eq. 13.4 of the present chapter.

Hence, it follows that Eq. 13.24 in Theorem 4 of Chi and Koch (2012) should be replaced by $\Sigma_{RD,o}^2 = \left[(\sigma_{C,o}^2 + \sigma_{T,o}^2)\left(1 + \frac{\delta_{RD,o}^2}{16\sigma_{C,o}^2\sigma_{T,o}^2}\right) + \frac{\delta_{RD,o}^2}{2}\right] - (1 - 2p_{C,o})\delta_{RD,o}$ which is given by Eq. 13.8 of the present chapter. In addition, in Theorem 4 of Chi and Koch (2012), in the expression for the variance $\Sigma_{LOR,o}^2$ given by Eq. 13.26, the variance $\Sigma_{SRD,\,o}^2$ in the first term should be as given above which is given by Eq. 13.4 of the present chapter.

Similarly, the same error appears in Chi (2013). In Theorem 1 of Chi (2012), the variance term $\Sigma_{RD,o}^2(p_{C,o}|H_o)$ in Eq. 13.15 should be replaced by $\Sigma_{RD,o}^2\left(p_{C,o}\ H_o\right) = \left[(\sigma_{C,o}^2 + \sigma_{T,o}^2)\left(1 + \frac{\delta_{RD,o}^2}{16\sigma_{C,o}^2\sigma_{T,o}^2}\right) + \frac{\delta_{RD,o}^2}{2}\right] - (1 - 2p_{C,o})\delta_{RD,o}$ which is given by Eq. 13.8 of this chapter.

References

Berry AC (1941) The accuracy of the Gaussian approximation to the sum of independent variates. Trans Am Math Soc 49:122–136

Bristol DR (1996) Determining equivalence and the impact of sample size in anti-infective studies: a point to consider. J Biopharm Stat 6(3):319–326

Byrne GD, Chi DNH (1972) Linear multistep formulas based on g-splines. SIAM J Numerical Anal 9:316–324

Chi GYH (2012) Inferiority index and the Behrens-Fisher problem for non-inferiority trials. In: 2012 Proceedings of the American Statistical Association, Biopharmaceutical Section, p 776–784

Chi GYH (2013) A hybrid design for non-inferiority trials with binary outcomes. In: 2013 Proceedings of the American Statistical Association, Biopharmaceutical Section, p 3728–3742

Chi GYH, Koch GG (2012) Inferiority index and margin function for non-inferiority trials with binary outcomes. In: 2013 Proceedings of the American Statistical Association, September 2012 FDA-Industry Workshop, p 4451–4465

de Boor C (2001) A practical guide to splines. Applied mathematical sciences series, vol. 27. New York, Springer-Verlag

Esseen CG (1942) On the Liapunoff limit of error in the theory of probability. Ark Mat Astron Fys A28:1–19

Garrett AD (2003) Therapeutic equivalence: fallacies and falsification. Stat Med 22:741–762

Kim MY, Xue X (2004) Likelihood ratio and a Bayesian approach were superior to standard non-inferiority analysis when the non-inferiority margin varied with the control event rate. J Clin Epidemiol 57:1253–1261

Li G, Chi GYH (2011) Inferiority index and margin in non-inferiority trials. Stat Biopharm Res 3(2):288–301

Munk A, Skipka B, Stratmann B (2005) Testing general hypotheses under binomial sampling: the two sample case—asymptotic theory and exact procedures. Comput Stat Data Anal 49:723–739

Phillips KF (2003) A new test of non-inferiority for anti-infective trials. Stat Med 22:201–212

Reinsch CH (1967) Smoothing by spline functions. Numerische Mathematik 10:177–183

Röhmel J (1998) Therapeutic equivalence investigations: statistical considerations. Stat Med 17:1703–1714

Röhmel J (2001) Statistical considerations of FDA and CPMP rules for the investigation of new anti-bacterial products. Stat Med 20:2561–2571

Senn S (2000) Consensus and controversy in pharmaceutical statistics (with discussion). J Roy Stat Soc Ser. D 49:135–176

Tu D (1998) On the use of the ratio or the odds ratio of cure rates in therapeutic equivalence clinical trials with binary endpoints. J Biopharm Stat 8(2):263–282

US Food and Drug Administration (1992) Anti-infective points to consider guidance, Office of Communication/Division of Drug Information/CDER/FDA, W051, Room 2001, 10903 New Hampshire Avenue, Silver Spring, MD, 20993

US Food and Drug Administration (2010) Guidance to industry: non-inferiority clinical trials, Office of Communication/Division of Drug Information/CDER/FDA, W051, Room 2001, 10903 New Hampshire Avenue, Silver Spring, MD, 20993

US Food and Drug Administration (2011) Anti-infective drugs advisory committee meeting materials, 3–4 Nov 2011, http://www.fda.gov/AdvisoryCommittees/CommitteesMeetingMaterials/Drugs/Anti-InfectiveDrugsAdvisoryCommittee/ucm242307.htm. Accessed 7 Feb 2013

U.S. Food and Drug Administration (2013) 'IND content and format', 21 CFR 312.23 (a)(6)(ii), www.accessdata.fda.gov/scripts/cdrh/cfdocs/cfcfr/cfrsearch.cfm?fr†=312.23. Accessed 3 Jan 2014

Weng CSW, Liu JP (1994) Some pitfalls in sample size estimation for an anti-infective study. In: 1994 Proceedings of the Pharmaceutical Section of the ASA, p 56–60

Zhang Z (2006) Non-inferiority testing with a variable margin. Biometrical J 48(6):948–965

Chapter 14
Group-Sequential Designs When Considering Two Binary Outcomes as Co-Primary Endpoints

Koko Asakura, Toshimitsu Hamasaki, Scott R. Evans, Tomoyuki Sugimoto and Takashi Sozu

Abstract We discuss group-sequential designs with two binary endpoints as co-primary. We derive the power and required sample size within two decision-making frameworks: (i) to evaluate whether superiority of a test intervention relative to control has been shown for both endpoints *at any interim time point, not necessarily simultaneously* and (ii) to evaluate whether superiority has been demonstrated for both endpoints *at the same interim time point* of the trial. We evaluate the utility of the method in practice using Monte Carlo simulation and investigate the behavior of the sample sizes with varying design characteristics. We provide a real example to illustrate the method. We also discuss sample size recalculation based on observed interim data. Lastly, we discuss a method for hierarchical hypothesis testing with adaptive type I error allocation in group-sequential designs with co-primary endpoints in order to improve the power of the methods.

14.1 Introduction

Clinical trials are often conducted with the objective of comparing a test intervention with a standard intervention based on several binary outcomes. For example, irritable bowel syndrome (IBS) is one of the most common gastrointestinal disorders and is characterized by symptoms of abdominal pain, discomfort, and altered bowel function (American College of Gastroenterology 2013; Grundmann and Yoon 2010). The comparison of the interventions to treat IBS is based on the proportions of participants with adequate relief of abdominal pain and discomfort, and improvements in urgency, stool frequency, and stool consistency. Traditionally, one important and

T. Hamasaki (✉) · K. Asakura
National Cerebral and Cardiovascular Center, 5-7-1 Fujishirodai, Suita, Osaka 565-8565, Japan
e-mail: toshi.hamasaki@ncvc.go.jp

S. R. Evans
Harvard School of Public Health, Boston, Massachusetts, USA

T. Sugimoto
Hirosaki University, Aomori, Japan

T. Sozu
Kyoto University School of Public Health, Kyoto, Japan

Z. Chen et al. (eds.), *Applied Statistics in Biomedicine and Clinical Trials Design*,
ICSA Book Series in Statistics, DOI 10.1007/978-3-319-12694-4_14

clinically relevant outcome is selected as the primary endpoint and is then used as the basis for the trial design, including sample size determination, interim monitoring, and final analyses. However, many recent clinical trials have utilized more than one endpoint as co-primary. "Co-primary" in this setting means that the trial is designed to evaluate whether the new intervention is superior to the control on all endpoints, thus evaluating the intervention's multidimensional effects. For example, the US Food and Drug Administration recommends the use of two endpoints for assessing IBS signs and symptoms: (1) pain intensity and (2) stool frequency (Food and Drug Administration 2012). The Committee for Medicinal Products for Human Use (2013) recommends the use of two endpoints for assessing IBS signs and symptoms: (1) global assessment of symptoms and (2) assessment of symptoms of abdominal discomfort/pain. Offen et al. (2007) provide other examples.

The resulting need for new approaches to the design and analysis of clinical trials with co-primary endpoints has been noted. Controlling the type I and type II error rates when the multiple co-primary endpoints are potentially correlated is nontrivial. When designing the trial to evaluate the joint effects on *all* of the endpoints, no adjustment is needed to control the type I error rate if each endpoint is tested at the same prespecified significance level. However, the type II error rate increases as the number of endpoints to be evaluated increases. Thus, sample size adjustment is needed to maintain the overall power. This often results in large and impractical sample sizes. In order to reduce the sample size, methods for clinical trials with co-primary endpoints have been discussed for fixed-sample designs by many authors (Chuang-Stein et al. 2007; Eaton and Muirhead 2007; Hamasaki et al. 2013; Julious and Mclntyre 2012; Kordzakhia et al. 2010; Offen et al. 2007; Senn and Bretz 2007; Sozu et al. 2010, 2011, 2012; Sugimoto et al. 2012, 2013; Xiong et al. 2005). These methods incorporate the correlations among the endpoints into sample size calculations. In practice, the correlations are usually unknown. The correlations may be estimated based on external or pilot data but such data are often unavailable.

Hung and Wang (2009) proposed a group-sequential design for clinical trials with co-primary endpoints because it offers the possibility to stop a trial early when evidence is overwhelming, thus offering efficiency (i.e., potentially fewer patients than the fixed-sample designs). The method also allows recalculation of the sample size based on the observed interim effect sizes. Recently, Asakura et al. (2014) discuss two decision-making frameworks associated with hypothesis testing in clinical trials with two continuous endpoints as co-primary in a group-sequential setting.

We extend the methods in Asakura et al. (2014) and discuss group-sequential designs in clinical trials with two binary outcomes as co-primary. As a foundation case, we consider a two-arm parallel-group trial designed to evaluate whether an experimental intervention is superior to a control based on two binary endpoints. The methods in Asakura et al. (2014) consist of prespecifying the type I error allocation for both endpoints, using any α-spending function methods. In order to improve the power, we discuss a method for hierarchical hypothesis testing with adaptive type I error allocation, which was proposed by Tsong et al. (2004). They discussed a three-arm clinical trial for the assessment of the efficacy and equivalence of a generic drug. This chapter is structured as follows: In Sect. 14.2, we describe the decision-making frameworks for group-sequential designs in clinical trials using two correlated binary outcomes evaluated as co-primary and define the corresponding power and sample size calculations based on the normal approximation method. In Sect. 14.3, we evaluate the practical utility of the normal approximation method by Monte Carlo simulation, and investigate the behavior of the required sample size with varying design parameters. In Sect. 14.4, we describe methods for sample size recalculation based on the observed interim effects. In Sect. 14.5, we discuss a method for hierarchical hypothesis testing with adaptive type I error allocation. In Sect. 14.6, we summarize the findings.

14.2 Group-Sequential Designs with Co-Primary Endpoints

14.2.1 Statistical Settings

Consider a randomized clinical trial designed to compare the test intervention with control intervention, with two binary outcomes being evaluated as co-primary endpoints ($k = 1,2$). n and rn participants are recruited and randomly assigned to the test intervention group (T) and the control intervention group (C), respectively, where r is the sample ratio ($r > 0$). Then, we have n binary outcomes $Y_{\mathrm{T}ki} (i = 1, \ldots, n; k = 1,2)$ for the test intervention group and rn outcomes $Y_{\mathrm{C}kj} (j = 1, \ldots, rn; k = 1,2)$ for the control group. Suppose $Y_{\mathrm{T}ki}$ and $Y_{\mathrm{C}kj}$ are independently binomial distributed with probabilities of success $p_{\mathrm{T}k}$ and $p_{\mathrm{C}k}$, i.e., $\mathrm{B}(1, p_{\mathrm{T}k})$ and $\mathrm{B}(1, p_{\mathrm{C}k})$, but the observations within pairs for the two interventions are correlated with a common correlation $\mathrm{corr}\,[Y_{\mathrm{T}1i}, Y_{\mathrm{T}2i}] = \mathrm{corr}\,[Y_{\mathrm{C}1j}, Y_{\mathrm{C}2j}] = \rho$. The range of the correlation ρ is restricted, depending on the marginal probabilities (Prentice 1988; Le Cessie and Houwelingen 1994).

Let $Y_{\mathrm{T}k} = \sum_{i=1}^{n} Y_{\mathrm{T}ki}$ and $Y_{\mathrm{C}k} = \sum_{j=1}^{rn} Y_{\mathrm{C}kj}$ denote the number of successes under the test and the control interventions, then $Y_{\mathrm{T}k} \sim \mathrm{B}(n, p_{\mathrm{T}k})$ and $Y_{\mathrm{C}k} \sim \mathrm{B}(rn, p_{\mathrm{C}k})$. We now have the two (observed) differences in proportions $\hat{\delta}_k = \hat{p}_{\mathrm{T}k} - \hat{p}_{\mathrm{C}k}$, where $\hat{p}_{\mathrm{T}k} = n^{-1} Y_{\mathrm{T}k}$ and $\hat{p}_{\mathrm{C}k} = (rn)^{-1} Y_{\mathrm{C}k}$. We are interested in conducting a hypothesis testing on the difference in proportions $\delta_k = p_{\mathrm{T}k} - p_{\mathrm{C}k}$ ($k = 1, 2$) to evaluate whether the intervention is superior to the control intervention, where a positive value of δ_k indicates a treatment benefit. Thus, the hypotheses are $\mathrm{H}_0 : \delta_1 \le 0$ or $\delta_2 \le 0$ versus $\mathrm{H}_1 : \delta_1 > 0$ and $\delta_2 > 0$. The H_0 is rejected if and only if both of the null hypotheses associated with each of the two primary endpoints are rejected at significance level α. Let (Z_1, Z_2) be the test statistics given by

$$Z_k = \frac{\sqrt{n}\hat{\delta}_k}{\sqrt{\hat{\bar{p}}_k\left(1 - \hat{\bar{p}}_k\right)(1+r)/r}},$$

where $\hat{\bar{p}}_k = (\hat{p}_{Tk} + r\hat{p}_{Ck})/(1+r)$. The rejection regions of H_0 are $[\{Z_1 > z_\alpha\} \cap \{Z_2 > z_\alpha\}]$, where z_α is the $100(1-\alpha)$th percentile of the standard normal distribution. For large samples, using the delta method, the distribution of (Z_1, Z_2) is approximately bivariate normal with correlation matrix $\boldsymbol{\rho}_Z$, where its off-diagonal element is

$$\rho_Z = \rho \frac{r\sqrt{p_{T1}q_{T1}p_{T2}q_{T2}} + \sqrt{p_{C1}q_{C1}p_{C2}q_{C2}}}{\sqrt{r\,p_{T1}q_{T1} + p_{C1}q_{C1}}\sqrt{r\,p_{T2}q_{T2} + p_{C2}q_{C2}}},$$

where $q_{Tk} = 1 - p_{Tk}$ and $q_{Ck} = 1 - p_{Ck}$. Note that ρ_Z is not free to range over $(-1,1)$. For large samples, as $\hat{p}_{Tk} \to p_{Tk}$, $\hat{p}_{Ck} \to p_{Ck}$, and $\hat{\bar{p}}_k \to \bar{p}_k$, therefore, the power function for the joint effect is approximately

$$1 - \beta = \text{Prob}\left[\bigcap_{k=1}^{2} \{Z_k > z_\alpha\} | \, \text{H}_1\right] \approx \text{Prob}\left[\bigcap_{k=1}^{2} \left\{Z_k^* > c_k\right\} \middle| \, \text{H}_1\right], \tag{14.1}$$

where

$$Z_k^* = \frac{\sqrt{rn}(\hat{p}_{Tk} - \hat{p}_{Ck} - \delta_k)}{\sqrt{r\,p_{Tk}q_{Tk} + p_{Ck}q_{Ck}}} \text{and } c_k = \frac{\sqrt{\bar{p}_k\bar{q}_k(r+1)}z_\alpha - \sqrt{rn}\delta_k}{\sqrt{r\,p_{Tk}q_{Tk} + p_{Ck}q_{Ck}}}.$$

The power (14.1) is, in general, referred as to complete power or conjunctive power (Senn and Bretz 2007). The power can be simply calculated by using the cumulative distribution function of the bivariate normal distribution, i.e., $1 - \beta = \Phi_2(-c_1, -c_2 | \boldsymbol{\rho}_Z)$. The sample size required for achieving the desired power $1 - \beta$ at the significance level α is given by the smallest integer not less than n satisfying the power (14.1). An iterative procedure is required to solve for the power and to calculate the sample size as no closed-form expression for the calculation is available. For details of the calculation, and extension to more than two endpoints, see Sozu et al. (2010, 2011) and Sugimoto et al. (2012).

14.2.2 The Decision-Making Frameworks, Stopping Rules, and Power

Now consider a randomized, group-sequential clinical trial comparing the test intervention with the control intervention based on two binary outcomes as co-primary endpoints. Suppose that a maximum of L analyses are planned, where the same number of analyses with the same information space are selected for both endpoints. Let n_l and rn_l be the cumulative number of participants on the test and the control intervention groups at the lth analysis ($l = 1, \ldots, L$), respectively. Hence, up to n_L and rn_L participants are recruited and randomly assigned to the test and the control intervention groups, respectively.

When evaluating the joint effects on both of the endpoints within the context of group-sequential designs, Asakura et al. (2014) discuss two decision-making frameworks associated with hypothesis testing. One is to reject H_0 if superiority is achieved for the two endpoints at any interim time point (i.e., not necessarily simultaneously) (DF-A). The other is to reject H_0 if and only if superiority is achieved for the two endpoints simultaneously (i.e., at the same interim time point of the trial) (DF-A'). We outline the two decision-making frameworks, and the corresponding stopping rules and powers as follows:

DF-A: If superiority is demonstrated on one endpoint at the interim, then the trial will continue but subsequent hypothesis testing is repeatedly conducted only for the previously nonsignificant endpoint until superiority is demonstrated. The stopping rule for DF-A is formally given as follows:

At the lth analysis ($l = 1, \ldots, L-1$)
If $Z_{1l} > c_{1l}$ and $Z_{2l'} > c_{2l'}$ for some $1 \leq l' \leq l$, then reject H_0 and stop the trial,
if $Z_{2l} > c_{2l}$ and $Z_{1l'} > c_{1l'}$ for some $1 \leq l' \leq l$, then reject H_0 and stop the trial,
otherwise, continue to the $(l+1)$th analysis,
at the Lth analysis
if $Z_{1L} > c_{1L}$ and $Z_{2l'} > c_{2l'}$ for some $1 \leq l' \leq L$, then reject H_0,
if $Z_{2L} > c_{2L}$ and $Z_{1l'} > c_{1l'}$ for some $1 \leq l' \leq L$, then reject H_0,
otherwise, do not reject H_0.

where Z_{1l} and Z_{2l} are the test statistics at the lth analysis, given by

$$Z_{kl} = \frac{\sqrt{n_l}\hat{\delta}_{kl}}{\sqrt{\hat{\bar{p}}_{kl}\left(1 - \hat{\bar{p}}_{kl}\right)(1+r)/r}}$$

with $\hat{\delta}_{kl} = \hat{p}_{\mathrm{T}kl} - \hat{p}_{\mathrm{C}kl}$, $\hat{p}_{\mathrm{T}kl} = n_l^{-1}\sum_{i=1}^{n_l} Y_{\mathrm{T}ki}$ and $\hat{p}_{\mathrm{C}kl} = (rn_l)^{-1}\sum_{j=1}^{rn_l} Y_{\mathrm{C}kj}$, and $\hat{\bar{p}}_{kl} = (\hat{p}_{\mathrm{T}kl} + r\hat{p}_{\mathrm{C}kl})/(1+r)$. Also, c_{1l} and c_{2l} are the critical values at the lth analysis, and they are prespecified separately, using any group-sequential methods such as the Lan–DeMets (LD) α-spending method (Lan and DeMets 1983) to control an overall type I error rate of α, as if they were a single primary endpoint, ignoring the other co-primary endpoint. The testing procedure for co-primary endpoints is conservative. For example, if a zero correlation between the two endpoints is assumed and each endpoint is tested at the one-sided significance level of 2.5 %, then the type I error rate is 0.0625 %. As shown in Sect. 14.3, the maximum type I error rate associated with the rejection region of the null hypothesis increases as the correlation goes toward one, but it is not greater than the targeted significance level.

Therefore, the power is

$$1 - \beta = \Pr\left[\left\{\bigcup_{l=1}^{L} A_{1l}\right\} \cap \left\{\bigcup_{l=1}^{L} A_{2l}\right\} \middle| \mathrm{H}_1\right], \tag{14.2}$$

where $A_{kl} = \{Z_{kl} > c_{kl}\}\,(k = 1,2; l = 1,\ldots,L)$. The power (14.2) can be numerically assessed by using multivariate normal integrals as for large samples. The joint distribution of $(Z_{11}, Z_{21}, \ldots, Z_{1L}, Z_{2L})$ is approximately multivariate normal with their correlations given by $\text{corr}\,[Z_{kl}, Z_{k'l'}] = \sqrt{n_{l'}/n_l}$ if $k = k'$; $\rho_Z\sqrt{n_{l'}/n_l}$ and if $k \neq k'$. For the detailed calculation, see Asakura et al. (2014).

DF-A offers the option of stopping measurement of an endpoint for which superiority has been demonstrated. Stopping measurement may be desirable if the endpoint is very invasive or expensive, although stopping measurement may also introduce operational difficulties into the trial. To avoid operational difficulties, a restriction on the condition of when H_0 is rejected and the trial is stopped, may be imposed.

DF-A′: is a special case of DF-A representing a restriction on the condition of when H_0 is rejected and the trial is stopped: If superiority is demonstrated on only one endpoint at an interim, then the trial continues, and the hypothesis testing is repeated for both endpoints until the joint significance for the two endpoints is established simultaneously. The stopping rule for DF-A' is formally given as follows:

At the lth analysis $(l = 1, \ldots, L-1)$
  If $Z_{1l} > c_{1l}$ and $Z_{2l} > c_{2l}$, then reject H_0 and stop the trial,
  otherwise, continue to the $(l+1)$th analysis,
at the Lth analysis
  if $Z_{1L} > c_{1L}$ and $Z_{2L} > c_{2L}$, then reject H_0,
  otherwise, do not reject H_0.

Therefore, the power is

$$1 - \beta = \Pr\left[\bigcup_{l=1}^{L}\{A_{1l} \cap A_{2l}\}\,\middle|\,H_1\right], \tag{14.3}$$

Similarly as in the power (14.2), the power can be calculated by using multivariate normal integrals. For the details, see Asakura et al. (2014).

As discussed in Asakura et al. (2014), the probability of making an inconsistent decision between DF-A and DF-A' is quite low, so that there is little practical difference in the power and sample size determinations for DF-A and DF-A'.

14.2.3 Sample Sizes

We discuss two sample size concepts, i.e., the maximum sample size (MSS) and the average sample number (ASN) based on the two decision-making frameworks, and the corresponding powers discussed in the previous section.

The MSS is the sample size required for the final analysis to achieve the desired power $1-\beta$. The MSS is given by the smallest integer not less than n_L satisfying the power (14.2) or (14.3) for a group-sequential design at the prespecified p_{Tk} and p_{Ck}, and ρ, with Fisher's information time for the interim analyses, $n_l/n_L (l = 1, \ldots, L)$. To find a value of n_L, an iterative procedure is required to numerically solve for the power (14.2) or (14.3). This can be accomplished by using a grid search to gradually increase n_L until the power under n_L exceeds the desired power, although this often requires considerable computing resources. To reduce the computational resources, the Newton–Raphson algorithm in Sugimoto et al. (2012) or the basic linear interpolation algorithm in Hamasaki et al. (2013) may be utilized.

The ASN is the expected sample size under a specific hypothetical reference. For example, given these prespecifications, for equally sized groups, i.e., $r = 1$, the ASN per intervention group for DF-A is

$$\mathrm{ASN} = n_L\left(1 + \sum\nolimits_{l=1}^{L-1} \Pr\left[\{\bar{A}_{11} \cap \cdots \cap \bar{A}_{1l}\} \cup \{\bar{A}_{21} \cap \cdots \cap \bar{A}_{2l}\}\right]\right) \Big/ L,$$

and then for DF-A',

$$\mathrm{ASN} = n_L\left(1 + \sum\nolimits_{l=1}^{L-1} \Pr\left[\{\bar{A}_{11} \cup \bar{A}_{21}\} \cap \cdots \cap \{\bar{A}_{1l} \cup \bar{A}_{2l}\}\right]\right) \Big/ L,$$

where $n_l = l n_1 (l = 1, \ldots, L)$. The MSS and ASN will depend on the design parameters including differences in proportions, the correlation structure between the endpoints, the testing procedure (e.g., O'Brien–Fleming (OF) testing procedure (O'Brien and Fleming 1979), Pocock (PC) testing procedure (Pocock 1977), the number of analyses, and the information time.

14.3 Evaluation of the Method Utility

14.3.1 Behavior of Empirical Power and Evaluation of the Type I Error Rate

The normal approximation discussed in the previous sections may not work well in the occurrence of extremely small event rates or small sample sizes as the joint distribution is not fully specified in the first- and second-order moments. There are more direct ways of calculating sample size without using a normal approximation. However, such methods are computationally difficult, particularly for a large number of analyses and outcomes, and thus can be impractical. In this section, we evaluate the utility of using the normal approximation.

In order to evaluate the utility of using the normal approximation, the power and type I error rate were evaluated by Monte Carlo simulation since no closed-form expression is available. The total numbers of 100,000 replications and 1,000,000 replications were selected for the assessments of power and type I error rate respectively, under given sample sizes (equally sized groups: $r = 1$) with two binary outcomes being evaluated as co-primary. Bivariate Bernoulli data for Monte Carlo simulation were generated by the method in Emrich and Piedmonte (1991). As there is no major difference in behaviors of the empirical powers and type I error rates between DF-A and DF-A', we only describe the result for DF-A'.

Figs. 14.1, 14.2 and 14.3 display behaviors of the empirical powers and the type I error rates for DF-A' under a given sample size using the normal approximation method with $L = 2$, 3, 4, and 5, in the cases of $\delta_1 = \delta_2 = \delta$ and $p_{C1} = p_{C2} = p_C$, and $\rho = 0.0$ and 0.8. The required sample size per group ($r = 1$) was calculated to detect a joint effect on both endpoints with the desired overall power of $1 - \beta = 80\,\%$ for a one-sided test at the significance level of $\alpha = 2.5\,\%$, where the critical values are determined by the three testing procedure combinations, i.e., (i) the OF for both endpoints (OF–OF), (ii) the OF for δ_1 and the PC for δ_2 (OF–PC), and (iii) the PC for both endpoints (PC–PC), with the LD α-spending method with equally spaced information level. For the type I error evaluation, two situations are considered, i.e., $\delta_1 \leq 0$ and $\delta_2 \leq 0$ (Fig. 14.2) and, i.e., $\delta_1 \leq 0$ and $\delta_2 > 0$ (Fig. 14.3). For all three testing procedure combinations, the empirical power achieves the targeted power of 80 %, but it is larger than the targeted power as δ is larger and p_C is higher. Especially when $\delta \geq 20\,\%$ with $p_C = 70\,\%$ or 80 %, the empirical power is greater than 90 %. For these situations, Cochran's condition regarding small expected frequencies (Cochran 1952) was not satisfied for each endpoint under the given sample size. The empirical power does not greatly vary with the number of analyses.

When $\delta_1 \leq 0$ and $\delta_2 \leq 0$, for all three testing procedure combinations, in case of $\boldsymbol{\rho} = 0.0$, the type I error rate is not greater than the nominal significance level of 2.5 %, but it is quite small. In the case of $\boldsymbol{\rho} = 0.8$, the type I error rate is increased compared with those of $\boldsymbol{\rho} = 0.0$, but is still not greater than the nominal significance level. On the other hand, when $\delta_1 \leq 0$ and $\delta_2 > 0$, the type I error rate is around the nominal significance level in both cases of $\boldsymbol{\rho} = 0.0$ and 0.8.

In addition, the sample sizes derived by the Monte Carlo simulation-based approach were compared with the sample sizes calculated using the normal approximation, where 100,000 replications were selected for the power evaluation. Figure 14.4 displays the ratio of the sample sizes calculated by the normal approximation to that determined by the Monte Carlo simulation-based approach. For all three testing procedure combinations, the ratio is roughly equal to 1 when δ is small, but it is larger than 1 when δ is larger, especially in $p_C = 0.8$. When Cochran's condition is not satisfied for each endpoint under the given sample size, the ratio is larger than roughly 1.2. As discussed in Landau and Stahl (2013), this result suggests that the use of the Monte Carlo simulation approach may be considered as an alternative to the normal approximation method because the Monte Carlo simulation approach in this instance leads to a saving in sample size. However, the Monte Carlo simulation approach requires expensive computation costs and technical programming skills. It is important to consider an appropriate number of replications for simulations to control simulation error in calculating the empirical power when using the Monte Carlo simulation approach.

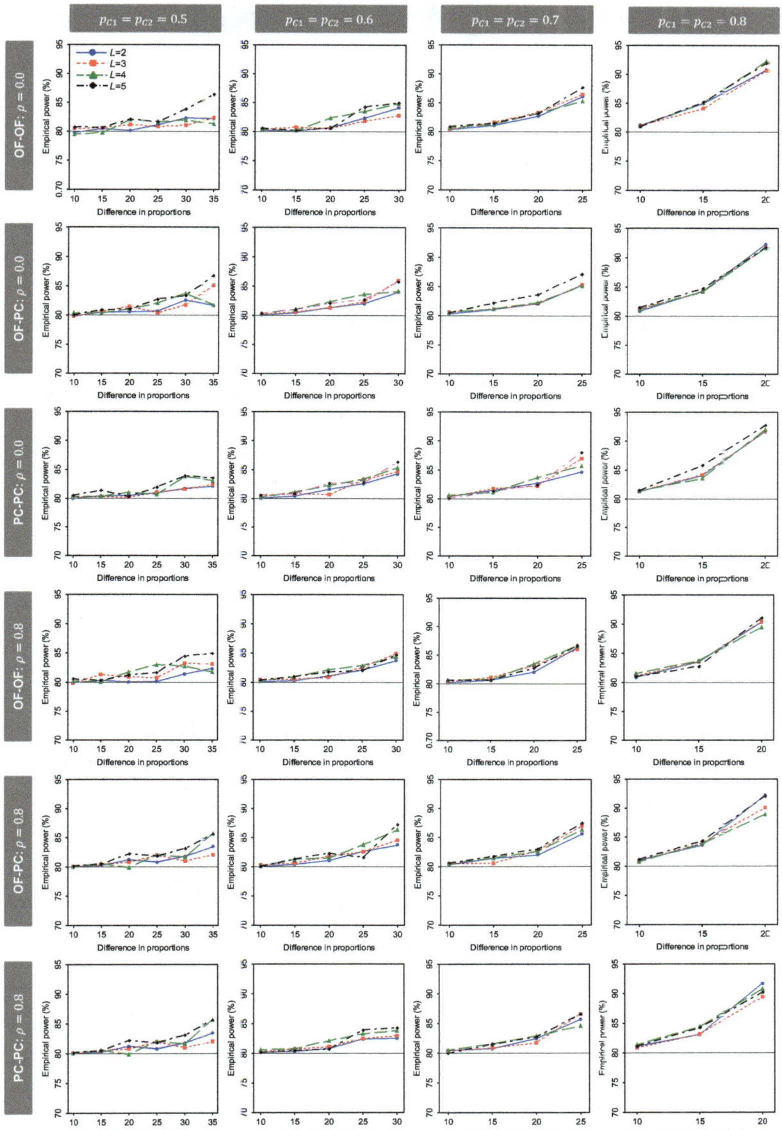

Fig. 14.1 Behaviors of the empirical powers for DF-A' with difference in proportions (test–control), based on the normal approximation method when $L = 2$, 3, 4, and 5, and $\rho = 0.0$ and 0.8, in the cases of $\delta_1 = \delta_2$ and $p_{C1} = p_{C2}$. The sample size (equally sized groups) was calculated to detect a joint effect on both endpoints with the desired overall power of $1-\beta = 80\,\%$ for a one-sided test at the significance level of $\alpha = 2.5\,\%$. The critical values are determined by the three testing procedure combinations, i.e., (i) the OF for both endpoints (OF–OF), (ii) the OF for δ_1 and the PC for δ_2 (OF–PC), and (iii) the PC for both endpoints (PC–PC), with the LD α-spending method with equally spaced information level. *DF-A'* at the same interim time point of the trial, *OF* O'Brien–Fleming, *PC* Pocock, *LD* Lan–DeMets

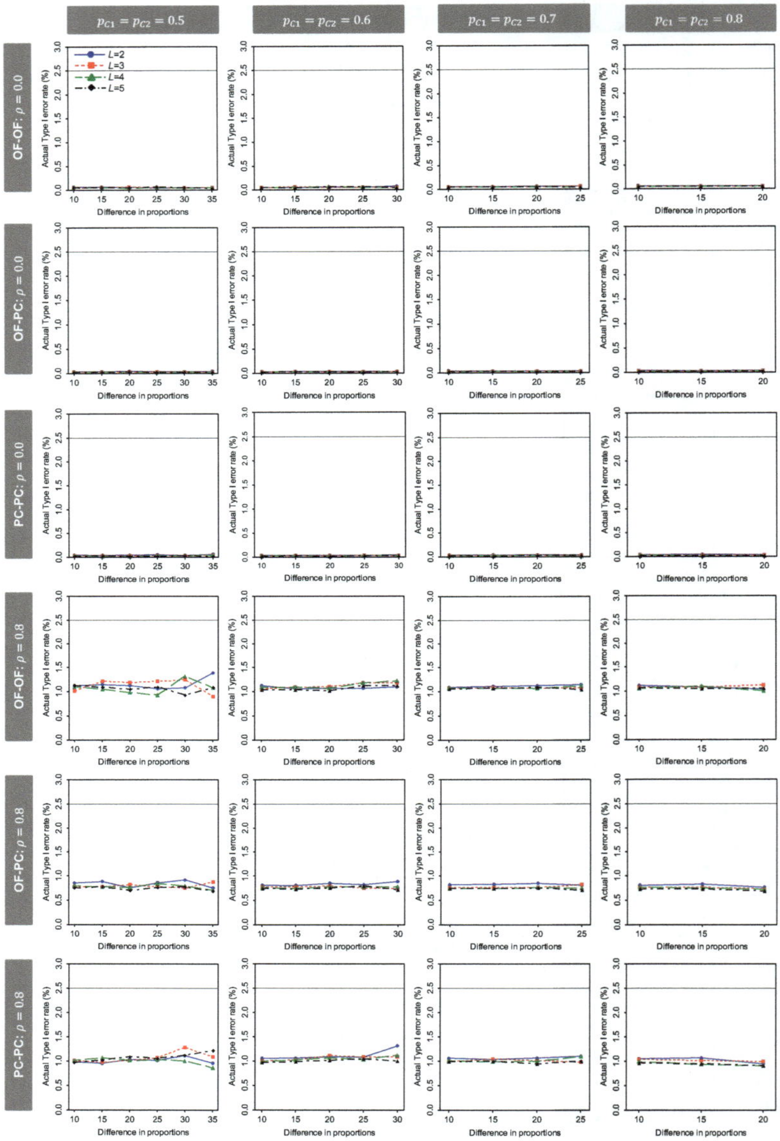

Fig. 14.2 Behaviors of the actual type I error rates ($\delta_1 \leq 0$ and $\delta_2 \leq 0$) for DF-A', with difference in proportions (test–control) based on the normal approximation method when $L = 2$, 3, 4, and 5, and $\rho = 0.0$ and 0.8, in the cases of $\delta_1 = \delta_2$ and $p_{C1} = p_{C2}$. The sample size (equally sized groups) was calculated to detect a joint effect on both endpoints with the overall power of $1 - \beta = 80\,\%$ for a one-sided test at the significance level of $\alpha = 2.5\,\%$. The critical values are determined by the three testing procedure combinations, i.e., (i) the OF for both endpoints (OF–OF), (ii) the OF for δ_1 and the PC for δ_2 (OF–PC), and (iii) the PC for both endpoints (PC–PC), with the LD α-spending method with equally spaced information level. *DF-A'* at the same interim time point of the trial, *OF* O'Brien–Fleming, *PC* Pocock, *LD* Lan–DeMets

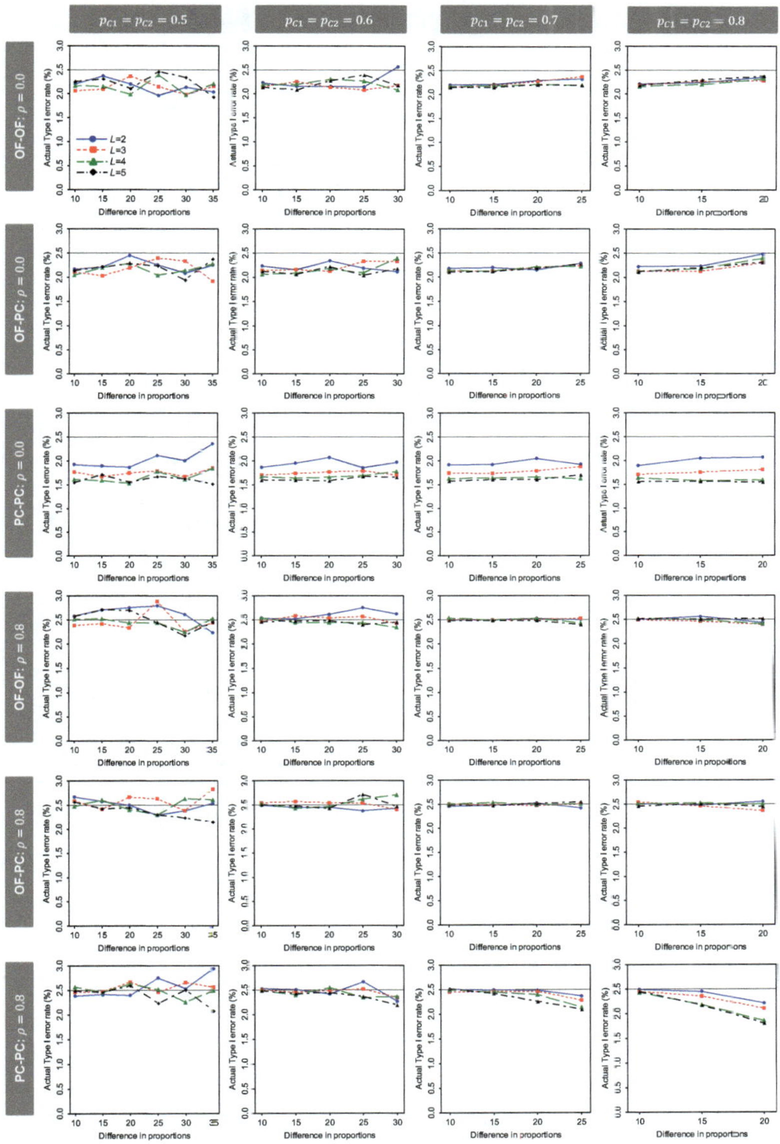

Fig. 14.3 Behaviors of the actual type I error rates ($\delta_1 \leq 0$ and $\delta_2 > 0$) for DF-A', with difference in proportions (test–control) based on the normal approximation method when $L = 2, 3, 4$, and 5, and $\rho = 0.0$ and 0.8, in the cases of $\delta_1 = \delta_2$ and $p_{C1} = p_{C2}$. The sample size (equally sized groups) was calculated to detect a joint effect on both endpoints with the desired overall power of $1 - \beta = 80\,\%$ for a one-sided test at the significance level of $\alpha = 2.5\,\%$. The critical values are determined by the three testing procedure combinations, i.e., (i) the OF for both endpoints (OF–OF), (ii) the OF for δ_1 and the PC for δ_2 (OF–PC), and (iii) the PC for both endpoints (PC–PC), with the LD α-spending method with equally spaced information level. *DF-A'* at the same interim time point of the trial, *OF* O'Brien–Fleming, *PC* Pocock, *LD* Lan–DeMets

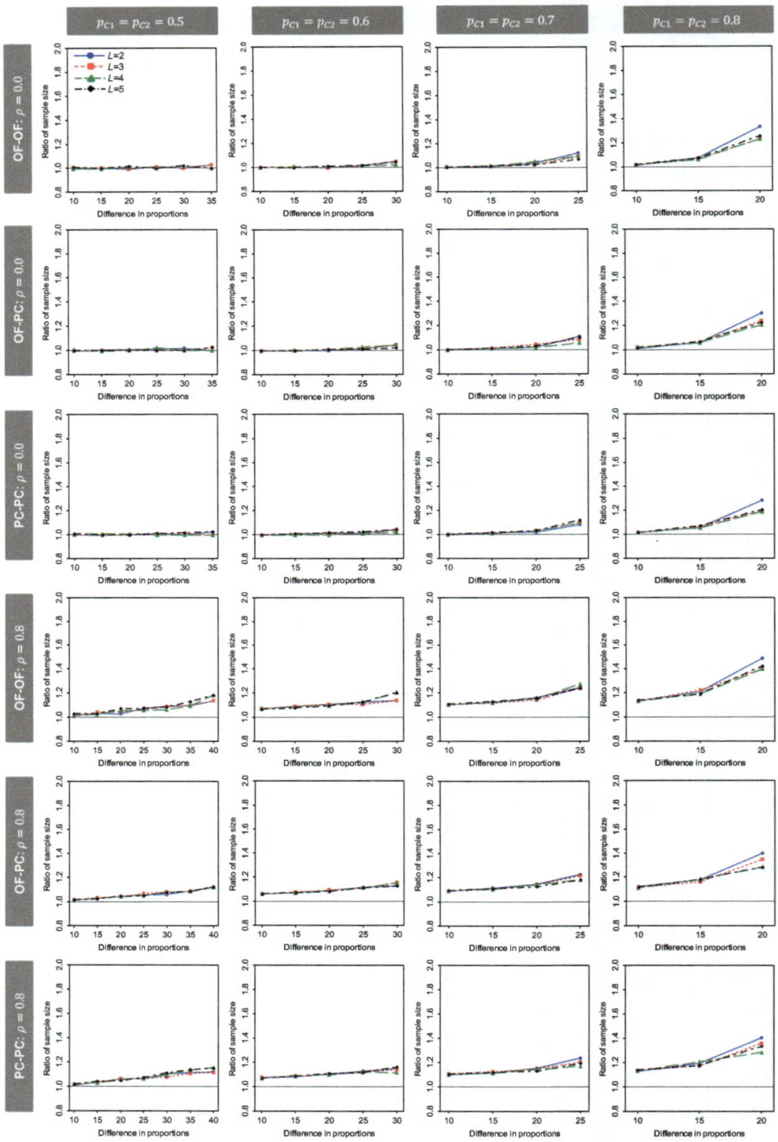

Fig. 14.4 The ratio of the sample size for DF-A' with difference in proportions (test–control), by the normal approximation method to that by the Monte Carlo simulation-based approach, when $L = 2$, 3, 4, and 5, and $\rho = 0.0$ and 0.8, in the cases of $\delta_1 = \delta_2$ and $p_{C1} = p_{C2}$. The sample size (equally sized groups) was calculated to detect a joint effect on both endpoints with the desired overall power of $1 - \beta = 80\,\%$ for a one-sided test at the significance level of $\alpha = 2.5\,\%$. The critical values are determined by the three testing procedure combinations, i.e., (i) the OF for both endpoints (OF–OF), (ii) the OF for δ_1 and the PC for δ_2 (OF–PC), and (iii) the PC for both endpoints (PC–PC), with the LD α-spending method with equally spaced information level. *DF-A'* at the same interim time point of the trial, *OF* O'Brien–Fleming, *PC* Pocock, *LD* Lan–DeMets

14.3.2 Illustration

We provide an example to illustrate the sample size methods discussed in the previous sections. Consider a double-blind, randomized, parallel group, placebo-controlled trial evaluating *lactobacilli* and *bifidobacteria* in the prevention of antibiotic-associated diarrhoea (AAD) in older people admitted to hospital (the PLACIDE study) (Allen et al. 2012, 2013). The study was designed to demonstrate that the administration of a probiotic comprising two strains of *lactobacilli* and two strains of *bifidobacteria* alongside antibiotic treatment prevents AAD. The co-primary outcomes were (1) the occurrence of AAD within 8 weeks and (2) the occurrence of *Clostridium difficile* diarrhoea (CDD) within 12 weeks of recruitment. The original sample size per intervention group of 1239 participants provided a power of 80 % to detect a 50 % reduction in CDD, in the probiotic group compared with the placebo group, by using a two-sided Fisher's exact test at 5 % significance level, assuming CDD frequencies of 4 % in placebo group and 2 % in probiotic group. Although Cochran's condition seems to be hold for this setting, the normal approximation method was not used for the sample size calculation, resulting in conservatively-calculated sample size. This sample size would provide a power of more than 99 % to detect a 50 % reduction in AAD, by using a two-sided Fisher's exact test at 5 % significance level, assuming AAD frequencies of 20 % in placebo group and 10 % in probiotic group as the normal approximation. The correlation between the two outcomes was not incorporated into the original sample size calculation.

Table 14.1 displays the MSS and ASN per intervention group (equally sized groups: $r = 1$) for DF-A and DF-A'. The sample size was derived using an alternative hypothesis of differences in proportions for AAD ($p_{T1} = 0.2$ and $p_{C1} = 0.4$) and CDD ($p_{T2} = 0.02$ and $p_{C2} = 0.04$) with the overall power of 80 % at the significance level of 2.5 % by one-sided test, using the normal approximation method discussed in the previous section, where $\rho = \rho_T = \rho_C = 0.0, 0.3, 0.5$, and 0.8; $L = 1, 2, 3, 4$, and 5. The critical values are determined by the four testing procedure combinations, i.e., (i) the OF for both endpoints (OF–OF), (ii) the OF for AAD and the PC for CDD (OF–PC), (iii) the PC for AAD and the OF for CDD (PC–OF), and (iv) the PC for both endpoints (PC–PC), with the LD α-spending method, with equally spaced information level.

Based on the selected parameters described in Allen et al. (2012), i.e., $L = 1$ and $\rho = 0.0$, the sample size per intervention group is calculated as 1143. If four interims and one final analysis are planned (i.e., $L = 5$) with DF-A', and conservatively assuming a zero correlation between the endpoints, then the MSS is 1170 for OF–OF, 1399 for OF–PC, 1170 for PC–OF, and 1387 for PC–PC, and the ASN is 943.5 for OF–OF, 975.5 for OF–PC, 941.2 for PC–OF, and 921.4 for PC–PC. On the other hand, even if the correlation is incorporated into the calculation, the MSS and ASN do not change as the correlation varies. This means that when one standardized effect size is relatively larger than the other, i.e., $\delta_1 > \delta_2$ or $\delta_1 < \delta_2$ with $p_{C1} \neq p_{C2}$, then there is little benefit in incorporating the correlation into sample size calculation.

Table 14.1 The MSS and ASN (equally sized groups). The MSS was calculated to detect the joint effect for both endpoints with the overall power of $1-\beta=80\,\%$ at the one-sided significance level of $\alpha=2.5\,\%$, based on the assumption from the PLACIDE study. The critical values are determined by the four testing procedure combinations, i.e., (i) the OF for both endpoints (OF–OF), (ii) the OF for AAD and the PC for CDD (OF–PC), (iii) the PC for AAD and the OF for CDD (PC–OF), and (iv) the PC for both endpoints (PC–PC), with the LD α-spending method with equally spaced information level.

			(i) OF–OF		(ii) OF–PC		(iii) PC–OF		(iv) PC–PC	
DF	ρ	L	MSS	ASN	MSS	ASN	MSS	ASN	MSS	ASN
DF-A	0.0	1	1143		1143		1143		1143	
		2	1146	1055.7	1282	982.2	1146	1052.7	1282	977.0
		3	1156	991.4	1336	978.1	1156	988.6	1336	939.4
		4	1164	959.8	1366	972.1	1164	958.1	1366	925.4
		5	1170	943.4	1385	956.0	1170	941.1	1385	917.8
	0.3	1	1143		1143		1143		1143	
		2	1146	1055.6	1282	982.2	1146	1052.7	1282	977.0
		3	1156	991.4	1336	977.8	1156	988.6	1336	939.3
		4	1164	959.7	1366	971.8	1164	958.1	1366	925.3
		5	1170	943.3	1385	955.9	1170	941.1	1385	917.7
	0.5	1	1143		1143		1143		1143	
		2	1146	1055.6	1282	982.2	1146	1052.7	1282	977.0
		3	1156	991.4	1336	977.8	1156	988.6	1336	939.3
		4	1164	959.7	1366	971.8	1164	958.1	1366	925.3
		5	1170	943.3	1385	955.9	1170	941.1	1385	917.7
	0.8	1	1143		1143		1143		1143	
		2	1146	1055.6	1282	982.2	1146	1052.7	1282	977.0
		3	1156	991.4	1336	977.8	1156	988.6	1336	939.3
		4	1164	959.7	1366	971.8	1164	958.1	1366	925.3
		5	1170	943.3	1385	955.9	1170	941.1	1385	917.7
DF-A’	0.0	1	1143		1143		1143		1143	
		2	1146	1055.7	1283	982.8	1146	1052.7	1282	977.0
		3	1156	991.5	1346	986.6	1156	988.6	1337	940.2
		4	1164	959.8	1380	989.4	1164	958.2	1368	927.6
		5	1170	943.5	1399	975.5	1170	941.2	1387	921.4
	0.3	1	1143		1143		1143		1143	
		2	1146	1055.0	1283	982.0	1146	1052.6	1282	976.9
		3	1156	991.0	1345	982.3	1156	988.5	1337	939.5
		4	1164	959.4	1380	986.7	1164	958.1	1368	925.9
		5	1170	943.0	1398	973.3	1170	941.1	1387	919.7
	0.5	1	1143		1143		1143		1143	
		2	1146	1055.0	1283	982.0	1146	1052.6	1282	976.9

Table 14.1 (continued)

			(i) OF–OF		(ii) OF–PC		(iii) PC–OF		(iv) PC–PC	
DF	ρ	L	MSS	ASN	MSS	ASN	MSS	ASN	MSS	ASN
		3	1156	991.0	1345	982.3	1156	988.5	1337	939.5
		4	1164	959.4	1380	986.7	1164	958.1	1368	925.9
		5	1170	943.0	1398	973.3	1170	941.1	1387	919.7
	0.8	1	1143		1143		1143		1143	
		2	1146	1055.0	1283	982.0	1146	1052.6	1282	976.9
		3	1156	991.0	1345	982.3	1156	988.5	1337	939.5
		4	1164	959.4	1380	986.7	1164	958.1	1368	925.9
		5	1170	943.0	1398	973.3	1170	941.1	1387	919.7

DF-A at the interim time point not necessarily simultaneously, *DF-A'* at the same interim time point of the trial, *MSS* maximum sample size, *ASN* average sample number, *AAD* antibiotic-associated diarrhoea, *CDD Clostridium difficile* diarrhoea, *OF* O'Brien–Fleming, *PC* Pocock, *LD* Lan–DeMets

When comparing DF-A to DF-A', there are no major differences in MSS and ASN for all of the testing procedure combinations, although DF-A provides a slightly smaller MSS and ASN than DF-A'. However, if the endpoint is very invasive, and thus stopping measurement may be ethically desirable, there is a benefit of using DF-A as DF-A offers the option of stopping measurement of an endpoint for which superiority has been demonstrated. For example, when $L = 5$ with DF-A, the average total numbers of measurements for two endpoints for each intervention group are 2887.1 for OF–OF, 2948.0 for OF–PC, 2493.0 for PC–OF, and 2486.4 for PC–PC when $\rho = 0.0$. They are relatively smaller than those for DF-A' as the average total numbers of measurements for DF-A' are 3260.5 for OF–OF, 2966.4 for OF–PC, 2493.0 for PC–OF and 2488.4 for PC–PC.

Figure 14.5 illustrates the probability of rejecting/not rejecting the null hypothesis for DF-A' and DF-A when $\rho = 0.0$ and $L = 5$. The figure shows that the method offers the possibility to stop a trial early if evidence is overwhelming, and thus offers potentially fewer patients than the fixed-sample designs. The expected analysis of stopping for DF-A' is 4.03 for OF–OF, 3.49 for OF–PC, 4.02 for PC–OF, and 3.32 for PC–PC, and, for DF-A, 4.03 for OF–OF, 3.45 for OF–PC, 4.02 for PC–OF, and 3.31 for PC–PC. In the OF–OF and PC–OF testing procedure combinations, it is more difficult to reject the null hypothesis at the earliest analyses, but easier later on. On the other hand, in the PC–PC and OF–PC testing procedure combinations, it is easier to reject the null hypothesis at the earliest analysis.

Table 14.2 displays the Monte Carlo simulation-based MSS and ASN per intervention group (equally sized groups: $r_r = 1$) for DF-A and DF-A'. The sample size was derived based upon an alternative hypothesis of differences in proportions for AAD ($p_{T1} = 0.2$ and $p_{C1} = 0.4$) and CDD ($p_{T2} = 0.02$ and $p_{C2} = 0.04$) with the overall power of 80 % at the significance level of 2.5 % by one-sided test, where 100,000 replications were selected for the empirical power evaluation and Bivariate

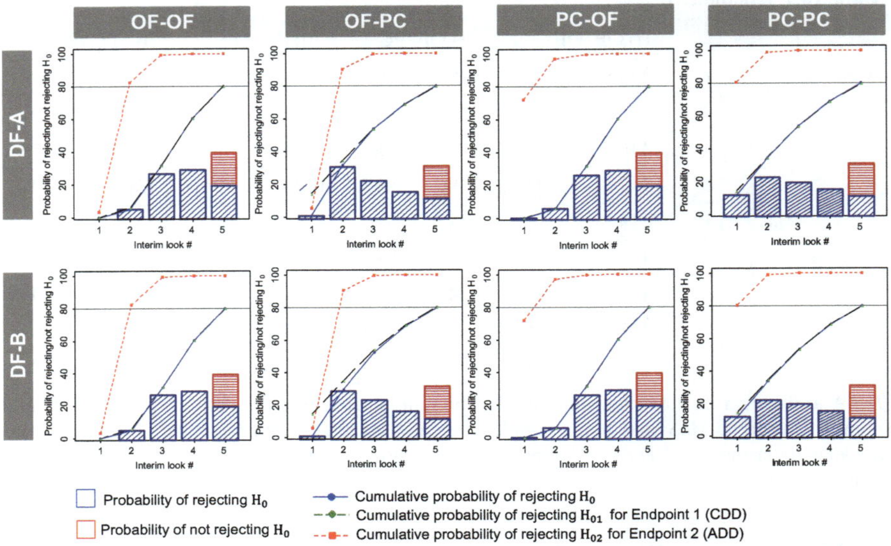

Fig. 14.5 The probability of rejecting/not rejecting the null hypothesis when four interim and one final analyses are planned with $\rho = 0.0$. The MSS were calculated to detect the joint effect for both endpoints with the overall power of $1 - \beta = 80\,\%$ at the one-sided significance level of $\alpha = 2.5\,\%$, based on the assumption from the PLACIDE study. The critical values are determined by the four testing procedure combinations, i.e., (i) the OF for both endpoints (OF–OF), (ii) the OF for AAD and the PC for CDD (OF–PC), (iii) the PC for AAD and the OF for CDD (PC–OF), and (iv) the PC for both endpoints (PC–PC), with the LD α-spending method with equally spaced information level. *DF-A'* at the same interim time point of the trial, *OF* O'Brien–Fleming, *PC* Pocock, *LD* Lan–DeMets, *AAD* antibiotic-associated diarrhoea, *CDD Clostridium difficile* diarrhoea

Bernoulli data for Monte Carlo simulation were generated by the method in Emrich and Piedmonte (1991). The Monte Carlo simulation approach always provides smaller sample size (roughly 20 to 30 smaller) than the sample sizes by the normal approximation methods.

14.4 Sample Size Recalculation

14.4.1 Test Statistics and Conditional Power

Clinical trials are designed based on assumptions often constructed based on prior data. However, prior data may be limited, or an inaccurate indication of future data, resulting in trials that are over/underpowered. Interim analyses provides an opportunity to evaluate the accuracy of the design assumptions and potentially make design adjustments (i.e., to the sample size) if the assumptions were markedly inaccurate. Group-sequential designs allow for decreasing the sample size when observed treatment effects are much larger than assumed. In this section, we discuss sample size

Table 14.2 The Monte Carlo simulated-based MSS and ASN (equally sized groups), where MSS was calculated to detect the joint effect for both endpoints with the overall power of $1-\beta=80\,\%$ at the one-sided significance level of $\alpha=2.5\,\%$, based on the assumption from the PLACIDE study. The critical values are determined by the four testing procedure combinations, i.e., (i) the OF for both endpoints (OF–OF), (ii) the OF for AAD and the PC for CDD (OF–PC), (iii) the PC for AAD and the OF for CDD (OF–PC), and (iv) the PC for both endpoints (PC–PC), with the LD α-spending method with equally spaced information level, where 100,000 replications were selected for the empirical power evaluation.

			(i) OF–OF		(ii) OF–PC		(iii) PC–OF		(iv) PC–PC	
DF	ρ	L	MSS	ASN	MSS	ASN	MSS	ASN	MSS	ASN
DF-A	0.0	1	1109		1115		1114		1113	
		2	1115	1037.6	1261	968.2	1122	1040.0	1257	961.2
		3	1129	974.1	1308	962.7	1128	971.7	1311	928.5
		4	1139	945.8	1336	956.7	1142	946.7	1335	914.6
		5	1151	932.9	1365	947.3	1146	928.3	1364	912.6
	0.3	1	1114		1116		1114		1116	
		2	1115	1035.8	1266	968.1	1115	1034.7	1266	966.3
		3	1125	968.9	1312	950.6	1130	973.4	1310	923.3
		4	1138	943.1	1343	951.8	1138	943.0	1339	910.8
		5	1153	932.5	1361	938.4	1150	931.0	1363	905.3
	0.5	1	1114		1113		1112		1117	
		2	1116	1035.3	1260	963.6	1114	1034.4	1259	962.1
		3	1128	972.3	1305	939.6	1129	973.1	1313	924.1
		4	1139	943.8	1340	945.8	1138	943.5	1343	911.3
		5	1152	932.6	1367	939.3	1149	929.1	1364	904.1
	0.8	1	1110		1116		1115		1113	
		2	1117	1036.6	1265	967.2	1113	1032.7	1258	961.2
		3	1127	971.9	1312	943.0	1130	973.4	1312	919.9
		4	1139	944.1	1340	945.8	1142	945.7	1341	910.9
		5	1154	932.8	1364	936.8	1154	932.3	1368	906.3
DF-A'	0.0	1	1113		1115		1113		1112	
		2	1119	1040.8	1258	966.3	1114	1034.4	1265	966.4
		3	1129	974.1	1314	969.3	1130	973.3	1309	925.0
		4	1126	938.4	1353	976.5	1137	942.5	1339	917.9
		5	1148	931.2	1380	966.0	1150	930.5	1363	914.0
	0.3	1	1115		1113		1115		1113	
		2	1115	1035.0	1262	966.2	1116	1035.1	1264	963.0
		3	1128	972.2	1321	956.5	1130	973.2	1314	925.4

Table 14.2 (continued)

DF	ρ	L	(i) OF–OF		(ii) OF–PC		(iii) PC–OF		(iv) PC–PC	
			MSS	ASN	MSS	ASN	MSS	ASN	MSS	ASN
		4	1144	948.3	1358	967.7	1142	945.4	1337	909.8
		5	1152	932.4	1378	958.3	1151	930.4	1367	909.7
	0.5	1	1114		1116		1116		1116	
		2	1113	1032.5	1263	964.7	1120	1037.9	1264	965.0
		3	1128	972.0	1319	951.1	1131	974.7	1309	921.3
		4	1143	946.9	1350	957.1	1139	942.1	1343	912.5
		5	1153	932.4	1380	954.9	1149	929.4	1368	906.9
	0.8	1	1116		1112		1112		1111	
		2	1117	1036.6	1262	966.2	1114	1032.2	1261	962.7
		3	1124	969.9	1325	952.8	1130	972.7	1311	922.1
		4	1142	945.9	1353	957.3	1141	944.4	1341	912.2
		5	1150	929.7	1377	952.5	1149	929.4	1363	906.5

DF-A at the interim time point not necessarily simultaneously, *DFA'* at the same interim time point of the trial, *MSS* maximum sample size, *ASN* average sample number, *AAD* antibiotic-associated diarrhea, *CDD Clostridium difficile* diarrhea, *OF* O'Brien–Fleming, *PC* Pocock, *LD* Lan–DeMets

recalculation based on the observed intervention's effects at an interim analysis with a focus on control of statistical error rates.

Suppose that the MSS is recalculated to n'_L based on the interim data at the Rth analysis. Suppose that n'_L is subject to $n_R < n'_L \leq \lambda n_L$, where λ is a prespecified constant for the maximum allowable sample size. Let $(\tilde{\delta}_1, \tilde{\delta}_2)$ and (δ_1^*, δ_2^*) be the differences in proportions used for planned sample size and for recalculated sample size, respectively. Note that the value of correlation assumed at the design stage is retained for the sample size recalculation, i.e., without updating based on observed correlation at the interim as the correlation is a nuisance parameter in hypothesis testing.

To preserve the overall type I error rate at a prespecified significance level even when the sample size is increased and conventional test statistics are used, we consider an extension of the Cui–Hung–Wang (CHW) statistics (Cui et al. 1999) for sample size recalculation in group-sequential designs with two co-primary endpoints.

$$Z'_{km} = \sqrt{\frac{n_R}{n_m}} Z_{kR} + \sqrt{\frac{n_m - n_R}{n_m}} \frac{\sum_{i=n_R+1}^{n'_m} Y_{\mathrm{T}ki} - \sum_{j=n_R+1}^{n'_m} Y_{\mathrm{C}kj}}{\sqrt{2(n'_m - n_R)\hat{\bar{p}}''_{km}(1 - \hat{\bar{p}}''_{km})}},$$

where $r = 1$, $n'_m = (n_m - n_R)(n'_L - n_R)/(n_L - n_R) + n_R$ and $\hat{\bar{p}}''_{km} = (\hat{p}''_{\mathrm{T}km} + \hat{p}''_{\mathrm{C}km})/2$ with $\hat{p}''_{\mathrm{T}km} = (n'_m - n_R)^{-1} \sum_{i=n_R+1}^{n'_m} Y_{\mathrm{T}ki}$ and $\hat{p}''_{\mathrm{C}km} = (n'_m - n_R)^{-1} \sum_{j=n_R+1}^{n'_m} Y_{\mathrm{C}kj}$ $(k = 1,2;\ R = 1, \ldots, L-1;\ m = R+1, \ldots, L)$. The same critical values utilized for the case without sample size recalculation are used.

The sample size is increased or decreased when the conditional power evaluated at the Rth analysis is lower or higher than the desired power $1-\beta$. Under the planned MSS and a given observed value of (Z_{1R}, Z_{2R}), for DF-A', the conditional power is defined by

$$CP = \Pr\left[\bigcup_{m=R+1}^{L} \{A_{1m} \cap A_{2m}\} \,|a_{1R}, a_{2R}\right] \tag{14.4}$$

if $Z_{1l} \leq c_{1l}$ or $Z_{2l} \leq c_{2l}$ for all $l = 1, \ldots, R$, where (a_{1R}, a_{2R}) is a given observed value of (Z_{1R}, Z_{2R}). On the other hand, the conditional power for DF-A is given by

$$CP = \begin{cases} \Pr\left[\bigcup_{m=R+1}^{L} A_{1m} \; a_{1R}, a_{2l'}\right] \\ \quad \text{if } Z_{1l} \leq c_{1l} \text{ for all } l = 1, \ldots, R \text{ and } Z_{2l'} > c_{2l'} \text{ for some } l' = 1, \ldots, R, \\ \Pr\left[\bigcup_{m=R+1}^{L} A_{2m} \,|a_{2R}, a_{1l'}\right] \\ \quad \text{if } Z_{2l} \leq c_{2l} \text{ for all } l = 1, \ldots, R \text{ and } Z_{1l'} > c_{1l'} \text{ for some } l' = 1, \ldots, R, \\ \Pr\left[\left\{\bigcup_{m=R+1}^{L} A_{1m}\right\} \cap \left\{\bigcup_{m=R+1}^{L} A_{2m}\right\} |a_{1R}, a_{2R}\right] \\ \quad \text{if } Z_{1l} \leq c_{1l} \text{ and } Z_{2l} \leq c_{2l} \text{ for all } l = 1, \ldots, R. \end{cases} \tag{14.5}$$

Since (δ_1, δ_2) is unknown, it is customary to substitute (δ_1^*, δ_2^*), the estimated mean differences at the Rth analysis $(\hat{\delta}_{1R}, \hat{\delta}_{2R})$ or the assumed mean differences during trial planning $(\tilde{\delta}_1, \tilde{\delta}_2)$. We consider the conditional power based on $(\delta_1^*, \delta_2^*) = (\hat{\delta}_{1R}, \hat{\delta}_{2R})$, which allows evaluation of behavior of power independent of $(\tilde{\delta}_1, \tilde{\delta}_2)$.

When recalculating the sample size, three options are possible: (a) only allowing an increase in the sample size, (b) only allowing a decrease in the sample size, and (c) allowing an increase or decrease in the sample size. For all the cases, we assign Z'_{km} and n'_m instead of Z_{km} and n_m in the conditional powers (14.4) and (14.5) for the conditional power with sample size recalculation. Consider the rule for determining the recalculated sample size n'_L, when the sample size may be increased only, which is:

$$n'_L = \begin{cases} n_L, & \text{if } CP \geq 1-\beta \text{ or } \min(\hat{\delta}_{1R}, \hat{\delta}_{2R}) \leq 0, \\ \min(n''_L, \lambda n_L), & \text{otherwise,} \end{cases}$$

where n''_L is the smallest integer $n'_L(> n_R)$, where the conditional power achieves the desired power $1-\beta$. When the sample size may be decreased only, the recalculated sample size n'_L is:

$$n'_L = \begin{cases} n''_L, & \text{if } CP > 1-\beta, \\ n_L, & \text{otherwise.} \end{cases}$$

When the sample size may be increased or decreased, then the recalculated sample size n'_L is:

$$n'_L = \begin{cases} n''_L, & \text{if } CP > 1-\beta, \\ n_L, & \text{if } CP = 1-\beta \text{ or } \min(\hat{\delta}_{1R}, \hat{\delta}_{2R}) \leq 0, \\ \min(n''_L, \lambda n_L), & \text{otherwise.} \end{cases}$$

14.4.2 Illustration

In this section, we provide an example to illustrate the sample size recalculation discussed in the previous section, using the PLACIDE study. For illustration, we consider a two-stage group-sequential design with one interim and final analyses. The test statistics based on independent samples at the interim and final analyses Z_{k1} and Z''_{k2} are given by

$$Z_{k1} = \frac{\sqrt{n_1}\hat{\delta}_{k1}}{\sqrt{2\hat{\bar{p}}_{k1}(1-\hat{\bar{p}}_{k1})}} \text{ and } Z''_{k2} = \frac{\sqrt{n'_2 - n_1}\hat{\delta}''_{k2}}{\sqrt{2\hat{\bar{p}}''_{k2}(1-\hat{\bar{p}}''_{k2})}},$$

where $\hat{\delta}''_{k2} = (n'_2 - n_1)^{-1}\left(\sum_{i=n_1+1}^{n'_2} Y_{\mathrm{T}ki} - \sum_{i=n_1+1}^{n'_2} Y_{\mathrm{C}kj}\right)$. Therefore, the CHW statistics are $Z'_{k2} = w_1 Z_{k1} + w_2 Z''_{k2}$, where $w_1 = \sqrt{n_1/n_2}$ and $w_2 = \sqrt{(n_2 - n_1)/n_2}$. As mentioned in Sect. 14.3.2, the MSS for DF-A and DF-A' is given as 1146 per intervention group, based on an alternative hypothesis of a difference for both AAD ($\delta_1 = -0.10$ with $p_{\mathrm{C}1} = 0.20$) and CDD ($\delta_2 = -0.02$ with $p_{\mathrm{C}2} = 0.04$), $\rho = 0.0, 0.3, 0.5,$ and 0.8, with an alternative hypothesis of differences in proportions for AAD ($p_{\mathrm{T}1} = 0.2$ and $p_{\mathrm{C}1} = 0.4$) and CDD ($p_{\mathrm{T}2} = 0.02$ and $p_{\mathrm{C}2} = 0.04$) with the overall power of 80 % at the significance level of 2.5 % by one-sided test, using the normal approximation method, where the critical values are determined by the OF for both endpoints, with the LD α-spending method with equally spaced information level.

Table 14.3 displays the recalculated sample sizes, conditional powers, and empirical conditional powers for DF-A and DF-A' under the five scenarios, i.e., (i) both differences in proportions, at the interim, are the same as those at the planning, (ii) both differences in proportions, at the interim, are smaller than those at the planning, (iii) both differences in proportions at the interim are larger than those at the planning, (iv) only the difference in proportions for AAD at the interim is smaller than that at the planning, and (v) only the difference in proportions for CDD at the interim is smaller than that at the planning. The sample size is recalculated when the conditional power evaluated at the interim analysis is lower or higher than the desired power $1-\beta$ under the three options of (a) only decreasing the sample size, (b) only increasing the sample size, and (c) increasing or decreasing the sample size, with a prespecified constant for the maximum allowable sample size $\lambda = 1.5$ and $\rho = 0.0$, where the critical values are determined by the OF for both endpoints, with the LD α-spending method with equally spaced information level.

Table 14.3 The recalculated sample sizes, conditional powers (CPs) and empirical conditional powers (ECP) for DF-A' and DF-A under the five scenarios, i.e., (i) both differences in proportions, at the interim, are the same as those at the planning, (ii) both differences in proportions, at the interim, are smaller than those at the planning, (iii) both differences in proportions, at the interim, are larger than those at the planning, (iv) only the difference in proportions for AAD at the interim is smaller than that at the planning, and (v) only the difference in proportions for CDD at the interim is smaller than that at the planning. The sample size is recalculated when the CP evaluated at the interim analysis is lower or higher than the desired power $1-\beta$, under the three options of (a) only decreasing the sample size, (b) only increasing the sample size, and (c) increasing or decreasing the sample size, with a prespecified constant for the maximum allowable sample size $\lambda = 1.5$ and $\rho = 0.0$, where the critical values are determined by the OF for both endpoints, with the LD α-spending method with equally spaced information level.

	Scenario-observed effect at the interim				Before recalculation		After recalculation		
DF	#	δ_1	δ_2	Options	CP(%)	ECP(%)	n_2'	CP(%)	ECP(%)
DF-A	(i)	0.1	0.02	(a)	88.2	88.7	1146	88.2	88.7
				(b)	88.2	88.7	967	80.2	80.5
				(c)	88.2	88.7	967	80.2	80.5
	(ii)	0.05	0.01	(a)	54.8	55.2	1719	82.8	83.3
				(b)	54.8	55.2	1146	54.8	55.2
				(c)	54.8	55.2	1719	82.8	83.3
	(iii)	0.15	0.025	(a)	96.3	96.2	1146	96.3	96.2
				(b)	96.3	96.2	669	73.1	72.6
				(c)	96.3	96.2	669	73.1	72.6
	(iv)	0.05	0.02	(a)	88.2	88.8	1146	88.2	88.8
				(b)	88.2	88.8	1074	85.5	85.9
				(c)	88.2	88.8	1074	85.5	85.9
	(v)	0.10	0.01	(a)	54.8	55.3	1719	82.8	83.6
				(b)	54.8	55.3	1146	54.8	55.3
				(c)	54.8	55.3	1719	82.8	83.6
DF-A'	(i)	0.1	0.02	(a)	88.2	88.8	1146	88.2	88.8
				(b)	88.2	88.8	968	80.2	80.8
				(c)	88.2	88.8	968	80.2	80.8
	(ii)	0.05	0.01	(a)	54.8	55.2	1719	82.8	83.3
				(b)	54.8	55.2	1146	54.8	55.2
				(c)	54.8	55.2	1719	82.8	83.3
	(iii)	0.15	0.025	(a)	96.3	96.2	1146	96.3	96.2
				(b)	96.3	96.2	669	73.1	72.7
				(c)	96.3	96.2	669	73.1	72.7

Table 14.3 (continued)

	Scenario-observed effect at the interim				Before recalculation		After recalculation		
DF	#	δ_1	δ_2	Options	CP(%)	ECP(%)	n_2'	CP(%)	ECP(%)
	(iv)	0.05	0.02	(a)	88.2	88.8	1146	88.2	88.8
				(b)	88.2	88.8	1074	85.5	85.9
				(c)	88.2	88.8	1074	85.5	85.9
	(v)	0.10	0.01	(a)	54.8	55.3	1719	82.8	83.6
				(b)	54.8	55.3	1146	54.8	55.3
				(c)	54.8	55.3	1719	82.8	83.6

DF-A at the interim time point not necessarily simultaneously, *DFA'* at the same interim time point of the trial, *AAD* antibiotic-associated diarrhoea, *CDD Clostridium difficile* diarrhoea, *OF* O'Brien–Fleming, *LD* Lan–DeMets

There is no major difference in conditional powers for sample size recalculation between DF-A and DF-A'. In all scenarios of observed effects at the interim, when only allowing an increase in the sample size, the conditional power (and empirical conditional power) is always higher than the desired power of 80 %. When allowing an increase or a decrease in the sample size, except for scenario (iii) of both differences in proportions at the interim are larger than those at the planning—the conditional powers are always larger than desired power of 80 %. On the other hand, when only allowing a decrease in the sample size, the conditional powers are always lower than the desired power. In this example, the sample size recalculation is supposed to be conducted at 50 % information time. As Asakura et al. (2014) discuss, the timing of sample size recalculation is important. The power is much lower than desired power if the sample size recalculation is conducted early in the study, especially when allowing for a decrease in the sample size.

14.5 Hierarchical Hypothesis Testing with Adaptive Type I Error Allocation

One limitation in the methods discussed in Sect. 14.2 is the requirement that the allocation of type I error to each interim analysis for both endpoints is prespecified, using an α-spending function. Tsong et al. (2004) discuss a method for hierarchical hypothesis testing with adaptive type I error allocation in group-sequential three-arm clinical trials for the assessment of equivalence and efficacy of a generic product, where the co-primary objectives of the study are to assess whether the generic and reference product are effective relative to placebo and whether it is equivalent to the reference product using a prespecified equivalence limit. One of their methods is to evaluate equivalence only after both the null hypotheses of efficacy are rejected and then to specify the type I error allocation, just before the equivalence evaluation is performed.

In this section, we discuss an extension to the hierarchical hypothesis testing with adaptive type I error allocation strategy. In this method, first, the order of the hypothesis testing, i.e., which endpoint is first tested, is determined, and then the type I error allocation for the first-tested endpoint is prespecified. If superiority has been established for the first-tested endpoint at lth analysis ($l = 1, \ldots, L$), then the type I error allocation for the second-tested endpoint is specified just before the hypothesis testing for the second-tested endpoint is performed, where L is a maximum of planned analyses. If superiority has been established for the second-tested endpoint at l^*th analysis ($l^* = l, \ldots, L$), then the null hypothesis H_0 is rejected and study is stopped. The stopping rule is formally given as follows:

For the first-tested endpoint, at the lth analysis ($l = 1, \ldots, L - 1$),
  if $Z_{1l} > c_{1l}$ and then evaluate the second-tested endpoint,
  otherwise, continue to the $(l + 1)$ th analysis,
at the Lth analysis,
  if $Z_{1L} > c_{1L}$ and then evaluate the second-tested endpoint,
  otherwise, do not reject H_0.
For the second-tested endpoint, at the l^*th analysis ($l^* = l, \ldots, L - 1$),
  if $Z_{2l^*} > c_{2l^*}$, then reject H_0 and stop the trial,
  otherwise, continue to the $(l^* + 1)$ th analysis,
at the Lth analysis
  if $Z_{2L} > c_{2L}$, then reject H_0,
  otherwise, do not reject H_0.

We provide an example to illustrate the method using the PLACIDE study. Table 14.4 displays the MSS and ASN per intervention group (equally sized groups: $r_{\cdot} = 1$) with the two hypothesis-testing orders, i.e., (1) AAD is first tested, then CDD is tested and (2) CDD is first tested and then AAD is tested. The sample size was derived using an alternative hypothesis of differences in proportions for AAD ($p_{T1} = 0.2$ and $p_{C1} = 0.4$) and CDD ($p_{T2} = 0.02$ and $p_{C2} = 0.04$) with the overall power of 80 % at the significance level of 2.5 % by the one-sided test, using the normal approximation method discussed in the previous section, where $\rho = \rho_T = \rho_C = 0.0, 0.3, 0.5$ and 0.8; $L = 1, 2, 3, 4$, and 5. The critical values are determined by the four testing procedure combinations, i.e., (i) the OF for both endpoints (OF–OF), (ii) the OF for AAD and the PC for CDD (OF–PC), (iii) the PC for AAD and the OF for CDD (PC–OF), and (iv) the PC for both endpoints (PC–PC), with the LD α-spending method, with equally spaced information level.

There is no major difference in MSS and ASN between the two hypothesis-testing orders, (1) first AAD, then CDD and (2) first CDD and then AAD when the same testing procedure is selected for both endpoints. The smallest MSS is given by when the AAD is first tested, or when the CDD is first tested, with the OF–OF or PC–OF testing procedure combination. The smallest ASN is given by when the AAD is first tested, or the CDD is first tested, with PC–PC testing procedure combination. Comparing the method to the methods with the prespecified type I error allocation,

Table 14.4 The MSS and ASN (equally sized groups). The MSS was calculated to detect the joint effect for both endpoints with the overall power of $1-\beta=80\,\%$ at the one-sided significance level of $\alpha=2.5\,\%$, based on the assumption from the PLACIDE study. The critical values are determined by the four testing procedure combinations, i.e., (i) the OF for both endpoints (OF–OF), (ii) the OF for AAD and the PC for CDD (OF–PC), (iii) the PC for AAD and the OF for CDD (PC–OF), and (iv) the PC for both endpoints (PC–PC), with the LD α-spending method with equally spaced information level.

Order of testing			(i) OF–OF		(ii) OF–PC		(iii) PC–OF		(iv) PC–PC	
	ρ	L	MSS	ASN	MSS	ASN	MSS	ASN	MSS	ASN
AAD → CDD	0.0	1	1143		1143		1143		1143	
		2	1146	1052.3	1281	975.8	1146	1052.3	1281	975.8
		3	1156	988.2	1336	936.4	1156	988.2	1336	936.1
		4	1164	957.8	1363	920.7	1164	957.7	1366	918.4
		5	1170	940.6	1377	913.3	1170	940.6	1384	908.7
	0.3	1	1143		1143		1143		1143	
		2	1146	1052.3	1281	975.8	1146	1052.3	1281	975.8
		3	1156	988.2	1336	936.3	1156	988.2	1336	936.1
		4	1164	957.7	1363	919.3	1164	957.7	1366	918.4
		5	1170	940.6	1376	910.4	1170	940.6	1384	908.6
	0.5	1	1143		1143		1143		1143	
		2	1146	1052.3	1281	975.8	1146	1052.3	1281	975.8
		3	1156	988.2	1336	936.3	1156	988.2	1336	936.1
		4	1164	957.7	1363	919.3	1164	957.7	1366	918.4
		5	1170	940.6	1376	910.4	1170	940.6	1384	908.6
	0.8	1	1143		1143		1143		1143	
		2	1146	1052.3	1281	975.8	1146	1052.3	1281	975.8
		3	1156	988.2	1336	936.3	1156	988.2	1336	936.1
		4	1164	957.7	1363	919.3	1164	957.7	1366	918.4
		5	1170	940.6	1376	910.4	1170	940.6	1384	908.6
CDD → AAD	0.0	1	1143		1143		1143		1143	
		2	1146	1052.3	1281	975.8	1146	1052.3	1281	975.8
		3	1156	988.2	1336	936.4	1156	988.2	1336	936.1
		4	1164	957.8	1366	923.9	1164	957.7	1366	918.4
		5	1170	940.6	1384	924.4	1170	940.6	1384	908.6
	0.3	1	1143		1143		1143		1143	
		2	1146	1052.3	1281	975.8	1146	1052.3	1281	975.8
		3	1156	988.2	1336	936.3	1156	988.2	1336	936.1
		4	1164	957.7	1366	922.7	1164	957.7	1366	918.4
		5	1170	940.6	1384	922.3	1170	940.6	1384	908.6

Table 14.4 (continued)

Order of testing			(i) OF–OF		(ii) OF–PC		(iii) PC–OF		(iv) PC–PC	
	ρ	L	MSS	ASN	MSS	ASN	MSS	ASN	MSS	ASN
	0.5	1	1143		1143		1143		1143	
		2	1146	1052.3	1281	975.8	1146	1052.3	1281	975.8
		3	1156	988.2	1336	936.3	1156	988.2	1335	936.1
		4	1164	957.7	1366	922.7	1164	957.7	1365	918.4
		5	1170	940.6	1384	922.3	1170	940.6	1384	908.6
	0.8	1	1143		1143		1143		1143	
		2	1146	1052.3	1281	975.8	1146	1052.3	1281	975.8
		3	1156	988.2	1336	936.3	1156	988.2	1335	936.1
		4	1164	957.7	1366	922.7	1164	957.7	1366	918.4
		5	1170	940.6	1384	922.3	1170	940.6	1384	908.6

MSS maximum sample size, *ASN* average sample number, *AAD* antibiotic-associated diarrhoea, *CDD Clostridium difficile* diarrhoea, *OF* O'Brien–Fleming, *PC* Pocock, *LD* Lan–DeMets

the method provides savings (i.e., 10 to 30 smaller) of the ASN than DF-A or DF-A', depending on the testing procedure combinations, although there is no major difference in MSS for all of the testing procedure combinations. Although the use of the method may be attractive in practice, however, further investigation of the method regarding the behavior of type I error rate is needed as discussed by Hung et al. (2007).

14.6 Summary

The determination of sample size and the evaluation of power are fundamental and critical elements in the design of a clinical trial. If a sample size is too small, then important effects may not be detected, while a sample size that is too large is wasteful of resources, and unethically puts more participants at risk than necessary. Recently, many clinical trials were designed with more than one endpoint considered as co-primary. Co-primary endpoints offer an attractive design feature as they capture a more complete characterization of the effect of an intervention. The effects of interventions are multidimensional requiring the measurement of several important clinical endpoints. However, co-primary endpoints create challenges in the evaluation of power and the calculation of sample size during trial design. Current methods often result in large and impractical sample sizes.

In this chapter, we discuss group-sequential designs in clinical trials with co-primary endpoints, where both endpoints are binary outcomes. To provide the fundamental foundation, we consider a two-arm parallel-group trial designed to evaluate whether an experimental intervention is superior to a control. We describe two decision-making frameworks for evaluating joint effects in group-sequential designs, and define the corresponding power and sample size calculations based on the normal approximation method. We evaluate the utility of using the normal approximation method in practice using Monte Carlo simulation, and investigate the behavior of the required sample size with varying design assumptions. We also discuss sample size recalculation based on the observed interim effects. Furthermore, we discuss a hierarchical hypothesis testing with adaptive type I error allocation for clinical trials with co-primary endpoints in order to improve power.

The Monte Carlo simulation results suggest that the normal approximation works well in most situations. However, in the occurrence of extremely small event rates or small sample sizes, the Monte Carlo simulation-based method or more direct methods may be more appropriate although this occurs at the expense of considerable computational resources.

As with group-sequential trials involving a single primary endpoint, designing group-sequential trials with co-primary endpoints can provide efficiencies by detecting trends prior to planned completion of the trial. It may also be prudent to evaluate design assumptions, at the interim, and potentially make design adjustments (i.e., sample size recalculation) if design assumptions were dramatically inaccurate.

The main objective of this chapter is to provide the fundamental foundation in group-sequential designs for co-primary endpoints. Our discussion is restricted to a superiority clinical trial comparing two interventions. The design allows for early stopping when large intervention differences are observed, i.e., rejecting a null hypothesis only. The PLACIDE study, mentioned in Sect. 14.3.2, failed to demonstrate a beneficial effect of probiotic on both AAD and CDD. The observed treatment effects were smaller than the assumed effects. Stopping a clinical trial, when the interim results suggest effect sizes are smaller than those deemed as clinically important, can also save resources that could be used on more promising research. The methodology discussed here can be extended to other situations such as evaluating futility or simultaneously evaluating both efficacy and futility.

Acknowledgments Research reported in this publication was supported by JSPS KAKENHI under Grant Number 26330038 and the National Institute of Allergy and Infectious Diseases of the National Institutes of Health under Award Numbers UM1AI104681 and UM1AI068634. The content is solely the responsibility of the authors and does not necessarily represent the official views of the National Institutes of Health.

References

Allen SJ, Wareham K, Bradley C, Harris W, Dhar A, Brown H, Foden A, Cheung WY, Gravenor MB, Plummer S, Phillips CJ, Mack D (2012) A multicentre randomised controlled trial evaluating lactobacilli and bifidobacteria in the prevention of antibiotic-associated diarrhoea in older people admitted to hospital: the PLACIDE study protocol. BMC Infect Dis 12:108

Allen SJ, Wareham K, Wang D, Bradley C, Hutchings H, Harris W, Dhar A, Brown H, Foden A, Gravenor MB, Mack D (2013) Lactobacilli and bifidobacteria in the prevention of antibiotic-associated diarrhoea and *Clostridium difficile* diarrhoea in older inpatients (PLACIDE): a randomised, double-blind, placebo-controlled, multicentre trial. The Lancet 382:1249–1257

American College of Gastroenterology website (2013) Understanding irritable bowel syndrome. www.patients.gi.org/gi-health-and-disease/understanding-irritable-bowel-syndrome leaving site icon. Accessed 4 Dec 2013

Asakura K, Hamasaki T, Sugimoto T, Hayashi K, Evans SR, Sozu T (2014) Sample size determination in group-sequential clinical trials with two co-primary endpoints. Stat Med 33:2897–2913

Chuang-Stein C, Stryszak P, Dmitrienko A, Offen W (2007) Challenge of multiple co-primary endpoints: a new approach. Stat Med 26:1181–1192

Cochran WG (1952) The χ^2 test of goodness of fit. Ann Math Stat 25:315–345

Committee for Medicinal Products for Human Use (2013) Guideline on the evaluation of medicinal products for 4 the treatment of irritable bowel syndrome. CPMP/EWP/785/97 Rev. 1

Cui L, Hung HMJ, Wang SJ (1999) Modification of sample size in group sequential clinical trials. Biometrics 55:853–857

Eaton ML, Muirhead RJ (2007) On multiple endpoints testing problem. J Stat Plan Inference 137:3416–3429

Emrich LJ, Piedmonte MR (1991) A method for generating high-dimensional multivariate binary variates. Am Stat 45:302–304

Food and Drug Administration (2012) Guidance for industry. Irritable bowel syndrome: clinical evaluation of products for treatment. Center for Drug Evaluation and Research, Food and Drug Administration, Rockville

Grundmann O, Yoon SL (2010) Irritable bowel syndrome: epidemiology, diagnosis, and treatment: an update for health-care practitioners. J Gastroenterol Hepatol 25:691–699

Hamasaki T, Sugimoto T, Evans SR, Sozu T (2013) Sample size determination for clinical trials with co-primary outcomes. Exponential event-times. Pharm Stat 12:28–34

Hung HMJ, Wang SJ (2009) Some controversial multiple testing problems in regulatory applications. J Biopharm Stat 19:1–11

Hung HMJ, Wang SJ, O'Neill R (2007) Statistical considerations for testing multiple endpoints in group sequential or adaptive clinical trials. J Biopharm Stat 17:1201–1210

Julious S, McIntyre NE (2012) Sample sizes for trials involving multiple correlated must-win comparisons. Pharm Stat 11:177–185

Kordzakhia G, Siddiqui O, Huque MF (2010) Method of balanced adjustment in testing co-primary endpoints. Stat Med 29:2055–2066

Lan KKG, DeMets DL (1983) Discrete sequential boundaries for clinical trials. Biometrika 70:659–663

Landau S, Stahl D (2013) Sample size and power calculations for medical studies by simulation when closed form expressions are not available. Stat Methods Med Res 22:324–345

Le Cessie S, van Houwelingen JC (1994) Logistic regression for correlated binary data. Appl Stat 43:95–108

O'Brien PC, Fleming TR (1979) A multiple testing procedure for clinical trials. Biometrics 35:549–556

Offen W, Chuang-Stein C, Dmitrienko A, Littman G, Maca J, Meyerson L, Muirhead R, Stryszak P, Boddy A, Chen K, Copley-Merriman K, Dere W, Givens S, Hall D, Henry D, Jackson JD, Krishen A, Liu T, Ryder S, Sankoh AJ, Wang J, Yeh CH (2007) Multiple co-primary endpoints: medical and statistical solutions. Drug Inf J 41:31–46

Pocock SJ (1977) Group sequential methods in the design and analysis of clinical trials. Biometrika 64:191–199

Prentice RL (1988) Correlated binary regression with covariates specific to each binary observation. Biometrics 44:1033–1048

Senn S, Bretz F (2007) Power and sample size when multiple endpoints are considered. Pharm Stat 6:161–170

Sozu T, Sugimoto T, Hamasaki T (2010) Sample size determination in clinical trials with multiple co-primary binary endpoints. Stat Med 29:2169–2179

Sozu T, Sugimoto T, Hamasaki T (2011) Sample size determination in superiority clinical trials with multiple co-primary correlated endpoints. J Biopharm Stat 21:1–19

Sozu T, Sugimoto T, Hamasaki T (2012) Sample size determination in clinical trials with multiple co-primary endpoints including mixed continuous and binary variables. Biometrical J 54:716–729

Sugimoto T, Sozu T, Hamasaki T (2012) A convenient formula for sample size calculations in clinical trials with multiple co-primary continuous endpoints. Pharm Stat 11:118–128

Sugimoto T, Sozu T, Hamasaki T, Evans SR (2013) A logrank test-based method for sizing clinical trials with two co-primary time-to-events endpoints. Biostatistics 14:409–421

Tsong Y, Zhang J, Wang SJ (2004) Group sequential design and analysis of clinical equivalence assessment for generic nonsystematic drug products. J Biopharm Stat 14:359–373

Xiong C, Yu K, Gao F, Yan Y, Zhang Z (2005) Power and sample size for clinical trials when efficacy is required in multiple endpoints: application to an Alzheimer's treatment trial. Clin Trials 2:387–393

Chapter 15
Issues in the Use of Existing Data: As Controls in Pre-Market Comparative Clinical Studies

Lilly Q. Yue

Abstract Randomized, well-controlled clinical trials have been viewed as the gold standard in the evaluation of medical products, and observational comparative clinical studies also play an important role in the evaluation in both premarket and postmarket settings. Such observational comparative studies could be concurrent or nonconcurrent depending on the timing when patients get treated. A nonconcurrent control group could be formed from patients with existing data, when indeed appropriate. For example, a control group could come from patients with historical data collected from earlier investigational device exemption (IDE) studies of previously approved medical products or selected from a well-designed and executed registry database. However, the construction of a control group from existing data presents extra challenges compared to the formation of a concurrent control group. In this chapter, some of the design challenges, such as validity of study design, historical control group selection and treatment group comparability, and identification of a control group from an applicable registry database, are discussed and illustrated with examples from regulatory perspectives.

15.1 Introduction

Carefully designed and well-conducted randomized controlled trials (RCTs) provide the highest level of evidence in the safety and effectiveness evaluation of medical products, but may not be feasible in some circumstances due to practical or ethical reasons. As an alternative, observational (nonrandomized) comparative studies play an important role in the medical product evaluations, in both premarket and postmarket regulatory settings. A comparator (control) used in such an observational comparative study could be concurrent or nonconcurrent in terms of timing when

No official support or endorsement by the Food and Drug Administration of this presentation is intended or should be inferred.

L. Q. Yue (✉)
Center for Devices and Radiological Health, US Food and Drug Administration,
10903 New Hampshire Avenue, Silver Spring, MD 20993, USA
e-mail: lilly.yue@fda.hhs.gov

Z. Chen et al. (eds.), *Applied Statistics in Biomedicine and Clinical Trials Design*,
ICSA Book Series in Statistics, DOI 10.1007/978-3-319-12694-4_15

patients get treated, and the patients in the control group could be enrolled in the current investigational study or obtained from existing data. For example, when deemed appropriate, a control group could be formed from patients with existing data collected from earlier investigational device exemption (IDE) studies of previously approved medical products or may be selected from an applicable high-quality registry database. The potential benefits in using existing data for controls include saving in cost or time of conducting clinical studies. However, statistical and regulatory issues also arise regarding the validity of study design and the interpretability of study results. In this chapter, some study design considerations will be given to the issues such as study design process, historical control selection and treatment group comparability, and control group construction from a registry database, illustrated with examples.

15.2 Study Design Process and Validity

One key advantage of RCT is that with randomization, the distributions of all baseline covariates, observed and unobserved, tend to be balanced across two treatment groups, and another critical feature of RCT is that the study is "prospectively" designed, i.e., it is designed without access to any outcome data from either treatment group. Rubin (2001, 2007, 2008) advocates that observational studies can and should be designed to approximate randomized experiments as closely as possible without access to any outcome data at the design stage. To do so, there are some matching methods developed to design observational study and perform outcome analysis. One example of such methods is propensity score methodology, introduced by Rosenbaum and Rubin (1983, 1984). Propensity score is the probability of receiving treatment rather than control, conditional on observed baseline covariates, and the methodology could be used to design observational studies in a way analogous to the way RCT is designed: without seeing any outcome data, and then to conduct outcome analysis based on the resulting study design. The design part refers to employing propensity scores to help create distributional balance of covariates between the two treatment groups, including *propensity score modeling and covariate balance assessment,* and to specifying statistical analysis plan (SAP) for the treatment comparison on outcomes. These activities have to be accomplished without access to any outcome data, as is the case in RCT. The analysis part refers to making treatment comparison on outcome data, adjusting for propensity scores.

In practice, however, sufficient attention has not been paid to the *prospective* design as it should. Oftentimes, an observational study is designed as if it were an RCT—prior to enrolling patients, selecting a control group, determining sample size, specifying covariates, etc., and after completing patient follow-up, performing outcome analysis adjusted for baseline covariates using traditional regression or propensity score methods with both outcome and covariate data in sight. Under such a practice, arguments in the statistical modeling and concerns with type I error arise, as the model-based analyses may be repeated to produce desired answers. Without a prospective design, Rubin (2001) points out that "It is essentially impossible to be objective when a variety of analyses are being done, each producing an answer, favorable, neutral, or unfavorable to the investigator's interests." Indeed, such a study design resulted in debates in the objectivity of study design and the concerns with the reliability and interpretability of outcome analyses. For example, Yue (2012) describes a premarket study with a historical control, in which, without a prospective study design, two fitted propensity score estimation models were submitted to the Food and Drug Administration (FDA)—one with 10 out of 35 covariates leading to a so-called significant outcome result and the other with 15 covariates but "insignificant" outcome result. As the propensity scores were estimated with both covariates and outcomes data in sight, it was hard to tell how many propensity score models had been tried, and therefore, there was no way to control for the type I error. Another problem encountered in a number of premarket observational studies is that the treatment group incomparability was discovered at the final outcome analysis stage, which left no time to identify a more appropriate control group for replacement. All of these issues led to challenges in the interpretation of study results and then difficulties in regulatory decision making.

To solve the problems discussed above, it is critical to follow the principle of prospective design: approximate RCT and balance covariates, design study without access to any outcome data; and, moreover, communicate with FDA and get agreement on the study design prospectively. In doing so, the following two-stage design is recommended for premarket observational comparative studies.

Stage I: Initial Study Planning by a Sponsor Stage I involves initial study planning performed by a sponsor, and begins before the investigational study starts. The tasks performed in this stage include, but are not limited to (1) identify a potential control group; (2) prespecify the inclusion/exclusion criteria so that the similar patient populations are being compared; (3) prespecify an appropriate set of baseline covariates to be collected in the study and utilized in propensity score modeling, based on prior clinical knowledge but not outcomes under consideration; (4) based on previous knowledge, make sure all clinically important covariates are measured similarly in the two treatment groups; (5) specify propensity score method(s) to be used and provide related details; and (6) perform preliminary sample size estimation. Some commitments are needed to: (1) identify an independent statistician, who is masked to the outcome data of treatment and control groups and will perform the study design in the stage II, and (2) establish firewalls to protect outcomes of treatment and control groups from leaking. There may be a need to change the control group if the treatment group incomparability is identified at the design stage II, or to increase the sample size if lower study power is noticed.

Stage II: Approximating RCT by the Independent Statistician Identified in Stage I The design stage II involves utilizing the propensity scores to create distributional balance of covariates between the two treatment groups (referring to propensity score modeling and covariates balance assessment) and specifying a SAP for the treatment comparison on outcome data. This design stage should start as soon as all patients are enrolled, and the design should be accomplished by the independent statistician identified in the design stage I, without access to any outcome data of either treatment group. In details, if some control patients were to be excluded from the study, provide the justification on the exclusion and information on how to exclude control patients; revisit sample size estimation and power; develop SAP on outcome data analysis, based on the resulting study design; communicate with the FDA and provide detailed information on the propensity score modeling and covariate balance assessment; and reach an agreement with the FDA on the final study design.

In the regulatory environment, the expected benefits of such a prospective study design include: (1) avoid arguments regarding "study design" at the final outcome analysis stage; (2) increase the integrity of study design and creditability of study results; (3) increase the consistency, transparency, and predictability of regulatory decision making; and (4) increase flexibility of study design, in terms of control group selection, sample size estimation, and propensity score method(s) to be used. In addition, there is saving in time for a sponsor to complete the study and submit it to the FDA for evaluation, as the design stage II takes place during the subject follow-up, and for the FDA to make regulatory decisions, as the number of review cycles is expected to be decreased.

15.3 Historical Control Selection and Treatment Group Comparability

One of the major benefits for utilizing a historical control is the potential saving in time or cost. However, the usage of historical control may present great challenges for the study design and interpretation of study results. Due to the change of medical practice and the rapid evolution of device technology, there may be significant differences between the two treatment groups in terms of patient population, definition and adjudication of clinical outcomes, treatment management, timing and length of patient follow-up, and collection of important baseline confounding covariates. Another challenge particularly involved in the study design is that the outcomes of historical control group are already available in designing the current investigational study, and therefore extra efforts would be needed to mask the outcomes to the study designers. In selecting a historical control for an investigational study, these challenges need to be carefully considered.

As discussed above, one major issue encountered in a number of device evaluations is the lack of treatment comparability, even after covariate adjustment. Yue (2007) provides an example where the enrollment time between the two treatment groups was minimally overlapped (Fig. 15.1) and some important patient characteristics were imbalanced between the two treatment groups. Two propensity score stratification models were fitted—one with the enrollment time and the other without, but neither of the models presented a reasonable overlap of propensity score distribution as indicated in Figs. 15.2 and 15.3. Particularly, it was noticed that the fifth propensity score quintile contained 30 % of the treated patients but did not have any control patients to compare with (Table 15.1). The findings led to a conclusion

Fig. 15.1 Patient enrollment time

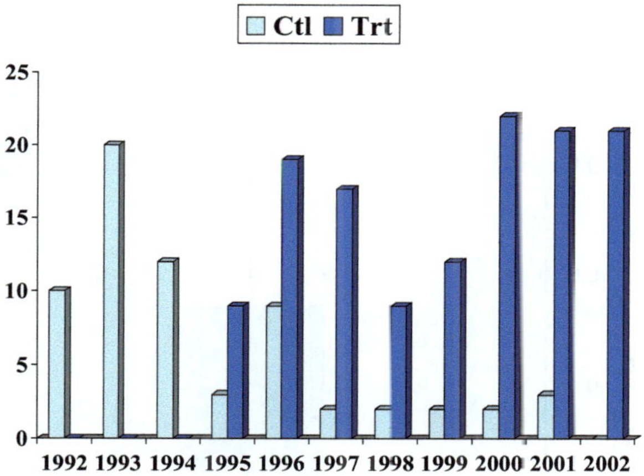

that the two treatment groups did not overlap sufficiently to allow a sensible treatment comparison, and therefore any treatment comparisons, adjusted or unadjusted for imbalanced covariates, were problematic and all resulting p values were uninterpretable. In such a situation, it may be wise to abandon the historical control group

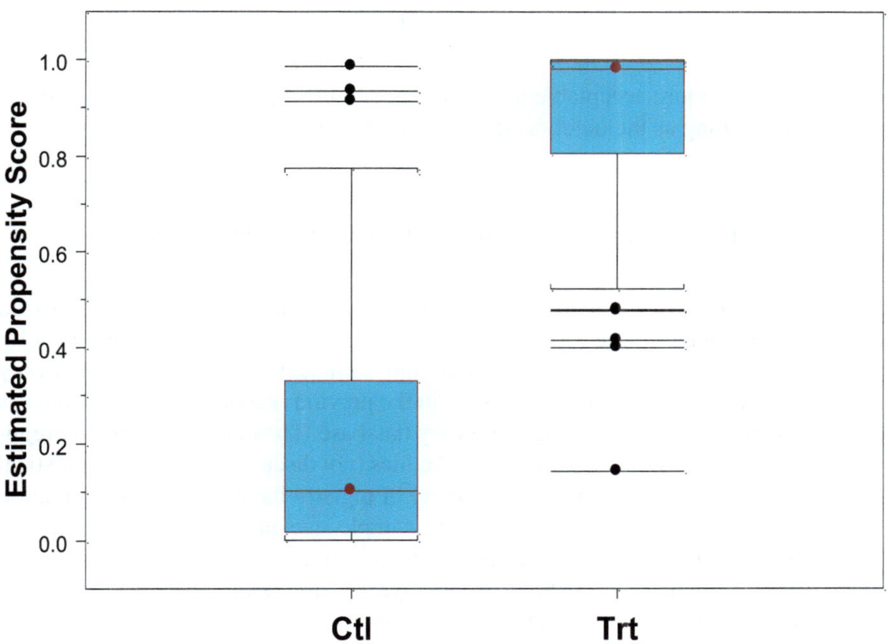

Fig. 15.2 Estimated propensity scores (with time)

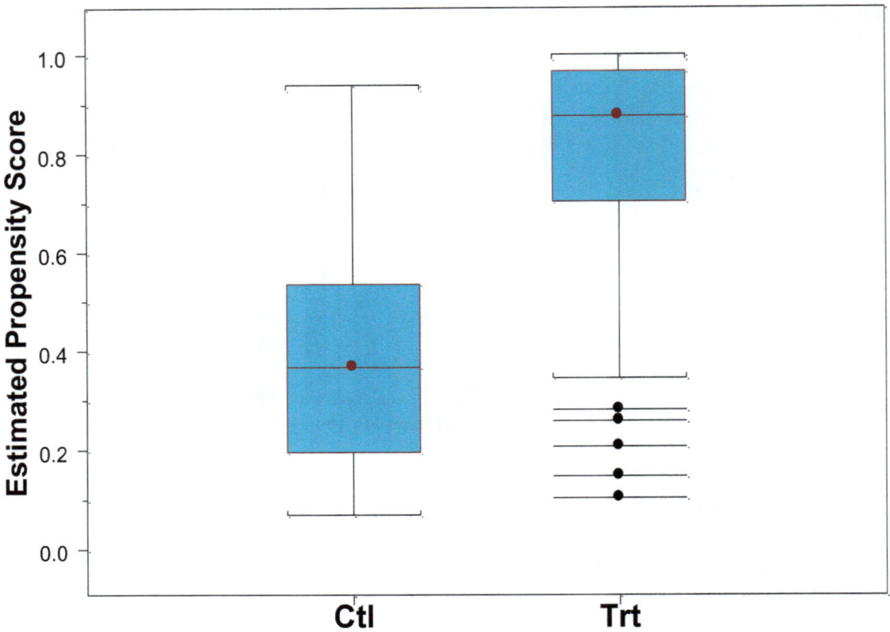

Fig. 15.3 Estimated propensity scores (without time)

and search for a more acceptable one. In doing so, the objectivity of study design is maintained as long as the outcome data are not involved.

15.4 Control Group Selection from Registry Database

A well-designed and implemented registry database may provide valuable real-world resources and could be used to form a control group in the evaluation of a new investigational device. However, a study design with such a control group not only proposes the similar challenges discussed in the previous section but also introduces additional ones unique to the use of registry database. The challenges include regulatory issues such as informed consent and ethics (not discussed here), and statistical study design issues, for example, the quality of registry database and the formation of control group from the registry database, sample size, and power consideration.

For a registry database to serve as an acceptable control for an investigational medical device, the registry data should be of high quality, comprehensive, complete, and reliable. The clinical comparability between registry database and investigational study needs to be demonstrated with respect to patient population, treatment management, patient follow-up, definition of endpoints, and the event adjudication.

To identify an appropriate control group from a registry database, a good selection strategy is needed. Unlike the sample size in a historical control obtained from a previously approved device, the number of available control patients may not be clear in the study design stage I, and sometimes not all of the potential control patients are comparable with the patients treated with a new device in the investigational study. As the first step, the same patient inclusion/exclusion criteria proposed for the investigational device could be used to identify potential control patients from the registry database, with the hope that the selected potential control group is comparable to the treated group with respect to baseline covariate distributions. And then, some matching methods, for example, propensity score matching or stratification, can be utilized to finalize control group selection. In doing so, some control patients may be reasonably discarded if they look nothing like any treated patients, with respect to propensity scores and then baseline covariates. However, any attempt of excluding treated patients could lead to a danger of changing the intended use of the device, and therefore the practice should be discouraged in premarket settings. A hard lesson has been learned as shown in the following example.

A new device was evaluated through the comparison to a control group obtained from a registry database, using propensity score matching. Fifteen baseline covariates were identified and a sample size of 250 was proposed for the investigational device. Using the same inclusion/exclusion criteria specified for the investigational device, 1000 potential control patients were initially selected from the registry. And then, 1:1 propensity score matching was performed with 12 out of 15 covariates included in the propensity score model, leading to a selection of 150 matched pairs—150 out of 1000 potential control patients and 150 out of 250 treated patients. The results raised concerns by excluding 40 % treated patients: (1) the target patient population may be changed. What patient population do the 60 % treated patients left in the study represent? (2) The patient population parameters being estimated may be changed. (3) What is the new indication for use with the device? (4) How to label the product? (5) How reliable are the study results with the post hoc selected target patient population?

The following hypothetical example provides a simple illustration on how a control group could be appropriately selected from a registry. A sample size of 250 for an investigational device was proposed and 15 covariates were specified at stage I. Using the same inclusion/exclusion criteria, 1000 potential control patients were selected. As preplanned, a propensity score stratification model with all 15 covariates was fitted in stage II, leading to a possible study design indicated in Table 15.2. However, in the first propensity score quintile, there were no treated patients, indicating the 250 potential control patients do not match any treated patients and therefore could be reasonably removed from the consideration. Based on the remaining 750 potential control patients and 250 treated patients, a repeated propensity score stratification model was fitted and the distribution of subjects by treatment group is listed in Table 15.3. This repeated modeling process may lead to an appropriate control group, if the covariate distribution balance between the two groups could be demonstrated. However, the iterative propensity score modeling process is valid if and only if outcome-free.

Table 15.1 Distribution of patients in propensity score quintiles

		1	2	3	4	5	Total
W/time	Ctl	39 (58 %)	19 (28 %)	8 (12 %)	1 (2 %)	*0 (0 %)*	67
	Trt	1 (0 %)	21 (16 %)	33 (25 %)	38 (29 %)	*40 (30 %)*	133
W/o time	Ctl	30 (45 %)	25 (37 %)	8 (12 %)	4 (6 %)	*0 (0 %)*	67
	Trt	11 (8 %)	14 (11 %)	32 (24 %)	36 (27 %)	*40 (30 %)*	133

Ctl control patients; *Trt* treated patients

Table 15.2 Distribution of patients at the five propensity score quintiles (1000 in control, 250 in investigational device)

	1	2	3	4	5	Total
Ctl	250	244	234	186	86	1000
Trt	0	6	16	64	164	250

Table 15.3 Distribution of patients at the five propensity score quintiles (750 in control, 250 in investigational device)

	1	2	3	4	5	Total
Ctl	196	193	172	128	61	1000
Trt	4	7	28	72	139	250

15.5 Summary

Premarket comparative studies using existing data need to be carefully and prospectively designed to approximate RCT. It is crucial to design such studies without access to any outcome data for the integrity and interpretability of study results. Propensity score methodology can play an important role in the study design and outcome data analysis.

Clinical comparability between the existing database and investigational study is essential. For a registry to serve as an acceptable control population for a new investigational product, the registry data must be of high quality, comprehensive, complete, and reliable. A good strategy is critically needed for the selection of control group from the registry database.

References

Rubin DB (2001) Using propensity scores to help design observational studies: application to the tobacco litigation. Health Serv Outcomes Res Methodol 2:169–188

Rubin DB (2007) The design versus the analysis of observational studies for causal effects: Parallel with the design of randomized trials. Stat Med 26:20–36

Rubin DB (2008) For objective causal inference, design trumps analysis. Ann Appl Stat 2(3):808–840

Rosenbaum PR, Rubin DB (1983) The central role of the propensity score in observational studies for causal effects. Biometrika 70(1):41–55

Rosenbaum PR, Rubin DB (1984) Reducing bias in observational studies using subclassification on the propensity score. JASA 79:516–524

Yue LQ (2007) Statistical and regulatory issues with the application of propensity score analysis to non-randomized medical device clinical studies. J Biopharm Stat 17:1–13

Yue LQ (2012) Regulatory considerations in the design of comparative observational studies using propensity scores. J Biopharm Stat 22:1272–1279

Chapter 16
A Two-Tier Procedure for Designing and Analyzing Medical Device Trials Conducted in US and OUS Regions for Regulatory Decision Making

Nelson Lu, Yunling Xu and Gerry Gray

Abstract The number of clinical trials conducted simultaneously in the USA and outside of the US (OUS) for medical device development has been increasing over the last decade. However, the presence of inherent regional differences in treatment effects poses a great challenge to the US regulatory agency's decision making. In this chapter, we propose a two-tier procedure for analyzing data from such trials for the US regulatory agency's decision making, allowing treatment effects to vary from region to region. We differentiate direct evidence from supporting evidence while using both to exemplify the advantage of such trials for the US regulatory agency's decision making. The contribution of the supporting evidence can be adjusted according to the expectation of the magnitude of regional differences and the statutory requirements in the USA. Examples are presented to illustrate the design and analysis based on our proposed procedure. Using the proposed two-tier procedure with an upfront explicit decision tree can increase the predictability and transparency of the regulatory decision making.

16.1 Introduction

In the past decade, more and more medical device sponsors have begun conducting clinical trials simultaneously in the USA and outside of the US (OUS) to support regulatory approval of their products in the USA. Such trials are referred as multi-regional clinical trials (MRCTs) in this chapter. Lu et al. (2011) reported that from 2006 to 2010, about 21 % (17/81) of approved premarket applications (PMAs) for therapeutic devices at the Center for Device and Radiological Health (CDRH) are based on MRCTs conducted in the USA and OUS. Both sponsors and the Food and Drug Administration (FDA) are embracing such a concept, hoping to speed up medical device development, and thus to provide earlier availability of effective medical

Y. Xu (✉) · N. Lu · G. Gray
Division of Biostatistics, Center for Devices and Radiological Health, Food and Drug Administration, 10903 New Hampshire Ave, Silver Spring, MD 20993, USA
e-mail: Yun-Ling.Xu@fda.hhs.gov

Z. Chen et al. (eds.), *Applied Statistics in Biomedicine and Clinical Trials Design*,
ICSA Book Series in Statistics, DOI 10.1007/978-3-319-12694-4_16

devices to patients in the USA. Nonetheless, statistical issues for design, conduct, monitoring, and analysis of medical device MRCTs are very challenging, especially in a regulatory setting. Such challenges may not be the same as the ones encountered in drug MRCTs due to the fundamental differences in the characteristics of the products and the regulatory requirements among regions.

In Sect. 2 of this chapter, we present the issues associated with the current framework for analyzing MRCTs for regulatory decision making regarding the US medical device approval. In Sect. 3, a two-tier procedure is proposed for analyzing MRCTs for regulatory decision making with close alignment with the US statutory requirements. Examples for analyzing medical device trials are presented in Sect. 4, followed by design considerations in Sect. 5. The chapter concludes with discussion in Sect. 6.

16.2 Issues with Current Practice in Analyzing Medical Device MRCTs for Regulatory Decision Making in the USA

The statutory requirements for medical devices' premarket approval may vary significantly in different jurisdictions. For example, in the European Union (EU), the demonstration of the device effectiveness is not required for the CE (*Conformité Européenne* or *Communauté Européenne*) marking (CE Mark 2012). For the approval of a Class III medical device in the USA, a reasonable assurance of safety and effectiveness has to be demonstrated as indicated by Section 513(a)(1)(C) of the Federal Food, Drug, and Cosmetic Act (FD and C Act). As set forth in the US FD & C Act 513(a)(2), the safety and effectiveness of a medical device should be determined: (A) with respect to the persons for whose use the device is represented or intended and (B) with respect to the conditions of use prescribed, recommended, or suggested in the labeling of the device (Food, Drug and Cosmetic Act 2012). These statutory provisions specify that a finding of reasonable assurance of safety and effectiveness must be supported by data relevant to the target population, and evaluated in light of the device labeling (Guidance on the Collection of Race and Ethnicity Data in Clinical Trials 2012).

Following the US statutory requirement, if a study is intended to eventually support a premarket submission in the USA, selected study subjects should adequately reflect the target population for the device. This means, ideally the study should be conducted in the USA. Apparently, not all subjects in an MRCT are from USA. Regardless of where a study is conducted, it should be relevant to understanding the safety and effectiveness of the device when used in US subjects with regard to subject demographics, standard of care, practice of medicine, and any cultural differences in terms of expectations regarding medical care. "The Secretary shall accept data from clinical investigations conducted outside of the United States, including the European Union, if the applicant demonstrates that such data are adequate under applicable standards."(FADASIA 2014)

Currently, statistical inference on the global estimate of treatment effect based on pooled data is often used for regulatory decision making in approval of a medical device in the USA based on an MRCT. Following International Conference on Harmonization (ICH) E5 Q&A #11 (2012), data from all regions are pooled together for analysis through prespecified hypothesis testing with a formal decision rule, and the treatment effect consistency across regions is assessed in a post hoc manner without a formal decision rule. There are notable difficulties associated with this current practice in analyzing MRCTs for regulatory decision making. To facilitate the discussion of these issues, let us set up a cell-mean model as follows:

For a randomized controlled superiority MRCT, let k index region: 1, 2, ..., K; l index treatment (t) and control (c); ${n_k}^l$ be the sample size in region k for treatment l; and N_k be the size of the intended population in region k; μ_k^l be the cell mean for the population in region k with treatment l; δ_k $(= {\mu_k}^t - {\mu_k}^c)$ be the treatment effect in region k. In a cell-mean model, the inference on the global mean of treatment effect in an MRCT is essentially to test the following hypothesis, where a larger μ indicates a better result:

$$H_0 : ({n_1}^t/n.^t){\mu_1}^t + \ldots + ({n_K}^t/n.^t){\mu_K}^t \leq ({n_1}^c/n.^c){\mu_1}^c + \ldots + ({n_K}^c/n.^c){\mu_K}^c$$

i.e., a test of treatment effect averaged across regions with a weight of ${n_k}^l/n.^l$; where $n.^l = n_1^l + \ldots + {n_K}^l$ attached to the region k. Please observe that:

1. If ${n_k}^l$ is not proportional to N_k within the MRCT and $\delta_1 = \ldots = \delta_K$ does not hold, the inference on the global estimate by the above test is based on a sample that does not match the population in any local region.
2. If ${n_k}^l$ is proportional to N_k within the MRCT and $\delta_1 = \ldots = \delta_K$ does not hold, the inference on the global estimate by the above test is for an intended population in the whole area covered by all the participated regions, which, however, does not match the population for any local region.
3. If $\delta_1 = \ldots = \delta_K$ holds, the inference on the global estimate by the above test is for an intended population, which matches the intended population in each of the local regions.

From the above observation, current practice in analyzing MRCTs for a local regulatory decision making is valid for that region only if the treatment effect is consistent across regions. There have been several papers discussing statistical methods for assessing treatment effect consistency across regions, for example, Chen et al. (2010), Hung et al. (2010), Quan et al. (2010), and Chen et al. (2012). Nonetheless, in a traditional hypothesis testing framework, it is inherently difficult to prove that $\delta_1 = \ldots = \delta_K$. The power for detecting treatment effect inconsistency among regions is generally fairly low when a study is only powered for testing the overall treatment effect.

A challenging regulatory issue is that, under the current framework, the regulatory decision becomes less predictable and less transparent when facing an observed state of heterogeneity in treatment effects. We believe that such an issue could be addressed with a prespecified decision tree, and our proposed statistical procedure in the next section should be able to serve this purpose.

16.3 A Two-Tier Procedure

For regulatory decisions regarding medical devices in the USA, the statutory requirement is that effectiveness be evaluated for the intended population identified in the labeling (Food, Drug and Cosmetic Act 2012). The intended population is usually characterized by its unique intrinsic and extrinsic factors, such as demographics, standard of care, practice of medicine, and any cultural differences in terms of expectations regarding medical care. As some of the intrinsic and extrinsic factors could be treatment effect modifiers, the effectiveness of a medical device should be evaluated as an estimate of efficacy for the intended population in the USA conditional on its unique intrinsic and extrinsic factors. In other words, potential regional difference must be taken into account when a regulatory decision in the USA on a medical device approval is made using MRCT data.

For medical devices, it is well known that physician's skill and accessibility of high-tech equipment contribute significantly to the effectiveness of a device in use, and this varies from region to region (Campbell 2008; Rothwell 2005). Tanaka (2010) discusses several US regulatory examples where regional treatment differences exist, and Tsou et al. (2010) discuss treatment effect differences from country to country in Asia. A similar pattern is observed in drug applications, as Hung et al. (2010) commented that "We have seen that many MRCTs suggest that there are regional differences in effect estimates."

To account for potential regional difference into an upfront decision tree, we here attempt to recast the issue of assessment on consistency of treatment effects across regions to an issue of information borrowing. The task is to incorporate effectiveness information from the OUS regions into the US regulatory decision making with acknowledgment that treatment effects may vary among regions. We propose a two-tier procedure for decision making in the US medical device approval based on MRCTs. The procedure is outlined in the following and displayed in Fig. 16.1. For convenience, region 1 is designated as the USA, the region of interest.

Step 1: Using data solely from region 1, test for H_{01}: $\delta_1 = 0$.
If the *p* value (p1) is less than a critical value c1, declare a tier 1 success in region 1; otherwise,
if p1 is less than a threshold value π ($\pi \geq$ c1), go to step 2;
otherwise, declare a failure in region 1.

Step 2: Using data from all regions, test for the effect of the variable treatment in the model, which has main effects treatment and regions, and the interaction term of treatment by region.
If the *p* value (p2) is less than a critical value c2, declare a tier 2 success in region 1; otherwise, declare a failure in region 1.

In the proposed two-tier procedure, direct evidence for the effectiveness of the product is evaluated in step 1 using data from region 1 only; and if warranted, supporting evidence is provided in step 2 using data from all regions. The null hypothesis listed in step 2 is that there is no treatment effect for the medical device

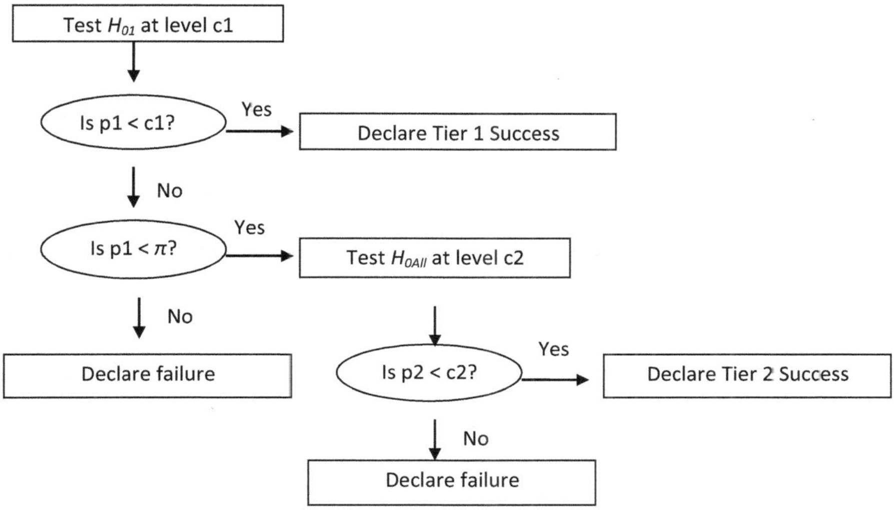

Fig. 16.1 Flow diagram of the two-tier procedure

based on a model that takes regions into consideration. For example, when testing a normally distributed endpoint, the null hypothesis is equivalent to H_{0all}: $\delta_1 + \delta_2 + \ldots \delta_K = 0$ when using type 3 sum of squares. In this case, the treatment effect is expressed as the average effectiveness across regions. Other statistical models may also be considered. Note that the distribution of the outcome measures can be of any type such as normal, binary, and censored failure time. A tier 1 success carries the most direct effectiveness evidence taking into account all the intrinsic and extrinsic factors associated with the intended population in the labeling; a tier 2 success is a synthesis of direct and supporting evidence from all regions by taking regional differences into account.

Note that the two-tier procedure (Fig. 16.1) is a decision procedure with an explicit decision tree, which can help the predictability of regulatory decision making in region 1. The false approval rate in region 1 is controlled at a level of c1 (for testing H_{01} in tier 1) plus $P_{HG1,H0all}$ (c1 < p1 < π, p2 < c2) (for testing H_{0all} in tier 2). A desirable false approval rate in region 1 could be controlled by appropriately chosen c1, π, c2, and group sample size in all regions (n_k^l). In analyzing and designing an MRCT with the two-tier procedure, these choices are of paramount importance to interpretation of the trial result and should be based on the totality of considerations from both statistical and local regulatory perspectives. In the following sections, the choices of these parameters will be discussed.

The CDRH often has certain requirements for a minimal US sample size for some products to ensure the applicability of the study conclusion to the USA. In general, substantial expected regional differences would warrant a substantial proportion of the total sample size allocated to the local region. Once n_k^l/n^l is decided, one possible alpha allocation to the direct evidence is $(n_k^l/n^l)\ \alpha$, where α is the probability of false

Table 16.1 Average infarct size for treatment and control across regions

	Treatment		Control	
Region	US	Europe	US	Europe
Average	30	33	40	31
Standard deviation	19	18	18	20
Sample size	77	132	24	48

approval in region 1. This reflects the extent of importance of direct evidence needed in the regulatory decision making. A small c1 implies using supporting evidence through the global test for H_{0all} unless the direct evidence is quite strong, whereas a larger c1 implies emphasizing direct evidence from the local region unless supporting evidence is necessary. Given the choice of c1, the critical value c2 could then be conservatively set equal to $\alpha-c1$. Alternatively, c2 can be obtained by simulation; the task is to find c2* such that the equation $(c1 + P_{H01,H0all}\,(c1 < p1 < \pi, p2 < c2^*)) = \alpha$ is satisfied. If the derived c2* is greater than α, c2 can be set at α and c1* can be derived by satisfying $(c1^* + P_{H01,H0all}\,(c1^* < p1 < \pi,\ p2 < \alpha)) = \alpha$. The threshold π specified in two-tier procedure is a design parameter, which determines when to use the supporting evidence. If π is set equal to c1, supporting evidence will never be used in the local regulatory decision making. If π is set equal to 1, supporting evidence will always be used in local regulatory decision making. Note that, when π is set equal to 0.5, supporting evidence can be used as long as the point estimate of treatment effect of the local region exhibits the desired direction. Depending on the expectation of the magnitude of regional difference and the willingness to use supporting evidence, π should be set between c1 and 0.5, say 0.15. This relatively small value for π means that supporting evidence will only be used if the result from tier 1 is "marginally" significant. This allows for the use of supporting evidence when warranted, while ensuring that a negative or poor outcome in a local region will not be overcome by results from other regions.

16.4 Examples for Analyzing Medical Device Trials

In this section, we illustrate how to analyze MRCTs data using the two-tier procedure with two hypothetical medical device premarket applications (by regulatory policy, we are not allowed to use real cases here). The first was an example of a cardiovascular interventional trial, and the primary endpoint was infarct size. The trial was a two-arm, randomized controlled study, and it was conducted in two regions: USA and Europe. Randomization was stratified by region. The descriptive result of the trial is shown in Table 16.1.

Suppose that the proposed two-tier procedure served as the decision rule in the USA with the rate of false approval (α) being set at 0.025. Based on the sample size within each region (Table 16.1), the critical value c1 is set at 0.009 $(=(n_i^l/n_\cdot^l)\alpha)$

Table 16.2 Observed clinical success rate for treatment and control across regions

	Treatment		Control	
Region	USA	Europe	USA	Europe
Clinical success rate	54.4 % (35/65)	52.4 % (37/71)	35.7 % (12/34)	26.7 % (10/36)

according to the prespecified rule. The threshold value π is set at 0.15 as suggested above.

A two-sample t-test for the null hypothesis δ_{us} $(=\mu^t_{us}\mu^c_{us}) \geq 0$ resulted in a p value (p1) of 0.0073, which is less than 0.009. Therefore, a tier 1 success is claimed; the direct evidence is strong enough for claiming a study success.

The second was an example of an ablation catheter to treat atrial fibrillation, and the primary endpoint was clinical success at 12 months. The trial was a two-arm, randomized controlled study with a treatment to control ratio of 2:1, and it was conducted in two regions: USA and Europe. Randomization was stratified by region. The descriptive result of the trial is shown in Table 16.2.

Suppose that the proposed two-tier procedure served as the decision rule in the USA with the rate of false approval (α) being set at 0.025. Based on the sample size within each region (Table 16.2), set critical value c1 = 0.012 $(=(n^l_i/n^l_.)\alpha)$ according to the prespecified rule. The threshold value π is set at 0.15.

A two-sample t-test for the null hypothesis δ_{us} $(=p^t_{us}-p^c_{us}) \geq 0$ using the US data only resulted in a p value (p1) of 0.041. As p1 is greater than c1 (0.012) but less than π (0.15), H_{0all}: $\delta_{US} + \delta_{EU} = 0$ is tested using both the US and EU data. The resulting p value (p2) is 0.002, which is less than 0.013 (α-c1). Therefore, a tier 2 success was claimed. That is, the marginally significant direct evidence plus significant supporting evidence would lead to the US approval for the device.

16.5 Design Considerations: Sample Size Planning and Operating Characteristics

With the traditional two-sample test assuming constant treatment effect across regions, the design for an MRCT is relatively straightforward. Instead, using the proposed two-tier procedure as a tool, the design for an MRCT requires careful considerations and extensive simulations. In this section, we first discuss the paradigm of sample size planning. Then, we illustrate the process with a hypothetical example.

Fig. 16.2 is a diagrammatic display of the process for planning the sample size of an MRCT.

Step 1: Define regulatory decision context The regulatory decision context is device specific, mainly considering the intended population and its public health impact in the USA. From our review experience, for some devices, the clinical performance may be highly dependent on surgeon skills, health care system, medical

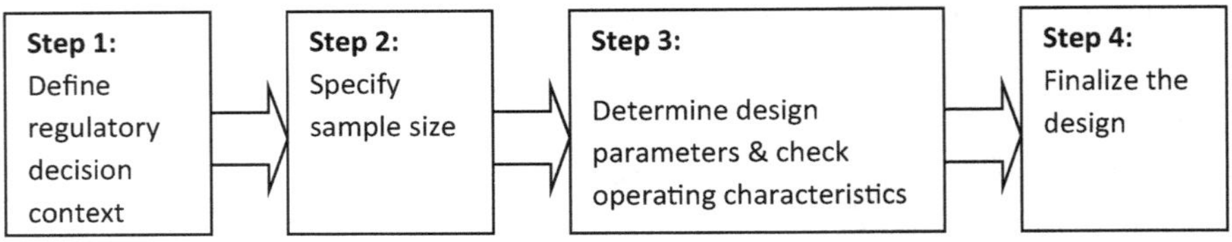

Fig. 16.2 Flow diagram of study design/sample size planning with the two-tier procedure

practice, and available ancillary surgical equipment in the country/region. In such cases, a larger sample size (or higher proportion) has often been called for with a consideration of the size of target population in the USA. Following our proposed paradigm, the direct evidence should be more valuable in the approval decision and thus the design parameter π should be set smaller. Considering that it is possible that the device works in other regions but has minimal effect in the USA, the false approval probability in the USA needs to be carefully considered.

Step 2: Specify sample size Within the defined regulatory decision context, the sample size can be specified with consideration of the sponsor's preference for the possible allocation of resources to the OUS regions.

Step 3: Determine design parameters and check operating characteristics Based on preliminary sample size allocation from step 2, the operating characteristics, such as the approval rates in the USA under different scenarios of true treatment effect in each region, δ_k, are examined via simulation. Meanwhile, the values of c1 and c2 (or c1* and c2*) will be determined per description in Sect. 3.

Step 4: Finalize the design There could be an iterative process between step 3 and step 2. When the statistical properties of the design, especially the false approval rate in the USA, are in alignment with the regulatory decision context and all stakeholders are in agreement, the sample size and all the design parameters are finalized.

In this hypothetical example, suppose that a two-arm, randomized controlled superiority MRCT is planned to be conducted in three regions (USA, region A, and region B) with a randomization ratio of 1:1 within each region. The clinical endpoint response follows a $N(\delta_k, 1)$ in the treatment arm and a $N(0, 1)$ in the control arm. A positive value of δ indicates a desirable outcome. Also, suppose that our proposed procedure is agreed upon between the CDRH and the sponsor.

A conventional way of designing such a trial serves as a good starting point. Assuming that the true treatment effect δ is 0.3 for all regions and that the data will be analyzed by pooling across regions, 174 subjects per arm are needed to have a power of 80 % with one-sided α of 0.025, using a two-sample t-test.

For illustration purpose, suppose that the CDRH calls for at least half (per regulatory decision context as discussed earlier in this section) of the sample size being from the USA. It is decided that the sample size is split roughly evenly in the other two OUS regions. Therefore, the sample size is allocated according to a 2:1:1 ratio, or roughly 87, 44, and 43 subjects per arm in the USA, region A, and region B, respectively.

The two-tier procedure is implemented as the following. In tier 1, the two-sample t-test is performed using the data in the USA only. The analysis of variance (ANOVA) model is used in tier 2. The model includes main effects of region and treatment, along with the treatment $\times$ region interaction term. The p value of the Wald test for main effect term of treatment is obtained by PROC GENMOD of statistical analysis system (SAS), using type 3 sum of squares.

Please note that the operating characteristics are multifaceted due to the fact that the regional treatment effects are allowed to differ by region. For this allocated sample size, the design operating characteristics are examined based on nine different scenarios of δ_i's via simulation for illustration purpose here. (In practice, as many scenarios as desired should be evaluated). In the first five scenarios (A–E), the true treatment effect exists in the USA, while in the remaining scenarios (F–I), the true treatment effect is 0 in the USA. For each scenario, eight cases of values (c1, π, c2) are specified. These parameters are selected such that the false approval rate (in the USA) of scenario F is controlled at 0.025. The parameter π is set to range from 0.1 to 0.5. In cases b through g, the parameters are derived following our recommendation in Sect. 3. The value π is set at 0.1 in both cases a and b. Unlike case b where c1* and c2* are derived to control the false approval probability at 0.025, in case a, the c2 is conservatively set equal to $\alpha - $c1 (Table 16.3).

Several observations can be made by examining the simulation results. First, the approval rate based on t-test is fairly consistent at around 80 % when the overall average of the treatment effect is around 0.3, regardless of whether $\delta_1 = 0$, by comparing cases A, B, D, and E. This means that the t-test tends to inflate the false approval rate in the USA above the nominal alpha. Second, in scenarios G, H, and I, it is indeed shown that the false approval rate in the USA using t-test is higher than that using our proposed method. Third, when the device does work in the USA, the approval rate is generally getting larger with increasing π, except for scenario C. Meanwhile, with increasing π, the false approval rates in scenarios G, H, and I are increasing relatively rapidly than in other scenarios. This suggests that a smaller π may work better in controlling the false approval rate in the USA. Finally, the result in scenario D indicates that the proposed two-tier procedure has a higher approval rate than the t-test when the device is hardly effective in OUS regions.

Another set of simulation was done to investigate the impact of varying c1 (and thus c2) with a fixed value of π ($\pi = 0.15$, 0.2, and 0.3). The results, which are not presented here, indicate that the approval probabilities do not vary much.

Let us further examine some details from the extensive simulation for (c1, π, c2*) = (0.015, 0.15, 0.025). Note that the approval probability in scenario A based on the two-tier procedure is reduced from 80 to 71.6 % comparing to the conventional two-sample t-test, in which the treatment effect is assumed to be constant across regions. Taking into account of the potential differences in treatment effect across regions, the assumption of $\delta_1 = \ldots = \delta_K$ is relaxed in our proposed two-tier procedure. The reduction in the approval probability is mainly due to this relaxation. If it is desired to maintain the probability of approval at 80 % under the assumption of consistent treatment effect δ of 0.3, the sample size needs to be increased. Certainly,

Table 16.3 Simulation results on design operating characteristics based on t-test and two-tier procedure

Sample size (87:44:43)		Approval probability							
		t-test	Parameter set# of two-tier procedure						
Scenario	$(\delta_{US}, \delta_A, \delta_B)$		a	b	c	d	e	f	g
A	(0.3, 0.3, 0.3)	0.801	0.626	0.678	0.716	0.738	0.750	0.748	0.744
B	(0.3, 0.4, 0.2)	0.795	0.617	0.663	0.698	0.716	0.730	0.728	0.724
C	(0.3, 0.0, 0.0)	0.278	0.414	0.477	0.455	0.433	0.427	0.423	0.421
D	(0.6, 0.0, 0.0)	0.785	0.956	0.969	0.964	0.958	0.957	0.957	0.957
E	(0.3, 0.6, 0.0)	0.800	0.555	0.597	0.613	0.618	0.634	0.639	0.640
F	(0.0, 0.0, 0.0)	0.025	0.017	0.025	0.025	0.025	0.025	0.025	0.025
G	(0.0, 0.3, 0.3)	0.284	0.070	0.082	0.116	0.145	0.185	0.219	0.244
H	(0.0, 0.3, 0.6)	0.535	0.093	0.097	0.143	0.187	0.266	0.337	0.408
I	(0.0, 0.0, 0.6)	0.270	0.068	0.080	0.112	0.143	0.186	0.215	0.270

#:
a: $c1 = 0.025/2$, $\pi = 0.1$, $c2 = 0.025/2$
b: $c1^* = 0.018$, $\pi = 0.1$, $c2^* = 0.025$
c: $c1^* = 0.015$, $\pi = 0.15$, $c2^* = 0.025$
d: $c1 = 0.025/2$, $\pi = 0.2$, $c2^* = 0.025$
e: $c1 = 0.025/2$, $\pi = 0.3$, $c2^* = 0.02$
f: $c1 = 0.025/2$, $\pi = 0.4$, $c2^* = 0.017$
g: $c1 = 0.025/2$, $\pi = 0.5$, $c2^* = 0.015$

there are numerous ways to allocate the extra needed subjects, based on the requirement of the regulatory agency and the resources of the sponsor. Suppose that all extra subjects are determined to be assigned to the USA. Through a trial-and-error process of simulations, it can be found that a total of 118 subjects per arm are required in the USA to achieve a probability of approval of 80 %, when the design parameters $(c1^*, \pi, c2^*) = (0.016, 0.15, 0.025)$.

In summary, evaluation of operating characteristics for a design with the two-tier procedure is inherently multifaceted as there are many ways to construct treatment effects varying across regions. A thorough exploring over many scenarios is of paramount importance to help understand the impact of anticipated and unexpected regional differences on the approval rate in the USA and to reach an agreement among stakeholders.

16.6 Discussion

Our proposed framework is devised to fit the situations that are common or relatively unique in the medical device trials. First, regulatory requirements for premarket approval may be different across regions, as discussed in Sect. 2. Consequently, the decision rule or the success criteria of a trial may be different across regions. Second, the number of regions in many medical device MRCTs is relatively small. This may be due to the overall smaller sample size resulting from generally larger effect size of medical devices (as compared to drugs). In some cases, the number of regions is limited due to the accessibility of high-tech equipment and the requirement of innovative or delicate surgical techniques. Third, the consistency of the treatment effect may be suspicious even in the design stage.

While the proposed two-tier procedure provides an explicit decision tree upfront, it requires increased rigor to demonstrate effectiveness in the local region of interest, which can lead to a greater sample size. As the direct and supporting evidence are defined in terms of p values from statistical tests, the proposed procedure is perhaps more meaningful and works better when the sample size in the local region is relatively large. Motivated by our regulatory review experience, in this chapter, we attempt to develop a procedure for use in the USA by closely following the US medical device law and we have noticed that a large proportion of the sample size are from the USA in many submissions to the CDRH. Note that this two-tier procedure does not need to be adopted in every region even within the same MRCT as the medical device laws vary significantly from region to region. Alternatively, the proposed two-tier procedure can also work with relatively small sample size in a local region by setting π close to 1. Considering judiciary independence in medical device approvals across regions, each region could adopt its own statistical analysis plan.

In a regulatory setting, it is necessary to predefine the regions in an MRCT and ideally to have randomization stratified by region to facilitate the all-region analysis. The geographic area under the US FDA jurisdiction would form the main region for effectiveness evaluation; OUS regions could be predefined by various criteria. One is to be formed according to judicial areas. Another is to be formed across judicial boundaries according to similarity in intrinsic and extrinsic factors, such as medical practice and healthcare policy in particular, as discussed by Binkowitz (2010).

An important design feature with the two-tier procedure is the adjustability of acceptable levels of direct versus supporting evidence to meet regulatory expectations. When less regional treatment effect difference is expected, a regulatory decision could be based more on significant supporting evidence through setting the design parameter π closer to 0.5 from below; when substantial regional treatment effect difference is expected, a regulatory decision should be based less on significant supporting evidence through setting the design parameter π closer to alpha from above. In an MRCT with the two-tier procedure, the false approval rate for a region (say region A, $\delta_A = 0$) is evaluated upfront at design stage under many scenarios (δother-region be any plausible values) to understand the impact of plausible regional difference on regulatory decision making and subsequently help all the stakeholders reach an agreement on a study design.

In summary, our proposed two-tier procedure represents a new paradigm in which an explicit decision tree is generated upfront to increase the transparency and predictability for regulatory decision making in contrast to the current paradigm in which there is no explicit decision tree for regulatory decision making when the consistency of regional treatment effects is in doubt. We feel that it is better aligned with the statutory requirements for medical device approval in the USA to have a regulatory decision making from analyses based on a careful evaluation to account for undesirable regional differences in treatment effect at the design stage.

Disclaimer No official support or endorsement by the Food and Drug Administration of this article is intended or should be inferred.

References

Binkowitz B (2010) Highlights from the PhRMA MRCT Key Issue Team & DIA MRCT Workshop. Presented at: the 4th Seattle Symposium in Biostatistics: Clinical Trials. Seattle, WA, 20–23 November

Campbell G (2008) Statistics in the world of medical devices: the contrast with pharmaceuticals. J Biopharm Stat 18:4–19

Chen J, Quan H, Binkowitz B et al (2010) Assessing consistent treatment effect in a multi-regional clinical trial: a systematic review. Pharm Stat 9:242–253

Chen J, Quan H, Gallo P et al (2012) An adaptive strategy for assessing regional consistency in multiregional clinical trials. Clin Trials 9:330–339

CE Mark (2012) http://eur-lex.europa.eu/LexUriServ/site/en/consleg/1993/L/01993L0042-20031120-en.pdf. Accessed 22 Oct 2012

FADASIA (2014) http://www.gpo.gov/fdsys/pkg/BILLS-112s3187enr/pdf/BILLS-112s3187enr.pdf. Accessed 3 Feb 2014

Food, Drug and Cosmetic Act (FD & C Act) (2012) www.fda.gov/RegulatoryInformation/Legislation/FederalFoodDrugandCosmeticActFDCAct/FDCActChapterVDrugsandDevices/ucm110188.htm. Accessed 25 May 2012

Guidance on the Collection of Race and Ethnicity Data in Clinical Trials (2012) http://www.fda.gov/RegulatoryInformation/Guidances/ucm126340.htm. Accessed 22 Oct 2012

Hung HMJ, Wang S-J, O'Neill RT (2010) Consideration of regional difference in design and analysis of multi-regional trials. Pharm Stat 9:173–178

International Conference on Harmonisation of Technical Requirements for Registration of Pharmaceuticals for Human Use. Q & A for the ICH E5 guideline on ethnic factors in the acceptability of foreign data (2012) www.ich.org/fileadmin/Public_Web_Site/ICH_Products/Guidelines/Efficacy/E5_R1/Q_As/E5_Q_As__R5_.pdf. Accessed 25 May 2012

Lu N, Nair R, Xu Y (2011)Decision rules and associated sample size planning for regional approval utilizing multi-regional clinical trials. Presented at: the 4th Annual FDA/MTLI Medical Device and IVD Statistical Issues Workshop, National Harbor, MD, 13-14 April, 2011

Quan H, Chen J, Gallo P et al (2010) Assessment of consistency of treatment effects in multiregional clinical trials. Drug Inf J 44:617–632

Rothwell P (2005) External validity of randomized controlled trials: to whom do the results of this trial apply?. Lancet 365:82–93

Tanaka Y (2010) Statistical considerations in multi-regional clinical trials. Presented at: the Biopharmaceutical Applied Statistics Symposium XVII, Hilton Head, SC, 5–9 November, 2010

Tsou H-H, Chow S-C, Lan KKG et al (2010) Proposals of statistical consideration to evaluation of results for a specific region in multi-regional trials—Asian perspective. Pharm Stat 9:201–206

Chapter 17
Multiplicity Adjustment in Seamless Phase II/III Adaptive Trials Using Biomarkers for Dose Selection

Pei Li, Yanli Zhao, Xiao Sun and Ivan S. F. Chan

Abstract In seamless phase II/III adaptive trials, multiple doses are often evaluated in the phase II part of the study and one or two doses are selected to continue into the phase III part. This setup introduces complicated multiplicity issues on the final efficacy analyses, especially when different endpoints are used in the two phases, such as biomarkers used in phase II for dose selection, and efficacy endpoints used in phase III. In addition, subjects in the dropped arms may not have efficacy follow-up in phase III. Potential type I error inflation on the final efficacy endpoint may arise due to various causes, such as the correlation between the biomarker and the efficacy endpoint. We first investigate the multiplicity issues related to such two-stage designs by assessing the potential factors for type I error inflation in various scenarios. Then, we propose two multiple testing methods (level-α test and first-stage Šidák procedure) that control the family-wise type I error rate for trials observing biomarkers in phase II and efficacy endpoints in phase III. Their performances are evaluated through simulations for different types of biomarker and efficacy endpoints.

17.1 Introduction

In recent years, adaptive designs have received widespread attention due to their potential to bring novel medicines to patients in a more expeditious and cost effective way. New statistical methodologies have been developed to allow for adaptation of some aspects of a trial design while the trial is still ongoing without compromising the integrity and validity of the drug development process.

A seamless phase II/III clinical trial is one type of adaptive designs where objectives traditionally addressed in separate phase II and phase III trials are evaluated in one single trial. It is carried out in two stages: Stage 1 is a phase II part, also called a

I. S. F. Chan (✉) · Y. Zhao · X. Sun
Late Development Statistics, Merck Research Laboratories, Upper Gwynedd, PA 19454, USA,
e-mail: ivan_chan@merck.com

P. Li
CRDM Clinical Research and Reimbursement, Medtronic, Mounds View, MN 55112, USA

Y. Zhao
MedImmune/Astrazeneca, Gaithersburg, MD 20878, USA

Z. Chen et al. (eds.), *Applied Statistics in Biomedicine and Clinical Trials Design*,
ICSA Book Series in Statistics, DOI 10.1007/978-3-319-12694-4_17

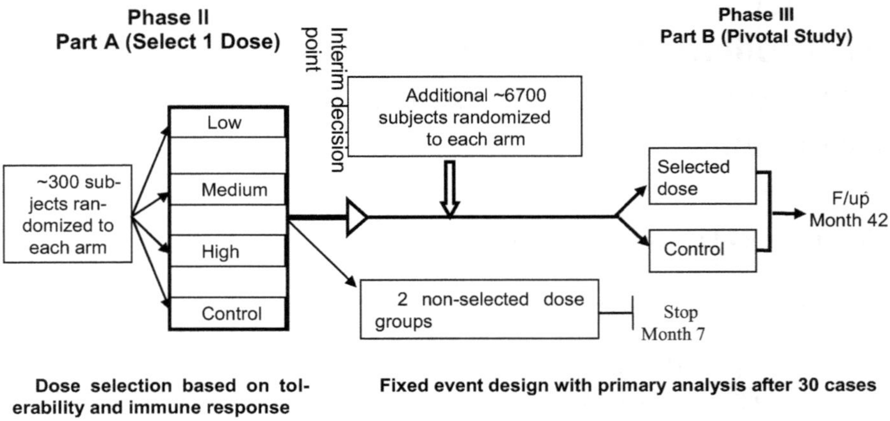

Fig. 17.1 Seamless phase II/III design with dose-selection for the human papilloma virus vaccine trial

learning phase, where multiple doses are often evaluated. An interim analysis is usually performed at the end of stage 1 in order to select a dose to carry forward. Stage 2 is a phase III part, also called a confirming phase, where the efficacy and safety of the selected dose are compared to a control group for the primary hypothesis testing. This type of design eliminates the time delay that would have occurred between the phase II and phase III trials had they been conducted separately, and it also allows for combining data from both phases for formal statistical testing in the final analyses. Therefore, it has potential advantages over separate phase II and phase III trials.

One such example is a recently completed Merck second-generation human papillomavirus (HPV) vaccine trial (Fig. 17.1). In the phase II part of this seamless phase II/III clinical trial, approximately 1200 subjects were randomized in a 1:1:1:1 ratio to one of three vaccine dose groups (low, medium, or high) or the control group. A dose was selected at an interim decision point based on the immunogenicity and tolerability results from phase II (efficacy endpoint remained blinded) and continued into phase III. The two nonselected dose groups were stopped at the end of phase II (month 7). In the phase III part, approximately 13,400 additional subjects were randomized in a 1:1 ratio to the selected dose group or the control group and followed for any occurrence of HPV-related high-grade cervical lesions, which is the primary efficacy endpoint. At the end of the trial, the formal assessment of vaccine efficacy was to test the reduction of the incidence rate of HPV-related high-grade cervical lesions. The subjects enrolled in the phase II part who received the selected dose or in the control arm would be combined with all subjects enrolled in the phase III part for the assessment of vaccine efficacy.

This kind of seamless phase II/III design may introduce complicated multiplicity issues on the final analysis, especially when different study endpoints are used in the two phases. For example, a biomarker (or a surrogate endpoint) may be used in phase II and a clinical disease endpoint may be used in phase III. The use of correlated biomarker and disease endpoints can increase the efficiency of study design and help guide the interpretation of the results from the entire trial. In the HPV vaccine trial example, since the disease endpoint, HPV-related high-grade cervical lesions, takes a long time to develop, it is only feasible to use the immunogenicity endpoint (biomarker for efficacy) for dose selection at the interim timepoint. Although the disease endpoint was never looked at in the interim analysis, a potential type I error inflation for the final efficacy analysis using aggregated phase II and III data might arise due to various reasons such as the correlation between the biomarker and the disease endpoint, the number of dose groups to choose from, the decision rules for dose selection, the relative sample size of phase II to phase III, and the choice of statistical test.

The majority of statistical literature for multiplicity adjustment in seamless phase II/III trials focuses on the trials where the same efficacy endpoint is used for both phase II and phase III and assumes the endpoint is observed for all subjects from all selected and dropped treatment groups in both phase II and III. Posch et al. (2005) described a general two-stage adjustment method which guarantees strong control of type I error and therefore is becoming an important regulatory consideration. The method utilizes two principles: (1) combining p values from different stages and (2) adopting a closed testing procedure to ensure strong control of the overall type I error.

In a two-stage design, the p values from the two stages are combined to yield a single global test for the final hypothesis. Examples of combination tests include: (1) the inverse χ^2 method proposed by Bauer (1989) and Bauer and Kohne (1994) and (2) the weighted inverse normal combination test proposed by Lehmacher and Wassmer (1999). Formula (17.1) shows the weighted inverse normal combination test, where p_1 and p_2 are the p values for the efficacy endpoint and N_1 and N_2 are the sample sizes on the selected dose or control group in phase II and III, respectively:

$$p_{12} = C(p_1, p_2) = 1 - \Phi(b_1 \Phi^{-1}(1 - p_1) + b_2 \Phi^{-1}(1 - p_2))$$
$$b_1 = \sqrt{\frac{N_1}{N_1 + N_2}}, b_2 = \sqrt{\frac{N_2}{N_1 + N_2}} \tag{17.1}$$

where $\Phi()$ is the cumulative distribution function of the standard normal distribution. To ensure strong control of type I error, a closed testing procedure is often utilized on the combined p values. Closed testing procedures require testing of intersection hypotheses of those single hypotheses. Any valid significance test can be used to test intersection hypotheses as long as its size does not exceed α at the hypothesis level.

In some settings such as the aforementioned Merck HPV vaccine trial, the above methodologies cannot be easily applied as different endpoints are used in phase II and phase III. In addition, the efficacy endpoint may not be observed for the phase II subjects in the dropped treatment arms of which follow-up was discontinued before phase III, which will make it difficult to apply the Simes test. The Bonferroni-adjusted p value described in Posch et al. (2005) provided a potential way to adopt. However, it can be ultraconservative for correlated endpoints.

In this chapter, we first evaluate the potential factors for type I error inflation in seamless phase II/III trials using biomarkers for dose selection and then propose two multiple testing methods to control the type I error. In Sect. 17.2, we examine the potential factors that are related to type I error inflation in such designs through simulations. In Sect. 17.3, we propose two testing methods to control the family-wise type I error rate in such setting. Their performances are evaluated by simulations in Sect. 17.4. Some discussions and concluding remarks are offered in Sect. 17.5.

17.2 Simulations to Examine the Potential Factors for Type I Error Inflation in Seamless Phase II/III Design Using Biomarkers for Dose Selection

In order to examine the potential type I error inflation in seamless phase II/III adaptive trials using biomarkers for dose selection, the following simulations were conducted. In the phase II stage, X is the biomarker endpoint measurement in m active treatment groups (each corresponding to a dose level) and one control group. Let Y be the clinical efficacy endpoint. Without loss of generality, we assume equal number of patients, N_1, in each group in phase II. Only one dose level with the maximum biomarker effect compared to control group will be selected to enter phase III. The other nonselected (m-1) treatment arms in phase II will be dropped at the end of phase II, and no efficacy endpoint (Y) will be observed in these dropped arms. In phase III, N_2 additional patients in the selected arm and the control group will be enrolled and followed for the efficacy endpoint (Y). The biomarker (X) and the efficacy endpoint (Y) are assumed to be correlated with the correlation parameter ρ. Let r denote the proportion of phase II sample size out of the total sample size combining phases II and III, i.e., $r = N_1/(N_1 + N_2)$. The studies are simulated under different scenarios regarding distributions of X and Y. Each simulation study is based on 100,000 simulation runs. The nominal type I error α is 0.025. The empirical type I error is defined as the percentage of simulation counts having $Z_y > Z_{1-a}$ out of 100,000 runs.

17.2.1 *Continuous Biomarker and Continuous Efficacy Endpoint*

Let observations of the phase II biomarker endpoint X be normally distributed with the means for the control and m dose arms be $m_{x0}, m_{xi}, i = 1, \ldots, m$, and a common variance across groups ${\sigma_x}^2$. The dose arm with the maximum effect is defined as the dose with the largest Z_x test statistic out of m pairwise Z_x test statistic comparing different doses versus the control. Suppose that a dose arm μ_{x1} is selected to enter phase III. Let observations of the phase III efficacy endpoint Y be normally distributed with the means for the control and the selected dose arm be (μ_{y0}, μ_{y1}), and a common variance ${\sigma_y}^2$: As noted previously, X and Y are correlated with the correlation

Table 17.1 Empirical type I error rate by correlation of normal biomarker and normal clinical endpoint, number of doses, and proportion of phase II in seamless phase II/III study with dose selection[a]

		$\rho=0.95$	$\rho=0.8$	$\rho=0.5$	$\rho=0.2$	$\rho=0.1$	$\rho=0$
Three dose arms + control in phase II	$N_2=0$ $(r=1)$	0.061	0.055	0.044	0.032	0.028	0.025
	$N_2=200$ $(r=1/2)$	0.050	0.046	0.039	0.030	0.028	0.025
	$N_2=1000$ $(r=1/6)$	0.039	0.036	0.033	0.027	0.027	0.025
	$N_2=2000$ $(r=1/11)$	0.035	0.034	0.030	0.027	0.026	0.025
Six dose arms + control in phase II	$N_2=0$ $(r=1)$	0.098	0.085	0.059	0.038	0.030	0.025
	$N_2=200$ $(r=1/2)$	0.074	0.063	0.048	0.032	0.028	0.025
	$N_2=1000$ $(r=1/6)$	0.049	0.046	0.038	0.030	0.027	0.025
	$N_2=2000$ $(r=1/11)$	0.041	0.039	0.034	0.029	0.027	0.025

[a]The simulation setup: $\mu_{x0}=\mu_{x1} = \ldots = \mu_{xm}=2$, $\mu_{y0}=\mu_{y1}=10$, $\sigma_x^2 = \sigma_y^2=1$, $N_1=200$, $\alpha=0.025$, $r=N_1/(N_1+N_2)$

parameter ρ. At the end of the study, the selected dose is claimed to be effective if $Z_y > Z_{1-a}$, where Z_y is the Z-test statistic for comparing the treatment difference between the selected dose and the control based on all the patients with observed Y, i.e., $N_1 + N_2$ patients for each of the selected dose and control groups. For type I error investigation, the simulations are set up such that $\mu_{x0} = \mu_{x1} = \ldots = \mu_{xm}$, *and* $\mu_{y0} = \mu_{y1}$. The simulation results by different correlations of X and Y (i.e., ρ), number of dose candidates, and proportion of phase II (r) are illustrated in Table 17.1 and Fig. 17.2.

At fixed r, the proportion of phase II sample size out of total study size, as correlation ρ increases, type I error inflation increases in a nearly linear fashion. The degree of type I error inflation also depends on the number of dose candidates and the proportion of phase II sample size. The larger the number of dose candidates and the higher proportion of phase II sample size, the larger the inflation. At $\rho=0$, i.e., the biomarker and efficacy endpoints are independent, the type I error is not inflated and remains at one-sided 0.025 level. With high correlation, type I error can inflate greatly if there is a large number of dose candidates and the size of the phase II stage dominates the study. For example, the type I error inflates from 0.025 to 0.098 at $\rho=0.95$ for a study with six doses and no phase III stage (extreme case). Similarly, at fixed correlation ρ, as the proportion of phase II sample size increases, type I error inflation increases. At fixed correlation ρ and proportion of phase II stage r, as the number of dose candidates in phase II increases, type I error inflation increases.

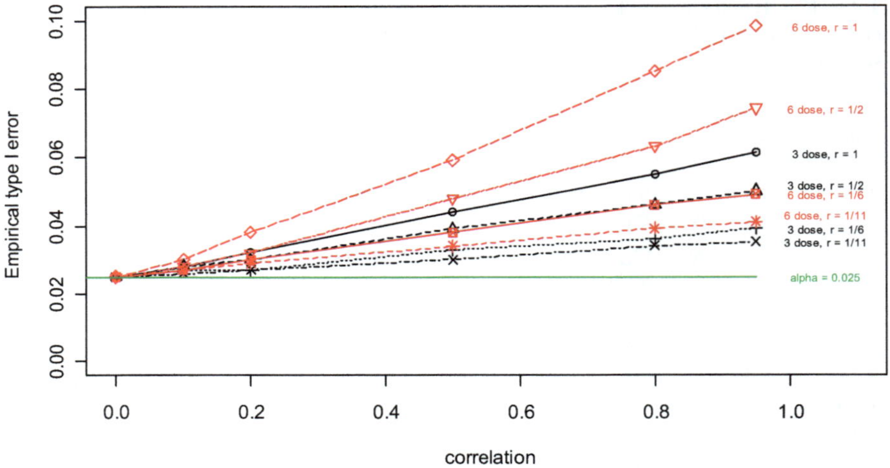

Fig. 17.2 Empirical type I error by correlation, number of doses, and proportion of phase II sample size

17.2.2 Continuous Biomarker and Binary Efficacy Endpoint

We also examined type I errors when the biomarker is continuously distributed and the efficacy endpoint is a binary variable. This occurs in practice when the efficacy endpoint in phase III stage is the incidence of a clinical event of interest, while the biomarker in phase II (such as antibody titer) is a continuous variable. The simulation setting for type I error investigation is that the efficacy outcome (Y) in phase III for both the selected dose and control groups follows binomial (N_2, p), where p is the incidence of clinical event at the end of phase III. The biomarker (X) in phase II is simulated from a normal distribution under the condition that $\mu_{x0} = \mu_{x1} = \ldots = \mu_{xm} = \mu_1 \text{if } Y = 1$ (event); otherwise, $\mu_{x0} = \mu_{x1} = \ldots = \mu_{xm} = \mu_0 \text{if } Y = 0$ (no event). The common variance across groups at phase II is still σ_x^2. Therefore, the correlation ρ between X and Y is a closed form function on $\mu_1, \mu_0, p, \sigma_x^2$ (Appendix A). In our simulation, $\mu_1 = 2, \mu_0 = 0, {\sigma_x}^2 = 1.44$. The dose selection criterion in phase II is the same as for normal/normal scenario described in Sect. 17.2.1. At the end of phase III, the unconditional asymptotic method by Miettinen and Nurminen (1985) was used to test the treatment effect based on the binary endpoint. The selected dose is claimed to be effective if $Z_y > Z_{1-a}$, where Z_y is the asymptotic Z statistic comparing the selected dose and the control based on $N_1 + N_2$ patients for each group. The results based on 100,000 simulation runs are included in Table 17.2.

At fixed r, the type I error inflation generally increases as the correlation ρ increases, except for the small incidence rates (p), which may be due to the insensitiveness of Miettinen and Nurminen method in dealing with small incidence rates. Similarly, at fixed correlation ρ, as the proportion of phase II size r increases, type I error inflation increases.

Table 17.2 Empirical type I error rate by correlation of normal biomarker and binary clinical endpoint and proportion of phase II in seamless phase II/III study with dose selection[a]

		$p=0.01$ ($\rho=0.16$)	$p=0.1$ ($\rho=0.45$)	$p=0.2$ ($\rho=0.55$)	$p=0.5$ ($\rho=0.64$)	$p=0.9$ ($\rho=0.45$)
Three dose arms + control in phase II	$N_2=0$ ($r=1$)	0.051	0.048	0.049	0.049	0.043
	$N_2=200$ ($r=1/2$)	0.031	0.039	0.039	0.042	0.036
	$N_2=1000$ ($r=1/6$)	0.028	0.028	0.033	0.034	0.033
	$N_2=2000$ ($r=1/11$)	0.031	0.028	0.030	0.031	0.029

[a] The simulation setup: $\mu_{x0}=\mu_{x1}=\ldots=\mu_{xm}=2$ (*if* $Y=1$), $\mu_{x0}=\mu_{x1}=\ldots=\mu_{xm}=0$ (*if* $Y=0$), $\sigma_x^2=1.44$, $N_1=200$, $\alpha=0.025$, $r=N_1/(N_1+N_2)$

17.2.3 Continuous Biomarker and Binary Efficacy Endpoint at Rare Incidence Using Exact Test

Since the incidence rate for the disease endpoint—HPV-related high-grade cervical lesions in the motivating vaccine trial is expected to be very low (e.g., $p=0.004$), for the continuous/binary scenario, we also examined the type I error rates in the situation where the disease endpoint at phase III is rare. The simulation setup is the same as in Sect. 17.2.2, except that ${\sigma_x}^2$ is not fixed, but rather changes from setting to setting to keep p and ρ fixed. The proportions of phase II sample size are also set to be small ($N_1=300$, $N_2=3000$, 6000, or 9000) to mimic the real-world situation. At the end of phase III, the exact method proposed by Chan and Bohidar (1998) was used to test for vaccine efficacy based on the rare binary endpoint, as in the HPV vaccine study. The empirical type I error is defined as the percentage of simulation counts having the exact p value $\leq \alpha$ out of 100,000 simulations. The results are summarized in Table 17.3.

Overall, the results show that the type I error rate was not inflated under the scenarios studied. At a fixed incidence p, the type I error increases as the correlation ρ increases, but in a small scale, the absolute type I errors are all less than or equal to 0.025 even at a high correlation ρ of 0.8. There is no obvious relationship between incidence and type I error change at a fixed correlation. The control of type I error may be a result of a combination effect of low incidence, very small proportion of phase II sample size, and the conservatism of the exact testing method.

Table 17.3 Empirical type I error rate by correlation of normal biomarker and binary clinical endpoint at rare incidence in seamless phase II/III study with dose selection using exact test[a]

			$p=0.2$	$p=0.1$	$p=0.01$	$p=0.004$
Three dose arms + control in phase II	$N_2=3000$ ($r=1/11$)	$\rho=0.8$	0.018	0.024	0.025	0.021
		$\rho=0.5$	0.017	0.022	0.022	0.018
		$\rho=0.1$	0.013	0.018	0.019	0.015
Three dose arms + control in phase II	$N_2=6000$ ($r=1/21$)	$\rho=0.8$	0.016	0.023	0.025	0.022
		$\rho=0.5$	0.016	0.022	0.023	0.021
		$\rho=0.1$	0.014	0.019	0.021	0.019
Three dose arms + control in phase II	$N2=9000$ ($r=1/31$)	$\rho=0.8$	0.016	0.023	0.025	0.023
		$\rho=0.5$	0.016	0.021	0.023	0.021
		$\rho=0.1$	0.014	0.019	0.021	0.018

[a] The simulation setup: $\mu_{x0} = \mu_{x1} = \ldots = \mu_{xm} = 2$ (if $Y=1$), $\mu_{x0} = \mu_{x1} = \ldots = \mu_{xm} = 0$ (if $Y=0$), $N_1=300$, $\alpha=0.025$, $r=N_1/(N_1+N_2)$

17.3 Two Proposed Testing Methods for Multiplicity Adjustment

We propose the following two adjustment methods to control the overall type I error in seamless phase II/III trials using biomarkers for dose selection.

17.3.1 Level-α Test

As shown in Sect. 17.2, using $Z_{1-\alpha} = 1.96$ for testing the final hypothesis at one-sided α of 0.025 will inflate the type I error. The critical cutoff value c for the rejection region needs to be adjusted upward. Proschan and Hunsberger (1995) and Li et al. (2002) gave a closed form expression for the worst-case type I error rate for indiscriminately extending a study when the sample size is reestimated during the midcourse of a clinical trial. The critical cutoff value c is properly adjusted to protect the type I error rate.

We apply an analogous strategy in the seamless phase II/III adaptive design where the sample size is predetermined, and the selected dose level to phase III is based on the maximum observed treatment effect of the biomarker in phase II.

The type I error α was derived as follows (details in Appendix B):

$$\begin{aligned}\alpha &= \Pr(Z_s > c) = E_w(\Pr(Z_s > c)|W)\\ &= \int \Phi\left(\frac{-c+\sqrt{r}\rho w}{\sqrt{r(1-\rho^2)+(1-r)}}\right) f(w)dw,\end{aligned}$$

where w is the maximum of m standard normal statistics, m is the number of treatment arms in phase II, ρ is the known correlation between the two continuous endpoints, $r = N_1/(N_1 + N_2)$, N_1 and N_2 are sample sizes (per group) in phase II and III, respectively, and c is the critical cutoff value. Note α is a monotone function for both parameters ρ and r at fixed c, as is shown in Fig. 17.3. Table 17.4 gives the critical cutoff value c that is obtained via Monte Carlo integration approximation and numerical search to attain the test level at α of 0.025 for known values of ρ and r.

17.3.2 First-Stage Šidák Method

Šidák test is another common adjustment method where the adjusted p value is defined as

$$p_{\text{sidak}} = 1\text{-}(1\text{-}\min(p_{\text{i}}))^{\text{m}}, i = 1, \ldots, m,$$

where m is the number of hypotheses. Šidák (1967) demonstrated that the size of this test does not exceed α when the individual test statistics are either independent or are absolute statistics of multivariate normal distribution. Holland and Copenhaver (1987) described that as long as the test statistics exhibit positive orthant dependence, the Šidák test controls the family-wise error rate.

We incorporate this procedure into seamless phase II/III design with dose selection in the following steps:

Step 1: Compute the p value $p_{1,\text{s}}$ testing the difference between the selected treatment group and the control group regarding the efficacy endpoint for the $2*N_1$ population enrolled in phase II.

Step 2: Conduct the multiplicity adjustment by the Šidák test and compute the first-stage (phase II)-adjusted p value as follows:

$$p_1 = 1\text{-}(1\text{-}p_{1,\text{s}})^{\text{m}},$$

where $p_{1,\text{s}}$ is the long-term efficacy p value between the selected treatment arm and the control among the subjects enrolled in phase II, and m is the number of treatment groups at phase II.

Step 3: Combine the p values from both stages using formula (17.1) in Sect. 17.1 and compare the global p value with the prespecified error level α.

This procedure is a bit more conservative than the general Šidák-adjusted p value, since the p values for the long-term efficacy endpoint in the dropped treatment arms may not be available and p_1 may not be the minimum among all groups. Therefore, the first-stage Šidák method can control the family-wise error rate in seamless phase II/III designs, as long as the test statistics are independent or exhibit positive orthant dependence. Note that the proposed first-stage Šidák method does not require assumptions on endpoint distributions and their correlation. As a result, it can be applied in general situations with different types of endpoints.

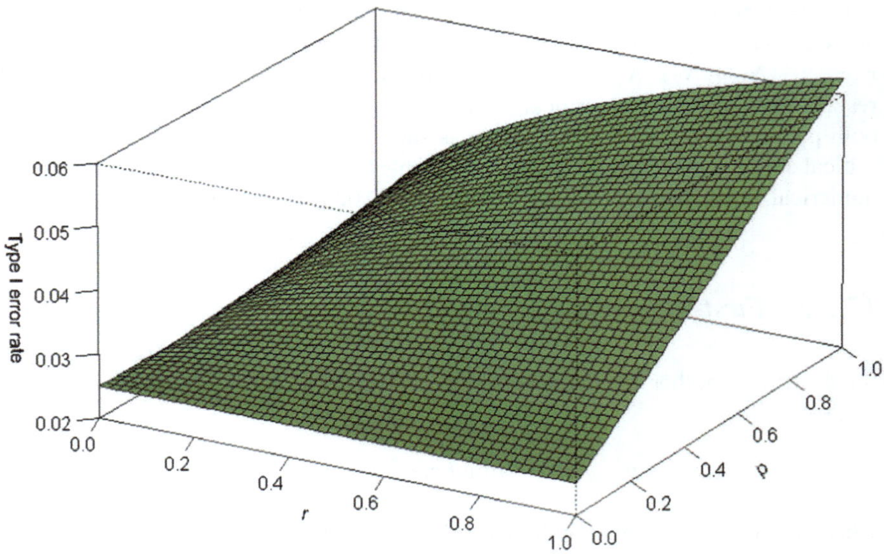

Fig. 17.3 Type I error rate α as a function with respect to r and ρ for the level-α test

Table 17.4 Critical cutoff value c associated with ρ and r to attain the level- α test at $\alpha = 0.025$ based on the maximum effective selection criterion

	$\rho = 0.95$	$\rho = 0.8$	$\rho = 0.5$	$\rho = 0.2$	$\rho = 0.1$	$\rho = 0$
$r = 1$	2.338	2.304	2.205	2.071	2.018	1.96
$r = 1/2$	2.267	2.232	2.144	2.040	2.001	1.96
$r = 1/6$	2.160	2.132	2.073	2.007	1.985	1.96
$r = 1/11$	2.113	2.092	2.046	1.995	1.977	1.96

As an alternative to the two proposed adjustment method, one might consider the simple Bonferroni adjustment on the pooled efficacy data in the end. The adjusted final p value will be calculated as the raw p value for the selected dose and control on the pooled efficacy data across phase II and III multiplied by the number of treatment arms for dose selection in phase II. Although the Bonferroni procedure protects the overall false positive rate, it may become too conservative when the number of treatment arms or the correlation between biomarker and efficacy endpoint increases.

17.4 Performance of Proposed Methods by Simulations

Simulations were conducted to evaluate the performance of our proposed methods relative to the naive approach without adjustment and the simple Bonferroni adjustment method. The simulation is set up where both the biomarker and the efficacy

Table 17.5 Type I error rate associated with naïve method and the proposed adjustment methods under scenario 1 X, Y are both continuous, $N_1 = 200$, $\alpha = 0.025$

	$\rho = 0.95$			$\rho = 0.5$			$\rho = 0.1$		
N_2	Naïve	Level-α	First-stage Šidák	Naïve	Level α	First-stage Šidák	Naïve	Level-α	First-stage Šidák
200	0.0502	0.0253	0.0204	0.0385	0.0256	0.0150	0.0280	0.0249	0.0101
1000	0.0387	0.0244	0.021	0.0325	0.0244	0.0148	0.0269	0.0244	0.0118
2000	0.0353	0.0251	0.0204	0.0301	0.0241	0.0162	0.0256	0.0254	0.0132

Table 17.6 Power associated with the proposed adjustment methods and the simple Bonferroni adjustment under scenario 1 X, Y are both continuous, $N_1 = 200$, $\alpha = 0.025$

	$\rho = 0.95$			$\rho = 0.5$			$\rho = 0.1$		
N_2	Bonferroni	Level-α	First-stage Šidák	Bonferroni	Level-α	First-stage Šidák	Bonferroni	Level-α	First-stage Šidák
1000	0.6091	0.7008	0.6654	0.5715	0.6887	0.6242	0.5343	0.6865	0.5777
2000	0.8623	0.9157	0.9028	0.846	0.9125	0.8834	0.8256	0.9144	0.8669
3000	0.9599	0.9806	0.9793	0.9532	0.9789	0.9718	0.9485	0.9802	0.9650

endpoints are continuous, $\mu_{x0} = \mu_{x1} = \ldots = \mu_{xm} = 2, \mu_{y0} = \mu_{y1} = 10, {\sigma_x}^2 = {\sigma_y}^2 = 1, N_1 = 200, \alpha = 0.025, r = N_1/(N_1 + N_2)$, same as in Sect. 17.2.1. The naive approach refers to the approach ignoring the multiplicity issue and using the usual $Z_{1-\alpha}$ critical cutoff for the final hypothesis. The unnegligible and undesirable type I error inflation by the naive approach has been demonstrated in Sect. 17.2.1. Table 17.5 shows the level-α test controls the type I error rate exactly at α up to some simulation errors, as expected. The first-stage Šidák approach can also effectively protect the type I rate at level α, especially when the naive approach leads to a significant type I error inflation when the between endpoints correlation is high. Table 17.6 shows both of the level-α test and the first-stage Šidák method that improved the statistical power over the simple Bonferroni adjustment. Due to the strict conservativeness of the Šidák test for treatment comparisons, the first-stage Šidák has slightly less statistical power than the level-α test. However, the level-α test requires the knowledge of the between endpoints correlation and the assumption of normal and constant variance assumption across groups. In contrast, the first-stage Šidák is statistically valid as long as the test statistics meet the broad set of assumptions needed by Šidák multiple test approach (Holland and Copenhaver 1987).

17.5 Discussion

Our research addressed some aspects of the complicated multiplicity issues arising in the seamless phase II/III trials using biomarkers for dose selection. The source of type I error inflation on the final efficacy endpoint analyses comes from various sources, such as the correlation between the biomarker and the efficacy endpoint, the number of dose groups, the decision rules for dose selection, the relative sample size of the subjects in phase II relative to phase III, and the statistical analysis methodology.

For the setting of continuous biomarker and binary efficacy endpoint for rare incidences where the exact test (Chan and Bohidar 1998) was used, the absolute type I errors tend to be small. Results from Table 17.3 show that for a four-arm dose-selection phase II/III trial, the type I errors were controlled at the 0.025 level even at a high correlation (ρ) of 0.8 across a range of disease incidence rates (0.004–0.2). This may be attributed to the low disease incidence rate, relatively small proportion of patients in phase II versus phase III, and importantly the already conservatism of the exact testing method. Such settings are common in vaccine trials of rare diseases, as in the motivating HPV vaccine trial, for which the simulations demonstrate that the overall type I error is not inflated in the final pooled analysis.

For other settings where potential type I error inflation may occur, two methods are proposed for adjustment. Among the two proposed methods, the level-α test is more powerful, but it is computationally complex and requires stronger assumptions on the endpoint distributions and known correlation between the biomarker and efficacy endpoints. In practice, the correlation is usually unknown. One could consider using a conservative upper bound estimate of the correlation from relevant historical data; however, it may not guarantee the strict control of type I error rate. In contrast, the first-stage Šidák method does not require assumptions on endpoint distributions and their correlation, and hence it can be used in general situations. Both of these two methods control the type I error rate and are more powerful than the simple Bonferroni method in seamless phase II/III trial designs with short-term continuous biomarkers for dose selection in phase II and long-term continuous efficacy endpoints in phase III.

The proposed multiplicity adjustment methods and simulations studies apply to settings where the dose selection at phase II is based on the maximum dose response of a biomarker and the efficacy endpoint is not available in subjects in the dropped treatment arms. In reality, other criteria such as safety may also be used in the dose selection, and the treatment arm with the maximum biomarker effect may not be selected. In this case, the overall type I error should be smaller and the proposed methods would still be valid.

We also examined the setting where the continuous biomarker is used in phase II for dose selection and the time to event survival endpoint is collected in phase III. The overall p value combines the adjusted p value on the survival endpoint in phase II between the selected treatment group and the control group using the Šidák test and the p value on the survival endpoint in phase III subjects. If survival endpoints in all subjects including those in the dropped arms are observed during phase III, the

Dunnett test (1955) can be used in place of the Šidák test to calculate the adjusted p value in the first stage. We conducted a simulation study (result not shown to save space) where all treatments including the dropped treatment groups had complete phase III endpoint measurements, and compared the performance of the Dunnett test and the first-stage Šidák method. The simulation results suggested that both methods adequately controls the overall type I error, and that Dunnett test is slightly more powerful than the first-stage Šidák method, but the difference is very small.

In trials such as the motivating vaccine study where the dropped treatment groups do not have phase III endpoint measurements, Dunnett's test cannot be easily implemented. This is because the critical values of the Dunnett test are computed from a multivariate normal or t distribution where the marginal statistics on the phase III endpoint for all pairs of active treatments versus control are needed for estimation of the covariance matrix. Friede et al. (2011) proposed that the test statistics corresponding to comparisons with treatment groups for which no data are available be set to $-\infty$ and then apply the Dunnett method and the closure principle to obtain the combination test. Their testing strategy controls the family-wise type I error rate in the strong sense but is often conservative with the level of conservatism depending on the correlation between the endpoints, effect size on the phase II endpoint, and the selection rule at phase II. Our simulation results suggested this adaptive Dunnett test is slightly less powerful than the classical Dunnett test assuming all treatment groups have efficacy data in phase III, but the power loss is minimal in our simulation settings. In general, the power of the adaptive Dunnett test is similar to that of the first-stage Šidák method.

Jenkins et al. (2011) proposed an adaptive seamless phase II/III design with subpopulation selection using correlated survival endpoints in an oncology setting. Their methodology allows the trial to continue in all patients but with both the subgroup and the full population as co-primary populations. While their adaptation is on subpopulation selection with different flexible decision rules rather than dose selection as in our research, both approaches control the type I error rate raised from adaptive selections by incorporating the correlation between early and final outcomes in the adjustment.

Posch et al. (2011) described two approaches to control the type I error rate in adaptive designs with sample size reassessment and/or treatment selection: (1) a simulation-based approach adjusts the critical value by Monte Carlo simulation and the type I error rate is controlled only when the underlying assumptions are not violated and (2) an adaptive Bonferroni–Holm test procedure (1979) based on conditional error rates of the individual treatment–control comparisons which controls the type I error rate even if under the deviation from a preplanned adaptation rule or the time point of such a decision.

Not all clinical development programs may be candidates for seamless phase II/III adaptive designs for dose selection. The decision as to whether such design is appropriate requires input from multiple functional areas, such as statistics, clinical research, regulatory, marketing, data management, drug supply, and clinical operations. The required technical details need to be carefully evaluated, including simulation studies to verify operating characteristics, specifically to demonstrate that the type I error is preserved at the intended level. In addition, it is important to make every effort to maintain blinding and minimize the chance of potential bias introduced by information leakage. Finally, it is equally important that the study team communicates with health authorities as clearly and as early as possible to ensure that regulatory agencies are in support of such adaptations in a phase III registration trial.

17.6 Appendix A

Correlation ρ between continuous biomarker X and binary efficacy endpoint Y

$$
\begin{aligned}
& Y \sim Bernouli(p) \\
& X|\,Y \sim \left\{ \begin{array}{ll} N(u_1, \sigma^2) & y = 1 \\ N(u_2, \sigma^2) & y = 0 \end{array} \right\} \\
& E(Y) = p; Var(Y) = p(1-p) \\
& E(X) = pu_1 + (1-p)u_2 \\
& Var(X) = E(\operatorname{var}(X)\,|Y) + (\operatorname{var}(E(X)\,|Y\,) \\
& \qquad\quad = \sigma^2 + {u_1}^2 p + {u_2}^2(1-p) - (pu_1 + (1-p)u_2)^2 \\
& \rho = Cor(X, Y) = \frac{Cov(X, Y)}{\sqrt{\operatorname{var}(X)\operatorname{var}(Y)}} = \frac{E(XY) - EXEY}{\sqrt{\operatorname{var}(X)\operatorname{var}(Y)}} \\
& \qquad = \frac{pu_1 - (pu_1 + (1-p)u_2)p}{\sqrt{p(1-p)}\sqrt{\sigma^2 + {u_1}^2 p + {u_2}^2(1-p) - (pu_1 + (1-p)u_2)^2}}
\end{aligned}
$$

17.7 Appendix B

Type I error derivation of the level-α test

$$
\begin{aligned}
& W = \max(w_1, w_2, w_3),\ W \sim f(w) \\
& F(W < w) = \Pr(w_1 < w, w_2 < w, w_3 < w) \\
& \qquad = \iiint_{-\infty < w_1, w_2, w_3 < w} g(w_1, w_2, w_3)\, dw_1 dw_2 dw_3 \\
& g(w_1, w_2, w_3) = MVN\left(\begin{pmatrix} 0 \\ 0 \\ 0 \end{pmatrix}, \begin{pmatrix} 1 & 0.5 & 1 \\ 0.5 & 1 & 0.5 \\ 0.5 & 0.5 & 1 \end{pmatrix} \right)
\end{aligned}
$$

$$T = \sqrt{\frac{N_1}{N_1 + N_2}} Z_{1i} + \sqrt{\frac{N_2}{N_1 + N_2}} Z_{2i}$$

$$Z_{1i} \middle| W \sim N(\rho W, 1 - \rho^2), Z_{2i} \sim N(0,1) \Rightarrow T \,|W \sim N \left(\sqrt{\frac{N_1}{N_1 + N_2}} \rho W, \frac{N_1(1 - \rho^2) + N_2}{N_1 + N_2} \right)$$

$$\Pr(T > c) = E_w(\Pr(T > c) \,|W)$$

$$= E_w \left(\Pr \left(\frac{T - \sqrt{\frac{N_1}{N_1 - N_2}} \rho W}{\sqrt{\frac{N_1(1-\rho^2)+N_2}{N_1+N_2}}} > \frac{c - \sqrt{\frac{N_1}{N_1+N_2}} \rho W}{\sqrt{\frac{N_1(1-\rho^2)+N_2}{N_1+N_2}}} \right) |W \right)$$

$$= E_w \left(\Phi \left(\frac{-c + \sqrt{\frac{N_1}{N_1+N_2}} \rho W}{\sqrt{\frac{N_1(1-\rho^2)+N_2}{N_1-N_2}}} \right) \middle| W \right) = \int \Phi \left(\frac{-c + \sqrt{r} \rho W}{\sqrt{r(1 - \rho^2) + (1 - r)}} \right) f(w)dw$$

References

Bauer P (1989) Multistage testing with adaptive designs (with discussion). Biometrie und Informatik in Medizin und Biologie 20:130–148

Bauer P, Kohne K (1994) Evaluation of experiments with adaptive interim analyses. Biometrics 50:1029–1041

Chan ISF, Bohidar NR (1998) Exact power and sample size for vaccine efficacy studies. Commun Stat Theory Methods 27:1305–1322

Dunnett CW (1955) A multiple comparison procedure for comparing several treatments with a control. J Am Stat Assoc 50:1096–1121

Friede T, Parsons N, Stallard N, Todd S, Marquez EV, Chataway J, Nicholas R (2011) Designing a seamless phase II/III clinical trial using early outcomes for treatment selection: an application in multiple sclerosis. Stat Med 30:1528–1540

Holland B, Copenhaver MD (1987) An improved sequentially rejective Bonferroni test procedure. Biometrics 43:417–423

Holm S (1979) A simple sequentially rejective multiple test procedure. Scand J Stat 6 65–70

Jenkins M, Stone A, Jennison C (2011) An adaptive seamless phase II/III design for oncology trials with subpopulation selection using correlated survival endpoint. Pharm Stat 10:347–356

Lehmacher W, Wassmer G (1999) Adaptive sample size calculations in group sequential trials. Biometrics 55:1286–1290

Li G, Shih WJ, Xie T, Lu J (2002) A sample size adjustment procedure for clinical trials based on conditional power. Biostatistics 3(2):277–287

Miettinen O, Nurminen M (1985) Comparative analysis of two rates. Stat Med 4:213–26

Posch M, Koenig F, Branson M, Brannah W, Dunger-Baldauf Bauer P (2005) Testing and estimation in flexible group sequential designs with adaptive treatment selection. Stat Med 24:3697–3714

Posch M, Maurer W, Bretz F (2011) Type I error rate control in adaptive designs for confirmatory clinical trials with treatment selection at interim. Pharm Stat 10:96–104

Proschan MA, Hunsberger SA (1995) Designed extension of studies based on conditional power. Biometrics 51:1315–1324

Šidàk Z (1967) Rectangular confidence region for the means of multivariate normal distributions. J Am Stat Assoc 62:626–633

Part IV
Modelling and Data Analysis

Chapter 18
Empirical Likelihood for the AFT Model Using Kendall's Rank Estimating Equation

Yinghua Lu and Yichuan Zhao

Abstract The accelerated failure time (AFT) model, also called censored linear regression has played a central role in survival analysis. Motivated by (Zhao, Stat Probab Lett 81:603bab, 2011), we make an empirical likelihood (EL) inference for the model using the monotone censored Kendall's rank-estimating equation. The limiting distribution of the EL ratio follows the Wilks theorem. In addition, we carry out extensive simulation studies to compare the EL for the Kendall's rank-regression estimator with Wald-type and EL interval estimators. The simulation shows the benefit of the proposed method for small sample sizes in most cases.

18.1 Introduction

In survival analysis, there are two very popular approaches for modeling of covariate effects on survival time. One of them is the accelerated failure time (AFT) model, which is also called censored linear regression. This model utilizes the natural logarithm of survival time $Y = ln(T)$ to convert positive survival time to observations on entire real line. Fygenson and Ritov (1994) proposed censored monotone Fygenson–Ritov (i.e., Gehan-type) estimating equations for right censored data, which produce a unique set of estimators for the regression parameters.

Owen (1988, 1990) proposed empirical likelihood (EL), which is one kind of nonparametric statistical inference method. Recently, Zhou (2005) proposed the censored EL based on Log-rank and Gehan estimators. Zhou and Li (2008) demonstrated that the censored EL based on Buckley–James estimator for the AFT model is better than the adjusted empirical likelihood (AEL) and empirical likelihood based on synthetic data (ELSD) in terms of coverage probability, where AEL is Li and Wang (2003)'s adjusted EL method and ELSD refers to the EL method of Li and Wang (2003) based on synthetic data.

Y. Zhao (✉)
Department of Mathematics and Statistics, Georgia State University, Atlanta, GA 30303, USA
e-mail: yichuan@gsu.edu

Y. Lu
Risk Lighthouse LLC, 950 East Paces Ferry Road NE, Atlanta, GA 30326, USA

Z. Chen et al. (eds.), *Applied Statistics in Biomedicine and Clinical Trials Design*,
ICSA Book Series in Statistics, DOI 10.1007/978-3-319-12694-4_18

As Jing et al. (2008) did, Zhao (2011) applied the EL to the AFT model based on Fygenson–Ritov estimating equation. Although the performance of Zhao's method is better than Wald-type methods in terms of coverage probability, it still encounters under-coverage problem. We note that the Fygenson–Ritov estimating equation and the Kendall's rank-estimating equation are very similar. But the Kendall's rank-regression estimator has excellent properties compared to the Fygenson–Ritov regression estimator. For example, "it is very robust against covariate outliers in contrast to other estimates" (see Heller 2007). In this chapter, we propose the EL method with a monotone Kendall's rank-estimating equation. The new EL method can produce better or comparable interval estimate to existing methods for the AFT model in terms of coverage probability most of the time.

The rest of the chapter is organized as follows. In Sect. 18.2, the empirical likelihood ratio statistic is constructed, and the EL confidence interval for the regression parameter is constructed. In Sect. 18.3, we conduct a simulation study to compare the EL-based method and other existing methods. The conclusion is given in Sect. 18.4.

18.2 Main Procedure

In this section, we first review the normal approximation (NA) method, which is very similar to Fygenson and Ritov (1994) and Zhao (2011). We adopt the same notations as in Zhao (2011) for convenience. Let $T_1, \ldots T_n$ be positive i.i.d. random variable. Suppose that $Z_{1,} \ldots, Z_n$ are their corresponding $(p \times 1)$ covariates vectors, the AFT model is defined as follows:

$$logT_i = \beta' Z_i + \epsilon_i,\ i = 1, \ldots, n \tag{18.1}$$

Where $\beta\ is\ a\ (p \times 1) I(\cdot)$ regression parameter and ϵ_i are errors. Consider the censoring times C_i, and denote $X_i = \min\,(T_i, C_i\,), \Delta_i = I(T_i \le C_i\,)$, where $I(\cdot)$ is an indicator function.

Denote $e_i(\beta) = \log X_i - \beta' Z_i,\ 1 \le i \le n.$ The censored Kendall's rank-estimating equation can be written as a U-Statistic,

$$S\,(\beta) = n^{-3/2} \sum_{i=2}^{n} \sum_{j=1}^{i-1} sgn(Z_i - Z_j)[\Delta_i I\left\{e_j(\beta) > e_i(\beta)\right\} - \Delta_j I\{e_i(\beta) > e_j\,(\beta)\}], \tag{18.2}$$

where $sgn(\times)$ is a sign function, which is equal to1 when the argument is positive, -1 when the argument is negative, and 0 when the argument is zero. Replacing $Z_i - Z_j$ in the Fygenson–Ritov estimating equation in Zhao (2011) with $sgn(Z_i - Z_j)$we obtain Kendall's rank estimating equation. Let $\hat{\beta}$ be the solution of the equation $S(\beta) = 0$, and β_0 be true parameter of β. Like Zhao (2011), we can prove $E[S(\beta_O)] = 0$. Similar to Fygenson and Ritov (1994), $n^{\frac{1}{2}}(\hat{\beta} - \beta_0)$ satisfies the asymptotic normality. As Zhao (2011), we can obtain a Wald-type confidence interval for β_0. We adopt the same notations as in Zhao to denote $U_i = (Z_i, X_i, \Delta_i)$ and $k(U_i, U_j; \beta) = sgn\,(Z_i - Z_j)\left\{\Delta_i I(e_j(\beta) > e_i(\beta)) - \Delta_j I(e_i(\beta) > e_j(\beta))\right\}$. Like Zhao (2011), one can define

$M_i(\beta) = \frac{1}{n-1} \sum_{j=1, j \neq i}^{n} \{k(U_i, U_j; \beta)\}$ for $i = 1, \ldots, n$. The EL ratio $R(\beta)$ at the value β is defined. We get the following standard formula like Owen (1988, 1990, 2001).

$$\hat{l}(\beta) = -2log\ R(\beta) = -2\sum_{i=1}^{n} log \left\{\frac{1}{1 + \lambda^T M_i(\beta)}\right\},$$

where λ satisfies the following nonlinear equation

$$\sum_{i=1}^{n} \frac{M_i(\beta)}{1 + \lambda^T M_i(\beta)} = 0.$$

Replacing $Z_i - Z_j$ with $sgn\ (Z_i - Z_j)$ in each term $W_i(\beta_0)$ of Zhao (2011), we obtain $M_i(\beta_0)$. Thus, along the same lines of proof in Theorem 1 of Zhao (2011), we have the following result since $S(\beta_0)$ is a U statistic with a kernel of 2 degrees.

Proposition 1 Under the regularity conditions as in p.735 of Fygenson and Ritov (1994) and Zhao (2011), $\hat{l}(\beta_0)$ converges to $4\chi_p^2$, where χ_p^2 is a chi-square distribution with p degrees of freedom.

An asymptotic $100(1-\alpha)\%$ confidence region for β is as follows

$$R_E = \left\{\beta : \hat{l}\,(\beta_0) \leq 4\chi_p^2\,(\alpha)\right\}, \tag{18.3}$$

where $\chi_p^2(\alpha)$ is the upper α-quantile of χ_p^2.

We are interested in constructing confidence region for the q-dimensional vector $\beta^{(1)}\ of\ \beta = (\beta^{(1)'}, \beta^{(2)'})'$. Define $\beta_0 = (\beta^{(1)'}, \beta^{(2)'})'$. As Zhao (2011), one can define the profile EL ratio $\hat{l}_{profile}(\beta^{(1)})$at $\beta^{(1)}$. The corresponding proposition is valid along the same lines of Zhao (2011).

Proposition 2 Under the regularity conditions as in p. 735 of Fygenson and Ritov (1994) and Zhao (2011), $\hat{l}_{profile}(\beta_0^{(1)})$ converges to $4\chi_q^2$. Thus, we obtain an asymptotic $100(1-\alpha)\%$ confidence region for $\beta^{(1)}$:

$$R_p = \left\{\beta^{(1)} : \hat{l}_{profile}(\beta^{(1)} \leq 4\chi_q^2(\alpha)\right\}, \tag{18.4}$$

where $\chi_q^2(\alpha)$ is the upper α-quintile of χ_q^2.

18.2.1 Simulation Study

In this section, we will do two comparisons. The first one is to compare the EL confidence interval with the normal approximation confidence interval, based on the

Kendall's rank-estimating equation. The second one is to compare the EL based on Kendall's rank-estimating equation with the EL based on Buckley–James, Log-rank, and Gehan estimating equations proposed by Zhou (2005) and Zhou and Li (2008).

18.2.2 EL CI Versus Wald-Type CI Based on Kendall's Rank-Estimating Equation

In this subsection, we compare performance of the empirical likelihood procedure and the Wald-type based (i.e., normal approximation) approach by using Monte Carlo simulation study in terms of coverage accuracy and average length of confidence intervals. For the model, $logT_i = \beta Z_i + \epsilon_i$, we consider two different models which have skewed error distribution and symmetric error distribution respectively. Both of them assume that there is only one covariate Z and that the true parameter $\beta_0 = 2$. They are the same models as those in Zhao (2011). We discuss the two models in settings with four different censoring rates (CR), 15 , 30, 45, and 60 %. We also consider the two models in the settings with three different sample sizes 30, 50, and 100. In order to make the results to be reliable, there are 10,000 repetitions for each of the data settings. The simulation was done with Matlab.

All the results of comparison between the Wald-type based methods and the EL methods are shown in Table 18.1 and Table 18.2. CP stands for the value of coverage probabilities. From the two tables, we find that, in general, both the Wald-type based method and the EL methods have improved coverage probabilities for 90, 95, and 99 % as the sample size increases. The heavy censoring rate means high information loss. Having more information lost, the accuracy of coverage probabilities will be reduced.

From the tables, we find that proposed EL method outperforms Zhao (2011)'s method in terms of coverage probability. A comparison between these two methods is the main purpose of our work. When the sample size is large, the two methods have very close performance in model 1, while in model 2, the EL method is better than the Wald-type method when the censoring rate is moderate or heavy. For moderate sample size ($n = 50$), the EL method works well under censoring rate 15, 30, and 45 %, respectively (except for CR = 60 % in model 1), while the Wald-type-based method shows some problems of under-coverage. For an even smaller sample size of $n = 30$, the under-coverage issue in the Wald-type methods becomes more significant. Because the Wald-type confidence interval needs to estimate the variance as well as the regression coefficients β, the EL based confidence region R_E has more accurate coverage probability than that of the Wald-type confidence region when the censoring rate is less or equal to 45 % and the sample size is relatively small most of time. From the tables, we find that the average length for the EL method is slightly longer than that for the Wald-type (normal approximation) based method.

Table 18.1 Coverage probability (CP) and average length (AL) of confidence intervals for the regression parameter β with model 1

			$1-\alpha=0.90$		$1-\alpha=0.95$		$1-\alpha=0.99$	
CR (%)	*n*		Wald	EL	Wald	EL	Wald	EL
0.15	30	CP	0.8686	0.8986	0.9221	0.9427	0.9731	0.9736
		AL	1.4354	1.5751	1.7102	1.9030	2.2477	2.4332
	50	CP	0.8856	0.9084	0.9338	0.9516	0.9796	0.9869
		AL	1.0857	1.1840	1.2936	1.4138	1.7001	1.9051
	100	CP	0.8937	0.9152	0.9425	0.9607	0.9871	0.9916
		AL	0.7520	0.8065	0.8960	0.9793	1.1776	1.2976
0.3	30	CP	0.8669	0.8946	0.9163	0.9366	0.9702	0.9712
		AL	1.6870	1.8175	2.0101	2.1739	2.6418	2.6881
	50	CP	0.8768	0.8984	0.9272	0.9452	0.9804	0.9853
		AL	1.2694	1.3635	1.5124	1.6253	1.9878	2.1632
	100	CP	0.8911	0.9108	0.9418	0.9594	0.9852	0.9904
		AL	0.8810	0.9479	1.0497	1.1352	1.3796	1.4878
0.45	30	CP	0.8494	0.8720	0.9081	0.9188	0.9625	0.9629
		AL	2.0324	2.1770	2.4216	2.5976	3.1826	3.2799
	50	CP	0.8699	0.8846	0.9233	0.9333	0.9726	0.9759
		AL	1.5241	1.5961	1.8160	1.9005	2.3867	2.4899
	100	CP	0.8879	0.9041	0.9394	0.9470	0.9832	0.9865
		AL	1.0555	1.1255	1.2576	1.3275	1.6529	1.7333
0.6	30	CP	0.8136	0.8382	0.8760	0.8865	0.9383	0.9350
		AL	2.6101	2.7787	3.1099	3.2616	4.0873	4.1763
	50	CP	0.8482	0.8492	0.9008	0.9028	0.9575	0.9568
		AL	1.9459	1.9870	2.3186	2.3588	3.0472	2.9894
	100	CP	0.8738	0.8807	0.9284	0.9275	0.9761	0.9760
		AL	1.3462	1.3824	1.6040	1.6210	2.1081	2.1143

18.2.3 Comparison Among Kendall, Buckley-James, Log-Rank, and Gehan Methods

In this subsection, we compare the Kendall's rank regression with the Buckley–James (B-J; Zhou and Li 2008), Gehan, and Log-rank methods (Zhou 2005) in terms of coverage probability and average length of confidence interval. We consider the third censored linear regression model that is specified as follows:

Model 3

- The covariate Z follows $N(1, 0.5^2)$.
- The C follows N(μ, 42), where $\mu = 6.1,\ 3.1,\ 1\ and -1.8$ respectively, which produce samples with censoring rate equal to 10, 30, 50, and 75 %, respectively.

Table 18.2 Coverage probability and average length of confidence intervals for the regression parameter β with model 2

			$1-\alpha=0.90$		$1-\alpha=0.95$		$1-\alpha=0.99$	
CR (%)	n		Wald	EL	Wald	EL	Wald	EL
15	30	CP	0.8539	0.9082	0.912	0.9504	0.9667	0.9797
		AL	2.3067	2.4421	2.7485	2.8872	3.6123	3.5427
	50	CP	0.8753	0.9162	0.9293	0.9612	0.9775	0.9918
		AL	1.7432	1.8874	2.077	2.251	2.7298	2.9642
	100	CP	0.888	0.9122	0.9409	0.9626	0.9837	0.9926
		AL	1.2158	1.2851	1.4486	1.5596	1.9039	2.0844
30	30	CP	0.852	0.9002	0.9065	0.9458	0.9632	0.9788
		AL	2.4348	2.5429	2.901	2.9912	3.8127	3.6071
	50	CP	0.876	0.9063	0.9238	0.9514	0.9777	0.989
		AL	1.843	1.9749	2.196	2.3563	2.8861	3.0619
	100	CP	0.8832	0.9091	0.938	0.9587	0.9855	0.9933
		AL	1.2805	1.3528	1.5257	1.6343	2.0052	2.1774
45	30	CP	0.8434	0.8828	0.8985	0.9328	0.9582	0.9675
		AL	2.669	2.8711	3.1801	3.4428	4.1795	4.4189
	50	CP	0.8698	0.8959	0.9207	0.9415	0.9741	0.9838
		AL	2.0308	2.1348	2.4197	2.5526	3.1802	3.3567
	100	CP	0.8875	0.9077	0.9367	0.9543	0.9837	0.9893
		AL	1.4077	1.4885	1.6773	1.7755	2.2044	2.3341
60	30	CP	0.8319	0.8634	0.8869	0.9093	0.9482	0.9501
		AL	3.016	3.1968	3.5935	3.7967	4.7229	4.8916
	50	CP	0.8705	0.8783	0.9179	0.9222	0.9697	0.9715
		AL	2.277	2.3433	2.713	2.7909	3.5657	3.5854
	100	CP	0.8808	0.8995	0.933	0.9422	0.9795	0.9825
		AL	1.5662	1.6452	1.8661	1.9422	2.4526	2.5333

- The error term has a normal distribution $N(0, 0.5^2)$.
- We used sample size of $n = 50$, 100, and 200. The coverage probabilities are based on 5000 simulation runs. Note that this setting for the AFT model is defined as
- $Y_i = \beta Z_i + \epsilon_i$, $i = 1, \ldots, n$, and the true value for the coefficient $\beta_0 = 1$. Therefore, in this setting, we observe $X_i = min(Y_i, C_i)$, $\Delta_i = I(Y_i \leq C_i)$ and Z_i, $i = 1, \ldots, n$.

The results in Table 18.3 suggest a good performance of the EL based on Kendall's rank-estimating equation, especially when the sample size is small and the censoring rate is heavy. Specifically, for the sample size of $n = 50$, in most cases, it is better than the Buckley–James (B–J) method in terms of coverage probability. Compared to the log-rank and the Gehan methods, it still shows advantages for small sample size data.

Table 18.3 Coverage probability of confidence intervals for the regression parameter β with model 3 based on the EL method

		Confidence level = 90 %			
CR (%)	n	B–J	Log-rank	Gehan	Kendall
10	50	0.8924	0.8879	0.8832	0.9110
	100	0.8888	0.8909	0.8904	0.9212
	200	0.8810	0.9059	0.8938	0.9012
30	50	0.8866	0.8869	0.8804	0.9078
	100	0.8936	0.8889	0.8870	0.9212
	200	0.8922	0.9139	0.8958	0.9108
50	50	0.8838	0.8798	0.8650	0.8978
	100	0.8926	0.8939	0.8820	0.9090
	200	0.8952	0.8929	0.8968	0.9142
75	50	0.8420	0.8350	0.8030	0.8556
	100	0.8818	0.8740	0.8536	0.8856
	200	0.8928	0.8860	0.8788	0.9012
		Confidence level = 95 %			
CR (%)	n	B–J	Log-rank	Gehan	Kendall
10	50	0.9406	0.9399	0.9356	0.9516
	100	0.9404	0.9479	0.9446	0.9630
	200	0.9458	0.9500	0.9446	0.9506
30	50	0.9374	0.9359	0.9290	0.9522
	100	0.9472	0.9410	0.9382	0.9596
	200	0.9468	0.9619	0.9440	0.9592
50	50	0.9324	0.9319	0.9226	0.9370
	100	0.9414	0.9519	0.9370	0.9538
	200	0.9482	0.9469	0.9424	0.9604
75	50	0.9042	0.8910	0.8628	0.8866
	100	0.9344	0.9300	0.9118	0.9340
	200	0.9438	0.9440	0.9358	0.9490

Also, we note that there are some over-coverage problems when the sample size is large and the censoring rate is low. The EL based on the Kendall's rank regression is still a competitive method.

In terms of the average length of confidence interval, the Kendall's rank method outperforms Gehan and log-rank methods when the number of observations is large ($n = 200$) and the censoring rate is from light to heavy (10, 30 or 50 %). In other cases, the Kendall's rank method generates slightly longer average length of confidence intervals. It is clear that the B–J method outperforms any other alternatives in all cases (Table 18.4).

Table 18.4 Average length of confidence intervals for the regression parameter β with model 3 based on the EL method

		Confidence level = 90 %			
CR (%)	n	B–J	Log-rank	Gehan	Kendall
10	50	0.1973	0.5464	0.5000	0.5424
	100	0.1411	0.3535	0.3192	0.3139
	200	0.0975	0.2448	0.2255	0.1847
30	50	0.2289	0.6235	0.5482	0.6415
	100	0.1587	0.4022	0.3706	0.3812
	200	0.1110	0.2798	0.2615	0.2303
50	50	0.2742	0.7420	0.6485	0.7802
	100	0.1881	0.4861	0.4370	0.4820
	200	0.1321	0.3243	0.2907	0.2593
75	50	0.4569	1.0413	0.8697	1.2357
	100	0.2966	0.7139	0.6357	0.7569
	200	0.2024	0.4748	0.4360	0.4516
		Confidence level = 95 %			
CR (%)	n	B–J	Log-rank	Gehan	Kendall
10	50	0.2361	0.6526	0.6008	0.6735
	100	0.1687	0.4227	0.3825	0.3959
	200	0.1164	0.2922	0.2697	0.2307
30	50	0.2741	0.7476	0.6585	0.7765
	100	0.1898	0.4804	0.4440	0.4936
	200	0.1325	0.3344	0.3125	0.2834
50	50	0.3288	0.8919	0.7776	0.9626
	100	0.2252	0.5833	0.5246	0.6034
	200	0.1579	0.3875	0.3478	0.3391
75	50	0.5469	1.2519	1.0480	1.6786
	100	0.3570	0.8607	0.7629	0.9404
	200	0.2426	0.5687	0.5219	0.6002

18.3 Conclusion

In the simulation studies, we compare two methods that estimate the confidence intervals of regression parameters based on Kendall's rank-estimating equation. The coverage probabilities of the EL are closer to the nominal levels than their counterparts in most cases. We also compare the proposed EL based on Kendall's rank-estimating equation with several other popular empirical likelihood methods. The simulation studies indicate that the proposed method is better than the

Buckley–James method in terms of the coverage probability when the sample size is very small, say $n = 50$, or the censoring rate is very heavy in most cases, while it still provides a competitive interval estimator when the sample size becomes larger and the censoring rate becomes lower.

In addition, Zhou (2005) proposed the censored EL based on log-rank and Gehan estimators. The log-rank method outperforms the Gehan method with better coverage probabilities most of the time. In the second part of our simulation study, the proposed method performs better than the log-rank method when the sample size is small and it is comparable in other cases most of the time. As for the average length of confidence intervals, the B–J method is the best in all the cases. The Kendall's rank method does the better job than the log-rank and Gehan methods do for the large number of observations ($n = 200$).

In conclusion, the proposed EL confidence intervals based on Kendall's rank-estimating equation have advantages over other approaches in terms of the coverage probability for the small sample size most of the time. And it has no clear advantages in terms of the average length of confidence intervals compared to the Buckley–James method.

Acknowledgments The authors are grateful to the reviewer for the useful comments. The authors would like to thank Maxime Boudoumou and Jenny Zhao for their help. Yichuan Zhao acknowledges partial support from the NSA grant and the IRG grant in the Georgia State University.

References

Fygenson M, Ritov Y (1994) Monotone estimating equations for censored data. Ann Statist 22:732–746

Jing BY, Yuan J, Zhou W (2008) Empirical likelihood for non-degenerate U-statistics. Stat Probab Lett 78:599–607

Heller G (2007) Smoothed rank regression with censored data. J Am Stat Assoc 102:552–559

Li G, Wang QH (2003) Empirical likelihood regression analysis for right censored data. Stat Sin 13:51–68

Owen A (1988) Empirical likelihood ratio confidence intervals for a single functional. Biom 75: 237–249

Owen A (1990) Empirical likelihood and confidence regions. Ann Statist 18:90–120

Owen A (2001) Empirical Likelihood. Chapman and Hall, London

Zhao Y (2011) Empirical likelihood inference for the accelerated failure time model. Stat Probab Lett 81:603–610

Zhou M (2005) Empirical likelihood analysis of the rank estimator for the censored accelerated failure time model. Biom 92:492–498

Zhou M, Li G (2008) Empirical likelihood analysis of the Buckley–James estimator. J Multivar Anal 99:649–664

Chapter 19
Analysis of a Complex Longitudinal Health-Related Quality of Life Data by a Mixed Logistic Model

Mounir Mesbah

Abstract We consider the context of a longitudinal study, where participants are interviewed about their health-related quality of life (HRQOL), at regular dates of visit, previously established. The interviews consist, to fulfill a questionnaire in which they are asked multiple choice questions, built in order to measure, at the time of the visit, the latent trait. We assume here unidimensionality of the latent trait. The issue of choosing a longitudinal model can be considered as one of the most important issue in latent regression models. In this work, we take the opportunity of a real longitudinal study of quality of life to present in detail the stages of the construction of a mixed logistic model. As, HRQOL is a latent variable, not directly observable, we use in this study, a measurement model from Rasch family to link the latent with item responses. We discuss the appropriate choice of interactions to include in the latent regression model.

19.1 Introduction

We consider the context of a longitudinal study, where participants are interviewed about their quality of life, at regular dates of visit, previously established. The interviews consist to fulfill a questionnaire in which patients are asked multiple choice questions, chosen in order to measure, at the time of the visit, the latent (unobserved) trait (quality of life). We focus here on one unidimensional latent trait. We suppose that the unique effect of time on the observations (evolution) occurs through latent components. So, we assume that measurement properties of the instrument (questionnaire) are not changing.

In this work, we are not building a longitudinal measurement model, i.e , a model built to evaluate longitudinal measurement properties of the instrument (as responsiveness for instance), but a longitudinal model to analyze change of the latent patient quality of life, not to analyze change of the instrument (questionnaire) used to observe the latent variable.

M. Mesbah (✉)
Université Pierre et Marie Curie, Paris, France
e-mail: mounir.mesbah@upmc.fr

Z. Chen et al. (eds.), *Applied Statistics in Biomedicine and Clinical Trials Design*,
ICSA Book Series in Statistics, DOI 10.1007/978-3-319-12694-4_19

The main motivation of this work was a real study, where two different instruments were sequentially used: the short form twelve (SF-12), a shortened version (12 items) of the medical outcomes study 36-items short-form health survey (SF-36), a generic well-known questionnaire and then, the World Health Organization quality of life (WHOQOL) HIV brief (WHB), which is a shortened version of the WHOQOL HIV, an HIV-specific questionnaire developed by the WHO.

The switch to a different instrument in the middle of the study was decided because the study investigators hoped that the second instrument, an HIV-specific instrument, was more responsive.

Despite this particular study, one can imagine many situations where, one needs to use two "different" instruments to measure the same latent trait. One of them, easy to understand, in a longitudinal context, is to prevent against memory bias. When a subject is asked a question at visit t, he or she, remembers the answer to the same question given at the previous visit $t-1$. So, using different questions at time $t-1$ and time t avoids such bias. Another context could be the context of meta-analyze of health-related quality of life (HRQOL) studies, where different instruments are used in each study, to measure the same latent trait. Our method applies, if, a subsample is available, with individual's responses to all questionnaires.

In Sect. 2, we explain how the backward reliability curve (BRC, REF) can be used, (i) to identify an unidimensional subset of items, and (ii) then, in Sect. 3, we develop a mixed longitudinal logistic model to describe the evolution of the latent component underlying the identified unidimensional subset of items. In our setting, the longitudinal aspect of our model is mainly described by the latent process.

In this work, we suppose that this latent component θ_t follows an autoregressive AR(1) process:

$$\theta(t) = c + \rho_L \theta(t-1) + \varepsilon(t),$$

where $\varepsilon(t)$ is gaussian random variable with zero mean and unknown constant variance σ^2, ρ_L an unknown autocorrelation parameter and c a real unknown parameter. In Sect. 4, we derive the marginal likelihood of the latent regression model. In Sect. 5, we discuss the practical resolution of the maximum likelihood equations, presenting different possibilities offered by major statistical software, or the option of writing an ad hoc program. Finally, we devote the last section to the discussion of our choice over other choices, and possible extensions of the current work.

19.2 The BRC to Identify Unidimensional Set of Items

In this work, we focus on: (i) the twelve items of the SF-12 and (ii) on five items of the psychological subdimension of the WHB. We assume that each of the two instruments include respectively a subset of items, S1 and S2, that constitute, when combined, a unidimensional set of items, i.e., the set S of items included in S1 or S2 is unidimensional.

Table 19.1 The questionnaires

Questions	Label	Contents
WHB	Wq1	How much do you enjoy your life?
WHB	Wq2	How satisfied are you with your ability to learn new information?
WHB	**Wq3**	Are you able to accept your bodily appearance?
WHB	Wq4	How much do you value yourself?
WHB	Wq5	How often do you have negative feelings, such a blue mood, despair, anxiety, depression?
SF12	**sf1**	In general, would you say your health is excellent, very good, good, fair, or poor?
SF12	**sf2**	How much did pain interfere with your normal work, including both work outside the home and housework?
SF12	**sf3**	Has your physical health or emotional problems interfere with your social activities?
SF12	sf4	Does your health now limit you in moderate activities such as moving a table, pushing a vacuum cleaner, ...
SF12	**sf5**	Climbing several flights of stairs. Does your health now limit you a lot, limit you a little, or not limit you at all?
SF12	sf6	During the past 4 weeks, have you accomplished less than you would like?
SF12	sf7	During the past 4 weeks, were you limited in the kind of work or other regular activities you do?
SF12	**sf8**	During the past 4 weeks, have accomplished less than you would like?
SF12	sf9	During the past 4 weeks, did you not do work or other regular activities as carefully as usual?
SF12	sf10	How much time during the past 4 weeks have you felt calm and peaceful?
SF12	sf11	How much of the time during the past 4 weeks did you have a lot of energy?
SF12	sf12	How much time during the past 4 weeks have you felt down?

WHB World Health Organization quality of life (WHOQOL) HIV brief, *SF12* short form twelve. The significance of bold entities is given in section 19.2.4

The unidimensionality is the first requirement in latent variable models. It is the most important property. When it is reached, it is possible to target other. In this work, we focused on unidimensionality.

The text of the questions are presented in Table 19.1 below. The SF-12 is a shortened version (twelve items) of the medical outcomes study SF-36. From the WHB, which is a shortened version of the WHOQOL HIV, an HIV-specific questionnaire developed by the WHO, we focus on the psychological subdimension. So, we start with seventeen (17) items. In this section, we present the theoretical motivations underlying the BRC and we explain how it can be used to find among the 12 questions SF12 and 5 Questions WHB, a unidimensional subset of questions. At the end of the section, we present our results, using the BRC methodology.

19.2.1 Classical Unidimensional Models for Measurement

Latent variable models involve a set of observable variables $A = \{\mathbf{X}_1, \mathbf{X}_2, \ldots, \mathbf{X}_k\}$ and a latent (unobservable) variable θ of dimension $d \leq k$. In such models, the dimensionality of A is captured by the dimension of θ, the value of d. When $d = 1$, the dimensionality of set A is called as unidimensional.

In a HRQOL study, measurements are taken with an instrument: the questionnaire, which consists of questions (or items). In such cases, the $\mathbf{X}_{ij}$ represents the random response of the jth question by the ith subject and the $\mathbf{X}_j$ denotes the random variable generating responses to the jth question.

The parallel model is a classical latent variable model describing the unidimensionality of a set $A = \{\mathbf{X}_1, \mathbf{X}_2, \ldots, \mathbf{X}_k\}$ of quantitative observable variables. Let $\mathbf{X}_{ij}$ be the measurement of subject i, given by a variable $\mathbf{X}_j$, $i = 1, \ldots, n$, $j = 1, \ldots, k$, then:

$$\mathbf{X}_{ij} = \tau_{ij} + \varepsilon_{ij}, \tag{19.1}$$

where τ_{ij} is the unknown true measurement corresponding to the observed measurement $\mathbf{X}_{ij}$ and ε_{ij} a measurement error. The model is called as a parallel model if the τ_{ij} can be divided as

$$\tau_{ij} = \beta_j + \theta_i,$$

where β_j is an unknown fixed parameter (non-random) representing the effect of jth variable, and θ_i is an unknown random parameter effect of the ith subject.

It is generally assumed that θ_i has zero mean and unknown standard deviation σ_θ. It should be noted that the zero-mean assumption is an arbitrary identifiability constraint with consequence on the interpretation of the parameter: its value must be interpreted comparatively to the mean population value. *In HRQOL setting, θ_i is the true latent Health Related Quality Of Life that clinician or health scientist want to measure and analyze.* It is a zero mean individual random part of all observed subject responses $\mathbf{X}_{ij}$, the same whatever is the variable $\mathbf{X}_j$ (in practice, a question j of a HRQOL questionnaire). It is also generally assumed that ε_{ij} are independent random errors with zero mean and standard deviation σ corresponding to the additional measurement error. Moreover, the true measure and the error are assumed to be uncorrelated, i.e., $\text{cov}(\theta_i, \varepsilon_{ij}) = 0$. This model is known as the parallel model, because the regression lines relating any observed item $\mathbf{X}_j$, $j = 1, \ldots, k$ and the true unique latent measure θ_i are parallel.

The model (1) can be obtained in an alternative way through modeling the conditional moments of the observed responses. Specifically, the conditional mean of $\mathbf{X}_{ij}$ can be specified as:

$$E[\mathbf{X}_{ij}|\theta_i; \beta_j] = \beta_j + \theta_i. \tag{19.2}$$

where β_j, $j = 1, \ldots, k$, are fixed effects and θ_i, $i = 1, \ldots, n$ are independent random effects with zero mean and standard deviation σ_θ. The conditional variance of $\mathbf{X}_{ij}$ is specified as:

$$Var[\mathbf{X}_{ij}|\theta_i; \beta_j] = Var(\varepsilon_{ij}) = \sigma^2. \tag{19.3}$$

The assumptions (2) and (3) are classical in experimental design. The model defines relationships between different kinds of variables: the observed score $\mathbf{X}_{ij}$, the true score τ_{ij}, and the measurement error ε_{ij}. It is interesting to make some remarks about the assumptions underlying this model. The random part of the true measure given by response by the ith individual does not vary with the question number j as the θ_i does not depend on j, $j = 1, \ldots, k$. The model is unidimensional in the sense that the random part of all observed variables (questions $\mathbf{X}_j$) is generated by the common unobserved variable (θ_i). More precisely, let $\mathbf{X}^*_{ij} = \mathbf{X}_{ij} - \beta_j$ be the calibrated version of the response to the jth item by the ith subject, then the model (2) and (3) can be rewritten as:

$$E[X^*_{ij}|\theta_i; \beta_j] = \theta_i, \quad \text{for } \forall j, \tag{19.4}$$

along with the same assumptions on β and θ and the conditional variance model (3).

When both θ_i and ε_{ij} are normally distributed, then we have so-called conditional independence property: whatever j and j', two observed items $\mathbf{X}_j$ and $\mathbf{X}_{j'}$ are independent conditional to the latent θ_i.

19.2.2 *Reliability of an Instrument: Cronbach Alpha Coefficient*

A measurement instrument yields values that we call observed measure. The reliability ρ of an instrument is defined as the ratio of two variances of the true over the observed measure. Under the parallel model, one can show that the reliability of any variable $\mathbf{X}_j$ (as an instrument to measure the true value) is given by

$$\rho = \frac{\sigma^2_\theta}{\sigma^2_\theta + \sigma^2}. \tag{19.5}$$

This coefficient is also known as the intra-class coefficient. The reliability coefficient, ρ, can be easily interpreted as a correlation coefficient between the true and the observed measure. When the parallel model is assumed, the reliability of the sum of k variables is

$$\tilde{\rho}_k = \frac{k\rho}{k\rho + (1-\rho)}. \tag{19.6}$$

This formula is known as the Spearman–Brown formula (Brown 1910; Spearman 1910).

The Spearman–Brown formula shows a simple relationship between $\tilde{\rho}_k$ and k, the number of variables. It is easy to see that $\tilde{\rho}_k$ is an increasing function of k

The maximum likelihood estimator of $\tilde{\rho}_k$, under the parallel model with normal distribution assumptions, is known as Cronbach's alpha coefficient (CAC) (Cronbach

1951; Bland and Altman 1997), which is denoted as α:

$$\alpha = \frac{k}{k-1}\left(1 - \frac{\sum_{j=1}^{k} S_j^2}{S_{\text{tot}}^2}\right), \tag{19.7}$$

where

$$S_j^2 = \frac{1}{n-1}\sum_{i=1}^{n}\left(X_{ij} - \overline{X_j}\right)^2$$

and

$$S_{\text{tot}}^2 = \frac{1}{nk-1}\sum_{i=1}^{n}\sum_{j=1}^{k}\left(X_{ij} - \overline{X}\right)^2.$$

Under the parallel model, the variance–covariance matrix of the observed items X_j and the latent trait θ is

$$V_{X,\theta} = \begin{pmatrix} \sigma_\theta^2 + \sigma^2 & \sigma_\theta^2 & \cdots & \cdots \sigma_\theta^2 & \sigma_\theta^2 \\ \sigma_\theta^2 & \sigma_\theta^2 + \sigma^2 & \sigma_\theta^2 & \cdots \sigma_\theta^2 & \sigma_\theta^2 \\ \vdots & \vdots & \vdots & \vdots & \vdots \\ \sigma_\theta^2 & \cdots & \sigma_\theta^2 & \sigma_\theta^2 + \sigma^2 & \sigma_\theta^2 \\ \sigma_\theta^2 & \cdots & \cdots & \sigma_\theta^2 & \sigma_\theta^2 \end{pmatrix},$$

and the corresponding correlation matrix of the observed items X_j and the latent trait θ is

$$R_{X,\theta} = \begin{pmatrix} 1 & \rho & \cdots & \cdots \rho & \sqrt{\rho} \\ \rho & 1 & \rho & \cdots \rho & \sqrt{\rho} \\ \vdots & \vdots & \vdots & \vdots & \vdots \\ \rho & \cdots & \rho & 1 & \sqrt{\rho} \\ \sqrt{\rho} & \cdots & \cdots & \sqrt{\rho} & 1 \end{pmatrix}.$$

The *marginal* covariance V_X and correlation matrix R_X of the k observed variables X_j, under the parallel model, are

$$V_X = \begin{pmatrix} \sigma_\theta^2 + \sigma^2 & \sigma_\theta^2 & \cdots & \cdots \sigma_\theta^2 \\ \sigma_\theta^2 & \sigma_\theta^2 + \sigma^2 & \sigma_\theta^2 & \cdots \sigma_\theta^2 \\ \vdots & \vdots & \vdots & \vdots \\ \sigma_\theta^2 & \cdots & \sigma_\theta^2 & \sigma_\theta^2 + \sigma^2 \end{pmatrix}$$

and

$$R_X = \begin{pmatrix} 1 & \rho & \cdots & \cdots \rho \\ \rho & 1 & \rho & \cdots \rho \\ \vdots & \vdots & \vdots & \vdots \\ \rho & \cdots & \rho & 1 \end{pmatrix}.$$

This structure is known as *compound symmetry* type. It is easy to show that the reliability of the sum of k items given in (7) can be expressed as:

$$\tilde{\rho}_k = \frac{k}{k-1}\left[1 - \frac{trace(V_X)}{J' V_X J}\right]. \tag{19.8}$$

with J a vector with all components being 1, and

$$\alpha = \frac{k}{k-1}\left[1 - \frac{trace(S_X)}{J' S_X J}\right]. \tag{19.9}$$

where S_X is the observed variance, empirical estimation of S_X. There is, in the literature, even recent, a comprehensible confusion between Cronbach alpha as a population parameter (theoretical reliability of the sum of items) or its sample estimate.

In addition, it is easy to show a direct connection between the CAC and the percentage of variance of the first component in principal component analysis (PCA) which is often used to assess unidimensionality. The PCA is mainly based on the analysis of the latent roots of V_X or R_X (or, in practice, their sample estimate). The matrix R_X has only two different latent roots, the greater root is $\lambda_1 = (k-1)\rho + 1$, and the other multiple roots are $\lambda_2 = \lambda_3 = \lambda_4 = \cdots = 1 - \rho = \frac{k-\lambda_1}{k-1}$. So, using the Spearman–Brown formula, we can express the reliability of the sum of the k variables as $\tilde{\rho}_k = \frac{k}{k-1}(1 - \frac{1}{\lambda_1})$.

This clearly indicates a monotonic relationship between $\tilde{\rho}_k$, which can be consistently estimated by the CAC and the first latent root λ_x, which in practice is naturally estimated by the corresponding observed sample correlation matrix and thus the percentage of variance of the first principal component in a PCA. So, CAC can also be considered as a measure of unidimensionality.

Nevertheless, such a measure is not very useful, because, it is easy to show, using the Spearman–Brown formula (Brown 1910; Spearman 1910) that, under the parallel model assumption, the reliability of the total score is an increasing function of the number of variables.

Therefore, *if the parallel model is true,* increasing the number of items will increase the reliability of a questionnaire. Moreover, the coefficient lies between 0 and 1. Zero value indicates a totally unreliable scale, while unit value means that the scale is perfectly reliable. Of course, in practice, these two scenarios never occur!

The Cronbach α-coefficient is an estimate of the reliability of the raw score (sum of item responses) of a person *if the model generating those responses is a parallel model.*

In Hamon and Mesbah (2002), the conclusion of intensive simulations shows that "the classical Cronbach alpha seems nevertheless to remain a good reliability coefficient under Rasch model assumptions."

The result can be used as a criterium for checking the unidimensionality of such responses when those item responses are *generated by a parallel model.*

In the next section, we show how to build and to use a more operational and more valid criterium to measure the unidimensionality of a set of items: the BRC (the α-curve).

19.2.3 Unidimensionality of an Instrument: BRC

Statistical validation of unidimensionality can be performed through a goodness of fit test of the parallel model or Rasch model. There is a great literature on the subject, see the review by Mesbah (2012). The goodness of fit tests generally do not have power because their null hypothesis are not focusing on unidimensionality: it includes indirectly other additional assumptions (for instance, the normality for parallel models, local independence for Rasch models, etc.) As a result, the departure from the null hypotheses is not necessarily an indication of the departure from a unidimensionality.

In the following, we describe a graphical tool, which is helpful for checking the unidimensionality of a set of variables. It draws a curve in a stepwise manner, using estimates of reliability of sub scores (total of a sub set included in the starting set).

In the first step, the CAC will be calculated with all the variables. Then, at every successive step, CAC will be calculated by deleting one variable each time, and the variable which deletion yields the maximum CAC value among those CAC values will be removed. This procedure is repeated until only two variables remain. If the parallel model is true, increasing the number of variables increases the reliability of the total score which can be consistently estimated by Cronbach's alpha. The number of variables and the CAC values can be plotted which would yield a curve. This procedure is named as BRC. If there is a decrease of such a curve after adding a variable, it would indicate strongly that the added variable does not constitute a unidimensional set with variables already in the curve.

Drawing the BRC of a set of *unidimensional items is an essential tool in the validation process of a HRQOL questionnaire.* When one develop a HRQOL questionnaire, the main goal is generally to measure some unidimensional latent subjective traits (such as sociability, mobility, etc). The use of the BRC in empirical data are very helpful for detection of non-unidimensional subsets of items. When the BRC is not an increasing curve, one can remove one or more items to obtain an increasing curve (Mesbah 2013). If the reduced set gives an increasing curve, it is in some sense, *more valid in term of unidimensionality* than the previous one.

There is often a big misunderstanding of our method: The goal of the proposed method is not to "maximizes Cronbachs alpha to derive the best model." The goal of the proposed method is to check an underlying fundamental property of the parallel model: "increasing the number of variables, increases the reliability of the total score, which can be consistently estimated by the Chonbach's alpha!" The consequence of this fundamental property is the "Spearman–Brown formula," which is a formula derived under the parallel model and characterizing it. The Spearman–Brown formula shows a simple relationship between the reliability of the sum of k variables and k, the number of variables. It is easy to see that this reliability is an increasing function of k, under the parallel model (i.e., if the parallel model holds!).

This relationship between the reliability of the sum of k variables and k, the number of variables, is deterministic. This result is derived using only underlying properties of the parallel model. The BRC is a "statistics curve" estimate of the theoretical Spearman–Brown curve. For each k, it is a consistent estimate of the true Spearman–Brown curve. For each k, it is possible to draw a confidence interval for the true reliability, under normal assumption of the errors (see Mesbah 2012), and then to test the null hypothesis, that the curve is nondecreasing.

19.2.4 Use the BRC to Identify an Unidimensional Subset of Items

The final set of items include eleven (11) items: four (4) from the WHB questionnaire and seven (7) from the SF-12 questionnaire. Figure 19.1 shows the final BRC of the original set of items. Six items (wq3, sf1, sf2, sf3, sf5, sf8) must be excluded to obtain a unidimensional set. The SF-12 psychological dimension is based on all the 12 items of the SF-12 form. A score is derived as a weighted sum of the 12 items. The psychological dimension of the WFB is built in order to measure some underlying psychological trait. Our method finds a set of unidimensional items chosen (by the BRC) from the two sets. It is interesting to note that the only WFB item excluded from the list is the more specific item to the HIV disease (are you able to accept your bodily appearance) and is close to the physical dimension. Items $sf1$, $sf2$, $sf3$, $sf5$, and $sf8$ are obviously more related to the physical than to the psychological dimension. There is some coherence in the contents of the final set of questions obtained.

In this step of the analysis, we did not use data from the main study (see Table 19.2). Only data from the pilot study were used. A direct consequence is that estimation of the parameters in the main analysis model will not be noised by the measurement instrument.

19.3 Choice of the Components of the Latent Regression Model

Specification of a latent variable model is usually done by the choice of two components:

- The measurement model: A measurement model is a conditional probability model linking the observed variables to the latent variables.
- The probability distribution for the latent variables.

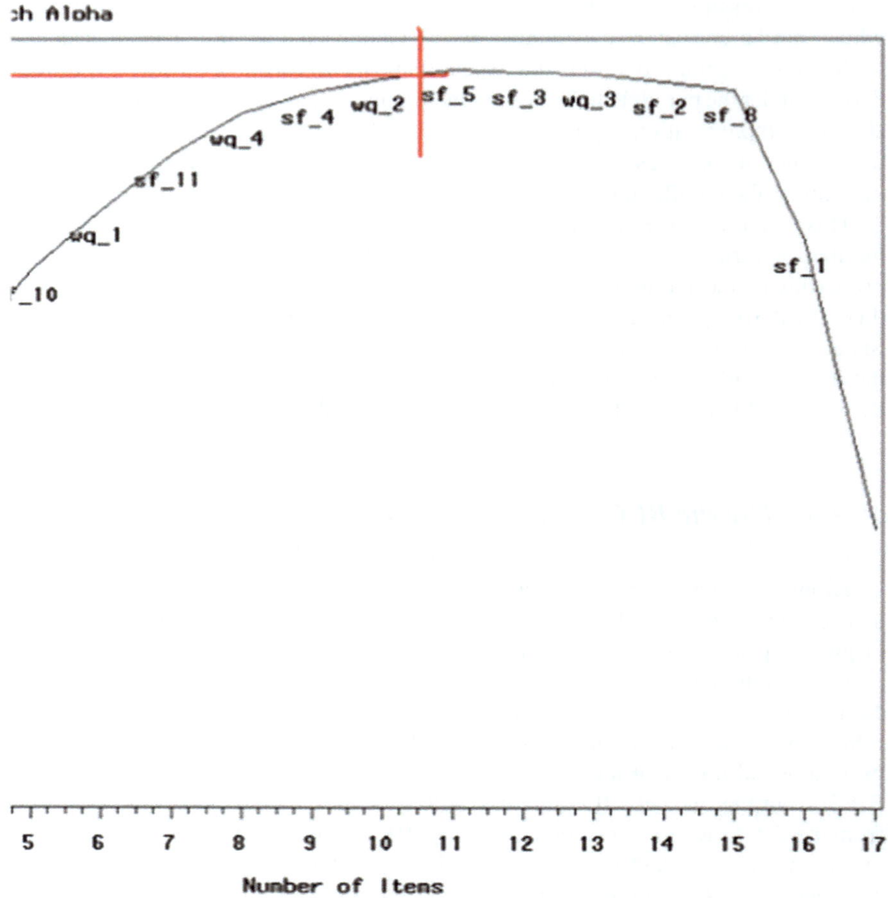

Fig. 19.1 The backward reliability curve (BRC) start with all 17 items. Items from the *right* must be excluded to obtain an increasing curve

In our setting,

- At a fixed time, the latent variable is a scalar.
- At a fixed time, the joint distribution of the observed items and the unobserved latent variable is described by its independence graph in Fig. 19.2.
- We assume that the instrument parameters, i.e., the parameters of the measurement model, are not changing over time.

The longitudinal aspect of our family of models is completely described by the independence graph of Fig. 19.3, the choice of the measurement model and the joint distribution of the latent process $(\Theta(1), \ldots, \Theta(T))$.

Table 19.2 The study design

Population and time	Questionnaires	Study type	Study size
Population A	SF12 and WHB	Pilot[a]	233
Population B, time M0	SF12	Main[b]	324
Population B, time M28	SF12	Main[b]	274
Population B, time M44	SF12	Main[b]	255
Population B, time M72	SF12 and WHB	Main[b]	263
Population B, time M84	WHB	Main[b]	258
Population B, time M96	WHB	Main[b]	269
Population B, time M108	WHB	Main[b]	215

[a] This is the pilot study done by INSERM in Marseille (France)
[b] This is the main study, done French ANRS (France). It is a multicentric cohort study, setup in 1997, aimed at describing clinical, immunological, virological and social-behavioral characteristics of HIV-1-infected patients who where beginning combination anti retro-viral therapy (HAART) that included a protease inhibitor (PI)
WHB World Health Organization quality of life (WHOQOL) HIV brief, *SF12* short form twelve

19.3.1 Choice of the Measurement Model

A large number of measurement models are possible. Item response theory is the field of psychometry devoted to that purpose. When the responses are ordinal, two reasonable choices could be the partial credit model (PCM) or the graded response model (GRM):

- Both are unidimensional models from the Rasch family of measurement models.
- Both own the nice property of independence of observed variables conditional to the latent (Fig. 19.2).
- Both are logistic model.
- The raw score (sum of item responses) of an individual is a sufficient statistic for the latent parameter under the PCM.
- The raw score of an individual is not a sufficient statistic for the latent parameter under the graded response mode.

19.3.1.1 The PCM

Let $X_j = x$ with $x = 0, \ldots, m$, the modalities of item j, and β_{jx} the parameter of modality x of item j. The PCM (Masters 1982) is defined as

$$\pi_{jx\theta} = Prob(X_j = x \mid \theta) = \frac{\exp\left(\sum_{l=0}^{x} (\theta - \beta_{jl})\right)}{\sum_{k=0}^{m} \exp \sum_{l=0}^{k} (\theta - \beta_{jl})}.$$

Constraints on the parameters are necessary to ensure the identifiability of parameters. This model is also known as model PCM at one parameter or polytomous Rasch model.

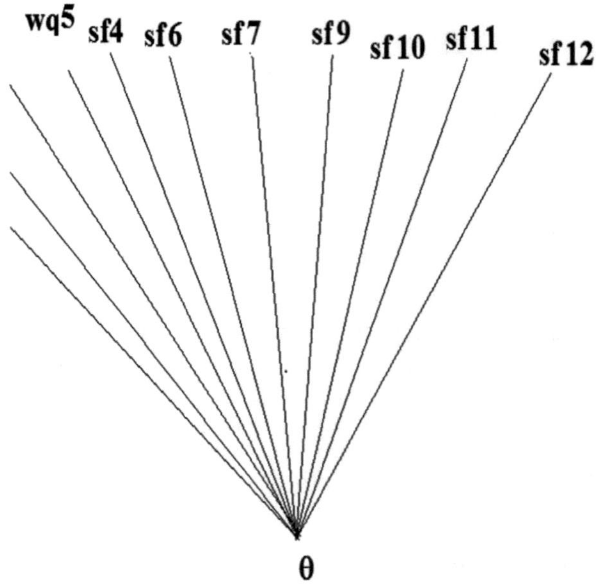

Fig. 19.2 Independence graph of a Rasch-type model at a fixed time

19.3.1.2 The GRM

The GRM (Samejima 1969) is defined as:

$$Prob(X_j \geq x \mid \theta) = \frac{\exp\left[(\theta - \beta_{jx})\right]}{1 + \exp\left[(\theta - \beta_{jx})\right]},$$

with $\beta_{j1} \leq \beta_{j2} \leq \ldots \leq \beta_{jm}$. For $x = 0$ and $x = m$, by definition $Prob(X_j \geq 0 \mid \theta) = 1$ and $Prob(X_j \geq m + 1 \mid \theta) = 0$, respectively. The probability of having item score x is given by the difference:

$$\begin{aligned}\pi_{jx\theta} &= Prob(X_j = x \mid \theta) = Prob(X_j \geq x \mid \theta) - Prob(X_j \geq x + 1 \mid \theta) \\ &= \frac{\exp\left[(\theta - \beta_{ix})\right]}{1 + \exp\left[(\theta - \beta_{ix})\right]} - \frac{\exp\left[(\theta - \beta_{i(x+1)})\right]}{1 + \exp\left[(\theta - \beta_{i(x+1)})\right]}\end{aligned}$$

19.3.2 Choice of the Latent Process Model

In this work, we suppose that this latent component $\theta(t)$ follows a Markovian process of order 1. A consequence is that: $\forall t, t > 0$, $\Theta(t-1)$, and $\Theta(t+1)$ are independent conditional to the current $\theta(t)$, the latent value at time t. Let us precise the distribution

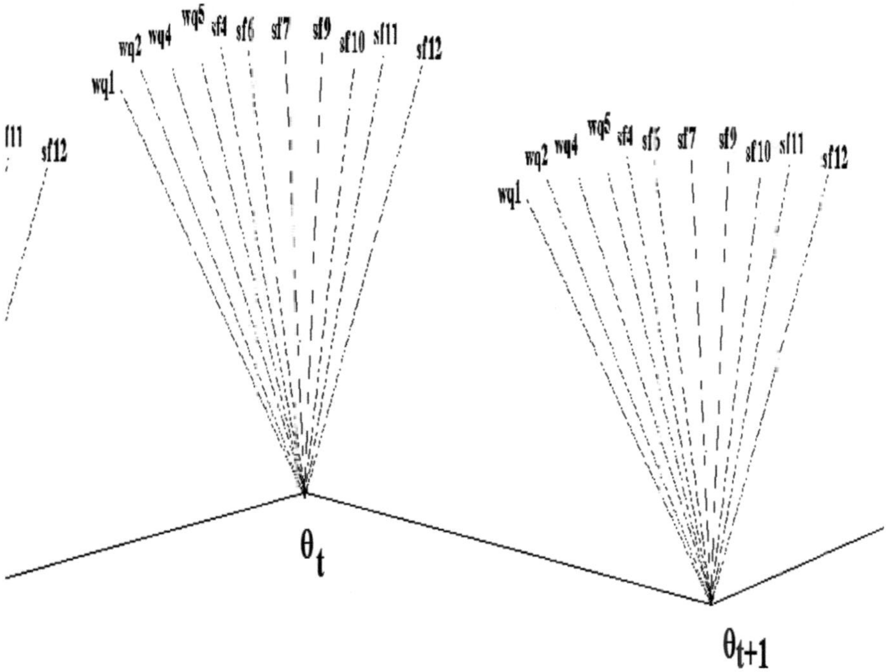

Fig. 19.3 Independence graph of a the longitudinal latent regression model

of Θ in such context:

$$\Theta(t) = c + \rho_L \Theta(t-1) + \varepsilon(t),$$

where $\varepsilon(t)$ is a gaussian white noise of variance σ^2 and ρ_L and c two real constants. It is easy to verify that this process is gaussian and defines a Markov chain of first order. Moreover, if $\mid \rho_L \mid < 1$, this process is stationary at the second order, of initial law the normal law with mean $\frac{c}{1-\rho}$ and variance $\frac{\sigma^2}{1-\rho_L^2}$ and the conditional probability of $\Theta(t)$ knowing $\Theta(t-1) = \theta(t-1)$ is gaussian of mean $c + \rho_L \times \theta(t-1)$ and variance σ^2. The joint law of variables $\Theta(1), \ldots, \Theta(T)$ is deduced easily:

$$g(\underline{\theta}) = \frac{\sqrt{1-\rho_L^2}}{\sqrt{(2\pi)^T.\sigma^T}} \exp\left\{-\frac{1}{2\sigma^2}[\left(1-\rho_L^2\right)\left(\theta(1) - \frac{c}{1-\rho}\right)^2 + \sum_{t=2}^{T} (\theta(t) - c - \rho_L \theta(t-1))^2]\right\} \tag{19.10}$$

where $\underline{\theta} = (\theta(1), \ldots, \theta(T))$.

19.4 The Marginal Likelihood of the Latent Regression Model

Let $(\underline{\mathbf{x}}(1), ..., \underline{\mathbf{x}}(T))$ be a trajectory of the observation process $(\underline{\mathbf{X}}(t)\colon 1 \leq t \leq T)$ relative to one individual only.

The process of observations $\{X_{i,j}(t)\}$ is supposed to have values in $\{1, 2, 3, ..., m\}$. The subscript i correspond to the patient, while j correspond to the item. The latent variable $\Theta_i(t)$ depends on the i patient only, it measures his level of HRQOL.

We note $\underline{\mathbf{X}}_i(t) = (X_{i,1}(t), ..., X_{i,q}(t))'$, the answer vector of the patient i at time t and by $\pi(x_{i,j}/\theta_i(t))$ the conditional probability $\mathbf{P}(X_{i,j}(t) = x_{i,j}(t)/\Theta_i(t) = \theta_i(t))$, $i = \overline{1, n}$, $j = \overline{1, q}$ and $t = \overline{1, T}$. Let us note $\underline{\mathbf{X}}_i$, the answer vector of the patient i for the whole period.

The probability of the answer vector of the patient i, in view of the observation during the whole period $\{1, ..., T\}$, can be written as:

$$p(\underline{\mathbf{X}}_i) = \int \cdots \int \prod_{j=1}^{q} \pi_{jx\theta} \times g(\theta(1), ..., \theta(T))\, d\theta(1) ... d\theta(T), \tag{19.11}$$

where g is the probability density of the latent vector $(\Theta(1), ..., \Theta(T))'$ chosen in the previous section and given by equation 10 and $\pi_{jx\theta}$ could indifferently chosen as the probability function of a PCM (Sect. 3.1) or a GRM (Sect. 3.2).

The formula 11, as a function of the unknown parameters is the likelihood function. Its maximization will let us to obtain estimates with optimal inferential properties. The design of the study is complex. In the analysis step, only data from the main study (population B) is used. In Table 19.2, we can see that seven time of visits were scheduled. At each visit, he patient is examined by a doctor, and asked to answer a HRQOL questionnaire. One of the main complexity is that the questionnaire that patients had to fulfill was not always the same in all these visit. The reason was that the clinicians decided to move to a more specific HRQOL after the third visit. This decision was taken because they were convinced, after analyzing data available at that time, that the HRQOL instrument (SF36) used until that visit was not sensitive enough to detect change. So, they decided to propose a new questionnaire, more specific (to the disease).

In this work, the main objective was to identify a unidimensional subset of items from the original two sets of questions, and then to build and analyze the following longitudinal latent model. The statistical analysis plan that we applied is a direct consequence of that goal.

The likelihood derived from formula (11) will be function of all available data. Only available observations will be used. Maximization of the likelihood will allow us, in a first step, to get consistent estimation of all item parameters, the auto-correlation parameter of the AR(1) latent process, and the constant c. Then, consistent prediction of the latent parameters will be obtained in a second step.

19.5 Practical Resolution of Maximum Likelihood Equations

The marginal likelihood function obtained from formula (11) is a nonlinear function of the vector of parameters $(\beta_{11}, ..., \beta_{1m}, ..., \beta_{qm}, c, \sigma^2, \rho_L)'$. There is no closed form for the exact maximum likelihood estimates (mles). The exact mles must be determined by numerically maximizing the exact log-likelihood function. Moreover, The expression of the exact log-likelihood function, contains integrals not analytically computable, which is often the case for similar latent variable model. Newton–Raphson-type algorithm with Gauss–Hermitte approximations of the integrals or Monte-Carlo Markov chain (MCMC) algorithm are the most commonly used solutions.

For the practical resolution of our problem, several solutions are possible, depending on the measurement model specified:

- (1) If this model is the GRM model, it is possible to use the GLIMMIX procedure of SAS which is an interesting generalization of the mixed procedure of SAS.
- (2) When the measurement model is the PCM model, it is not possible to use the GLIMMIX procedure, because the corresponding logit is not available in the link option. Another procedure of SAS is available, the NLMIXED procedure, which also use Gauss–Hermitte approximations, but need development of specific programming statements.
- (3) Another option is to develop an ad hoc program using Fortran or R language. With this this option, we can fit any model: GRM or PCM for the measurement model, and more complex AR model for the latent process.

19.6 Conclusion

In this work, the main objective was to identify a unidimensional subset of items from the original two sets of questions, and then to build and analyze the following longitudinal latent model. The statistical analysis plan that we applied is a direct consequence of that goal.

The likelihood derived from formula (11) will be function of all available data. Only available observations will be used. Maximization of the likelihood will allow us, in a first step, to get consistent estimation of all item parameters, the autocorrelation parameter of the AR(1) latent process, and the constant c. Then, consistent prediction of the latent parameters will be obtained in a second step.

Choice of the measurement model is an important step in the development of a HRQOL latent regression model. GRM or PCM for ordinal data? GRM-type models based on cumulative logits link were preferred by Mac Cullagh (1980), while PCM and Rasch-type models based on adjacent logits were preferred by Anderson (1984), mainly because they satisfy the sufficiency property for the latent parameter (Andersen 1977).

All these measurement models assume unidimensionality of the set of items. CAC is the maximum likelihood estimate of the reliability of the sum of k items if the true model underlying the data are the parallel model, which is a strong model for unidimensionality. In such case, it can be used as a measure of the reliability. But, if the true model underlying the data are not the parallel model, the CAC is a bad estimate of the reliability. The BRC allow us to check graphically the Spearman–Brown formula which is a consequence of the parallel model, then to confirm that a subset of items is unidimensional.

Choice of the latent process model is another challenge. Of course, the proposed model is adaptable to when the latent component does not follow an AR(1)! The AR(1) model is, apart from the model of mutual independence of the latent components, the simplest model that we can specify. This model is interesting because it is a model of short individual memory. The correlation between $\Theta(t)$ and $\Theta(t+s)$ will go to zero when s increase. One can imagine other kind of individual memory. Another work in progress, where the latent process is assumed to be a long memory process. The complexity of the model is due to the fact that for each specification of the latent distribution, one need to write the likelihood and to develop and adapted numerical program to get the estimates.

Longitudinal HRQOL belongs to the family of real data that must be analyzed by latent variable models. In this work, we have proposed some ways of thinking and some models that we have applied to a complex real trial.

References

Andersen EB (1977) Sufficient statistics and latent trait models. Psychometrika 42:69–81
Anderson JA (1984) Regression and ordered categorical variables. J R Statist Soc B 46(1): 1–30
Bland JM, Altman DG (1997) Statistics notes: Cronbach's alpha. BMJ 314:572
Brown W (1910) Some experimental results in the correlation of mental abilities. British J Psychol 3: 296–322
Cronbach, LJ (1951) Coefficient alpha and the internal structure of tests. Psychometrika 16:297–334
Hamon A, Mesbah M (2002) Questionnaire reliability under the Rasch model. In: Mesbah M, Cole BF, Lee MLT (eds) Statistical methods for quality of life studies. Kluwer Academic Publishing, Dordrecht, 155–168
Hemker BT, Sijtsma K, Molenaar IW, Junker BW (1996) Polytomous IRT models and monotone likelihood ratio of total score. Psychometrika 61, 679–693
Mac Cullagh P (1980) Regression models for ordinal Data. J R Statist Soc B 42(2), 109–142
Masters GN (1982) A Rasch model for partial credit scoring. Psychometrika 47:149–174
Mesbah M (2012) Measurement and analysis of quality of life in epidemiology. In: Chakraborty R, Rao CR, Sen PK (eds) Handbook of statistics, vol 28: BioInformatics in human health and heredity. North Holland, Amsterdam. (Chapter 15)
Mesbah M (2013) From measurement to analysis. In: Christensen KB, Kreiner S, Mesbah M (eds) Rasch models in health. Wiley, London. (Chapter 13)
Samejima F (1969) Estimation of ability using a response pattern of graded scores. Psychometrika Monograph, Né17
Spearman C (1910) Correlation calculated from faulty data. British J Psychol 3:271–295

Chapter 20
Goodness-of-Fit Tests for Length-Biased Right-Censored Data with Application to Survival with Dementia

Pierre-Jérôme Bergeron, Ewa Sucha and Jaime Younger

Abstract Cross-sectional surveys are often used in epidemiological studies to identify subjects with a disease. When estimating the survival function from the onset of disease, this sampling mechanism introduces bias, which must be accounted for. If the onset times of the disease are assumed to be coming from a stationary Poisson process, this bias, which is caused by the sampling of prevalent rather than incident cases, is termed length bias. One-sample goodness-of-fit tests are proposed for right-censored length-biased data based on Kolmogorov and Cramér–von-Mises criteria. Approximate critical values, power, and behavior are investigated using Weibull, lognormal, and log-logistic models through simulation. Algorithms detailing how to efficiently generate right-censored length-biased survival data of these parametric forms are given. Finally, the test is used to evaluate the goodness of fit using length-biased survival data of patients with dementia from the Canadian study of health and aging. Evidence for different parametric forms between men and women is found, suggesting course of disease to vary between genders.

20.1 Introduction

The sampling of prevalent cases is common in epidemiological studies as logistical constraints often prevent the recruitment of incident cases. The ideal setting for survival data are studies in which individuals are observed at the initiation of the event, or immediately after, and subsequently followed until the event or censoring occurs. These studies can be termed *incident studies*. Due to issues such as time and

P.-J. Bergeron (✉) · E. Sucha
Department of Mathematics and Statistics, University of Ottawa,
585 King Edward Avenue, Ottawa, ON K1N 6N5, Canada
e-mail: pbergero@uottawa.ca

E. Sucha
e-mail: ewa.sucha1@gmail.com

J. Younger
Toronto General Research Institute, University Health Network,
7-504, 610 University Avenue, Toronto, ON Canada M5G 2M9
e-mail: Jaime.Younger@uhnresearch.ca

Z. Chen et al. (eds.), *Applied Statistics in Biomedicine and Clinical Trials Design*,
ICSA Book Series in Statistics, DOI 10.1007/978-3-319-12694-4_20

cost, it is not always possible to capture individuals in this manner. Oftentimes, the subjects have experienced the initiation of the event prior to the initiation of the study, and these lifetimes are said to be left truncated. When subjects are identified cross-sectionally, the onset of disease (initiation of event) has already occurred. Under this type of sampling scheme, individuals who are longer lived have a higher probability of being selected into the study, and hence the recruited sample is not representative of the incident population. Sampling from a prevalent cohort is a form of selection bias that leads to an overestimation of the survival function if the truncation of lifetimes is not properly taken into account. When there has been no epidemic of disease, the incidence rate of the disease can be assumed to be constant over time. Under this scenario, the probability of sampling a subject is directly proportional to the disease duration, and the sampled lifetimes are said to be *length-biased*.

A one-sample goodness-of-fit test is one in which the discrepancy between a nonparametric estimator and some hypothesized parametric distribution is quantified. For length-biased survival data subject to right-censoring, a nonparametric estimator has been developed by Vardi (1989), which provides the nonparametric maximum likelihood estimator (NPMLE) of the survival function correcting for length bias. In order to test several specific parametric models for a particular set of data, we seek a versatile one-sample test, one that is adaptable to numerous distributions. The choice of a parametric model allows the use for simulations, aids in ease of interpretation, and for the development of regression models, and thus, choosing the best-adapted parametric model requires a proper test. In this chapter, we present two one-sample goodness-of-fit tests for length-biased right-censored data that can be applied to any suitable parametric model. The first is based on the Kolmogorov criterion, the second on Cramér–von-Mises criterion (Anderson 1962).

This chapter is organized as follows: Sect. 20.2 introduces notation and some preliminary remarks. The goodness-of-fit tests for length-biased data are constructed in Sect. 20.3. Section 20.4 provides the necessary algorithms to implement the tests, as well as power simulations. In Sect. 20.5, the methods are illustrated with survival data on dementia collected as part of the Canadian study of health and aging (CSHA) using Weibull, lognormal, and log-logisitic distributions. Finally, discussion of the results is offered in Sect. 20.6.

20.2 Preliminaries and Notation

20.2.1 Length Bias

Suppose we have a random variable, X, with corresponding *cdf* $F_U(x)$. X represents the true, unbiased event times. The length-biased distribution of X, $F_{LB}(x)$, is defined as (Cox 1969)

$$F_{LB}(x) = \frac{1}{\mu} \int_0^x y dF_U(y) \tag{20.1}$$

where $\mu = \int_0^\infty y dF_U(y) < \infty$. F_{LB} arises when a X, with *cdf* F_U, is observed with probability proportional to its length. In the case where F_U has a density f_U the length-biased density can be written as

$$f_{LB}(x) = \frac{x f_U(x)}{\mu} \qquad x \geq 0. \tag{20.2}$$

Suppose we obtain a sample from F_{LB}, $X_1, \ldots, X_n$. The X_i's can be thought of as sampled prevalent (i.e., already diseased) cases, where incidence follows a stationary Poisson process and thus the truncation distribution is uniform over lifetime. An informal test for stationarity was investigated by Asgharian et al. (2006), and the first formal test for stationarity of the incidence rate in prevalent cohort studies was proposed by Addona and Wolfson (2006).

Lifetimes can be split into two segments: the time from disease onset until recruitment into the study (truncation time, T) and the time from study recruitment until the event occurs (residual lifetime, R). Since it is not always possible to follow every individual under study until the event occurs, define C_i to be random residual censoring variables with cdf $F_C(c)$. The observed residual lifetime is such that only the minimum of R_i and C_i is observed, and therefore the ith observed or censored lifetime, X_i, can be represented as

$$X_i = T_i + R_i \wedge C_i. \tag{20.3}$$

δ, the censoring variable can be written as

$$\delta_i = \begin{cases} 1 & \text{if } R_i \leq C_i \\ 0 & \text{if } R_i > C_i. \end{cases} \tag{20.4}$$

Suppose the goal is to nonparametrically estimate $S_U = 1 - F_U$, using a set of full observations (the $(X_i, \delta_i = 1)$ pairs) and censored observations (the pairs $(X_i, \delta_i = 0)$). The likelihood for this setting, derived in Vardi (1989) is

$$L(f_U) = \prod_{i=1}^{n} \left(\frac{f_U(x_i)}{\mu} \right)^{\delta_i} \left(\int_{w \geq x_i} \frac{f_U(w)}{\mu} \right)^{1-\delta_i}, \tag{20.5}$$

where μ is the mean of f_U. An expectation–maximization (EM) algorithm is used to obtain nonparametric point masses at each unique observed time (censored or not), correcting for length bias, which in turn, properly summed, give the NPMLE of $S_U(x)$ (equivalently $F_U(x)$), namely $\hat{S}_V(x)$ ($\hat{F}_V(x)$). Unlike the Kaplan–Meier estimator, it is defined over the entire real line and provides something closer in behavior to the empirical distribution for the purposes of estimation and testing. The same likelihood can be adapted to parametric estimation, by including a family with parameter θ and maximized numerically to obtain $\hat{\theta}$.

For real data analysis, the maximum likelihood estimators arising from length-biased data with right-censoring $\hat{S}_V(x)$ and $\hat{\theta}$ can be obtained through the R package `lbiassurv` (Bergeron et al. 2013). As the nonparametric estimator is consistent for the true distribution (Asgharian et al. 2002) and the parametric estimator is consistent for a correctly specified model (Bergeron et al. 2008), they can be used together to assess goodness of fit of a parametric model.

20.3 Methods

The hypotheses of interest for the goodness-of-fit tests are

$$\begin{aligned} H_0 &: S_U(x) = S^*(x) \\ H_1 &: S_U(x) \neq S^*(x), \end{aligned} \tag{20.6}$$

where $S_U(x)$ is the true (unbiased) survival function from which the data arise and $S^*(x)$ is the hypothesized distribution. In this chapter, we do not assume that $S^*(x)$ is fully specified, only to belong to a particular family but with unspecified parameters, thus $S^*(x) = S^*_\theta(x)$ with θ unknown, though fitting a fully specified distribution is trivially implementable.

The one-sample goodness-of-fit tests we propose can use any suitable parametric model, and three models will be assessed here for the purpose of illustration and implementation: Weibull, lognormal, and log-logistic. The Weibull distribution has survival function:

$$S_{\lambda,\alpha}(x) = \exp\left(-\,(\lambda x)^{\alpha}\right), \quad x, \lambda, \alpha > 0. \tag{20.7}$$

The lognormal distribution survival function:

$$S_{\mu,\sigma^2}(x) = 1 - \Phi\left[\frac{\log x - \mu}{\sigma}\right], \quad x, \sigma^2 > 0, \tag{20.8}$$

where $\Phi(x)$ is the standard normal *cdf*. Finally, the log-logistic distribution has survival function:

$$S_{\lambda,\alpha}(x) = \frac{1}{1 + (\lambda x)^{\alpha}}, \quad x, \lambda, \alpha > 0. \tag{20.9}$$

20.3.1 Kolmogorov Criterion

The Kolmogorov criterion is based on the maximum distance between two distribution functions, and provides a mathematical basis for a graphical assessment: the point of maximum distance can be evaluated visually. With length-biased data, the idea is simply to extend the Kolmogorov statistic, which is defined as the maximum absolute distance between empirical and hypothesized *cdf,* to length-biased data using survival functions.

The proposed Kolmogorov statistic is expressed as

$$D = \sup_x |\hat{S}_V(x) - S^*_{\hat{\theta}}(x)|. \tag{20.10}$$

Obtaining an approximate distribution for D under the null hypothesis becomes a matter of simulating from the length-biased distribution associated with $S^*_{\hat{\theta}}$, taking into account the truncation and censoring mechanisms.

20.3.2 Cramér–von-Mises Criterion

The Cramér–von-Mises criterion is based on integrated squared distance between two curves, in our context yielding the variable:

$$W = n \int_{-\infty}^{\infty} \left[\hat{F}_V(x) - F^*_{\hat{\theta}}(x)\right]^2 dF^*_{\hat{\theta}}(x). \tag{20.11}$$

Equation 20.11 cannot be simplified using order statistics, but it has explicit form for observed data. Suppose the observed times can be expressed as the unique points $x_1 < x_2 < \cdots < x_h$, with NPMLE point masses $\hat{p}_j > 0,\ j = 1, \ldots, h$, $\sum_{j=1}^h \hat{p}_j = 1$. Then we can express the nonparametrically estimated cumulative distribution function by

$$\hat{F}_V(x) = \sum_{j:x_j \le x} \hat{p}_j, \tag{20.12}$$

and let $\hat{F}_j = \hat{F}_V(x_j)$. The Cramér–von-Mises statistic reduces to

$$W = n\left(\frac{1}{3} + F^{*2}_{\hat{\theta}}(x_h) - F^*_{\hat{\theta}}(x_h) + \sum_{j=1}^{h-1} \hat{F}_j \left(F^*_{\hat{\theta}}(x_{j+1}) - F^*_{\hat{\theta}}(x_j)\right)\left(\hat{F}_j - F^*_{\hat{\theta}}(x_{j+1}) - F^*_{\hat{\theta}}(x_j)\right)\right) \tag{20.13}$$

20.4 Approximating the Distributions of D and W

To find critical values for D and W and assess the power of the tests under different conditions, some simulations are necessary.

20.4.1 Algorithms

Efficient simulation of length-biased distributions can be done using transformations for a number of models. For the models of Sect. 20.3, the length-biased Weibull distribution can be obtained through a gamma distribution (Correa and Wolfson 1999), the length-biased lognormal distribution can be obtained through a normal distribution (Patil and Rao 1978), and the length-biased two-parameter log-logistic distribution can be obtained through a beta distribution.

Correa and Wolfson (1999) show how to generate length-biased log-logistic samples, under a one-parameter form reciprocal to (20.9). Below is the algorithm generated from (20.9).

Algorithm 1 Generating Length-Biased Log-Logistic Data

- Generate a $beta(1 - \frac{1}{\alpha}, 1 + \frac{1}{\alpha})$ random variable, Z.
- Take $Y = \left(\frac{1-Z}{\lambda^{\alpha} Z}\right)^{1/\alpha}$.

The random variable Y follows a length-biased log-logistic distribution with parameters α and λ.

See Appendix for details of the proof of this result.

Generating length-biased left-truncated and right-censored data require more steps. As in Asgharian et al. (2002), length-biased sampling is equivalent to uniform left truncation. Generating censoring times can be done in various ways, particularly to match real data. Three different approaches are considered here to investigate how censoring may affect the goodness-of-fit tests. The first is fixed censoring, which takes $C = c$ for some given c, and for NPMLE of $S_U(x)$ this is enough (Vardi 1989). A second approach is to use some known (essentially positive) distribution. In the application of the methods to the CSHA data, the choice taken was a normal distribution with parameters chosen to avoid negative values. The third censoring scheme used relies on nonparametric estimation of the distribution of residual censoring times from the real data set, using Kaplan–Meier estimator.

Algorithm 2 Generating Uniformly Left-Truncated, Right-Censored Data

- Use the data to obtain $\hat{\boldsymbol{\theta}}$, depending on the chosen model. Let n be the original data sample size.
- Generate n length-biased times, $y_1, \ldots, y_n$, from the chosen model.
- For each y_i, generate a truncation time t_i from a $U(0, y_i)$.
- Compute the residual lifetime, r_i, for each observation as $r_i = y_i - t_i$.
- Generate the residual censoring times, $c_1, \ldots, c_n$, using the desired method. Note: this step can be done in parallel to the previous ones.
- Let $x_i = t_i + r_i \wedge c_i$ and $\delta_i = I[r_i \leq c_i]$.

During analysis, it is not necessary to keep track of t_i and r_i, and so the generated data can be reduced to the form (x_i, δ_i).

Note that, under fully specified H_0 with $\theta = \theta_0$ known, one can reduce the length-biased variable generation to a beta (2, 1) (the length-biased distribution associtated

Table 20.1 Approximated critical values

Model	Weibull			Lognormal			Log-logistic		
Sample size	$\alpha =$ 0.10	$\alpha =$ 0.05	$\alpha =$ 0.01	$\alpha =$ 0.10	$\alpha =$ 0.05	$\alpha =$ 0.01	$\alpha =$ 0.10	$\alpha =$ 0.05	$\alpha =$ 0.01
30	0.290	0.345	0.479	0.186	0.203	0.237	0.198	0.220	0.269
100	0.199	0.227	0.369	0.117	0.130	0.151	0.121	0.135	0.170
250	0.136	0.162	0.261	0.074	0.081	0.096	0.077	0.087	0.107
500	0.106	0.125	0.203	0.052	0.058	0.066	0.056	0.063	0.079
1000	0.080	0.092	0.130	0.038	0.042	0.050	0.040	0.044	0.055

with the uniform(0,1)) via the probability integral transform. For large samples, as censoring appears to have negligible effect, using constant censoring giving the desired censoring rate will reduce computation time. Also, for fully specified models, the smaller D or W, the better the fit. With unspecified parameters, the null distributions of these statistics are no longer distribution free and require simulations based on $\hat{\theta}$ fitted from the data.

20.4.2 Critical Values

Using algorithm 2, $\hat{S}_V(x)$ and $S^*_{\hat{\theta}}(x)$ (equivalently, $\hat{F}_V$ and $F^*_{\hat{\theta}}$ for W) and thus d_j or w_j for $j = 1, \ldots, K$ for some large K, can be obtained. One can then pick the appropriate critical value based on the order statistic of $d_1, \ldots, d_K$ $(w_1, \ldots, w_K)$ and compare with the data.

Note that the critical values will depend not only on sample size (and theoretically censoring scheme) but also on $\hat{\theta}$ if θ is estimated, and will vary from model to model and from different data sets. This may affect power, as it is shown for different shape parameters of the Weibull in Sect. 20.6.

20.4.2.1 Kolmogorov Test

To illustrate this, Table 20.1 gives approximate critical values for different significance levels for Weibull, lognormal, and log-logistic distributions, using samples with approximately 20 % of censored observations and $\hat{\theta}$ taken from the CSHA data. Sample sizes of 30, 100, 250, 500, and 1000 were considered.

Censoring schemes giving 5 and 50 % censored observations were implemented, but it seemed to have little effect on the critical values; thus, the tables are omitted. It can be noted that the Weibull distribution has the largest critical values for all sample sizes which would reduce the power of the test.

Table 20.2 Approximate critical values for W

Sample size	Weibull data			Lognormal data		
	$\alpha = 0.10$	$\alpha = 0.05$	$\alpha = 0.01$	$\alpha = 0.10$	$\alpha = 0.05$	$\alpha = 0.01$
30	0.495	0.696	1.407	0.171	0.208	0.327
100	0.719	1.049	4.131	0.177	0.215	0.280
250	0.883	1.384	3.474	0.170	0.208	0.309
500	1.000	1.518	3.334	0.181	0.223	0.332
1000	1.085	1.658	4.870	0.179	0.214	0.316

20.4.2.2 Cramér–von-Mises Test

For Weibull and lognormal models (log-logistic skipped, see Remarks), Table 20.2 approximated critical values for the Cramér–von-Mises statistic under similar scenarios.

We notice here that, since the statistic is normalized by sample size, the critical values increase with sample size with the Weibull distribution. For lognormal distribution, they appear quite stable. Again, the Weibull critical values are much larger, so a worse visual fit may not translate to a worse actual fit.

20.4.3 Power Computations

To obtain power estimates, one needs to obtain $\hat{\theta}$ and the critical values from the null hypothesis, but generate data from an alternative distribution. Simulations were performed using $\hat{\theta}$ from the CSHA data and the sample size and critical values from the previous section. The following tables give power estimates at different significance levels for chosen null distributions against "true" alternatives. Since these tables are not distribution free, they are constrained to scenarios with approximately 20 % censoring, though scenarios with light and heavy censoring were implemented as well. Generally, power decreases with amount of censoring.

20.4.3.1 Kolmogorov Test

Tables 20.3–20.5 provide some approximated power levels at different sample sizes for Kolmogorov test.

20.4.3.2 Cramér–von-Mises Test

Table 20.6 gives approximate power for the Cramér–von-Mises test for Weibull and lognormal null hypothesis when the true distributions are lognormal and Weibull.

Table 20.3 Power of Kolmogorov test when H_0 is Weibull

Weibull H_0	Lognormal data			Log-logistic data		
Sample size	$1-\beta_{0.10}$	$1-\beta_{0.05}$	$1-\beta_{0.01}$	$1-\beta_{0.10}$	$1-\beta_{0.05}$	$1-\beta_{0.01}$
30	0.675	0.608	0.462	0.866	0.822	0.680
100	0.966	0.953	0.901	0.998	0.996	0.994
250	1.000	1.000	0.998	1.000	1.000	1.000
500	1.000	1.000	1.000	1.000	1.000	1.000
1000	1.000	1.000	1.000	1.000	1.000	1.000

Table 20.4 Power of Kolmogorov test when H_0 is lognormal

Lognormal H_0	Weibull data			Log-logistic data		
Sample size	$1-\beta_{0.10}$	$1-\beta_{0.05}$	$1-\beta_{0.01}$	$1-\beta_{0.10}$	$1-\beta_{0.05}$	$1-\beta_{0.01}$
30	0.116	0.067	0.018	0.234	0.150	0.068
100	0.198	0.113	0.014	0.447	0.327	0.143
250	0.443	0.241	0.024	0.780	0.647	0.383
500	0.731	0.474	0.045	0.960	0.902	0.666
1000	0.983	0.991	0.336	0.999	0.996	0.979

Table 20.5 Power of Kolmogorov test when H_0 is log-logistic

Log-logistic H_0	Weibull data			Lognormal data		
Sample size	$1-\beta_{0.10}$	$1-\beta_{0.05}$	$1-\beta_{0.01}$	$1-\beta_{0.10}$	$1-\beta_{0.05}$	$1-\beta_{0.01}$
30	0.200	0.121	0.033	0.179	0.122	0.048
100	0.454	0.274	0.034	0.253	0.170	0.067
250	0.860	0.643	0.075	0.571	0.464	0.212
500	0.990	0.939	0.224	0.848	0.753	0.569
1000	1.000	1.000	0.965	0.986	0.957	0.849

Table 20.6 Approximate power of Cramér–von-Mises test

	Weibull H_0, lognormal data			Lognormal H_0, Weibull data		
Sample size	$1-\beta_{0.10}$	$1-\beta_{0.05}$	$1-\beta_{0.01}$	$1-\beta_{0.10}$	$1-\beta_{0.05}$	$1-\beta_{0.01}$
30	0.625	0.538	0.392	0.077	0.044	0.012
100	0.951	0.931	0.888	0.164	0.084	0.011
250	0.999	0.998	0.994	0.437	0.215	0.021
500	1.000	1.000	1.000	0.798	0.504	0.043
1000	1.000	1.000	1.000	0.995	0.970	0.275

The simulation results are generally as expected. Power increases with sample size, and a Weibull survival curve will not fit log-logistic and lognormal data well at any sample size. Both tests appear to have similar power under the same scenarios. However, the tests have low power for testing a lognormal distribution against Weibull data, even at large sample size, and distinguishing between lognormal and log-logistic is difficult for even relatively large sample sizes. Fortunately, power appears to be satisfactory for sample sizes similar to that of the phase 1 CSHA data.

20.5 CSHA Data Analysis

The CSHA was a longitudinal study of the epidemiology of dementia and other health problems affecting the elderly across Canada. The CSHA had many aims, including estimating the prevalence and incidence of dementia among the elderly, investigating the risk factors for Alzheimer's disease, as well as estimating the survival distribution from onset of those with dementia. The study has undergone three phases, with the first phase beginning in 1991 (CSHA-1), the second phase in 1996 (CSHA-2), and the third phase in 2001 (CSHA-3).

During the first phase, 10,263 individuals aged 65 and above were recruited cross-sectionally. Those who screened positive for dementia were included in the final sample of prevalent cases and then followed until the second phase of the study in 1996. The final sample included 816 possibly censored survival times. The phase 1 portion of the CSHA was used here. The approximate date of onset of dementia, date of death or censoring, as well as the death indicator were used in estimating the survival function. Stationarity assumption was verified by both Asgharian et al. (2006) and Addona and Wolfson (2006), neither could reject length bias. Wolfson et al. (2001) reported an adjusted median survival of 3.3 years when correcting for length bias (this was done using Kaplan–Meier for truncated data, the NPMLE yields a median survival of 3.95 years correcting for length bias, and more in line with incident studies of dementia such as Xie et al. (2008), contrasted with median survival times varying from 5 to 9.3 years as suggested by previous studies.

Figure 20.1 shows both the unbiased and length-biased nonparametric survival estimates, using Vardi's algorithm. The importance of correcting for length bias is readily observed.

Weibull, lognormal, and log-logistic models were fitted for the CSHA data. Table 20.7 contains the d and w values, estimated model parameters, along with their standard deviation and confidence intervals, for each model. The graph of the survival curves is in Fig. 20.2.

Note that the median lifetimes are 3.57, 3.97, and 4.22 years for the Weibull, lognormal and log-logistic models, respectively. Figure 20.2 shows the nonparametric estimate for the CSHA data with each fitted parametric curve, for survival up to 15 years.

From a pure, Kolmogorov distance or Cramér–von-Mises criterion point of view, the lognormal model is the closest to the nonparametric curve with the smallest values

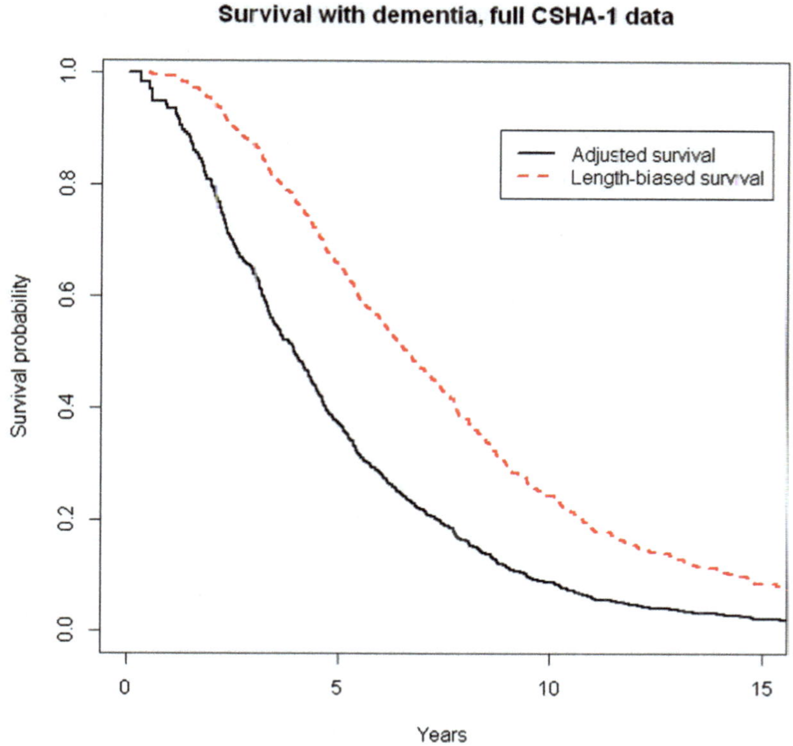

Fig. 20.1 Biased and unbiased nonparametric estimates of $S(x)$

Table 20.7 Canadian study of health and aging (CSHA) parameter estimates

Model	d	w	Estimate	SD	CI
Weibull	0.096	1.956	$\lambda = 0.207$	0.009	(0.189, 0.225)
			$\alpha = 1.215$	0.046	(1.125, 1.305)
Lognormal	0.065	0.744	$\mu = 1.378$	0.033	(1.313, 1.443)
			$\sigma = 0.679$	0.018	(0.644, 0.715)
Log-logistic	0.124	3.044	$\lambda = 0.237$	0.007	(0.223, 0.250)
			$\alpha = 2.808$	0.075	(2.660, 2.955)

SD standard deviation, *CI* confidence interval

of D and W. Here, estimated p values are presented using 10,000 simulated data sets for each model and censoring scheme using five different censoring schemes. Two simulations used a fixed censoring scheme with values of $c_1 = 5.2$ and $c_2 = 5.8$ years representing a constant follow-up from beginning of study. The next two scenarios used a random normal censoring with $\mu_1 = 5.2$, $\sigma_1 = 0.3$ and $\mu_2 = 5.8$, $\sigma_2 = 0.6$, respectively. This reflects actual variation in recruitment date and end of follow-up

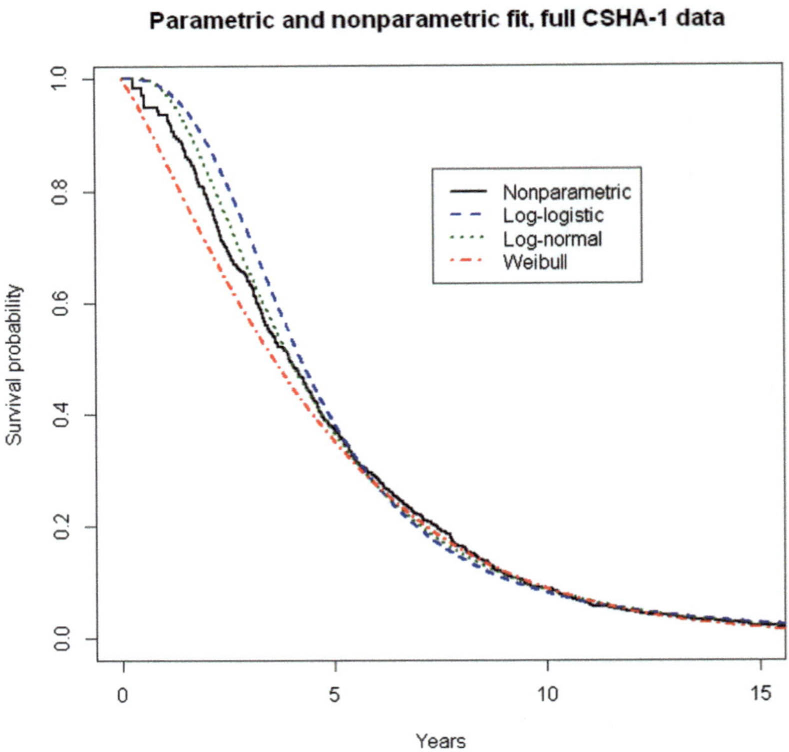

Fig. 20.2 Nonparametric and parametric survival curves

Table 20.8 p Values estimated by simulation for Kolmogorov test

Censoring approach	Weibull	Lognormal	Log-logistic
Fixed C=5.2	0.0556	0.0015	0.0000
Fixed C=5.8	0.0576	0.0008	0.0000
Normal (5.2,0.3)	0.0550	0.0011	0.0000
Normal (5.8,0.3)	0.0544	0.0010	0.0000
KM	0.0550	0.0007	0.0000

KM Kaplan–Meier

of the CSHA. The mean values were based on the data, where 5.2 is closer to average follow-up, but yields higher censoring proportion in simulated samples, while 5.8 years provides censoring proportion similar to that of CSHA-1. The fifth censoring scheme samples values from the real residual censoring times in the CSHA data based on Kaplan–Meier estimate of the residual censoring distribution. Results are given in Table 20.8.

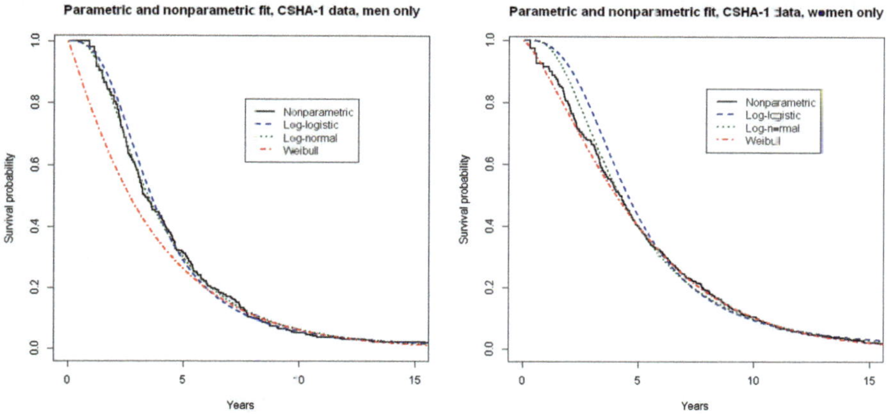

Fig. 20.3 Nonparametric and parametric survival curves by gender

Table 20.9 Canadian study of health and aging (CSHA) parameter estimates for men only subsample

Model	*d*	*w*	Estimate	SD	CI
Weibull	0.222	3.799	$\lambda = 0.265$	0.026	(0.215, 0.315)
			$\alpha = 1.053$	0.071	(0.913, 1.192)
Lognormal	0.033	0.039	$\mu = 1.244$	0.063	(1.120, 1.369)
			$\sigma = 0.692$	0.034	(0.625, 0.758)
Log-logistic	0.076	0.268	$\lambda = 0.277$	0.015	(0.243, 0.307)
			$\alpha = 2.756$	0.129	(2.503, 3.009)

SD standard deviation, *CI* confidence interval

From Table 20.8, lognormal and log-logistic models do not fit the data. However, at a 5 % significance level the Weibull model cannot be rejected, but it is a borderline result. It is also clear from the simulation results that the different approaches to censoring have negligible effects. Similarly, for Cramér–von-Mises, estimated p values are approximately 0.077 for Weibull and < 0.0001 for lognormal. The paradoxical result of closest visual fit for lognormal, but Weibull having the largest p value demands further investigation. As data on the gender of each patient was available, it was decided to perform separate analyses for men and women. There were 237 men and 579 women in CSHA-1. Fitting all three models on each, the best fit (smallest distance and largest p value) were Weibull for women (approximate p value 0.57) and lognormal for men ($p \approx 0.97$). The survival curves for each group are given in Fig. 20.3, while the parameter estimates are in Tables 20.9 and 20.10.

There are two different distributions, the mixture of which could explain the paradoxical results for the full sample: women outnumber men, which would pull the overall survival curve towards the Weibull model, but the shorter lived lognormal men better capture the early part of the survival curve, thus giving the closer Kolmogorov

Table 20.10 Canadian study of health and aging (CSHA) parameter estimates for women only subsample

Model	*d*	*w*	Estimate	SD	CI
Weibull	0.049	0.216	$\lambda = 0.187$	0.009	(0.169, 0.204)
			$\alpha = 1.313$	0.059	(1.196, 1.429)
Lognormal	0.094	0.999	$\mu = 1.440$	0.038	(1.365, 1.516)
			$\sigma = 0.668$	0.021	(0.626, 0.709)
Log-logistic	0.155	3.087	$\lambda = 0.220$	0.007	(0.205, 0.234)
			$\alpha = 2.871$	0.090	(2.694, 3.048)

SD standard deviation, *CI* confidence interval

distance and smaller Cramér–von-Mises statistic of the lognormal fit on the whole sample. Seeing different distributions by gender also falls within epidemiological conventional wisdom of treating men and women separately, and would suggest further investigation of how dementia affects the different genders.

20.6 Remarks

1. The proposed one-sample goodness-of-fit tests for length-biased survival data are based on simple extensions of the Kolmogorov test and Cramér–von-Mises statistic. They rely heavily on computational techniques and simulations which are easily implemented using statistical software, particularly the `lbiassurv` package in R. The illustration using the CSHA data carries one main message: *a good visual fit is not sufficient*. While Bergeron et al. (2008) had used a Weibull model based on visual fit, the new proposed test suggests that further investigation was required, and performing separate analyses for different genders may be warranted. It should be noted, however, for the CSHA, that separating by gender made two smaller samples out of the original large sample, and that for the subsample of men, the power to distinguish between lognormal curve on Weibull data is quite low. However, testing for a Weibull model gives an approximate p value of 0.022; thus, the power issue may no bet so essential in this case. A larger sample size would be needed to confirm.
2. It should be noted that simulating from the length-biased log-logistic distribution can sometimes yield unrealistically small observations that result in two problems. First, the NPMLE for such a sample is no longer representative of the true distribution as the length-bias correction makes the survival function's first step to be a large drop close to time zero. Second, in the presence of such outlying observations, maximizing the parametric likelihood may not work using standard numerical optimization, and will result in crash of the null distribution simulation program if not accounted once the simulated data are generated. A simple remedy to that is to always check for tiny outliers in simulated data sets and to resample

them before estimation. This correction will influence approximated quantities making them less volatile than the truth, but a slightly flawed approximation is better than none.

3. The flexibility of the Weibull model for the tests brings its own issues, mainly with respect to power and sampling from the left-hand tail of the distribution. When the shape parameter α is close to (or below) 1, there is constant (or decreasing) hazard that results in a fast-dropping survival function which may be well below the NPMLE, or have an NPMLE well below the fitted parametric curve for simulated data sets as short even times are possible even with length-biased sampling due to the shape of the hazard. This translates to more volatility of the Kolmogorov and Cramér–von-Mises statistics under the null. For example, for a sample size of 100 with 20 % censoring, at a given rate and significance level of 0.05, the approximate critical value for the Kolmogorov test goes from 0.51 to 0.27 and 0.14 as the shape parameter doubles from 0.5 to 1.0 and 2.0. Doubling the rate at a fixed shape, however, raises the critical value on the order of 0.01 instead. Since the CSHA data have estimated Weibull shape parameter in the upper vicinity of 1, not quite an exponential distribution but not that far from constant hazard, it is not surprising that we observe large deviation between the NPMLE and the Weibull estimated curve.
4. That separate parametric forms are obtained for men and women from the CSHA data suggests that one should be careful in implementing regression models, as it suggests nonproportional hazard between the two groups. Weibull naturally conforms to both proportional hazards (PH) and accelerated failure time (AFT) models, the former allowing elimination of the parametric assumption on the baseline in favor of a semiparametric Cox model adapted for length-biased data as in Qin and Shen (2010). The lognormal model only works well with AFT. Further discussion of how AFT models are naturally suited for length-biased data can be found in Mandel and Ritov (2010).
5. Development and extensions of the tests are possible. Using a mixture model with a fixed covariate, taking into account covariate bias (Bergeron et al. 2008), could perhaps improve performing separate analyses for the gender subsamples. Development of an Anderson–Darling test (Anderson and Darling 1954) using Vardi's NPMLE would be straight forward, but including a weight of $[F(x)(1 - F(x))]^{-1}$ that increases in the tails should be carefully considered with length-biased data, as the left-hand tail will be subject to more variability than the right-hand tail, where most of the data will be, as short observed times have more impact on the bias correction. Adaptation of weights similar to Harrington–Fleming (Harrington and Fleming 1982) may yield better results.

20.7 Appendix

20.7.1 Length-Biased Log-Logistic

The two parameter log-logistic has the following pdf and mean:

$$f(x) = \frac{\alpha\lambda^{\alpha}x^{\alpha-1}}{[1+(\lambda x)^{\alpha}]^2}. \tag{20.14}$$

$$\mu = \frac{\pi \csc\left(\frac{\pi}{\alpha}\right)}{\alpha\lambda}. \tag{20.15}$$

The mean, μ, can be represented using the gamma function if $\alpha > 1$:

$$\mu = \frac{\pi \csc\left(\frac{\pi}{\alpha}\right)}{\alpha\lambda} = \frac{\pi}{\alpha\lambda \sin\left(\frac{\pi}{\alpha}\right)} = \frac{\frac{1}{\alpha}\Gamma\left(\frac{1}{\alpha}\right)\Gamma\left(1-\frac{1}{\alpha}\right)}{\lambda} = \frac{\Gamma\left(1+\frac{1}{\alpha}\right)\Gamma\left(1-\frac{1}{\alpha}\right)}{\lambda}. \tag{20.16}$$

The length-biased density for a log-logistic random variable is given by

$$F_Y(t) = \int_0^t \frac{\alpha\lambda \exp[\alpha \log(\lambda x)]}{\Gamma\left(1+\frac{1}{\alpha}\right)\Gamma\left(1-\frac{1}{\alpha}\right)(1+\exp[\alpha\log(\lambda x)])^2}\,dx \tag{20.17}$$

Taking $z = \alpha \log(\lambda x)$, we obtain

$$F_Y(t) = \int_{-\infty}^{\alpha\log(\lambda t)} \frac{\exp\left(z(1+\frac{1}{\alpha})\right)}{\Gamma(1+\frac{1}{\alpha})\Gamma(1-\frac{1}{\alpha})(1+\exp(z))^2}\,dz \tag{20.18}$$

Letting $u = (1+e^z)^{-1}$, we obtain

$$F_Y(t) = \int_{(1+\exp[\alpha\log(\lambda t)])^{-1}}^{1} \frac{u^{-1/\alpha}(1-u)^{1/\alpha}}{\Gamma\left(1+\frac{1}{\alpha}\right)\Gamma\left(1-\frac{1}{\alpha}\right)}\,du \tag{20.19}$$

$F_Y(t)$ can be written as $F_Z(h(t))$, where F_Z is the distribution of a beta$(1-\frac{1}{\alpha}, 1+\frac{1}{\alpha})$ random variable and $h(t) = (1+\exp[\alpha\log(\lambda t)])^{-1} = \frac{1}{1+(\lambda x)^{\alpha}}$. $h(t)$ is nonnegative, strictly decreasing, and continuous. Its inverse is given by

$$g(s) = \frac{\left(\frac{1-s}{s}\right)^{1/\alpha}}{\lambda}. \tag{20.20}$$

Acknowledgments The data used in this chapter were collected as part of the Canadian Study of Health and Aging. The core study was funded by the Seniors' Independence Research Program, through the National Health Research and Development Program (NHRDP) of Health Canada (project no. 6606-3954-MC(S). Additional funding was provided by Pfizer Canada Incorporated through the Medical Research Council/Pharmaceutical Manufacturers Association of Canada Health Activity Program, NHRDP (project no. 6603-1417-302(R)), Bayer Incorporated, and the British Columbia Health Research Foundation (projects no. 38 (93-2) and no. 34 (96-1)). The study was coordinated through the University of Ottawa and the Division of Aging and Seniors, Health Canada.

References

Addona V, Wolfson DB (2006) A formal test for stationarity of the incidence rate using data from a prevalent cohort study with follow-up. Lifetime Data Anal 12:267–284

Anderson TW, Darling DA (1954) A test of goodness-of-fit. J Am Stat Assoc 49:765–769

Anderson TW (1962) On the distribution of the two-sample Cramér-von-Mises criterion. Ann Math Stat 33:1148–1159

Asgharian M, MLan CE, Wolfson D (2002) Length-biased sampling with right censoring: an unconditional approach. J Am Stat Assoc 97:201–209

Asgharian M, Wolfson DB, Zhang X (2006) Checking stationarity of the incidence rate using prevalent cohort survival data. Stat Med 25:1751–1767

Bergeron P-J, Ashgarian M, Wolfson DB (2008) Covariates bias induced by length-biased sampling of failure times. J Am Stat Assoc 103:737–742

Bergeron P-J, Partovi Nia V (2013) lbiassurv: length-biased correction to survival curve estimation. http://cran.r-project.org/web/packages/lbiassurv/index.html. Accessed 13 Aug 2014

Correa JA, Wolfson DB (1999) Length-bias: some characterizations and applications. J Stat Comput Sim 64:209–219

Cox DR (1969) Some sampling problems in technology. In: Johnson NL, Smith H Jr (eds) New developments in survey sampling, pp 506–527. Wiley-Interscience, New York

Harrington DP, Fleming TR (1982) A class of rank test procedures for censored survival data. Biometrika 69:133–143

Mandel M, Ritov Y (2010) The accelerated failure time model under biased sampling. Biometrics doi:10.1111/j.1467-9868.2010.00742.x

Patil GP, Rao CR (1978) Weighted distributions and size-biased sampling with applications to wildlife population and human families. Biometrics 34: 179–189

Qin J, Shen Y (2010) Statistical methods for analyzing right-censored length-biased data under Cox model. Biometrics 66:382–392

Vardi Y (1989) Multiplicative censoring, renewal processes, deconvolution and decreased density: nonparametric estimation. Biometrika 76:751–761

Wang MC (1991) Nonparametric estimation from cross-sectional survival data. J Am Stat Assoc 86:130–143

Wolfson C, Wolfson DB, Asgharian M, M'Lan CE, Ostbye T, Rockwood K, Hogan DB (2001) A reevaluation of the duration of survival after the onset of dementia. New Engl J Med 344:1111–1116

Xie J, Brayne C, Matthews FE (2008) Survival times in people with dementia: analysis from population based cohort study with 14 year follow-up. Brit Med J 336:258–262

Chapter 21
Assessment of Fit in Longitudinal Data for Joint Models with Applications to Cancer Clinical Trials

Danjie Zhang, Ming-Hui Chen, Joseph G. Ibrahim, Mark E. Boye, and Wei Shen

Abstract Joint models for longitudinal and survival data have now become increasingly popular in clinical trials or other studies for assessing a treatment effect while accounting for longitudinal measures such as patient-reported outcomes or tumor response. Most studies in the existing literature primarily focus on reducing the bias and improving efficiency in the estimate of the treatment effect in the joint modeling of survival and longitudinal data. Global fit indices such as Akaike information criterion (AIC) or Bayesian information criterion (BIC) can be used to assess the overall fit of the joint model. However, these indices do not provide separate assessments of each component of the joint model. In this chapter, we develop new model assessment criteria using a novel decomposition of AIC and BIC (i.e., $\text{AIC} = \text{AIC}_{\text{Surv}} + \text{AIC}_{\text{Long}|\text{Surv}}$ and $\text{BIC} = \text{BIC}_{\text{Surv}} + \text{BIC}_{\text{Long}|\text{Surv}}$) to assess the contribution of the survival data to the model fit of the longitudinal data. We apply the proposed methodology to the analysis of a real dataset from a cancer clinical trial in mesothelioma.

D. Zhang (✉)
Gilead Sciences, Inc.,
333 Lakeside Drive, Foster City, CA 94404, USA
e-mail: danjie.zhang@gilead.com

M.-H. Chen
Department of Statistics, University of Connecticut,
215 Glenbrook Road, U-4120, Storrs, CT 06269, USA
e-mail: ming-hui.chen@uconn.edu

J. G. Ibrahim
Department of Biostatistics, University of North Carolina,
McGavran Greenberg Hall, CB#7420, Chapel Hill, NC 27599, USA
e-mail: ibrahim@bios.unc.edu

M. E. Boye · W. Shen
Eli Lilly and Company, Lilly Corporate Center,
Indianapolis, IN 46285, USA
e-mail: boyema@lilly.com

W. Shen
e-mail: shen@lilly.com

Z. Chen et al. (eds.), *Applied Statistics in Biomedicine and Clinical Trials Design*,
ICSA Book Series in Statistics, DOI 10.1007/978-3-319-12694-4_21

21.1 Introduction

Joint modeling of longitudinal and survival data has now established a long history and is becoming a well-accepted standard in analyzing time to event data with longitudinal outcomes that are potentially associated with a time to event such as overall survival (OS) or progression-free survival in oncology studies, for example. Longitudinal outcomes such as patient reported outcomes (PROs) in oncology studies (Rothman et al. 2009) are now routinely collected to help assess a patient's quality of life (QOL), especially when toxic chemotherapies are administered. Such information is crucial in helping to assess the QOL versus efficacy benefit in such studies. Longitudinal and survival data are also collected in vaccine trials, where patients are administered a vaccine longitudinally and the goal is to determine the relationship between the immune response and the time to event such as OS (Brown and Ibrahim 2003a; Brown and Ibrahim 2003b; Chen et al. 2004; Ibrahim et al. 2004). Such data are also collected in HIV vaccine trials, where the focus is on jointly modeling of survival data and univariate or multivariate longitudinal CD4 counts (Pawitan and Self 1993; DeGruttola and Tu 1994; LaValley and DeGruttola 1996). Often in these joint modeling settings, the longitudinal outcome is viewed as a surrogate and the hope is that it will be highly associated with the time to event in order to reduce bias and yield higher efficiency in the estimate of the treatment effect.

There has been a substantial literature on joint models in which the goal is to incorporate the longitudinal marker in order to assess the association between the longitudinal marker and a time to event for the purposes of planning future trials, to develop a better understanding of the biology of the disease, and to also help reduce bias and yield greater efficiency in assessing the treatment effect. See the papers by Hsieh et al. (2006), Ibrahim et al. (2010), Chen et al. (2011), Hatfield et al. (2011), Wang et al. (2012), and Hatfield et al. (2012) for a discussion of this. However, very little has been done in assessing the goodness of fit of a joint model, which is a crucial issue in joint modeling, since there are so many assumptions and modeling components in these models. First, there is the assumption of the form of the longitudinal mixed model along with assumptions about its error distribution, random effects structure, and the covariates. Second, there is the crucial assumption regarding the form of the survival model: (i) whether it is parametric or semiparametric, (ii) the form of the hazard, whether it is proportional or nonproportional hazards, (iii) the choice of random effects and covariate structure in the survival model, and (iv) the form of the association parameters between the longitudinal and survival model. Related to all this, there are also the important issues of assessing the goodness of fit for the individual contributions of the joint model, that is, assessing the fit of the longitudinal and survival components separately, as well as assessing the gain in fit of the survival component given the longitudinal component and vice versa. All of these issues need to be carefully examined through the development of appropriate goodness of fit statistics and model diagnostic measures. Such model diagnostic measures have been proposed in Zhu et al. (2012).

There has been very little development on goodness-of-fit statistics for joint models addressing the above-mentioned issues. In this chapter, we use the well-known criteria Akaike information criterion (AIC) and Bayesian information criterion (BIC) to help assess the fit of a joint model. To help assess the individual components in a joint model, we employ a novel decomposition of these measures by appropriately factoring the joint density of the longitudinal and survival outcome in such a way that allows us to assess the contribution of the survival data to the model fit of the longitudinal data. This will yield a decomposition of AIC (BIC) as $\text{AIC} = \text{AIC}_{\text{Surv}} + \text{AIC}_{\text{Long}|\text{Surv}}$ ($\text{BIC} = \text{BIC}_{\text{Surv}} + \text{BIC}_{\text{Long}|\text{Surv}}$). These decompositions are novel and quite useful in assessing the contributions of each component in a joint model. This type of decomposition is most useful in the setting where the main goal is to make inferences on the parameters in the longitudinal model while using the information in the survival model. Thus, in this context, the hope is that the inclusion of the survival model may improve the inferences and result in a better goodness of fit in the longitudinal model compared to fitting the longitudinal model alone. Similarly, one can also perform the decomposition the other way in which $\text{AIC} = \text{AIC}_{\text{Long}} + \text{AIC}_{\text{Surv}|\text{Long}}$ and $\text{BIC} = \text{BIC}_{\text{Long}} + \text{BIC}_{\text{Surv Long}}$, and in this case, the main goal is to make inferences about the parameters in the survival model while using the information in the longitudinal model. Thus, in this context, the hope is that the inclusion of the longitudinal data may improve the inferences and result in better goodness of fit in the survival model compared to fitting the survival model alone (see Zhang et al. 2014).

The rest of this chapter is organized as follows. In Sect. 21.2, we give the general layout of the joint model by giving general forms of the longitudinal and survival components of the model, and also give the form of the likelihood function of the joint model. In Sect. 21.3, we derive the novel decompositions of AIC and BIC and discuss their advantages and their use in practice. In Sect. 21.5, we present a detailed analysis of a randomized lung cancer clinical trial in mesothelioma where the goal is to assess several PRO measures and their association with progression-free survival. A detailed analysis of these data helped us identify which PRO measures yield the most improved fit in the longitudinal model when the survival data are included in the model. We conclude the chapter with some discussion in Sect. 21.6.

21.2 The Joint Models of Longitudinal and Survival Data

Let $Y(a)$ denote the longitudinal measure at time a for $a \geq 0$, where $Y(0)$ corresponds to the baseline value. Let T denote the failure time. In addition, let z denote the treatment indicator with $z = 1$ for the treatment and $z = 0$ for the control, and let x denote the p-dimensional vector of covariates. We consider the joint model for $(Y(a), T)$, which consists of the longitudinal component and the survival component presented in following subsections.

21.2.1 The Longitudinal Component of the Joint Model

We assume a mixed effects regression model for the longitudinal outcome $Y(a)$, which is given by

$$Y(a) = \theta_R' g(a) + \gamma_1 z + \gamma_2' x + \varepsilon(a), \tag{21.1}$$

where $g(a) = (1, a, a^2, \ldots, a^q)'$ is a polynomial vector of order q, θ_R is a $(q+1)$-dimensional vector of random effects, and γ_2 is a p-dimensional vector of regression coefficients. In (21.1), we further assume

$$\theta_R \sim N(\theta, \Sigma),$$

where θ is the $(q+1)$-dimensional vector of overall effects, Σ is a $(q+1)\times(q+1)$ positive definite covariance matrix, $\varepsilon(a) \sim N(0, \sigma^2)$, and θ_R and $\varepsilon(a)$ are independent. We note that in (21.1), if $q = 1$, $g(a) = (1, a)'$ and $\theta_R' g(a)$ represents a linear trajectory, and if $q = 2$, $g(a) = (1, a, a^2)'$ and $\theta_R' g(a)$ leads to a quadratic trajectory.

21.2.2 The Survival Component of the Joint Model

For the failure time T, the hazard function is assumed to be of the general form:

$$\begin{aligned} &\lambda(t|\lambda_0, \beta, \alpha, \theta_R, g(t), \gamma, z, x) \\ &= \lambda_0(t) \exp\{h(\beta, \theta_R, g(t), \gamma_1 z, \gamma_2' x) + \alpha_1 z + \alpha_2' x\}, \end{aligned} \tag{21.2}$$

where $\lambda_0(t)$ is the baseline hazard function, $h(\cdot)$ is a linear function of θ_R, $g(t)$, $\gamma_1 z$, and $\gamma_2' x$ with β being a vector of the corresponding regression coefficients, $\gamma = (\gamma_1, \gamma_2')'$, and $\alpha = (\alpha_1, \alpha_2')'$. Note that in (21.2), θ_R, $g(t)$, γ_1, and γ_2 are the parameters or the functions from the longitudinal component of the joint model in (21.1), and λ_0, β, α_1 and α_2 are the fixed effects parameters pertaining to the survival component. When

$$h(\beta, \theta_R, g(t), \gamma_1 z, \gamma_2' x) = h^*(\beta, \theta_R' g(t), \gamma_1 z, \gamma_2' x), \tag{21.3}$$

where $h^*(\cdot)$ is a linear function of $\theta_R' g(t)$, $\gamma_1 z$, and $\gamma_2' x$, (21.2) leads to the trajectory model (TM). In this case, the hazard function depends on θ_R and g only through $\theta_R' g$. When h does not depend on $g(t)$, that is, $h(\beta, \theta_R, g(t), \gamma_1 z, \gamma_2' x) = h^*(\beta, \theta_R, \gamma_1 z, \gamma_2' x)$, where $h^*(\cdot)$ is a linear function of θ_R, $\gamma_1 z$, and $\gamma_2' x_i$, (21.2) reduces to the shared parameter model (SPM).

In (21.2), we take $\lambda_0(t)$ to be piecewise constant, i.e.,

$$\lambda_0(t) = \lambda_k, \quad t \in (s_{k-1}, s_k] \text{ for } k = 1, \ldots, K, \tag{21.4}$$

where $0 = s_0 < s_1 < s_2 < \ldots < s_{K-1} < s_K = \infty$ is a finite partition of the time axis.

21.2.3 The Likelihood Functions

Suppose there are n subjects. For the ith subject, the observed longitudinal measures are denoted by $Y_i = (Y_i(a_{i1}), \ldots, Y_i(a_{im_i}))'$, where $a_{i1} = 0 < a_{i2} < \cdots < a_{im_i}$ and $m_i > 1$. Let t_i and δ_i denote the failure time and the censoring indicator, respectively, where $\delta_i = 1$ if t_i is a failure time and 0 if t_i is right censored for the ith subject. In addition, let z_i, x_i, and θ_{Ri} be the treatment indicator, the p-dimensional vector of covariates, and the $(q + 1)$-dimensional vector of random effects. Write $W_i = ((g(a_{ij})', z_i, x_i')', j = 1, \ldots, m_i)'$. Then, given θ_{Ri}, the complete data likelihood function of the longitudinal outcomes can be written as

$$
\begin{aligned}
&L(\gamma, \sigma^2 | Y_i, W_i, \theta_{Ri}) \\
&= \frac{1}{(2\pi\sigma^2)^{\frac{m_i}{2}}} \exp\Big\{-\frac{1}{2\sigma^2}(Y_i - W_i(\theta_{Ri}', \gamma')')'(Y_i - W_i(\theta_{Ri}', \gamma')')\Big\}
\end{aligned} \tag{21.5}
$$

and the complete data likelihood function for the survival component is given by

$$
\begin{aligned}
L(\lambda, \beta, \alpha | t_i, \delta_i, z_i, x_i, \theta_{Ri}, g, \gamma) &= [\lambda(t_i | \lambda_0, \beta, \alpha, \theta_{Ri}, g(t_i), \gamma, z_i, x_i)]^{\delta_i} \\
&\times \exp\left\{-\int_0^{t_i} \lambda(u | \lambda_0, \beta, \alpha, \theta_{Ri}, g(u), \gamma, z_i, x_i) du\right\},
\end{aligned} \tag{21.6}
$$

where $\lambda = (\lambda_1, \ldots, \lambda_K)'$ and $\lambda(t | \lambda_0, \beta, \alpha, \theta_{Ri}, g(t), \gamma, z_i, x_i)$ is given in (21.2). The density of θ_{Ri} takes the form

$$
f(\theta_{Ri} | \theta, \Sigma) = \frac{|\Sigma|^{-\frac{1}{2}}}{(2\pi)^{\frac{q+1}{2}}} \exp\Big\{-\frac{1}{2}(\theta_{Ri} - \theta)' \Sigma^{-1} (\theta_{Ri} - \theta)\Big\}. \tag{21.7}
$$

Let $\varphi = (\gamma, \sigma^2, \theta, \Sigma, \lambda, \beta, \alpha)$ denote the collection of parameters in the longitudinal and survival components of the joint model. Using (21.5), (21.6), and (21.7), the observed data likelihood function for $(Y_i, t_i, \delta_i, z_i, x_i)$ for the ith subject is given by

$$
\begin{aligned}
&L(\varphi | Y_i, t_i, \delta_i, z_i, x_i, W_i, g) \\
&= \int L(\lambda, \beta, \alpha | t_i, \delta_i, z_i, x_i, \theta_{Ri}, g, \gamma) L(\gamma, \sigma^2 | Y_i, W_i, \theta_{Ri}) f(\theta_{Ri} | \theta, \Sigma) d\theta_{Ri},
\end{aligned} \tag{21.8}
$$

for $i = 1, \ldots, n$. Letting $D_{obs} = \{(Y_i, t_i, \delta_i, z_i, x_i),\ i = 1, \ldots, n\}$ denote the observed data, the joint likelihood function for all n subjects is given by

$$
L(\varphi | g, D_{obs}) = \prod_{i=1}^{n} L(\varphi | Y_i, t_i, \delta_i, z_i, x_i, W_i, g). \tag{21.9}
$$

Let $\hat{\varphi} = (\hat{\gamma}, \hat{\sigma}^2, \hat{\theta}, \hat{\Sigma}, \hat{\lambda}, \hat{\beta}, \hat{\alpha})$ denote the maximum likelihood estimate (MLE) of φ from the joint model. Then the AIC (Akaike 1973) for the joint model is given by

$$
\text{AIC} = -2\log L(\hat{\varphi} | g, D_{obs}) + 2\dim(\varphi), \tag{21.10}
$$

and the BIC (Schwarz 1978) is defined as

$$\text{BIC} = -2\log L(\hat{\varphi}|g, D_{obs}) + \dim(\varphi)\log n. \tag{21.11}$$

21.3 Criteria for Assessing Model Fit in Longitudinal Data Using Decompositions of AIC and BIC

21.3.1 Decompositions of AIC and BIC

To assess the contribution of the survival data to the fit of the longitudinal data, we decompose AIC in (21.10) into two parts: one part for the survival data and the other part for the longitudinal data conditional on the survival data. Write $\varphi_1 = (\gamma, \sigma^2, \theta, \Sigma)$ and $\varphi_2 = (\lambda, \beta, \alpha)$. Let $\hat{\varphi}_1$ and $\hat{\varphi}_2$ denote the MLEs of φ_1 and φ_2, respectively, so that $\hat{\varphi} = (\hat{\varphi}_1, \hat{\varphi}_2)$. Recall that the likelihood function corresponding to the distribution of (t_i, δ_i) conditional on the random effects θ_{Ri} and the marginal distribution of the random effects are given by (21.6) and (21.7), respectively. Let $[A|B]$ denote the conditional distribution of A given B and let $[B]$ denote the marginal distribution. Then, the joint distribution $[(t_i, \delta_i), \theta_{Ri}]$ can be expressed as $[t_i, \delta_i|\theta_{Ri}][\theta_{Ri}]$ or $[\theta_{Ri}|t_i, \delta_i][t_i, \delta_i]$. Mathematically, we have the identity

$$\begin{aligned} &L(\varphi_2|t_i, \delta_i, z_i, x_i, \theta_{Ri}, g, \gamma) f(\theta_{Ri}|\theta, \Sigma) \\ &= L(\lambda, \alpha|t_i, \delta_i, z_i, x_i, g, \gamma, \theta, \Sigma, \beta) f(\theta_{Ri}|t_i, \delta_i, g, \gamma, \theta, \Sigma, \varphi_2), \end{aligned} \tag{21.12}$$

where $L(\lambda, \alpha|t_i, \delta_i, z_i, x_i, g, \gamma, \theta, \Sigma, \beta) = \int L(\varphi_2|t_i, \delta_i, z_i, x_i, \theta_{Ri}, g, \gamma) f(\theta_{Ri}|\theta, \Sigma)$ $d\theta_{Ri}$ is the likelihood function corresponding to the marginal distribution of (t_i, δ_i), and $f(\theta_{Ri}|t_i, \delta_i, g, \gamma, \theta, \Sigma, \varphi_2) = L(\varphi_2|t_i, \delta_i, z_i, x_i, \theta_{Ri}, g, \gamma) f(\theta_{Ri}|\theta, \Sigma)/L(\lambda, \alpha|t_i,$ $\delta_i, z_i, x_i, g, \gamma, \theta, \Sigma, \beta)$ is the conditional density of the random effects θ_{Ri} given the survival data (t_i, δ_i). The key identity in (21.12) leads to a useful likelihood factorization for $L(\varphi|g, D_{obs})$ given in (21.9). Specifically, we have

$$\begin{aligned} L(\varphi|g, D_{obs}) =& \prod_{i=1}^{n} \int L(\varphi_2|t_i, \delta_i, z_i, x_i, \theta_{Ri}, g, \gamma) L(\gamma, \sigma^2|Y_i, W_i, \theta_{Ri}) f(\theta_{Ri}|\theta, \Sigma) d\theta_{Ri} \\ =& \prod_{i=1}^{n} L(\lambda, \alpha|t_i, \delta_i, z_i, x_i, g, \gamma, \theta, \Sigma, \beta) \\ & \times \prod_{i=1}^{n} \int L(\gamma, \sigma^2|Y_i, W_i, \theta_{Ri}) f(\theta_{Ri}|t_i, \delta_i, g, \gamma, \theta, \Sigma, \varphi_2) d\theta_{Ri}. \end{aligned} \tag{21.13}$$

The above likelihood factorization is the key step towards establishing the decompositions of AIC and BIC. We formally state the results in the following theorem.

Theorem 1 *AIC in (21.10) has the following decomposition:*

$$\text{AIC} = \text{AIC}_{\text{Surv}} + \text{AIC}_{\text{Long}|\text{Surv}}, \tag{21.14}$$

where $\text{AIC}_{\text{Surv}} = -2\sum_{i=1}^{n} \log L(\hat{\lambda}, \hat{\alpha}|t_i, \delta_i, z_i, x_i, g, \hat{\gamma}, \hat{\theta}, \hat{\Sigma}, \hat{\beta}) + 2\text{dim}(\lambda, \alpha)$ *and*

$$\begin{aligned}\text{AIC}_{\text{Long}|\text{Surv}} = & -2\sum_{i=1}^{n} \log \int L(\hat{\gamma}, \hat{\sigma}^2|Y_i, W_i, \theta_{Ri}) f(\theta_{Ri}|t_i, \delta_i, g, \hat{\gamma}, \hat{\theta}, \hat{\Sigma}, \hat{\varphi}_2) d\theta_{Ri} \\ & + 2\text{dim}(\varphi_1, \beta).\end{aligned}$$

The proof of Theorem 1 directly follows the likelihood factorization in (21.13). BIC in (21.11) has a similar decomposition which is stated in the following corollary.

Corollary 1 *BIC in (21.11) can be decomposed as*

$$\text{BIC} = \text{BIC}_{\text{Surv}} + \text{BIC}_{\text{Long}|\text{Surv}}, \tag{21.15}$$

where $\text{BIC}_{\text{Surv}} = \text{AIC}_{\text{Surv}} + \text{dim}(\lambda, \alpha)(\log n - 2)$, *and* $\text{BIC}_{\text{Long}|\text{Surv}} = \text{AIC}_{\text{Long}|\text{Surv}} +$ *dim*$(\varphi_1, \beta)(\log n - 2)$.

AIC_{Surv} in (21.14) (BIC_{Surv} in (21.15) measures the contribution of the total AIC (BIC) due to the survival data while $\text{AIC}_{\text{Long}|\text{Surv}}$ ($\text{BIC}_{\text{Long}|\text{Surv}}$) quantifies the contribution of the total AIC (BIC) due to the longitudinal data with the additional information from the survival data.

Remark 1 Zhang et al. (2014) consider an alternative likelihood factorization of $L(\varphi|g, D_{obs})$ as

$$\begin{aligned}L(\varphi|g, D_{obs}) = \prod_{i=1}^{n} L(\varphi_1|Y_i, W_i) \prod_{i=1}^{n} \int & L(\varphi_2|t_i, \delta_i, z_i, x_i, \theta_{Ri}, g, \gamma) \\ & \times f(\theta_{Ri}|Y_i, W_i, \varphi_1) d\theta_{Ri},\end{aligned}$$

where $L(\varphi_1|Y_i, W_i) = \int L(\gamma, \sigma^2|Y_i, W_i, \theta_{Ri}) f(\theta_{Ri}|\theta, \Sigma) d\theta_{Ri}$ and $f(\theta_{Ri}|Y_i, W_i, \varphi_1) = L(\gamma, \sigma^2|Y_i, W_i, \theta_{Ri}) f(\theta_{Ri}|\theta, \Sigma)/L(\varphi_1|Y_i, W_i)$. Using the above likelihood factorization, Zhang et al. (2014) propose an alternative decomposition of AIC given by

$$\text{AIC} = \text{AIC}_{\text{Long}} + \text{AIC}_{\text{Surv}|\text{Long}}, \tag{21.16}$$

where $\text{AIC}_{\text{Long}} = -2\sum_{i=1}^{n} \log L(\hat{\varphi}_1|Y_i, W_i) + 2\text{dim}(\varphi_1)$ and

$$\begin{aligned}\text{AIC}_{\text{Surv}|\text{Long}} = & -2\sum_{i=1}^{n} \log \int L(\hat{\varphi}_2|t_i, \delta_i, z_i, x_i, \theta_{Ri}, g, \hat{\gamma}) f(\theta_{Ri}|Y_i, W_i, \hat{\varphi}_1) d\theta_{Ri} \\ & + 2\text{dim}(\varphi_2).\end{aligned}$$

In addition, Zhang et al. (2014) develop the decomposition of BIC as

$$\text{BIC} = \text{BIC}_{\text{Long}} + \text{BIC}_{\text{Surv}|\text{Long}}, \tag{21.17}$$

where $\text{BIC}_{\text{Long}} = \text{AIC}_{\text{Long}} + (\varphi_1)(\log n - 2)$, and

$$\text{BIC}_{\text{Surv|Long}} = \text{AIC}_{\text{Surv|Long}} + \dim(\varphi_2)(\log n - 2).$$

Remark 2 The decompositions of AIC and BIC given by (21.14) and (21.15) are most useful in the setting where the main goal is to make inferences on the parameters in the longitudinal model using the information in the survival model. Similarly, if the primary goal is make inferences on the parameters in the survival model using the information in the longitudinal model, then the decompositions of AIC and BIC given by (21.16) and (21.17) are better suited for this goal.

21.3.2 ΔAIC_{Long} and ΔBIC_{Long} Criteria

We are interested in how much the survival data can contribute to the fit of the longitudinal component in the joint model. Towards this goal, we let $(\hat{\gamma}_L, \hat{\sigma}_L^2, \hat{\theta}_L, \hat{\Sigma}_L)$ denote the MLE of $(\gamma, \sigma^2, \theta, \Sigma)$ with respect to the likelihood function,

$$\prod_{i=1}^{n} \int L(\gamma, \sigma^2 | Y_i, W_i, \theta_{Ri}) f(\theta_{Ri} | \theta, \Sigma) d\theta_{Ri},$$

for the longitudinal data alone. Then, AIC and BIC based on the longitudinal data alone can be written as

$$\text{AIC}_{\text{Long,alone}} = -2 \sum_{i=1}^{n} \log \int L(\hat{\gamma}_L, \hat{\sigma}_L^2 | Y_i, W_i, \theta_{Ri}) f(\theta_{Ri} | \hat{\theta}_L, \hat{\Sigma}_L) d\theta_{Ri} + 2\dim(\varphi_1)$$

and

$$\begin{aligned} \text{BIC}_{\text{Long,alone}} = & -2 \sum_{i=1}^{n} \log \int L(\hat{\gamma}_L, \hat{\sigma}_L^2 | Y_i, W_i, \theta_{Ri}) f(\theta_{Ri} | \hat{\theta}_L, \hat{\Sigma}_L) d\theta_{Ri} \\ & + \dim(\varphi_1) \log n. \end{aligned}$$

Based on the decomposition of AIC in (21.14) and BIC in (21.15), we propose new model assessment criteria $\Delta\text{AIC}_{\text{Long}}$ and $\Delta\text{BIC}_{\text{Long}}$ as

$$\begin{aligned} \Delta\text{AIC}_{\text{Long}} &= \text{AIC}_{\text{Long,alone}} - \text{AIC}_{\text{Long|Surv}}, \\ \Delta\text{BIC}_{\text{Long}} &= \text{BIC}_{\text{Long,alone}} - \text{BIC}_{\text{Long|Surv}}. \end{aligned} \tag{21.18}$$

$\Delta\text{AIC}_{\text{Long}}$ ($\Delta\text{BIC}_{\text{Long}}$) in (21.18) quantifies the trade-off between improvement of fit in the longitudinal component due to the survival data and the dimension penalty for the additional parameters in the longitudinal component of the joint model. A model with a large value of $\Delta\text{AIC}_{\text{Long}}(\Delta\text{BIC}_{\text{Long}})$ is more preferred.

To make the $\Delta\text{AIC}_{\text{Long}}$'s or $\Delta\text{BIC}_{\text{Long}}$'s more comparable across different longitudinal datasets, we introduce the relative $\Delta\text{AIC}_{\text{Long}}$ and the relative $\Delta\text{BIC}_{\text{Long}}$, which are defined as

$$\begin{aligned} \text{R}\Delta\text{AIC}_{\text{Long}} &= \frac{\Delta\text{AIC}_{\text{Long}}}{\text{AIC}_{\text{Long,alone}}}, \\ \text{R}\Delta\text{BIC}_{\text{Long}} &= \frac{\Delta\text{BIC}_{\text{Long}}}{\text{BIC}_{\text{Long,alone}}}. \end{aligned} \tag{21.19}$$

We illustrate the application of $\text{R}\Delta\text{AIC}_{\text{Long}}$ and $\text{R}\Delta\text{BIC}_{\text{Long}}$ in the next sections.

21.4 A Simulation Study

The objective of this simulation study is to evaluate the empirical performance of $\Delta\text{AIC}_{\text{Long}}$ and $\text{R}\Delta\text{AIC}_{\text{Long}}$ in identifying the longitudinal measure that the survival data are most related to. We independently simulate 500 datasets with $n = 400$ subjects each. For each subject, seven time points $(a_{ij}, j = 1, \ldots, 7)$ for the longitudinal measures are chosen to be $(0, 21, 42, 63, 84, 105, 126)/(365.25/12)$, and the treatment indicator z_i is generated from a Bernoulli (0.5) distribution. The design values of the parameters are given as $\Sigma_{00} = 0.7$, $\Sigma_{10} = -0.03$, $\Sigma_{11} = 0.06$, $\sigma^2 = 0.3$, $\theta_0 = 0.2$, $\theta_1 = 0.1$, $\gamma = -0.1$, $\beta_1 = 0.3$, $\beta_2 = 1.2$, $\alpha = -0.4$, and $\lambda = 0.18$. The longitudinal data are simulated from a $N(\mu_i(a_{ij}), \sigma^2)$ distribution with linear trajectory $\mu_i(a_{ij}) = (\theta_0 + \theta_{0i}) + (\theta_1 + \theta_{1i})a_{ij} + \gamma z_i$. For the survival data, we generate $t_i^* = [-\lambda \exp\{\beta_1\theta_{0i} + \beta_2\theta_{1i} + \alpha z_i\}]^{-1} \log(1 - U)$, where $U \sim U(0, 1)$, and the censoring time C_i is sampled from an exponential distribution with mean 20. Then the failure time and censoring indicator are computed as $t_i = \min\{t_i^*, C_i\}$ and $\delta_i = 1$ if $t_i^* \leq C_i$ and 0 otherwise. The resulting censoring percentage is about 25%. The above longitudinal and survival datasets sampled from the true model are denoted by D_{Long} and D_{Surv}, respectively, and the joint dataset is written as $D_{\text{Long}} + D_{\text{Surv}}$. Two additional sets of longitudinal data are generated by adding different amounts of noise to the true longitudinal measures. More specifically, they are simulated from a $N(\mu_{\ell i}(a_{ij}), \sigma^2)$ distribution with linear trajectories $\mu_{\ell i}(a_{ij}) = (\theta_0 + \theta_{0i} + \tau_{\ell 0i}) + (\theta_1 + \theta_{1i} + \tau_{\ell 1i})a_{ij} + \gamma z_i$, where $(\tau_{\ell 0i}, \tau_{\ell 1i})' \sim N(0, \kappa_\ell^2 I_2)$, $\kappa_1 = 0.5$, and $\kappa_2 = 1$. Combining these two longitudinal datasets with the survival data D_{Surv} leads to two additional datasets, namely, $D_{\text{Long1}} + D_{\text{Surv}}$ and $D_{\text{Long2}} + D_{\text{Surv}}$.

We fit shared parameter model with linear trajectory (SPML) to each of the three joint datasets $D_{\text{Long}} + D_{\text{Surv}}$, $D_{\text{Long1}} + D_{\text{Surv}}$, and $D_{\text{Long2}} + D_{\text{Surv}}$, and the corresponding results are denoted as Long, Long1, and Long2, respectively. The means of $\Delta\text{AIC}_{\text{Long}}$ and $\text{R}\Delta\text{AIC}_{\text{Long}}$ as well as the frequencies of ranking each dataset as best are reported in Table 21.1. Note that $\text{R}\Delta\text{AIC}_{\text{Long}}$ is multiplied by 1000. From Table 21.1, we see that Long has the largest means of $\Delta\text{AIC}_{\text{Long}}$ and $\text{R}\Delta\text{AIC}_{\text{Long}}$, which are 29.83 and 4.77, and gets ranked as number one with 497 and 500 times out of 500 by $\Delta\text{AIC}_{\text{Long}}$ and $\text{R}\Delta\text{AIC}_{\text{Long}}$, respectively. We also observe that the mean and frequency corresponding to Long1 are higher than those of Long2, which is

Table 21.1 Means of ΔAIC_{Long} and $R\Delta AIC_{Long}$ and frequencies of ranking each dataset as best based on ΔAIC_{Long} and $R\Delta AIC_{Long}$

	ΔAIC_{Long}		$R\Delta AIC_{Long}$[a]	
Data	Mean	Frequency	Mean	Frequency
Long	*29.83*	*497*	*4.77*	*500*
Long1	9.89	3	1.42	0
Long2	3.26	0	0.43	0

[a]R ΔAIC_{Long} is multiplied by 1000
AIC Akaike information criterion

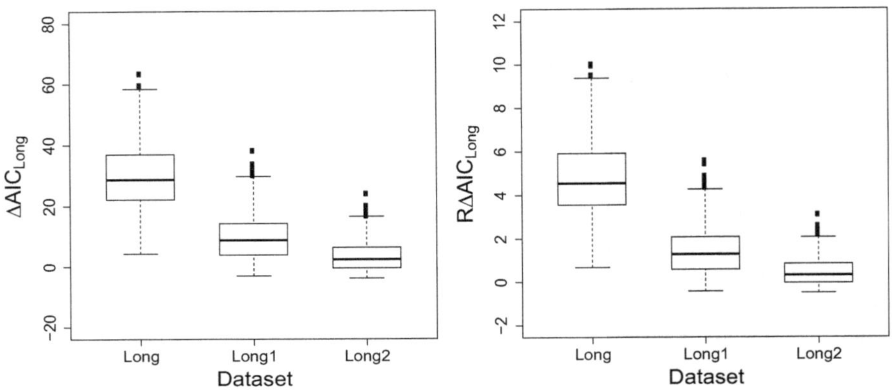

Fig. 21.1 Boxplots of the ΔAIC_{Long}'s and $R\Delta AIC_{Long}$'s for Long, Long1, and Long2. *AIC* Akaike information criterion

expected as κ_2 is greater than κ_1. Figure 21.1 shows the boxplots of the ΔAIC_{Long}'s and $R\Delta AIC_{Long}$'s for Long, Long1, and Long2. We see from these boxplots that Long has the largest medians of ΔAIC_{Long} and $R\Delta AIC_{Long}$, while Long2 has the smallest medians of ΔAIC_{Long} and $R\Delta AIC_{Long}$. These results empirically show that both ΔAIC_{Long} and $R\Delta AIC_{Long}$ can correctly identify the true longitudinal data that the survival data are most highly associated with.

21.5 Application to the EMPHACIS Data

21.5.1 The EMPHACIS Data

We consider a subset of the dataset from a multicenter, randomized, single-blind, EMPHACIS lung cancer clinical trial (Evaluation of Multi-Targeted Antifolate (MTA) in Mesothelioma in a Phase III Study with Cisplatin). The study drug was MTA pemetrexed (PEM) given in combination with cisplatin (Cis) (the PEM/Cis arm), and the active-treatment comparator was cisplatin alone (the Cis arm). The treatment for both arms was structured as six 21-day cycles of therapy. Patients receiving the treatment benefit could receive additional cycles based on investigator discretion. In our analysis, the time to event is the progression-free survival (PFS) time, which is defined as the time from randomization to the time until documented progression or death from any cause. A detailed description of this study can be found in Vogelzang et al. (2003).

This phase 3 first-line registration study of PEM in malignant pleural mesothelioma (MPM) included evaluation of PROs throughout the course of treatment. Most studies that incorporate the Lung Cancer Symptom Scale (LCSS) questionnaire (Patricia et al. 2006) use a single assessment to evaluate one or more cycles, over a period of 3 or more weeks, whereas this study balanced the limited span of the 24-h instrument recall period with more frequent PRO assessments; PRO administration was scheduled for each week versus, for example, once every 6 weeks (Hollen et al. 1997). The PROs considered here are five items, i.e., anorexia, cough, dyspnea, fatigue, and pain, from the disease-specific patient-reported LCSS, which were collected in the EMPHACIS trial. Our study cohort consists of 425 patients with at least one post-baseline value of each longitudinal measure and seven binary covariates, including race ($x_{i1} = 1$ if white), gender ($x_{i2} = 1$ if male), age ($x_{i3} = 1$ if age ≥ 65), Karnofsky status ($x_{i4} = 1$ if Karnofsky status is high), baseline stage of disease ($x_{i5} = 1$ if stage I/II), vitamin supplementation ($x_{i6} = 1$ if full vitamin supplementation), and treatment assignment ($z_i = 1$ if the ith patient is in the PEM/cisplatin arm). In all of the computations, we standardized these five LCSS measures to make them more comparable to each other and at the same time to improve numerical stability. The LCSS original-scaled item means (standard deviations) were 30.79 (27.19), 11.48 (17.93), 31.41 (26.33), 39.38 (27.06), and 24.64 (24.90) for anorexia, cough, dyspnea, fatigue, and pain, respectively. The total numbers of longitudinal measures (i.e., $\sum_{i=1}^{n} m_i$) including the baseline measures were 5504, 5544, 5553, 5530, and 5546 for anorexia, cough, dyspnea, fatigue, and pain, respectively.

21.5.2 Analysis of the EMPHACIS Data

Let D_{anorexia}, D_{cough}, D_{dyspnea}, D_{fatigue}, and D_{pain} denote the five observed longitudinal datasets and also let D_{Surv} denote the observed PFS data. Then the five different datasets are denoted by $D_{\text{anorexia}} + D_{\text{Surv}}$, $D_{\text{cough}} + D_{\text{Surv}}$, $D_{\text{dyspnea}} + D_{\text{Surv}}$, $D_{\text{fatigue}} + D_{\text{Surv}}$, and $D_{\text{pain}} + D_{\text{Surv}}$.

We first fit the joint models with linear and quadratic trajectories to each of the five longitudinal datasets, D_{anorexia}, D_{cough}, D_{dyspnea}, D_{fatigue}, and D_{pain}, to obtain the corresponding $\text{AIC}_{\text{Long,alone}}$'s. We then fit the SPMs as well as the TMs with linear and quadratic trajectories denoted by SPML, SPMQ, TML, and TMQ, respectively, to each of $D_{\text{anorexia}} + D_{\text{Surv}}$, $D_{\text{cough}} + D_{\text{Surv}}$, $D_{\text{dyspnea}} + D_{\text{Surv}}$, $D_{\text{fatigue}} + D_{\text{Surv}}$, and $D_{\text{pain}} + D_{\text{Surv}}$. We computed the corresponding quantities under the decomposition of AIC and BIC given in Sect. 21.3 to quantify the contribution of the PFS data to the fit of the longitudinal data. The results are summarized in Table 21.2. For all the models, we used the piecewise constant hazard model given in (21.4) with $K = 2$ for

Table 21.2 AICs and BICs

Model		Anorexia	Cough	Dyspnea	Fatigue	Pain
SPML	AIC	14205.13	14451.48	12101.25	13184.26	13030.38
	AIC_{Surv}	2208.54	2206.75	2208.91	2209.82	2214.45
	$AIC_{Long\|Surv}$	11996.60	12244.74	9892.34	10974.44	10815.93
	$AIC_{Long,alone}$	12017.59	12248.25	9911.72	11004.89	10867.45
	ΔAIC_{Long}	20.99	3.51	19.38	30.45	51.52
	$R\Delta AIC_{Long}$[a]	1.75	0.29	1.95	2.77	4.74
	BIC	14302.38	14548.73	12198.50	13281.52	13127.63
	BIC_{Surv}	2245.00	2243.22	2245.38	2246.29	2250.92
	$BIC_{Long\|Surv}$	12057.38	12305.52	9953.12	11035.22	10876.71
	$BIC_{Long,alone}$	12070.27	12300.93	9964.39	11057.57	10920.12
	ΔBIC_{Long}	12.89	−4.59	11.27	22.34	43.41
	$R\Delta BIC_{Long}$[b]	1.07	−0.37	1.13	2.02	3.98
SPMQ	AIC	14123.05	14250.06	11908.16	13058.62	12778.40
	AIC_{Surv}	2208.24	2206.79	2207.70	2208.84	2212.27
	$AIC_{Long\|Surv}$	11914.81	12043.28	9700.45	10849.78	10566.12
	$AIC_{Long,alone}$	11933.19	12046.45	9713.88	10873.74	10609.10
	ΔAIC_{Long}	18.38	3.18	13.42	23.97	42.98
	$R\Delta AIC_{Long}$	1.54	0.26	1.38	2.20	4.05
	BIC	14240.56	14367.57	12025.67	13176.13	12895.91
	BIC_{Surv}	2244.71	2243.25	2244.17	2245.31	2248.74
	$BIC_{Long\|Surv}$	11995.85	12124.32	9781.50	10930.82	10647.17
	$BIC_{Long,alone}$	12002.08	12115.34	9782.76	10942.63	10677.99
	ΔBIC_{Long}	6.23	−8.98	1.26	11.81	30.82
	$R\Delta BIC_{Long}$	0.52	−0.74	0.13	1.08	2.89
TML	AIC	14204.92	14449.26	12106.26	13185.81	13038.62
	AIC_{Surv}	2205.43	2207.63	2204.57	2205.37	2208.92
	$AIC_{Long\|Surv}$	11999.49	12241.64	9901.68	10980.44	10829.71
	$AIC_{Long,alone}$	12017.59	12248.25	9911.72	11004.89	10867.45
	ΔAIC_{Long}	18.09	6.61	10.04	24.45	37.74
	$R\Delta AIC_{Long}$	1.51	0.54	1.01	2.22	3.47
	BIC	14298.12	14542.46	12199.45	13279.01	13131.82
	BIC_{Surv}	2241.90	2244.10	2241.04	2241.84	2245.39
	$BIC_{Long\|Surv}$	12056.22	12298.36	9958.41	11037.17	10886.44
	$BIC_{Long,alone}$	12070.27	12300.93	9964.39	11057.57	10920.12
	ΔBIC_{Long}	14.04	2.56	5.98	20.40	33.69
	$R\Delta BIC_{Long}$	1.16	0.21	0.60	1.84	3.08

Table 21.2 (continued)

Model		Anorexia	Cough	Dyspnea	Fatigue	Pain
TMQ	AIC	14118.40	14244.30	11904.93	13049.48	12773.67
	AIC_{Surv}	2205.73	2208.05	2204.73	2205.32	2208.74
	$\text{AIC}_{\text{Long}\mid\text{Surv}}$	11912.67	12036.25	9700.20	10844.16	10564.92
	$\text{AIC}_{\text{Long,alone}}$	11933.19	12046.45	9713.88	10873.74	10609.10
	$\Delta\text{AIC}_{\text{Long}}$	20.53	10.20	13.67	29.59	44.18
	$\text{R}\Delta\text{AIC}_{\text{Long}}$	1.72	0.85	1.41	2.72	4.16
	BIC	14227.80	14353.70	12014.34	13158.88	12883.07
	BIC_{Surv}	2242.20	2244.52	2241.20	2241.79	2245.21
	$\text{BIC}_{\text{Long}\mid\text{Surv}}$	11985.60	12109.19	9773.14	10917.10	10637.86
	$\text{BIC}_{\text{Long,alone}}$	12002.08	12115.34	9782.76	10942.63	10677.99
	$\Delta\text{BIC}_{\text{Long}}$	16.48	6.15	9.62	25.53	40.13
	$\text{R}\Delta\text{BIC}_{\text{Long}}$	1.37	0.51	0.98	2.33	3.76

[a] $\text{R}\Delta\text{AIC}_{\text{Long}}$ is multiplied by 1000
[b] $\text{R}\Delta\text{BIC}_{\text{Long}}$ is multiplied by 1000
BIC Bayesian information criterion, *AIC* Akaike information criterion, *SPML* shared parameter model with linear trajectory, *SPMQ* shared parameter model with quadratic trajectory, *TML* trajectory model with linear trajectory, *TMQ* trajectory model with quadratic trajectory

the baseline hazard, and the partition intervals were constructed based on the median of the PFS times. Note that $K = 2$ gave the best fit of the PFS data according to AIC for all five longitudinal and survival datasets. As discussed in Sect. 21.5.2, the total numbers of observations for these five PROs were different, implying that $\Delta\text{AIC}_{\text{Long}}$ and $\Delta\text{BIC}_{\text{Long}}$ were not directly comparable for the EMPHACIS data. Therefore, we consider the relative $\Delta\text{AIC}_{\text{Long}}$ and $\Delta\text{BIC}_{\text{Long}}$ defined in (21.19). In Table 21.2, the values of $\text{R}\Delta\text{AIC}_{\text{Long}}$ and $\text{R}\Delta\text{BIC}_{\text{Long}}$ were multiplied by 1000. From Table 21.2, we see that pain had the largest relative improvement in terms of both $\text{R}\Delta\text{AIC}_{\text{Long}}$ and $\text{R}\Delta\text{BIC}_{\text{Long}}$ under all four joint models, namely, SPML, SPMQ, TML, and TMQ. We also see from Table 21.2 that pain had the largest $\Delta\text{AIC}_{\text{Long}}$ and $\Delta\text{BIC}_{\text{Long}}$ under SPML, SPMQ, TML, and TMQ. In addition, fatigue had the second largest values of $\Delta\text{AIC}_{\text{Long}}$ and $\Delta\text{BIC}_{\text{Long}}$ as well as $\text{R}\Delta\text{AIC}_{\text{Long}}$ and $\text{R}\Delta\text{BIC}_{\text{Long}}$, while cough had the smallest values of $\Delta\text{AIC}_{\text{Long}}$ and $\Delta\text{BIC}_{\text{Long}}$ as well as $\text{R}\Delta\text{AIC}_{\text{Long}}$ and $\text{R}\Delta\text{BIC}_{\text{Long}}$ under SPML, SPMQ, TML, and TMQ. Thus, for the EMPHACIS data, $\Delta\text{AIC}_{\text{Long}}$ and $\Delta\text{BIC}_{\text{Long}}$ yielded results consistent with $\text{R}\Delta\text{AIC}_{\text{Long}}$ and $\text{R}\Delta\text{BIC}_{\text{Long}}$. These results indicate that the PFS data led to the most gain in fitting the longitudinal data D_{pain} while the same PFS data had the least contribution to the fit of the longitudinal data D_{cough}. These results also imply that the PFS time was most highly associated with the LCSS pain symptom and was least associated with the LCSS cough symptom.

Finally, we mention that AIC and BIC were not able to determine the contribution of the PFS data in fitting these five sets of LCSS longitudinal measures under the joint modeling framework. We observe from Table 21.2 that the smallest values of AIC and BIC were attained by dyspnea under SPML, SPMQ, TML, and TMQ. After examining $AIC_{Long|Surv}$ and $BIC_{Long|Surv}$, we found that dyspnea had the smallest values of $AIC_{Long|Surv}$ and $BIC_{Long|Surv}$. Thus, $AIC_{Long|Surv}$ and $BIC_{Long|Surv}$ were the main contributions to the small values of AIC and BIC for dyspnea. These results indicate that AIC, BIC, $AIC_{Long|Surv}$, and $BIC_{Long|Surv}$ cannot be used to quantify the contribution of the survival data to the fit of the longitudinal data.

The parameter estimates (Ests), the standard errors (SEs), and the p values are shown in Table 21.3 for the longitudinal component of TMQ and Table 21.4 for the survival component of TMQ, respectively. From these tables, we see that treatment had a large p value in the longitudinal submodel for each of the five LCSS symptoms, indicating that treatment was not statistically significant at the 0.05 level in the longitudinal submodel. However, for the survival submodel, the treatment effect was highly significant with a p value of < 0.0001 for each LCSS symptom. We note that the parameter β captures the association between the survival time and the PRO measure under TMQ. From Table 21.4, we see that β was highly significant for all five LCSS symptoms. From Tables 21.2 and 21.4, we observe that the order of the estimates of β was also consistent with the order of the values of ΔAIC_{Long} and $R\Delta AIC_{Long}$ for five LCSS symptoms.

21.6 Discussion

In this chapter, we developed a novel decomposition of AIC and BIC to individually assess the contributions of each component in joint models of longitudinal and survival data, and used $R\Delta AIC_{Long}$ and $R\Delta BIC_{Long}$, as well as ΔAIC_{Long} and ΔBIC_{Long} to determine the contribution of the survival data to the fit of the longitudinal data. We conducted a simulation study to examine the empirical performance of ΔAIC_{Long} and $R\Delta AIC_{Long}$ and carried out a detailed analysis of the EMPHACIS data from a cancer clinical trial in mesothelioma. The empirical results shown in Sect. 21.5.2 are quite promising since the proposed model assessment criteria ΔAIC_{Long} and ΔBIC_{Long} were able to determine the contribution of the survival data to the fit of the longitudinal data.

All of the computations in Sects. 21.4 and 21.5 were done in SAS and Fortran 95 software with double precision and IMSL subroutines. SAS macros were developed to fit the joint models. We use the Monte Carlo method to calculate AIC_{Surv}, and then $AIC_{Long|Surv}$ is given by $AIC - AIC_{Surv}$. Macros are available upon request.

There are several potential extensions of the proposed method. The proposed methodology would be quite useful in situations where we wish to simultaneously jointly model a longitudinal marker and several time-to-event outcomes such as PFS and OS. The proposed ΔAIC_{Long} and ΔBIC_{Long} can be very useful in this context as they can tell us about the overall contribution of the multivariate survival data to the fit of the longitudinal data. Although the proposed model assessment criteria are developed under the joint model in Sect. 21.2, they can be easily extended to models for other types of data such as longitudinal binary/ordinal response or count data as well as other types of survival models such as cure rate models, nonproportional

Table 21.3 Parameter estimates (longitudinal component) of TMQ

Parameter (Variable)		Anorexia	Cough	Dyspnea	Fatigue	Pain
Σ_{00}	Est	0.473	0.655	0.598	0.480	0.624
	SE	0.045	0.057	0.048	0.042	0.052
	p value	< 0.0001	< 0.0001	< 0.0001	< 0.0001	< 0.0001
Σ_{10}	Est	−0.081	−0.142	−0.095	−0.070	−0.139
	SE	0.031	0.040	0.030	0.029	0.037
	p value	0.0085	0.0005	0.0017	0.0155	0.0003
Σ_{11}	Est	0.231	0.384	0.294	0.278	0.440
	SE	0.034	0.048	0.034	0.036	0.050
	p value	<0.0001	<0.0001	<0.0001	<0.0001	<0.0001
Σ_{20}	Est	0.006	0.008	0.010	0.006	0.019
	SE	0.006	0.009	0.006	0.006	0.008
	p value	0.37	0.3902	0.134	0.2805	0.0194
Σ_{21}	Est	−0.039	−0.078	−0.056	−0.050	−0.088
	SE	0.007	0.011	0.007	0.008	0.011
	p value	< 0.0001	< 0.0001	<0.0001	< 0.0001	< 0.0001
Σ_{22}	Est	0.008	0.019	0.012	0.010	0.020
	SE	0.002	0.003	0.002	0.002	0.003
	p value	< 0.0001	< 0.0001	< 0.0001	< 0.0001	< 0.0001
σ^2	Est	0.373	0.352	0.220	0.290	0.257
	SE	0.008	0.008	0.005	0.006	0.006
	p value	< 0.0001	< 0.0001	<0.0001	< 0.0001	< 0.0001
θ_0	Est	0.371	0.710	0.260	0.179	0.615
	SE	0.156	0.168	0.172	0.160	0.176
	p value	0.0177	< 0.0001	0.1297	0.2637	0.0005
θ_1	Est	0.135	−0.069	0.093	0.163	0.023
	SE	0.035	0.040	0.034	0.035	0.040
	p value	0.0001	0.0862	0.0062	< 0.0001	0.5625
θ_2	Est	−0.026	0.009	−0.014	−0.027	0.001
	SE	0.007	0.009	0.008	0.007	0.009
	p value	0.0004	0.3438	0.0731	0.0004	0.8926
γ_1 (treatment)	Est	0.105	0.036	−0.106	0.008	−0.080
	SE	0.068	0.073	0.075	0.070	0.077
	p value	0.1211	0.6249	0.1566	0.9129	0.2992
γ_2 (race)	Est	0.273	−0.362	0.211	0.408	−0.092
	SE	0.125	0.135	0.138	0.129	0.141
	p value	0.0293	0.0075	0.1268	0.0016	0.5125

Table 21.3 (continued)

Parameter (Variable)		Anorexia	Cough	Dyspnea	Fatigue	Pain
γ_3 (gender)	Est	−0.418	−0.067	0.011	−0.338	−0.191
	SE	0.087	0.094	0.096	0.090	0.098
	p value	< 0.0001	0.480	0.9076	0.0002	0.0529
γ_4 (age)	Est	0.130	0.022	−0.006	0.154	−0.048
	SE	0.070	0.076	0.077	0.072	0.079
	p value	0.0657	0.7708	0.9351	0.0342	0.542
γ_5 (Karnofsky)	Est	−0.569	−0.265	−0.779	−0.651	−0.581
	SE	0.069	0.074	0.076	0.070	0.077
	p value	< 0.0001	0.0004	<0.0001	< 0.0001	< 0.0001
γ_6 (stage)	Est	−0.152	−0.188	−0.042	0.007	−0.102
	SE	0.082	0.087	0.090	0.084	0.092
	p value	0.0642	0.0314	0.6382	0.9345	0.2688
γ_7 (vitamin)	Est	−0.088	−0.024	0.057	−0.066	0.116
	SE	0.078	0.084	0.085	0.080	0.087
	p value	0.2619	0.7784	0.5049	0.4088	0.1853

Est estimate, *SE* standard error, *TMQ* trajectory model with quadratic trajectory

hazards models, and competing risks models discussed in (Ibrahim et al. 2001; Klein et al. 2013). Oncology applications of these modeling extensions would provide robust evidence to support the use of PFS as a surrogate end point for patient-reported measures as well as OS (Booth and Eisenhauer 2012).

Table 21.4 Parameter estimates (survival component) of TMQ

Parameter (Variable)		Anorexia	Cough	Dyspnea	Fatigue	Pain
α_1 (treatment)	Est	−0.500	−0.443	−0.420	−0.468	−0.422
	SE	0.104	0.103	0.103	0.103	0.103
	p value	< 0.0001	<0.0001	<0.0001	<0.0001	< 0.0001
α_2 (race)	Est	0.002	0.221	0.057	−0.069	0.202
	SE	0.192	0.193	0.191	0.194	0.191
	p value	0.9898	0.2523	0.7639	0.724	0.2894
α_3 (gender)	Est	0.214	0.087	0.088	0.202	0.158
	SE	0.139	0.136	0.136	0.137	0.137
	p value	0.1232	0.5232	0.5148	0.1413	0.2496
α_4 (age)	Est	−0.086	−0.068	−0.070	−0.121	−0.006
	SE	0.107	0.106	0.106	0.107	0.107
	p value	0.4176	0.5241	0.5118	0.2565	0.9561
α_5 (Karnofsky)	Est	−0.180	−0.266	−0.152	−0.121	−0.178
	SE	0.109	0.105	0.111	0.110	0.107
	p value	0.0986	0.0113	0.1695	0.2722	0.0957
α_6 (stage)	Est	−0.391	−0.416	−0.464	−0.463	−0.406
	SE	0.132	0.132	0.131	0.131	0.131
	p value	0.0031	0.0017	0.0004	0.0004	0.0021
α_7 (vitamin)	Est	−0.034	−0.085	−0.116	−0.059	−0.156
	SE	0.116	0.115	0.115	0.115	0.116
	p value	0.7679	0.4611	0.3139	0.6069	0.179
λ_1	Est	0.172	0.169	0.186	0.183	0.150
	SE	0.041	0.040	0.044	0.044	0.037
	p value	< 0.0001	< 0.0001	< 0.0001	< 0.0001	< 0.0001
λ_2	Est	0.299	0.285	0.313	0.322	0.274
	SE	0.073	0.069	0.075	0.079	0.068
	p value	< 0.0001	< 0.0001	< 0.0001	< 0.0001	< 0.0001
β	Est	0.344	0.214	0.257	0.397	0.408
	SE	0.072	0.064	0.062	0.071	0.060
	p value	< 0.0001	0.0009	< 0.0001	< 0.0001	< 0.0001

Est estimate, *SE* standard error, *TMQ* trajectory model with quadratic trajectory

References

Rothman M, Burke L, Erickson P, Leidy NK, Patrick DL, Petrie CD (2009) Use of existing patient-reported outcome (PRO) instruments and their modification: the ISPOR good research practices for evaluating and documenting content validity for the use of existing instruments and their modification PRO task force report. Value Health 12:1075–1083

Brown ER, Ibrahim JG (2003a) A Bayesian semiparametric joint hierarchical model for longitudinal and survival data. Biometrics 59:221–228

Brown ER, Ibrahim JG (2003b) Bayesian approaches to joint cure rate and longitudinal models with applications to cancer vaccine trials. Biometrics 59:686–693

Chen MH, Ibrahim JG, Sinha D (2004) A new joint model for longitudinal and survival data with a cure fraction. J Multivar Anal 91:18–34

Ibrahim JG, Chen MH, Sinha D (2004) Bayesian methods for joint modeling of longitudinal and survival data with applications to cancer vaccine studies. Statistica Sinica 14:863–883

Pawitan Y, Self S (1993) Modeling disease marker processes in AIDS. J Am Stat Assoc 88:719–726

DeGruttola V, Tu XM (1994) Modeling progression of CD4-lymphocyte count and its relationship to survival time. Biometrics 50:1003–1014

LaValley MP, DeGruttola V (1996) Model for empirical Bayes estimators of longitudinal CD4 counts. Stat Med 15:2289–2305

Hsieh F, Tseng Y, Wang J (2006) Joint modeling of survival and longitudinal data: likelihood approach revisited. Biometrics 62:1037–1043

Ibrahim JG, Chu H, Chen LM (2010) Basic concepts and methods for joint models of longitudinal and survival data. J Clin Oncol 28:2796–2801

Chen LM, Ibrahim JG, Chu H (2011) Sample size and power determination in joint modeling of longitudinal and survival data. Stat Med 30:2295–2309

Hatfield LA, Boye ME, Carlin BP. Joint modeling of multiple longitudinal patient-reported outcomes and survival. J Biopharm Stat 21:971–991

Wang P, Shen W, Boye ME (2012) Joint modeling of longitudinal outcomes and survival using latent growth modeling approach in a mesothelioma trial. Health Serv Outcomes Res Methodol 12:182–199

Hatfield LA, Boye ME, Hackshaw MD, Carlin BP (2012) Multilevel Bayesian models for survival times and longitudinal patient-reported outcomes with many zeros. J Am Stat Assoc 107: 875–885

Zhu H, Ibrahim JG, Chi Y, Tang N (2012) Bayesian influence measures for joint models of longitudinal and survival data. Biometrics 68:954–964

Zhang D, Chen MH, Ibrahim JG, Boye ME, Wang P, Shen W (2014) Assessing model fit in joint models of longitudinal and survival data with applications to cancer clinical trials. Stat Med 33(27):4715–4733

Akaike H (1973) Information theory and an extension of the maximum likelihood principle. In Petrov BN, Csaki F (eds) Proceedings of the Second International Symposium on Information Theory. Akademiai Kiado, Budapest, pp 267–281

Schwarz G (1978) Estimating the dimension of a model. Ann Stat 6:461–464

Vogelzang NJ, Rusthoven JJ, Symanowski J, Denham C, Kaukel E, Ruffie P, Gatzemeier U, Boyer M, Emri S, Manegold C, Niyikiza C, Paoletti P (2003) Phase III study of pemetrexed in combination with cisplatin versus cisplatin alone in patients with malignant pleural mesothelioma. J Clin Oncol 21:2636–2644

Patricia HJ, Gralla RJ, Liepa AM, Symanowski JT, Rusthoven JJ (2006) Measuring quality of life in patients with pleural mesothelioma using a modified version of the Lung Cancer Symptom Scale (LCSS): psychometric properties of the LCSS-Meso. Support Care Cancer 14:11–21

Hollen PJ, Gralla RJ, Cox C, Eberly SW, Kris MG (1997) A dilemma in analysis: issues in the serial measurement of quality of life in patients with advanced lung cancer. Lung Cancer 18:119–136

Ibrahim JG, Chen MH, Sinha D (2001) Bayesian survival analysis. Springer, New York

Klein JP, van Houwelingen HC, Ibrahim JG, Scheike TH (eds) (2013) Handbook of survival analysis. Chapman & Hall, Boca Raton

Booth CM, Eisenhauer EA (2012) Progression-free survival: meaningful or simply measurable? J Clin Oncol 30:1030–1033

Chapter 22
Assessing the Cumulative Exposure Response in Alzheimer's Disease Studies

Jianing Di, Xin Zhao, Daniel Wang, Ming Lu and Michael Krams

Abstract To assess long-term cumulative benefit of a treatment, relationship between cumulative drug exposure and outcomes could be explored to understand the dose response. However, cumulative exposure corresponds to the longitudinal profile of an outcome, which is often heavily confounded with natural disease progression and missing data. A model-based approach is developed to account for the confounding factors. In particular, the observed measures are adjusted by the projected disease progression at the corresponding time points before exposure response is assessed. The proposed approach introduces new insights to the interpretation of exposure data. In the presented case study, the proposed method identified various degrees of potential efficacy trend favoring higher level of cumulative exposure in active drug.

22.1 Introduction

During drug development, two of the most typical questions are "how high" the dose and "how long" the treatment duration need to be. These questions are naturally answered by assessing the relationship between cumulative drug exposure and cumulative treatment effect (Lee 2003; Hutmacher et al. 2007). However, in clinical

---

J. Di (✉)
Janssen R&D, LLC, 3210 Merryfield Row, San Diego, CA 92128, USA
e-mail: jdi@its.jnj.com

X. Zhao
Janssen R&D, LLC, 6500 Paseo Padre Parkway Fremont, CA 94555, USA
e-mail: xzhao2@its.jnj.com

D. Wang
Janssen R&D, LLC, 6500 Paseo Padre Parkway Fremont, CA 94555, USA
e-mail: dwang@its.jnj.com

M. Lu
Janssen R&D, LLC, 1400 McKean Rd, Spring House, PA 19002, USA
e-mail: mlu7@its.jnj.com

M. Krams
Janssen R&D, LLC, Trenton Harbourton Rd, Titusville, NJ 08560, USA
e-mail: mkrams@its.jnj.com

Z. Chen et al. (eds.), *Applied Statistics in Biomedicine and Clinical Trials Design*,
ICSA Book Series in Statistics, DOI 10.1007/978-3-319-12694-4_22

trials, understanding the real cumulative treatment effect is often difficult because the longitudinal profile of the observed outcome is always a mixture of multiple factors:

- Drug effect: The actual treatment difference over naïve treatment.
- Natural disease progression: The deterioration observed under naïve treatment.
- Missing data impact: Greater deterioration observed in early dropouts.

This complexity is particularly clear for a clinical trial of the neurodegenerative disease. For example, clinical trials for the Alzheimer's disease (AD) are usually conducted with elderly patients and last for years. During the course of a lengthy AD trial, the disease condition of the trial participants, who often have complex concomitant medical conditions, deteriorates dramatically. Consequently, there is often a large portion of early dropouts that invalidates the direct interpretation of the cumulative exposure. As a result, when assessing the effect of cumulative exposure, it is critical to adjust for the impact of these confounding factors.

We have proposed a model-based approach to account for the confounding factors. This approach provides a way to adjust for the impact of the confounding factors and undercover the true treatment benefit associated with the drug exposure. This method introduces important new insights to the interpretation of study exposure data. In particular, in the presented case study, the proposed modeling approach suggests that there are various degrees of potential efficacy trend favoring higher level of cumulative exposure in active drug, based on selected clinical and biomarker end points.

The rest of the chapter is organized as follows: in Sect. 22.2, the proposed approach is introduced with details; in Sect. 22.3, a case study is presented to illustrate its use; Sect. 22.4 concludes and offers some discussion.

22.2 Method

The rationale of the proposed approach can be illustrated using an example of two hypothetical subjects who have received active treatment in an AD clinical trial. The trial plans to record six consecutive post-baseline cognitive measurements, but only one of these two subjects finished the trial (the other early terminated after the fifth measurement). The observed longitudinal outcomes of these two subjects are displayed by the solid curves in Fig. 22.1. As a piece of evidence for informative dropout, subject 2 exhibited slightly faster deterioration as compared to subject 1. In addition, assume the real disease progression for these two subjects without treatment is given by the *dashed* lines of the corresponding color, then the real drug response is represented by the distance between the observation and the potential disease progression under naïve treatment. This formulates the observed outcome as

$$R_{\text{Observed}}(t) = E(t) + P(t),\ t = 1, 2, ..., T, \tag{22.1}$$

where R is the response, E is the real effect of cumulative exposure, and P is the natural disease progression. It should be noted that, while the observed responses are

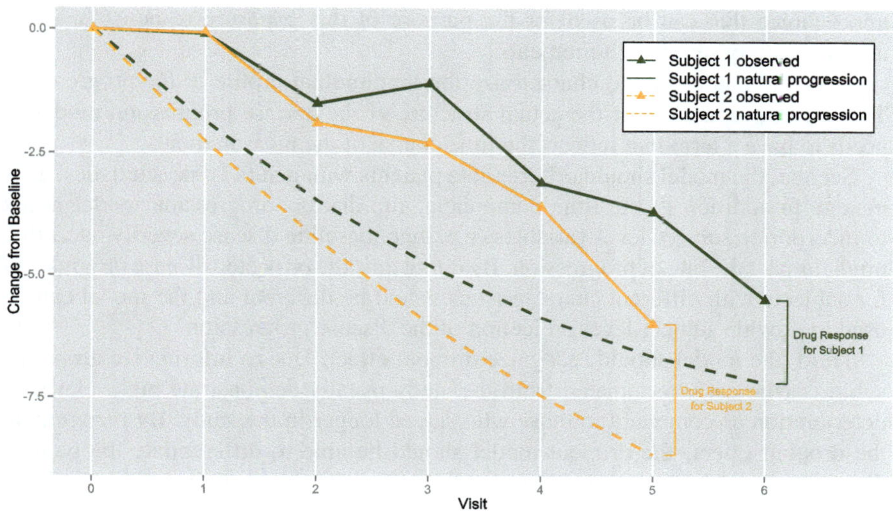

Fig. 22.1 Subject level response adjustment

also impacted by dropout, the missing data effect should be used to more accurately describe the disease progression and thus is not formulated as a separate component outside P. By Eq. 22.1, the true effect of drug exposure is given by

$$E(t) = R_{\text{Observed}}(t) - P(t) = R_{\text{Adjusted}}(t), \; t = 1, 2, ..., T. \qquad (22.2)$$

This leads to the proposed three-step approach in evaluating the real effect of cumulative exposure:

1. A disease progression model is constructed to represent the natural disease progression over the time course of the trial, where subject-level characteristics and dropout timing are taken into consideration.
2. The observed outcome measures are adjusted by the projected disease progression at the corresponding time points.
3. The resulting model-adjusted outcome measures are linked with the level of cumulative exposure (i.e., total area under the pharmacokinetics (PK) concentration curve).

22.2.1 Disease Progression Model

A disease progression model reflects the amount of deterioration over time under naïve treatment. Being used as the basis of the adjustment made to the observed data, the disease progression model is a critical part of the proposed approach. While a disease progression model can be established following multiple approaches, a good choice that can be used for the purpose of this exposure response analysis needs to satisfy several requirements.

First, the model should characterize the longitudinal profile of the progression. This means, regardless of the actual structure of the disease progression model, it needs to have a term that reflects the time course of the measurements.

Second, the model should differentiate patients with distinct characteristics. This means, in addition to the time component, the disease progression model needs to incorporate subject-level variables (e.g., age, baseline disease severity, etc.) that might impact the rate of progression. By doing this, the projected disease progression for subjects with different characteristics would be different and the model can be used to provide subject-level projection of the disease progression.

Third, the model should recognize dropout effect. Due to informative dropouts, subjects who early terminated from the study usually demonstrate higher level of deterioration as compared to those who stayed longer in the study. By recognizing the dropout effect, the dropout model should be able to differentiate the path of disease progression between a study early terminator and a study completer. With that, consider two patients with identical characteristics but one completed the study and one early terminated before completion, the dropout model should give different projected disease worsening paths for these two subjects.

The disease progression model we considered is a mixed-effect model for repeated measures (MMRM). In any study with longitudinal measurements, such model can be established by using all observed response of the placebo-treatment subjects. In particular, our MMRM includes the observed response as the dependent variable, and a set of model covariates such as subject demographics (e.g., age), baseline disease severity, time (visit) corresponding to each observed response, and several interaction terms as appropriate. It should also be noted that, to recognize the different progression trajectory of subjects with different disposition profile, the model also includes time to dropout as a covariate.

22.2.2 *Subject-Level Model-Based Adjustment*

After a disease progression model is constructed, all observed response could be adjusted by subtracting the model-projected disease progression. Several points should be noted to ensure that the adjusted responses are interpretable.

First, the model-projected disease progression should be calculated at the subject level. That means, for a given subject, the disease progression should be estimated by considering that particular subject's information as required by the disease progression model. With that, subjects are compared with their own path of natural disease progression.

Second, while the disease progression model provides the entire path of the disease progression for any given subject, the adjustment should be made only at the matching time point.

Third, although the main interest of exposure response analysis focuses on subjects treated by the active drug, it is important that observations from placebo-treated subjects are adjusted in the same way. There are at least two reasons for this. First of all, without including placebo data in the analysis, the performance of the exposure response at lower end of the exposure level can be overly impacted by responses at higher level of exposure. In particular, depending on the method used to establish the relationship between cumulative exposure and adjusted responses (see Sect. 22.2.3), the result might imply hard-to-interpret effect of low exposure level. Second, by including placebo data, the method will fully appreciate the variability in placebo-treated subjects. In this case, because the disease progression model itself is constructed using the placebo data, the adjusted response of placebo-treated subjects should represent a set of random noise that centers at 0.

22.2.3 *Exposure Response Modeling*

The relationship of interest is the one between adjusted response and corresponding cumulative exposure level. Once every single observed response has been adjusted, an analysis that links the cumulative exposure and adjusted response at corresponding time point could be performed. Such analysis could be as simple as a correlation analysis utilizing only a single data point from each subject, or as complicated as a model that includes all information (i.e., multiple records provided by the same subject) as an analysis for repeated measures.

However, it is worth to point out that, since the adjustment is made based on the matching time point, the adjusted response is no longer impacted by time. In other words, an adjusted response at visit five can now be compared to an adjusted response at visit six, and the only factor that differentiates these two records would be the cumulative exposure level. For example, as we will further discuss in the case study in Sect. 22.3, the final exposure–response analysis is performed by using each subject's last available measurement, even though those observations could be collected at different time points due to early dropouts. Also, if multiple records from the same subject are included in the analysis, the underlying correlation between those repeated measurements should not be described using a time series structure (e.g., AR(p)).

22.3 A Case Study

As a case study, we considered data from two recently finished phase 3 clinical studies in testing the safety and efficacy of bapineuzumab IV in patients with mild to moderate AD.

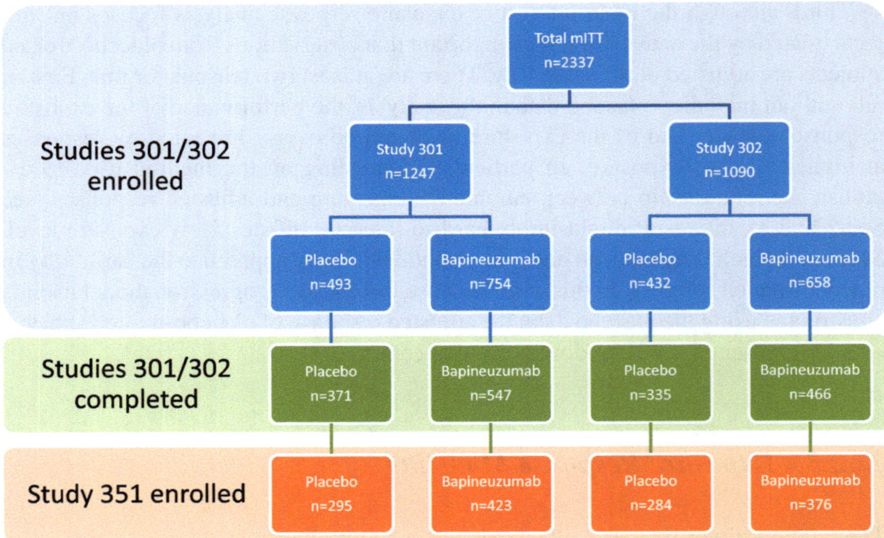

Fig. 22.2 Sample size in bapineuzumab IV phase 3 studies

22.3.1 Bapineuzumab

While the real cause of AD is yet to be confirmed, the most commonly accepted explanation is given by the amyloid hypothesis which suggests that the disease develops when clumps of abnormal proteins (beta amyloid) grow in the brain. Bapineuzumab is a humanized monoclonal antibody, which binds to and clears beta amyloid peptide, and is designed to provide antibodies to beta amyloid directly to the patient.

Two phase 3 placebo-controlled clinical trials were conducted to evaluate the safety and efficacy of bapineuzumab in patients with mild to moderate AD. The first study (study ELN115727-301 or simply study 301) enrolled only patients who are apolipoprotein E $\varepsilon 4$ gene noncarriers. Patients were to receive six quarterly IV injections of placebo or bapineuzumab at 0.5 or 1.0 mg/kg dose levels. The second study (study ELN115727-302 or simply study 302) enrolled only patients who are apolipoprotein E $\varepsilon 4$ gene carriers. Enrolled patients followed the same dosing scheme as study 301 patients, but only 1 bapineuzumab dose (0.5 mg/kg) was tested. An open-label extension study (study ELN115727-351 or simply study 351) was conducted where completers of the double-blind parent studies (study 301 or study 302) might be enrolled to receive only bapineuzumab. A diagram is given in Fig. 22.2 to illustrate the sample size in each study.

The co-primary clinical end points were lost of cognitive and functional abilities as measured by Alzheimer's Disease Assessment Scale-Cognitive (ADAS-Cog)/11 total score and disability assessment for dementia (DAD) total score. In addition, brain amyloid load was also assessed via positron emission tomography (PET) imaging.

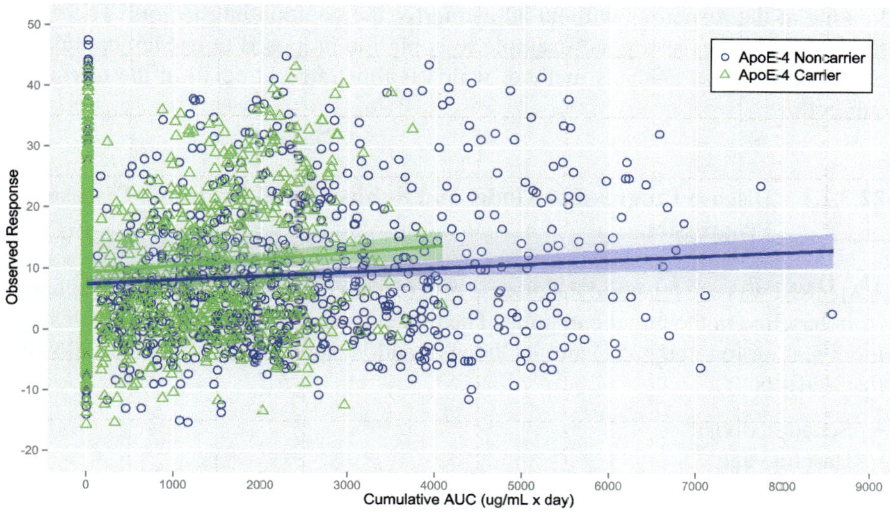

Fig. 22.3 Observed response Alzheimer's Disease Assessment Scale-Cognitive (ADAS-Cog)/11 total score versus cumulative exposure area under the curve (AUC)

Finally, compared to placebo, tested doses of bapineuzumab did not demonstrate statistically significant treatment effect based on co-primary clinical end points, but statistically significant treatment effect on brain amyloid in ApoE $\varepsilon 4$ carriers was observed.

22.3.2 *Cumulative Exposure Analysis*

The proposed cumulative exposure analysis was performed as a post hoc analysis to explore whether or not higher level of cumulative exposure has potentially larger treatment benefit. Fig. 22.3 shows a simple scatter plot of cumulative drug exposure in area under the curve (AUC; ug/mL × day) and the observed response, defined as change from baseline in ADAS-Cog/11 total score at the last visit. Two trend lines are superimposed to indicate the clear upward trend in both ApoE $\varepsilon 4$ carriers and noncarriers. For ADAS-Cog/11 total score, larger value means greater impairment, therefore Fig. 22.3 seems to suggest that higher level of exposure causes greater amount of deterioration.

Such counter-intuitive observation is a direct consequence of confounding factors discussed in Sect. 22.1. To see this, it should be noted that subjects with high level of cumulative exposure are generally those who stayed longer in the study. However, due to natural disease progression, subjects who stayed longer in the study had a longer time period for disease deterioration. This natural disease progression is strong enough to offset the drug effect and cause an apparent upward trend when looking at the responses without adjusting for the confounding factors. Therefore, this dataset serves as a good example to apply the proposed three-step cumulative exposure response analysis method, which is illustrated in detail in the next three subsections.

22.3.2.1 Disease Progression Model and Subject Level Projected Disease Progression

A MMRM was used to build the disease progression model that measures the change from baseline in the target end point. The model used only placebo data (with slight modification for study 351) and included a random subject effect and the following fixed effects:

- Scheduled visit
- Baseline age
- Randomization strata
  - Baseline mini mental state examination (MMSE; low or high)
  - Use of baseline AD medication (yes or no)
  - Number of ApoE $\epsilon 4$ allele (1 or 2, carrier study only)
- Baseline value of the corresponding end point
- Time to dropout
- Baseline value versus visit interaction

In addition, to appreciate the difference in disease progression between different patient populations, the model was constructed separately for ApoE $\varepsilon 4$ carriers and ApoE $\varepsilon 4$ noncarriers, and then for the double-blind period and open-label extension period. Thus, the final model is a combination of 4 submodels.

To illustrate the structure of the model, the estimated terms for the double-blind period based on ADAS-Cog/11 total score are given in Table 22.1. It is worth to note that, while not always being statistically significant, the coefficients for the term "time to dropout" were negative for both the noncarrier and carrier populations. This intuitively reflects the fact that subjects who early terminated from the study often demonstrated greater amount of deterioration (for ADAS-Cog/11, larger score means greater impairment).

With the fitted disease progression models, each subject's own projected disease progression is estimated by plugging in the subject level values of the fixed effect terms.

22.3.2.2 Adjusted Response

Based on the MMRM-based disease progression model specified in Sect. 22.3.2.1, each subject's last observed outcome is adjusted by subtracting the model projected disease progression at the corresponding time point. For example, subject 1 was a study completer, therefore his projected disease progression at the sixth post-baseline

Table 22.1 Fitted disease progression model for ADAS-Cog/11 total score

ApoE ε4 noncarrier			ApoE ε4 carrier		
Model terms	Coefficient estimate (SE)	*p* value	Model terms	Coefficient estimate (SE)	*p* value
Intercept	5.6499 (2.2179)	0.0111	Intercept	7.8834 (2.6256)	0.0028
Baseline	0.2271 (0.0481)	<0.0001	Baseline	0.2300 (0.0558)	< 0.0001
Age	−0.0443 (0.0216)	0.0412	Age	−0.0470 (0.0273)	0.0861
Time to dropout	−0.0196 (0.0117)	0.0939	Time to dropout	−0.0265 (0.0125)	0.0352
MMSE: Low	2.8437 (0.5386)	<0.0001	MMSE: Low	1.9702 (0.5427)	0.0003
AD Med: No	−1.9626 (0.7593)	0.0100	AD Med: No	−1.2737 (0.9078)	0.1613
ApoE Allele: 1	NA (NA)	NA	ApoE Allele: 1	−0.6596 (0.5268)	0.2112
Week: 13	1.1309 (0.9812)	0.2498	Week: 13	0.2257 (1.2464)	0.8564
Week: 26	−0.0966 (0.8937)	0.9141	Week: 26	−1.4345 (1.1145)	0.1989
Week: 39	−0.5595 (0.7890)	0.4787	Week: 39	−1.7955 (1.0306)	0.0824
Week: 52	−1.5227 (0.7093)	0.0325	Week: 52	−0.3949 (0.9196)	0.6679
Week: 65	−0.0160 (0.7082)	0.9820	Week: 65	−1.3741 (0.8406)	0.1031
Baseline × week: 13	−0.3528 (0.0443)	<0.0001	Baseline × Week: 13	−0.3349 (0.0505)	< 0.0001
Baseline × week: 26	−0.2413 (0.0387)	< 0.0001	Baseline × Week: 26	−0.2271 (0.0454)	< 0.0001
Baseline × week: 39	−0.1633 (0.0344)	<0.0001	Baseline × Week: 39	−0.1230 (0.0422)	0.0038
Baseline × week: 52	−0.0597 (0.0311)	0.0554	Baseline × Week: 52	−0.1172 (0.0379)	0.0022
Baseline × week: 65	−0.0597 (0.0311)	0.0554	Baseline × Week: 65	−0.0103 (0.0347)	0.7678

MMSE mini mental state examination, *SE* standard error, *AD* Alzheimer's disease

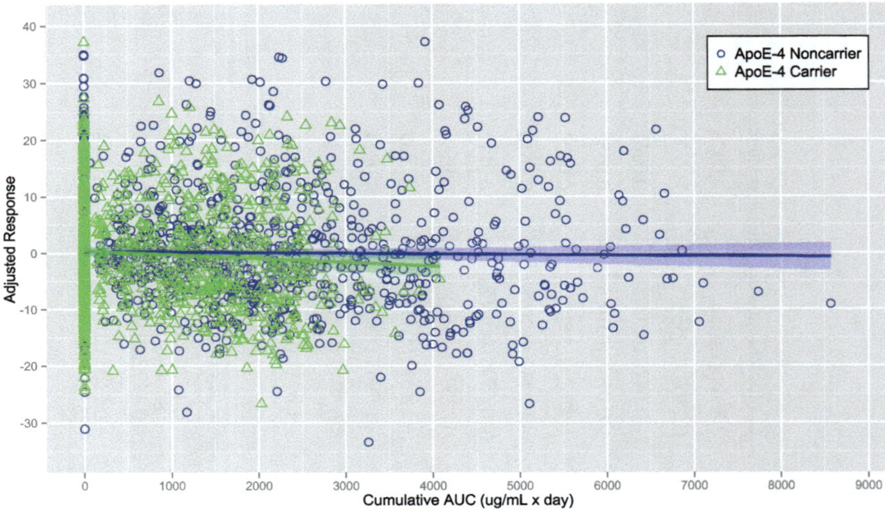

Fig. 22.4 Adjusted response Alzheimer's Disease Assessment Scale-Cognitive (ADAS-Cog)/11 total score versus cumulative exposure area under the curve (*AUC*)

visit was subtracted from his last observed response. On the other hand, subject 2 early terminated after the fourth dose, therefore her projected disease progression at the third post-baseline visit was subtracted from her last observed response.

Figure 22.4 illustrates a scatter plot of cumulative drug exposure in AUC (ug/mL $\times$ day) and the adjusted response. Similar to Fig. 22.3, two trend lines are also superimposed. However, this time it is easy to see there is a downward trend in both ApoE $\varepsilon 4$ carrier and noncarrier populations.

22.3.2.3 Cumulative Exposure Response Modeling

Based on the scatter plot (Fig. 22.4), for simplicity, a linear regression was performed to demonstrate the relationship between cumulative drug exposure and the adjusted response:

$$R_{\text{Adjusted}} = \alpha + \beta \cdot E. \tag{22.3}$$

However, other approaches might be preferred under various considerations. For example, from a typical dose-response point of view, an *E*Max type of model might be fit to recognize the potential "ceiling effect" of high exposure level

$$R_{\text{Adjusted}} = \alpha + \frac{\beta \cdot E}{\gamma + E}. \tag{22.4}$$

Also, a nonparametric approach (e.g., LOESS) might be applied if specific parametric shapes of the dose response cannot be identified at priori.

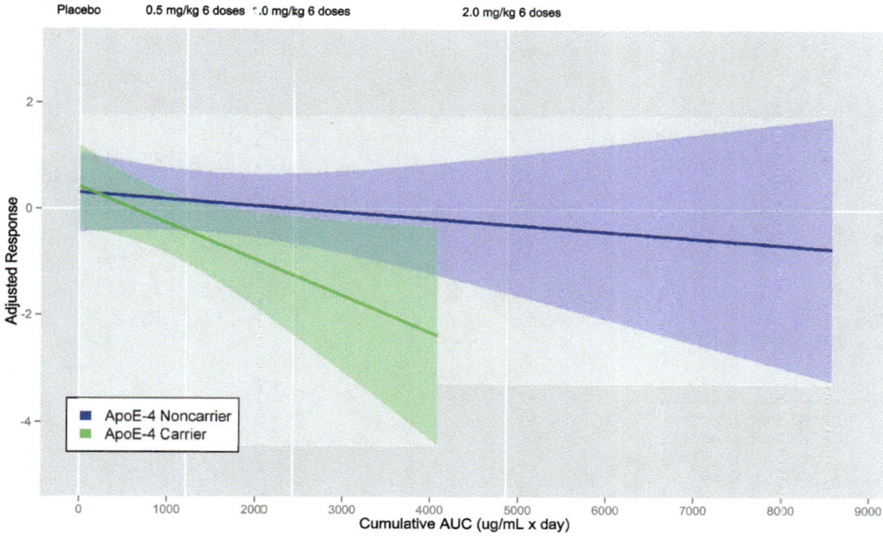

Fig. 22.5 Adjusted response in Alzheimer's Disease Assessment Scale-Cognitive (ADAS-Cog)/11 by cumulative area under the curve (*AUC*)

Figure 22.5 shows the exposure response for ADAS-Cog/11 total score based on simple linear regression. The two trend lines are identical to the trend lines in Fig. 22.4 but, to better illustrate the trend signal, scatter plot is not provided. Several vertical reference lines are provided to show the cumulative exposure level of a study completer from each treatment group with typical body weight. The exposure response in both patient populations exhibit certain level of downward trend, suggesting stronger treatment effect associated with higher level of cumulative drug exposure. Also, the left tail of both trend lines are at the zero level, suggesting no treatment effect of placebo.

Similarly, Fig. 22.6 shows the exposure response for PET amyloid load (Florbetapir PET global cortical average SUVr). Similar to that of the ADAS-Cog/11 total score, the exposure response for PET amyloid load also exhibits a downward trend for both patient populations, with the signal in the ApoE e4 carrier population a bit stronger.

22.4 Summary and Discussion

In this chapter, we introduced a model-based approach to assess the treatment effect of cumulative drug exposure. Such approach accounts for several confounding factors that are typically experienced in longitudinal studies of chronic neurodegenerative disease. The proposed approach has three steps: first, a disease progression model is constructed to represent the natural disease progression over the time course of the

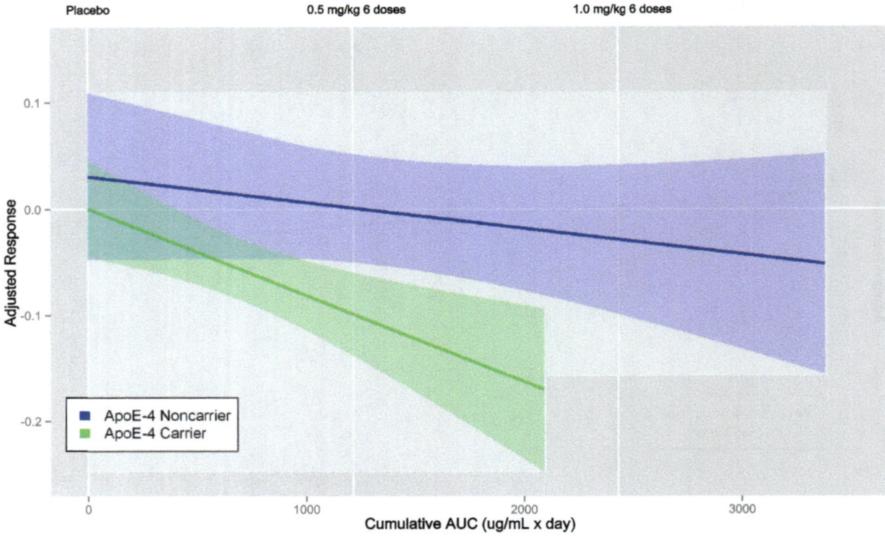

Fig. 22.6 Adjusted response in positron emission tomography (*PET*) global cortical average standard uptake value ratio (GCA SUVr) by cumulative area under the curve (*AUC*)

trial, where subject-level characteristics and dropout timing are taken into consideration; then, the observed outcome measures are adjusted by the projected disease progression at the matching time points; finally, the model-adjusted outcome measures are linked with the level of cumulative exposure (AUC). In the case study, the proposed method seems to suggest various degrees of efficacy trend favoring higher level of cumulative exposure in active drug, based on selected clinical and biomarker end points.

While this approach is demonstrated for analyzing the effect of cumulative drug exposure, it can be in principle applied in all situations where the confounding impacts of time course need to be adjusted. The key component of the approach is the construction of disease progression model. Such a model can be established using different approaches, but in all cases its appropriateness needs to be validated via methods such as visual predictive checking (VPC). Figure 22.7 compares the observed ADAS-Cog/11 total score mean placebo response during parent and extension periods with that is suggested by the proposed disease progression model. The VPC suggests that the MMRM-based disease progression model well captures the natural disease deterioration in the overall population and in subpopulations defined by baseline disease severity.

Finally, despite of its potentially wide application, the proposed approach has certain limitations that need to be emphasized

- Interpretation of cumulative exposure. The cumulative exposure (AUC) is jointly impacted by multiple factors (e.g., dose level, number of doses, clearance, body weight, etc.); therefore, it is difficult to identify the marginal effect of a single

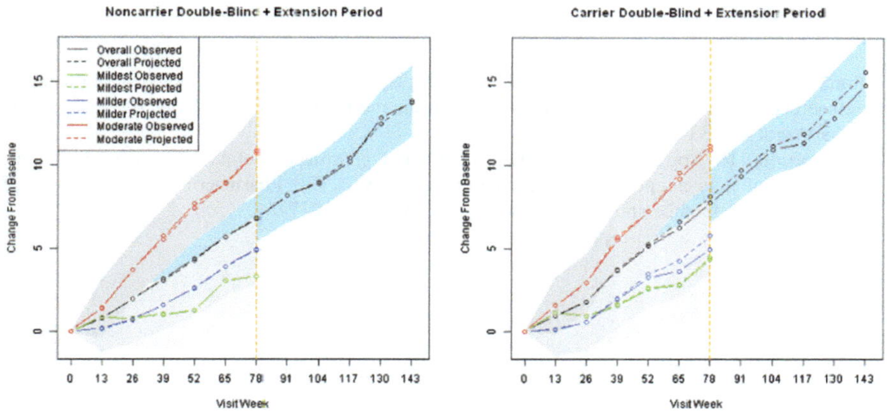

Fig. 22.7 Visual predictive check: disease progression model Alzheimer's Disease Assessment Scale-Cognitive (ADAS-Cog/11)

factor. For example, when higher level of cumulative exposure is beneficial, unless additional control is applied, it is impossible to determine if the benefit comes from higher dose level or longer treatment duration.

- Due to the purpose and hence the design of the study, subjects' allocation to different exposure levels is generally not random. For example, low cumulative exposure is to some extent confounded with early dropouts, while the efficacy performance of the early terminated subjects is almost always observed to be worse than the general population.
- The adjustment of natural disease progression is performed based on a specific disease progression model. Therefore, the results could be sensitive to model misspecification. For example, informative dropouts may create bias in modeling the disease progression. Although related factors (e.g., time to dropout) could be included in the disease progression model, this might not be sufficient in completely capturing the missing data impact, especially when missing data are missing not at random (Rubin 1976).
- The exposure–response is modeled using specific parametric functions, which assume particular curve shapes and add certain restrictions and limitations in representing the relationship.

Acknowledgement This work was sponsored by Janssen Alzheimer Immunotherapy Research & Development, LLC, and Pfizer Inc.

References

Hutmacher M, Nestorov I, Ludden T et al (2007) Modeling the exposure-response relationship of etanercept in the treatment of patients with chronic moderate to severe plaque psoriasis. J Clin Pharmacol 47:238–248

Lee H, Kimbo H, Rogge M et al (2003) Population pharmacokinetic and pharmacodynamic modeling of etancercept using logistic regression analysis. Clin Pharmacol Ther 73(4):348–365

Rubin B (1976) Inference and missing data. Biometrika 63:581–592

Chapter 23
Evaluation of a Confidence Interval Approach for Relative Agreement in a Crossed Three-Way Random Effects Model

Joseph C. Cappelleri and Naitee Ting

Abstract We specify a three-factor random effects model from a reliability study, where the effects of subjects, raters, and items are random. The reliability measure of interest is an intraclass correlation coefficient that measures the relative agreement of a single measurement on an individual from a randomly selected rater on a randomly selected item. Our objective is to evaluate and illustrate an approximate confidence interval for this intraclass correlation coefficient based on Satterthwaite's approximation (Wong and McGraw, Educational and Psychological Measurement, 59:270–288, 1999). In doing so, we perform Monte Carlo simulations and provide an illustration. Overall, the actual coverage of one-sided 95 % lower bounds and upper bounds, along with two-sided 90 % confidence intervals, for this particular intraclass correlation coefficient aligns with the nominal coverage for the commonly applied settings evaluated. This methodological evaluation is, to our knowledge, the first to validate the method.

23.1 Introduction

Reliable measurements are fundamental to medical research, especially when judgments are made by humans. Unreliable or imprecise measurement may have serious undesirable consequences (Fleiss 1986). Because measurement error can impair an analysis and its interpretation, it is important to quantify the amount of measurement error by reliability coefficients such as intraclass correlation coefficients. The intraclass correlation coefficient (ICC) may be defined as the proportion of some overall variance that is attributable to the variance of interest (e.g., between-subject variance; Armitage and Berry 1994). Several versions of the intraclass correlation

J. C. Cappelleri (✉)
Pfizer Inc, 445 Eastern Point Road, MS 8260-2502, Groton, CT 06340, USA
Tel.: (860) 441-8033
e-mail: joseph.c.cappelleri@pfizer.com

N. Ting
Boehringer Ingelheim Pharmaceuticals, Inc, Ridgefield, CT 06877, USA
Tel.: (203) 798-4999
e-mail: naitee.ting@boehringer-ingelheim.com

Z. Chen et al. (eds.), *Applied Statistics in Biomedicine and Clinical Trials Design*,
ICSA Book Series in Statistics, DOI 10.1007/978-3-319-12694-4_23

exist for different models and objectives (Müller and Büttner 1994; McGraw and Wong 1996; St. Laurent 1998; Perisic and Rosner 1999). The appropriate version is dictated by the specific situation defined by the experimental design and conceptual intent of the reliability study. This chapter concentrates on a particular type of intraclass correlation that measures reliability of measurements for quantitative data.

Specifically, we consider a reliability study of a randomly selected rater on a randomly selected item, in which each of K raters assesses each of J subjects on each of I items. For example, each of four raters could assess the muscle strength on each of eight subjects with rotator cuff dysfunction by using four items on a manual muscle test (which assess elevation, external rotation, internal rotation, and hand behind back lift-off maneuver; Hayes et al. 2002), with each item graded from 1 to 5 in terms of muscle strength, in order to assess the reliability of a single measurement made by a rater on an item.

For the balanced two-factor random design with one observation per subject–rater cell, in which the interaction term cannot be separated from the error term, confidence intervals for interrater reliability have been presented by several authors including Fleiss and Shrout (1978), Shrout and Fleiss (1979), Arteaga et al. (1982), McGraw and Wong (1996), Zou and McDermott (1999), Cappelleri and Ting (2003), Rousson et al. (2003), and Tian and Cappelleri (2004). In a general discussion of ICCs, Adamec and Burdick (2003) propose a Satterthwaite approach and Hamada and Weerahandi (2000) propose a generalized confidence interval approach.

This chapter centers on assessing the confidence interval for a particular ICC—specifically, the relative agreement of a single measurement on a subject made by a randomly selected rater on a randomly selected item, thereby giving the degree of consistency or relative standing or ranking among measurements made on the same person. Raters, subjects, and items are assumed to be randomly selected from their respective populations. Given this, and given that all subjects are rated by the same set of raters on the same set of items, the experimental design involves a crossed and balanced three-way random effects model with one observation per subject–rater–item cell. The set of items is assumed to be measuring different aspects of the same concept (such as items on the extent of bathing, walking, and running for measuring the concept of physical functioning).

Limited work has been performed on constructing a confidence interval on three-way random effects models in general (Adamec and Burdick 2003; Wong and McGraw 1999). In extending on the work of Fleiss and Shrout (1978) and Shrout and Fleiss (1979), which used Satterthwaite's method, Wong and McGraw (1999) constructed a confidence interval for ICC to measure relative agreement (consistency) among measurements, as well as to measure other types of ICCs. Because little research has been performed on evaluating the extent of the actual or true coverage (relative to the stated or nominal coverage) for this confidence interval, this chapter investigates such an assessment as it relates to ICC as a measure of reliability in a particular context: relative agreement of measurements from a randomly selected rater evaluating a randomly selected item on the same individual, with subjects, raters, and items taken as random factors in a crossed and balanced three-way analysis of variance model with one observation per cell. Section 23.2 provides a review of

Table 23.1 Data matrix for the crossed three-way random effects model (one observation per cell)

Subject	Rater 1 Item: 1...*i*....I	*k* 1...*i*...*I*	*K* 1...*i*...*I*
1	$Y_{111} \ldots Y_{I11}$	...	...
j	...	$Y_{1jk} \ldots Y_{Ijk}$	...
J	...	...	$Y_{1JK} \ldots Y_{IJK}$

Table 23.2 Analysis of variance table for the three-way random effects model

Source of variation	Sum of square	Degrees of freedom	Mean square	Expected mean square
Subject	SS_S	$n_1 = J - 1$	S_1^2	$\theta_1 = \sigma_e^2 + I\,\sigma_{SR}^2 + K\,\sigma_{TS}^2 + IK\,\sigma_S^2$
Item	SS_T	$n_2 = I - 1$	S_2^2	$\theta_2 = \sigma_e^2 + K\,\sigma_{TS}^2 + J\,\sigma_{TR}^2 + JK\,\sigma_T^2$
Rater	SS_R	$n_3 = K - 1$	S_3^2	$\theta_3 = \sigma_e^2 + J\,\sigma_{TR}^2 + I\,\sigma_{SR}^2 + IJ\,\sigma_R^2$
T × S	SS_{TS}	$n_4 = (I - 1)(J - 1)$	S_4^2	$\theta_4 = \sigma_e^2 + K\,\sigma_{TS}^2$
T × R	SS_{TR}	$n_5 = (I - 1)(K - 1)$	S_5^2	$\theta_5 = \sigma_e^2 + J\,\sigma_{TR}^2$
S × R	SS_{SR}	$n_6 = (J - 1)(K - 1)$	S_6^2	$\theta_6 = \sigma_e^2 + I\,\sigma_{SR}^2$
Error	SS_e	$n_e = (I - 1)(J - 1)(K - 1)$	S_e^2	$\theta_e = \sigma_e^2$

the methodology. Section 23.3 describes the Monte Carlo simulation procedure to examine the degree of coverage on the confidence intervals. Section 23.4 presents the results. Section 23.5 presents an illustration. Section 23.6 provides a discussion and Sect. 23.7 concludes with a summary.

23.2 Methodology

Table 23.1 contains the data layout. Table 23.2 contains the analysis of variance table for the three-way random effects model being considered, which includes three two-way interactions among the three factors. In this model, the score on the *i*th item from the *j*th rater on the *k*th subject may be represented as

$$Y_{ijk} = \mu + S_j + T_i + R_k + ST_{ij} + SR_{jk} + TR_{ik} + \varepsilon_{ijk}, \tag{23.1}$$

where $i = 1, \ldots, I$; $j = 1, \ldots, J$; $k = 1, \ldots, K$; $S, \sim T$, and R symbolize variation due to subjects, items and raters, respectively; μ is the overall mean; $S_j \sim N(0, \sigma_S^2)$; $T_i \sim N(0, \sigma_T^2)$; $R_k \sim N(0, \sigma_R^2)$; $ST_{ij} \sim N(0, \sigma_{ST}^2)$; $SR_{jk} \sim N(0, \sigma_{SR}^2)$; $TR_{ik} \sim N(0, \sigma_{TR}^2)$; and $\varepsilon_{ijk} \sim N(0, \sigma_e^2)$.

It can be shown that, as a measure of reliability, the intraclass coefficient

$$\rho = \frac{\sigma_S^2}{\sigma_S^2 + \sigma_{SR}^2 + \sigma_{TS}^2 + \sigma_e^2} = \frac{\theta_1 - \theta_4 - \theta_6 + \theta_e}{\theta_1 + (I-1)\theta_4 + (K-1)\theta_6 + (I-1)(K-1)\theta_e} \tag{23.2}$$

(with the θs defined Table 23.2) gives the population reliability of a single measurement on a subject made by a randomly selected rater on a randomly selected item—specifically, the degree of consistency or relative agreement among measurements on a single subject (Wong and McGraw 1999). The corresponding sample estimator (based on the analysis of variance framework in Table 23.2) becomes

$$\hat{\rho} = \frac{S_1^2 - S_4^2 - S_6^2 - S_e^2}{S_1^2 + (I-1) + S_4^2 + (K-1)S_6^2 + (I-1)(K-1)S_e^2}. \tag{23.3}$$

Wong and McGraw (1999) derived a one-sided $100(1-\alpha)$ % lower confidence limit L_{WM} and a one-sided $100(1-\alpha)$ % upper confidence limit U_{WM} using Satterthwaite's method (Satterthwaite 1946; Kirk 1995) as follows:

$$L_{WM} = \frac{S_1^2 - F_{\alpha;n_1,\upsilon}(S_4^2 + S_6^2 - S_e^2)}{S_1^2 + F_{\alpha:n_1,\upsilon}[(I-1)S_4^2 + (K-1)S_6^2 + (I-1)(K-1)S_e^2]} \tag{23.4}$$

and

$$U_{WM} = \frac{S_1^2 - F_{1-\alpha;n_1,\upsilon}(S_4^2 + S_6^2 - S_e^2)}{S_1^2 + F_{1-\alpha:n_1,\upsilon}[(I-1)S_4^2 + (K-1)S_6^2 + (I-1)(K-1)S_e^2]}, \tag{23.5}$$

where

$$\upsilon = \frac{(aS_4^2 + bS_6^2 + cS_e^2)^2}{\frac{a^2S_4^4}{n_1n_2} + \frac{b^2S_6^4}{n_1n_3} + \frac{c^2S_e^4}{n_1n_2n_3}}, \tag{23.6}$$

With $n_1 = J-1, n_2 = l-1, and\, n_3 = K-1$ (from Table 23.2); $\hat{\rho}$ is defined in Eq. 23.3; $a = 1 + (l-1)\hat{\rho}$; $b = 1 + (K-1)\hat{\rho}$; and $c = -1 + (l-1)(K-1)\hat{\rho}$. In addition, for L_{WM}, $F_{\alpha;n_1,\upsilon}$ represents the F-value with n_1 and ν degrees of freedom that has α to the right; for U_{WM}, $F_{1-\alpha;n_1,\upsilon}$represents the F-value with n_1 and νdegrees of freedom that has $(1-\alpha)$ to the right.

Bounds on the two-sided $100(1-2\alpha)$% interval correspond exactly to bounds on the two one-sided $100(1-2\alpha)$% intervals. As such, the same F critical values ($F_{\alpha;n_1,\upsilon}$ *and* $F_{1-\alpha:n_1,\upsilon}$) are used also for the two-sided $100(1-2\alpha)$% interval.

23.3 Simulation Procedure

An empirical study using Monte Carlo simulation was undertaken to examine the coverage probabilities of the confidence bounds for ρ. Several designs on the sample size mix were considered: 2, 5, and 10 raters evaluating 10, 25, 50, and 100 subjects on 2, 3, 5, 7, and 10 items. Nominal significance levels were 0.05 for a one-sided lower confidence interval (one-sided 95 % lower bound) and 0.10 for a two-sided confidence interval (two-sided 90 % bounds). Interval widths for the two-sided interval are calculated as the difference between the upper limit and the lower limit.

In the simulation procedure, we defined $r_1 = \theta_1/(\theta_1 + \theta_4 + \theta_6 + \theta_\varepsilon)$, $r_4 = \theta_4/(\theta_1 + \theta_4 + \theta_6 + \theta_\varepsilon)$, $r_6 = \theta_6/(\theta_1 + \theta_4 + \theta_6 + \theta_\varepsilon)$, and $r_\varepsilon = 1 - r_1 - r_4 - r_6$. Without loss of generality, we defined $\theta_1 + \theta_4 + \theta_6 + \theta_\varepsilon = 1$ so that $r_1 = \theta_1$, $r_4 = \theta_4$, $r_6 = \theta_6$, and $r_\varepsilon = \theta_\varepsilon$. The distributional assumptions were $S_1^2 \sim r_1 Q_1/df_1$, $S_4^2 \sim r_4 Q_4/df_4$, $S_6^2 \sim r_6 Q_6/df_6$, and $S_\varepsilon^2 \sim r_\varepsilon Q_\varepsilon/df_\varepsilon$ where Q_1, Q_4, Q_6, and Q_ε represented a set of jointly independent chi-square random variables with df_1, df_4, df_6, and df_ε degrees of freedom, respectively. (In the context of the analysis of variance model, note that $df_1 = J - 1$, $df_4 = (I - 1)(J - 1)$, $df_6 = (J - 1)(K - 1)$, and $df_\varepsilon = (I - 1)(J - 1)(K - 1)$ represented the degrees of freedom, respectively, for between-subject, item by subject, subject by rater, and residual variation.) These four chi-square random variables were generated using the RANGAM function in Statistical Analysis System (SAS; SAS Institute Inc. 2011).

For each possible combination of (r_1, r_4, r_6, r_ε), a total of 25,000 sets of (S_1^2, S_4^2, S_6^2, S_ε^2) were simulated for each design. Simulated values for the mean squares were substituted into the appropriate formulas (from Sect. 23.2) and intervals were computed. Confidence coefficients were determined by counting the number of intervals that contained ρ and then dividing by 25,000. Mean percent coverage across the parameter space of all possible parameter value combinations were computed for one-sided intervals and two-sided intervals. In addition, mean interval widths were calculated across these combinations for two-sided intervals, where each combination had an average interval width that was computed as the sum of the 25,000 interval widths divided by 25,000.

All computations throughout were performed in SAS (SAS Institute Inc. 2009).

23.4 Results of Simulation: Coverage Probabilities and Interval Widths

Based on the simulation procedure described in Sect. 23.3, the results for coverage of the one-sided 95 % lower bound, one-sided 95 % upper bound, and two-sided 90 % intervals appear in Tables 23.3, 23.4, and 23.5, respectively. Regarding the one-sided 95 % lower bound (Table 23.3), the true or actual coverage of the Wong–McGraw approach aligned with the purported or nominal coverage of 95 % or gave

Table 23.3 Mean percent coverage of approximate lower 95 % confidence bounds of relative agreement reliability (ρ) across parameter sets (25,000 simulations)

Raters	Subjects	Items				
		2	3	5	7	10
2	10	94.30	94.28	94.35	94.36	94.32
	25	94.59	94.56	94.59	94.53	94.52
	50	94.63	94.69	94.70	94.67	94.68
	100	94.80	94.78	94.82	94.71	94.74
5	10	93.16	94.44	94.81	94.90	94.94
	25	93.98	94.69	94.93	94.88	94.95
	50	94.27	94.76	94.86	94.94	94.99
	100	94.49	94.83	94.96	94.96	95.03
10	10	93.04	94.30	94.76	94.90	94.97
	25	93.88	94.62	94.89	94.95	94.94
	50	94.19	94.74	94.94	94.98	94.99
	100	94.50	94.78	94.96	94.98	94.92

Table 23.4 Mean percent coverage of approximate upper 95 % confidence bounds of relative agreement reliability (ρ) across parameter sets (25,000 simulations)

Raters	Subjects	Items				
		2	3	5	7	10
2	10	95.70	95.80	95.87	95.90	95.99
	25	95.55	95.48	95.51	95.56	95.55
	50	95.40	95.33	95.34	95.35	95.41
	100	94.80	94.78	94.82	95.28	95.26
5	10	96.23	95.48	95.20	95.13	95.15
	25	95.75	95.30	95.09	95.10	94.99
	50	95.61	95.23	95.05	95.09	95.05
	100	95.46	95.17	95.03	95.07	95.02
10	10	96.34	95.53	95.21	95.08	95.10
	25	95.88	95.33	95.10	95.06	95.06
	50	95.62	95.21	95.10	94.99	95.02
	100	95.51	95.20	95.03	95.04	95.02

slightly liberal coverage ($<94.73\,\%$ after accounting for simulation error). Mild liberal coverage was most evident for two raters or two items, whose actual coverage approached and eventually converged to the nominal coverage as the number of subjects increased.

Table 23.5 Mean percent coverage (and mean interval width) of approximate 90 % two-sided intervals of relative agreement reliability (ρ) across parameter sets with two, five, and ten raters (25,000 simulations)

Raters	Subjects	Items				
		2	3	5	7	10
2	10	90.00 (0.55)	90.01 (0.48)	90.23 (0.43)	90.27 (0.43)	90.31 (0.40)
2	25	90.14 (0.39)	90.04 (0.33)	90.10 (0.28)	90.08 (0.27)	90.07 (0.25)
2	50	90.03 (0.30)	90.02 (0.24)	90.04 (0.20)	90.02 (0.19)	90.08 (1.7)
2	100	90.09 (0.22)	90.03 (0.18)	90.05 (0.14)	89.99 (0.13)	89.99 (0.12)
5	10	89.39 (0.47)	89.92 (0.42)	90.01 (0.38)	90.04 (0.36)	90.09 (0.34)
5	25	89.73 (0.33)	89.99 (0.28)	90.02 (0.24)	89.98 (0.22)	89.99 (0.21)
5	50	89.88 (0.24)	89.99 (0.20)	89.90 (0.17)	90.03 (0.16)	90.04 (0.15)
5	100	89.95 (0.18)	90.00 (0.14)	89.98 (0.12)	90.03 (0.11)	90.05 (0.10)
10	10	89.38 (0.45)	89.83 (0.40)	89.97 (0.36)	89.98 (0.34)	90.07 (0.33)
10	25	89.76 (0.31)	89.96 (0.26)	89.99 (0.23)	90.01 (0.21)	90.00 (0.20)
10	50	89.88 (0.24)	89.99 (0.20)	89.90 (0.17)	89.97 (0.15)	90.01 (0.14)
10	100	90.01 (0.16)	89.98 (0.13)	89.99 (0.11)	90.02 (0.10)	89.95 (0.10)

Regarding the one-sided 95 % upper bound (Table 23.4), the actual coverage of the approach maintained the nominal coverage or gave slightly conservative coverage ($>$ 95.27 % after accounting for simulation error). Mild conservative coverage was most evident for two raters or two items, whose actual coverage approached and eventually converged to the nominal coverage (95 %) as the number of subjects increased.

Regarding the two-sided 90 % intervals (Table 23.5), the actual coverage was largely congruent with the nominal coverage. After accounting for simulation error ($<$ 89.69 % for lower limit, $>$ 90.31 % for upper limit), slight underestimation was found with ten subjects and two items having five raters and ten raters. Otherwise, the actual coverage gave the nominal coverage. The average interval width decreased, as expected, with an increase in the number of items (for a fixed number of raters and

Table 23.6 Data layout for illustrative example with 40 persons measured on eight items by three raters

	Rater 1								Rater 2								Rater 3							
Items	1	2	3	4	5	6	7	8	1	2	3	4	5	6	7	8	1	2	3	4	5	6	7	8
Persons																								
1	7	6	6	5	6	6	7	5	6	7	7	5	7	7	7	7	7	7	8	8	7	6	6	7
.																								
.																								
.																								
40	4	4	4	5	5	5	6	4	4	5	4	6	4	7	8	7	6	5	5	6	6	6	7	5

Table 23.7 Sum of squares and mean squares for illustrative example

Source	Sum of squares	Degrees of freedom	Mean square
Persons	439.96	39	11.28
Items	68.57	7	9.80
Raters	89.75	2	44.88
Persons × items	336.30	273	1.23
Persons × raters	118.42	78	1.52
Items × raters	14.35	14	1.02
Residual	666.15	546	1.22

subjects), number of subjects (for a fixed number of raters and items), and number of raters (for a fixed number of subjects and items).

23.5 Illustrative Example

Consider a study with 40 persons being evaluated on eight items by three raters or judges. The resulting three-way random effects analysis of variance model can also be considered a three (raters)-by-eight (items) repeated measures analysis of variance model on 40 individuals. The data layout is presented in Table 23.6 and the complete data are provided in Wong and McGraw (1999). Table 23.7 gives the corresponding sum of squares, degrees of freedom, and mean squares for the seven sources of variation. Based on the information given in this chapter, relative agreement reliability and confidence intervals for it can be calculated for these data. Relative agreement reliability of 0.24 was estimated for a single measurement made by a randomly selected rater on a randomly selected item; the limit of the approximate lower one-sided 95 % confidence interval was 0.16; the limit of the approximate upper one-sided 95 % confidence interval was 0.36; and the approximate two-sided 90 % interval was therefore between 0.16 and 0.36.

23.6 Discussion

In this chapter, attention is focused on a crossed design having every person to be evaluated on each item by each rater, where all three sources of variation are considered random. Interest centered on evaluating the actual or true coverage of a confidence interval on a particular intraclass correlation: relative agreement of a single measurement from a randomly selected rater on a randomly selected item taken on the same person. In what follows, several worthy points of distinction are made (for more details, see Shavelson and Webb 1991; Brennan 2001).

First, it should be emphasized that a reliability coefficient (and its confidence interval) is not restricted to the three particular sources of variation highlighted. For example, instead of items, occasions (time) can be used in order to estimate the reliability of a single measurement on an individual from a randomly selected rater at a randomly selected occasion.

Second, a reliability coefficient (and its confidence interval) is not restricted to all sources of variation being random (only variation due to subjects need be random). For instance, items can be taken as a fixed source of variation (analogous to a fixed factor in an analysis of variance model) when interest centers only on the particular items selected, which are not considered exchangeable with other items in the population. Confidence intervals for ICCs—including for relative agreement in a three-way crossed design—based on three-way mixed effects models, with one fixed factor and two random factors, are provided elsewhere (Zhou et al. 2011).

Third, a reliability coefficient (and its confident interval) is not restricted to a single measurement. In the special case of the three-way random effects design, for example, reliability of a person's average score (and its confidence interval) can be obtained by averaging scores across a random sample of multiple raters and multiple items (not necessarily the same number of raters and items given in the study). As the number of raters and items that go into the average score increase, so does the reliability. For the illustrative example given in the chapter, the relative agreement coefficient was 0.86 (with 95 % confidence interval from 0.76 to 0.93) when a person's score is averaged across three raters who each used eight items, compared with 0.24 (0.16–0.26) for a single measurement.

Fourth, the reliability coefficient (and its confidence interval) used in this chapter concerns relative agreement or consistency of scores grounded in relative interpretations that address how much better one individual performed than another. For relative decisions, measurement error is defined as all variance components that influence the relative standing of individuals. For the three-way design in this chapter, these components are the interactions of the item source of variation and the rater source of variation with persons, the object of measurement, as well as residual error.

An alternative reliability coefficient (and its confidence interval) involves absolute agreement, which addresses decisions about how well an individual can perform, regardless of the performance of others. For absolute decisions, not only do changes in the ranking of individuals contribute to error but the actual levels of their performance also depend on the characteristics of the factors such as whether the items are easy or difficult and whether the raters are lenient or strict. Thus, all variance components except the person variance component contribute to error (e.g., variance components from items, raters, and items by raters, as well as from patient by items, patient by raters, and residual error). Absolute agreement generally implies relative agreement, but the reverse is not true. As such, absolute agreement reliability is generally less than relative agreement reliability. In the illustrative example, absolute agreement reliability of a single measurement was 0.22, compared with 0.24 for relative agreement reliability.

Fifth, the formula for a reliability coefficient (and its confidence interval construction) depends on the type of research design. In addition to the crossed design where every person is evaluated on each item by each rater, several other types of three-way random factor designs are available. Among them is the design where items are nested within raters, as would occur when different items are used by different raters, with persons crossed with both items and raters, and the design where each person is measured by each rater but that the items are both person and rater specific (i.e., for each person–rater combination, a different set of items is used).

Using Satterthwaite's method, Wong and McGraw (1999) actually provided construction of confidence intervals for the relative agreement coefficient and the absolute agree coefficient for a single measurement score and average score in different types of three-way random effects designs. This chapter is limited to the evaluation of a confidence interval for the relative agreement coefficient for a single measurement score from the fully crossed (and balanced) three-way random effects designs. Although it is beyond the current scope of this chapter to evaluate all of the confidence intervals derived in Wong and McGraw (1999), further research is encouraged in assessing the coverage of other confidence intervals. While only one-sided 95 % bounds and two-sided 90 % confidence intervals were investigated in this chapter, there is no reason to believe that the results and conclusions would differ for other confidence intervals such as one-sided 99 % bounds.

23.7 Summary

Overall, the actual coverage probability of one-sided 95 % lower bounds and upper bounds, along with two-sided 90 % confidence intervals, for relative agreement reliability aligns with the nominal coverage within most of the commonly applied settings. Any understated (liberal) coverage probability for the one-sided 95 % lower bound is only slight and likely to be inconsequential in most circumstances. The same can be said about the slightly overstated (conservative) coverage of the one-sided 95 % upper bound. This methodological evaluation is, to our knowledge, the first to validate the coverage probability of this particular confidence interval and to show that its actual coverage is close or equal to the stated coverage.

Acknowledgments This chapter was presented as an invited oral presentation on innovative methods in multivariate analysis at the International Chinese Statistical Association and the International Society for Biopharmaceutical Statistics Joint Statistical Conference, Bethesda, MD, USA June 9–12, 2013. The authors thank Kelly Zou (Pfizer Inc) for organizing the invited session. We also thank Tom Abernathy (Pfizer Inc) for help with execution of the simulation program.

References

Adamec E, Burdick R (2003) Confidence intervals for a discrimination ratio in a gauge R&R study with three random factors. Qual Eng 15(3):283–389
Armitage P, Berry G (1994) Statistical methods in medical research, 3rd edn. Blackwell, Oxford
Arteaga C, Jeyaratnam S, Graybill FA: (1982) Confidence intervals for proportions of total variance in the two-way cross component of variance model. Comm Stat Theor M 11(15):1643–1658
Brennan RL (2001) Generalizability theory. Springer, New York
Cappelleri JC, Ting N (2003) A modified large-sample approach to approximate interval estimation for a particular intraclass correlation coefficient. Stat Med 22(11):1861–1877
Fleiss JL, Shrout PE (1978) Approximate interval estimation for a certain intraclass correlation coefficient. Psychometrika 43(2):259–262
Fleiss JL (1986) The Design and analysis of clinical experiments. Wiley, New York
Hamada M, Weerahandi S (2000) Measurement system assessment via generalized inference. J Qual Tech 32(3):241–253
Hayes K, Walton JR, Szomor ZL, Murrell GAC (2002) Reliability of 3 methods for assessing shoulder strength. J Shoulder Elb Surg 11(1):33–39
Kirk RE (1995) Experimental design: procedures for the behavioral sciences. Brooks/Cole, Pacific Grove
McGraw KO, Wong SP (1996) Forming inferences about some intraclass correlation coefficients. Psychol Methods 1(1):30–46
Müller R, Büttner P (1994) A critical discussion of intraclass correlation coefficients. Stat Med 13(23–24):2465–2476
Perisic I, Rosner B (1999) Comparisons of measures of interclass correlations: the general case of unequal group size. Stat Med 18(12):1451–1466
Rousson V, Gasser T, Seifert B (2003) Confidence intervals for intraclass correlation in inter-rater reliability. Scand J Stat 30(3):617–624
SAS Institute Inc. (2009) SAS/STAT® 9.2 user's guide, 2nd ed. SAS Institute, Cary
SAS Institute Inc. (2011) SAS® 9.2 language reference: dictionary, 4th ed. SAS Institute, Cary
Satterthwaite PE (1946) An approximate distribution of estimates of variance components. Biometrics 2(6):110–114
Shavelson RJ, Webb NM (1991) Generalizability theory. SAGE, Newbury Park
Shrout PE, Fleiss J (1979) Intraclass correlation: uses in assessing rater reliability. Psychol Bull 86(2):420–428
St. Laurent RT (1998) Evaluating agreement with a gold standard in method comparison studies. Biometrics 54(2):537–545
Tian L, Cappelleri JC (2004) A new approach for interval estimation and hypothesis testing of a certain intraclass correlation coefficient: the generalized variable method. Stat Med 23(13):2125–2135

Wong SP, McGraw KO (1999) Confidence intervals and F tests for intraclass correlations based on three-way random effects models. Educ Psychol Meas 59(2):270–288

Zhou H, Muellerleile P, Ingram D, Wong SP (2011) Confidence intervals and F tests for intraclass correlation coefficients based on three-way mixed effects models. J Educ Behav Stat 36(5): 638–671

Zou KH, McDermott MP (1999) Higher-moment approaches to approximate interval estimation for a certain intraclass correlation coefficient. Stat Med 18(15):2051–2061

Part V
Personalized Medicine and Subgroup Analysis

Chapter 24
Assessment of Methods to Identify Patient Subgroups with Enhanced Treatment Response in Randomized Clinical Trials

Richard C. Zink, Lei Shen, Russell D. Wolfinger and H. D. Hollins Showalter

Abstract In contrast to the "one-size-fits-all" approach of traditional drug development, the need to identify subjects with an enhanced treatment effect is a critical component for tailored therapeutics or personalized medicine. Typically, the goal is to determine which patient receives additional benefit from the treatment in terms of an efficacy response. Alternatively, finding subgroups based on the important safety endpoints could be considered to identify those individuals experiencing a reduced risk of key adverse events, or to identify subjects for whom the new therapy may be inappropriate. A number of methods for identifying subgroups with enhanced treatment response have been developed recently, and it is natural to expect many more in the coming years. In order for the development programs for tailored therapeutics to be successful, it is imperative to identify the best method(s) for subgroup identification to be applied in practice. Further, it is likely that no single method will be optimal across all scenarios, so fully characterizing the properties of each methodology is of the utmost importance. To accomplish these goals, the researchers who develop every new and existing method should ideally make use of the same set of simulated data scenarios and report their findings using the same performance measures. We outline and describe the key attributes and scenarios for simulated data as well as the performance measures to enable consistent and rigorous assessment of subgroup identification methods.

R. C. Zink (✉) · R. D. Wolfinger
JMP Life Sciences, SAS Institute Inc, Cary, NC, USA
e-mail: richard.zink@jmp.com

R. D. Wolfinger
e-mail: russ.wolfinger@jmp.com

L. Shen · H. D. H. Showalter
Eli Lilly & Company, Indianapolis, IN, USA
e-mail: shen_lei@lilly.com

H. D. H. Showalter
e-mail: showalter_howard_daniel_h@lilly.com

Z. Chen et al. (eds.), *Applied Statistics in Biomedicine and Clinical Trials Design*,
ICSA Book Series in Statistics, DOI 10.1007/978-3-319-12694-4_24

24.1 Introduction

Drug development has traditionally focused on comparing the average response of patients on an experimental treatment to the average response of patients receiving either placebo or standard of care. Assuming no meaningful changes in the safety profile, should the treatment effect based on these average responses meet the criteria for clinical and statistical significance, the trial would be deemed a success with the experimental treatment being interpreted as the "better" choice for the patient population. However, this interpretation is often an oversimplification of what has actually occurred within the clinical trial. If one were to examine the data further, there are usually instances where patients on the experimental treatment failed to respond, and where patients on the standard of care (and sometimes even placebo!) exhibited a preferential response to their treatment. When it comes to the treatment response for these individuals, the "mean doesn't mean as much anymore" (Ruberg et al. 2010). The goal for tailored therapeutics or personalized medicine is to identify the best treatment for each patient based upon their personal and disease characteristics.

Understanding this heterogeneity of treatment response is itself no easy task—after all, human beings are extraordinarily complex! Response to treatment may be influenced by demographic characteristics, medical and treatment history, genetic factors, local environment, or other co-occurring disease. The disease itself may be extremely complex; there may be variations or characteristics of the disease that can impact the level of treatment response. One oft-cited example in oncology is trastuzumab which has been shown to be an effective treatment for breast cancer only when the tumor is HER2 positive (Baselga et al. 2006). Cystic fibrosis patients with at least one G551D mutation in the cystic fibrosis transmembrane conductance regulator protein have been shown to receive benefit from ivacaftor (Ramsey et al. 2011). Diseases collectively known as "dry eye" have varying mechanisms of action; the tear film may be unstable or produced in insufficient quantities (evaporative versus aqueous deficient) (Bron 2001). Identifying biomarkers that influence response is necessary to tailor an appropriate treatment for each individual patient.

For the present discussion, it is important to draw a distinction between *prognostic* and *predictive* biomarkers. Prognostic biomarkers are those characteristics that impact an outcome independent of the treatment received. In a regression model, this can be interpreted as a shift in the intercept for marker-positive patients (left panel of Fig. 24.1). These biomarkers help us determine the prognosis of patients, but are not related to any additional benefit of the drug compared to the standard of care for marker-negative patients. In other words, the treatment effect is the same for either marker group. Predictive biomarkers, on the other hand, indicate an enhanced outcome that is specific to the particular treatment being received. In terms of a regression model, this can be interpreted as a treatment by marker interaction (right panel of Fig. 24.1). Such biomarkers may be reported in the drug label, and could potentially be codeveloped with a companion diagnostic. Within the remainder of this manuscript, the term *biomarker* refers to *predictive biomarkers*.

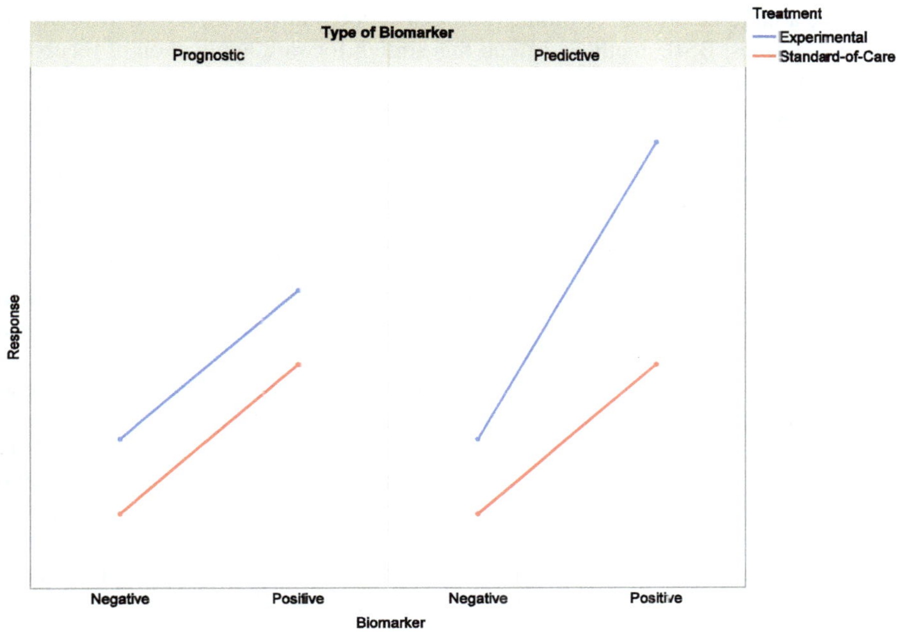

Fig. 24.1 Graphical presentation of *prognostic* versus *predictive* biomarkers. *Prognostic* biomarkers have enhanced effect independent of the treatment, but *predictive* biomarkers show enhanced effect with a particular treatment, i.e., interact with the treatment

Treatment response can be summarized within subgroups defined by important patient and disease characteristics (biomarkers), and this exercise is often performed as part of the secondary objectives of single trials or the integrated summary of efficacy (ISE) for new drug applications within the USA. However, there are some drawbacks with this approach. First, based on the emerging understanding of the disease, covariates that may be predictive of enhanced response could go overlooked. Second, waiting until the ISE to understand the treatment response within subgroups fails to take advantage of any efficiency that could be gained in the development process by enriching trials with responsive subpopulations.

Identifying these responsive subpopulations early in the development process has numerous benefits. Enriching studies with these patients could result in smaller clinical trials either through a larger possible treatment effect or through a reduced variability of response. Further, responsive patients may require smaller doses of drug to illicit a beneficial response which could benefit the safety profile. Finally, understanding which subjects may respond negatively to the novel treatment has benefits for the safety profile, as well as being ethical for maintaining these patients on their current or alternate treatment regimes.

The literature for biomarker subgroup identification (BSID) methods typically falls within one of two camps. Recursive partitioning methods are a natural way to analyze a large number of covariates and assess potentially complex interactions of these variables. BSID methods extend this straightforward application of recursive partitioning to an endpoint since the quantity of interest is the treatment effect, that is, the mean difference in that endpoint between two groups (Battioui et al. 2013; Foster et al. 2011; Loh 2011; Lipkovich and Dmitrienko 2014; Lipkovich et al. 2011; Negassa et al. 2005). The other set of methods involves tests of treatment by biomarker interactions in regression models, often testing each biomarker separately from the others (though adjustment for other covariates is possible) (Su et al. 2008; Su et al. 2009; Radcliffe and Surry 2011; Dusseldorp and Mechelen 2014). Similar to recursive partitioning methods, binary splits of continuous biomarkers are often used in the interaction models for the purposes of defining a subgroup. An illustrative example is presented in Sect. 24.2.

The BSID problem is closely related to, but not the same as, the optimal treatment regime (OTR) problem, as described, for example, in (Zhang et al. 2012; Zhao et al. 2012). The latter focuses on finding the best treatment assignment for each patient, whereas the former tries to find a subset of patients with enhanced treatment response. One difference between the two problems is illustrated in Fig. 24.1. If we assume a larger response is more desirable and that all plotted mean responses are clinically meaningful with sharp differences, then the OTR solution for all patients would be the experimental arm (blue line), regardless of whether the left panel or right panel represents the truth, because the blue line is always above the red line. However, for BSID, the left panel is a case in which there are no subgroups identified by the biomarker, but the right panel is a case in which the biomarker does identify a subgroup. BSID is effectively a search for biomarker-by-treatment interactions, whereas OTR typically builds on a full response model and does not need to distinguish between prognostic and predictive biomarkers. While this chapter focuses on BSID, many of the proposals discussed can be applied or extended to OTR as well.

With increasing interest in personalized medicine, it is natural to expect that the literature for BSID (and OTR) methods will proliferate over time. Given the inherent problems in subgroup analysis and the tendency of researchers to over-interpret findings (Rothwell 2005), it is of paramount importance to outline a strategy to determine the best method(s) for subgroup identification to be used in practice. An important part of any method is to minimize the likelihood of a false-positive finding—identifying subgroups based on apparently predictive biomarkers that fail to bear fruit with further testing. Further, it is likely that no single method will be optimal across all scenarios, so fully characterizing the properties of each methodology is vital.

The purpose of this chapter is to describe a strategy to (1) determine the best BSID method(s) to be used in practice for tailored therapeutics and (2) fully characterize the properties of these methods so that they are used appropriately in practice based on the characteristics of the clinical trial and disease under investigation. In Sect. 24.2, we present an illustrative example of an interaction-based BSID method to motivate the discussion. In Sect. 24.3, we describe the Predictive Biomarker Project (PBP) which details a prospective approach to rigorously and consistently assess new BSID methods as they are developed. We summarize our insights in Sect. 24.4.

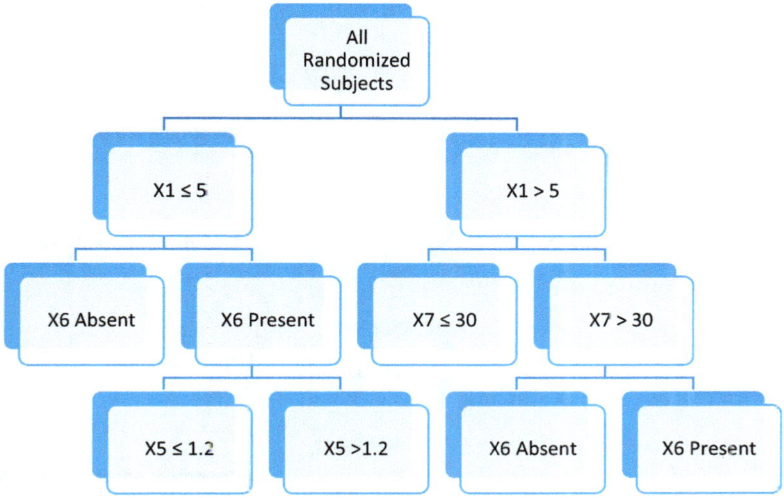

Fig. 24.2 Example of a subgroup tree based on binary splits from an interaction model

24.2 Illustrative Example

Here, we describe an example BSID method to motivate the proposal described in Sect. 24.3. Figure 24.2 presents a subgroup tree based on binary splits of a population of randomized subjects from a hypothetical clinical trial. Such a tree is the natural result of recursive partitioning; subsets are produced based on the ability to best predict the continuous or categorical endpoint of interest. However, in recursive partitioning, splits are not based on the treatment effect of the endpoint of interest. To generate a tree when trying to find enhanced treatment effects, the following model could be fit at a node for each covariate to determine whether splitting was appropriate:

$$f\left(y_i\right) = \beta_0 + \beta_1 x_i + \beta_2 \text{Treatment}_i + \beta_3 \text{Treatment}_i * x_i. \qquad (24.1)$$

Here, x_i represents a binary covariate, which could refer to the presence or absence of an allele for a particular genetic biomarker, or value exceeding a meaningful threshold (or not) for a continuous biomarker. In general, a single biomarker could generate multiple variables to review (e.g., a continuous covariate could be split at each of the three quartiles), though the number of splits is often limited based on the sample sizes of the resulting subgroups. A significant interaction for β_3 in model (1) implies differential treatment effects between subgroups defined by the binary covariate x_i. At a given node, the split is made based on the most "significant" interaction term present across all covariates, should such an interaction exist. This general description applies to the interaction trees methodologies (Su et al. 2008; Su et al. 2009; Radcliffe and Surry 2011; Dusseldorp and Mechelen 2014).

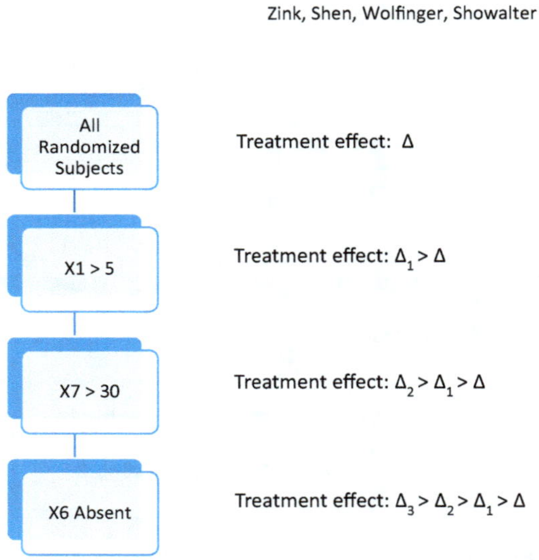

Fig. 24.3 Example of a subgroup tree using the PAYGO algorithm. *PAYGO* prune as you go

Completed trees require "pruning" to prevent a model that over-fits the data. One potential simplification to the above algorithm is to prune the tree as each split occurs (prune as you go, PAYGO). This suggestion is based on the idea that the significant interaction for β_3 in model (1) produces one subgroup with an enhanced treatment response compared to the parent node, while the other subgroup produces a weaker or potentially negative treatment effect compared to the parent node. From this point on, the "weaker" subgroup can be "ignored" resulting in a tree with reduced effort in terms of computation. A similar approach was implemented in (Lipkovich and Dmitrienko 2014) using recursive partitioning methodologies. Further, the treatment effects are necessarily larger at each subsequent level (Fig. 24.3). An additional benefit is that the subgroup problem is now sequential. Once a nonsignificant level is reached, no further splitting is performed.

The best way to handle what is "significant" at each level is up for debate. A large number of comparisons may be performed to assess the strongest split. Strict application of Bonferroni correction could be applied to these tests, though this could greatly affect the power for finding significant interactions. More powerful methods for control of type I error rate such as Hochberg (Hochberg 1988) can be used in practice. Alternatively, with a large number of covariates, the false discovery rate (FDR) method of Benjamini and Hochberg (Benjamini and Hochberg 1995) could be applied, though this method does not strongly control for the family-wise error rate. When a large number of continuous biomarkers are analyzed, many of these tests will be highly correlated with one another, so more stringent adjustment may be needed. One possibility is to permute the treatment assignment and re-perform the splitting exercise a large number of times to generate a distribution of the "best-split"

p values. Then, the p value from the original data can be compared to this distribution to assess how extreme the resulting interaction test truly was.

We shall make one final point about this example. The interaction models above are fit using one covariate at a time. Other possible predictive models allow one to fit a number of covariates greater than the number of observations in the data (e.g., LASSO, elastic net). However, final estimates of the treatment effect within the subgroup(s) of interest are necessary for planning future studies. After each split, the distribution of covariates could differ substantially between treatments, and these differences could contribute to the observed treatment effect. Without accounting for the distribution of the other covariates within the model, treatment effects within the subgroups could be biased. One possibility is to apply propensity-scoring methodologies (Xu and Kalbfleisch 2010) and adjust model (1) with propensity scores p_i obtained from a logistic regression model with the treatment as the outcome:

$$f(y_i) = \beta_0 + \beta_1 p_i + \beta_2 x_i + \beta_3 \text{ Treatment}_i + \beta_4 \text{ Treatment}_i * x_i \qquad (24.2)$$

This model would be reestimated at each level.

It is well known that the variance of the mean is inversely proportional to 1/N; we present an example in the context of subgrouping methodology to show how covariates can become increasingly different between treatments within smaller subgroups. We present an example in Fig. 24.4 from a simulated data set of 300 observations and 74 standard normal covariates, a normal outcome with mean 33 and standard deviation 25, and 1:1 randomization between a test and reference treatment. For each covariate, the data were randomly split to divide the 300 observations into two subgroups. Within each subgroup, the standardized difference was calculated between the treatments and plotted against the size of subgroup. This exercise was repeated 10 times for each covariate. Figure 24.4 illustrates that covariates that were initially balanced in the full population can exhibit larger differences between treatments as the group size decreases.

While the above method seems reasonable to identify interesting subgroups, how is it possible to directly compare the performance of PAYGO against other completed methodologies and those currently under development? Further, how can researchers keep informed of the properties of the best-performing method(s) so that the optimal approaches are used in practice? The proposed PBP in Sect. 24.3 addresses these concerns.

24.3 Predictive Biomarker Project

24.3.1 Overview

In order to assess the performance, developers of a subgroup identification method typically rely on applying the particular method to simulated data sets, where the "interesting" subgroup(s) are known. However, simulation studies as they are currently presented in the literature are insufficient to identify the best BSID methods for

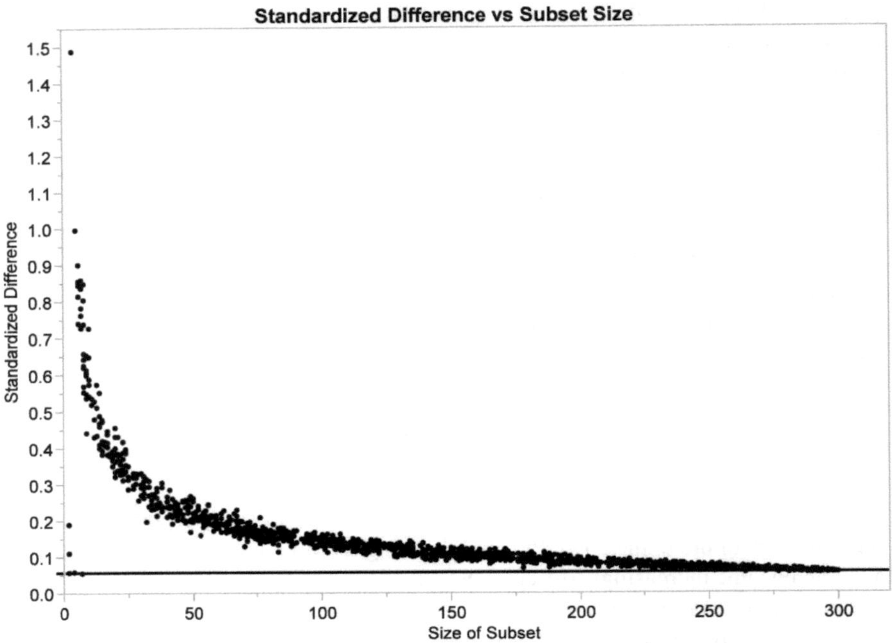

Fig. 24.4 Standardized difference of a N(0,1) covariate between treatments by subset size. The reference line indicates the standardized difference from the original data, where standardized difference = |mean(treatment)—mean(control)|/(pooled standard deviation)

use in practice. The simulations reported may highlight scenarios where a particular method performs best, or may not account for important analysis considerations, such as the correlation among covariates, missing data patterns, or the number and distribution of covariates. Further, reproducing simulations for new research based on the available description in the literature is difficult at best. Finally, even if simulated data sets could be reproduced, how one chooses to compare the performance of the methods under investigation could vary, which could make comparisons across several manuscripts challenging. The goal of the proposed PBP is to define important and relevant scenarios and summary criteria so that the performance of a method, such as the one described in the previous section, can be assessed in a consistent manner as it is developed. Additionally, maintaining an environment, such as a PBP web portal, where individuals can collaborate and track the performance of available methods, could be immensely valuable.

The above proposal suggests a major change to the conventional way in which statistical research is performed. Often, several methods to solve a particular problem are introduced into the literature. This may include methods that are refinements of earlier published algorithms, or entirely new approaches. As frequently occurs, once several methods become available, the key question then becomes which of the available methods is the best. Certain publications may compare a subset of

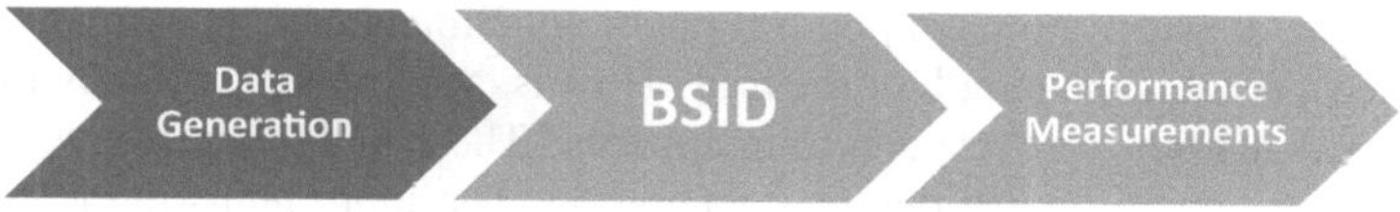

Fig. 24.5 The three components of the Predictive Biomarker Project (*PBP*)

the methods, but rarely would a definitive study of the methods be available. This necessitates additional research to compare the methods in a single large simulation study. Even here, all interesting simulation scenarios may not be considered, and certain methods may be excluded due to limitations of available software. Newer methods will be excluded from this study until a new simulation study is performed. This research paradigm also slows the progress due to the time needed to publish methods and results before comparisons are made.

The goal of the PBP exercise is to identify the best method(s) for subgroup identification in a given setting to be applied in practice for tailored therapeutics. In order to be successful, there are three components to consider (Fig. 24.5). Data generation is to ensure consistent inputs, as well as inputs that cover a wide range of scenarios. Ideally, the interface of the PBP web portal will provide data sets (or the code) in which to generate the data. The BSID component can be considered the "open" part of the process in which researchers would apply their methodologies. Here, it would be advantageous to get consistent output from the methods in order to compute a standard set of reports for a complete set of performance metrics. In this way, a consistent summary is generated to compare across the available methodologies as the candidate method is being developed. There is no need to wait for the publication, or hunt down the needed software for comparator methods. In the following section, we provide the additional information for the suggested components of the PBP web portal.

24.3.2 *Data Generation*

For generating data sets, the first goal is to outline the key attributes necessary to cast as wide a net as possible to cover the situations likely to occur in practice. At a minimum, this includes the distributions and moments of the outcome and covariates (as well as censoring mechanism for time-to-event endpoints), a range of sample sizes and treatment allocations to be expected in phase II or III trials, the number of covariates, as well as the magnitude of predictive and prognostic effects (including null effects). More complex simulation criteria could include the presence of outliers among one or more covariates, levels of correlation among the covariates, and missing data patterns.

Once key attributes are defined, various combinations of these criteria can be combined to define likely scenarios. These scenarios should best represent the conduct of trials for the therapeutic area(s) where the BSID methodology is to be applied.

For example, consider a typical phase II oncology clinical trial. How many patients are studied? What is the length of the trial? How is dropout appropriately modeled? How do patients typically respond to treatments? These and other questions are the important considerations for the data generation. The more realistic the simulated data are, the more useful the assessment of the BSID methods would be.

To ensure completeness of the simulation, it may be necessary to recruit a panel of experts to outline an initial set of parameters with the corresponding range of values. The current literature on BSID methods may provide a reasonable starting place, and therapeutic area knowledge will likely provide further suggestions for simulation criteria. Initially, scenarios may focus on finding subgroups within single trials. However, more complicated examples including multiple trials of varying sizes and durations or simulated development programs could be considered for the future. It is not expected that all factors will be initially identified; researchers should be able to suggest additional areas to the simulation factor space.

It is important that clear identifiers are available so that the simulation characteristics of the data are easily interpretable. These identifiers should be flexible enough so that additions or changes to the simulation criteria do not alter the meaning of past labels. These identifiers will aid in the reporting of the simulations at the PBP web portal as well as within individual publications. These identifiers should be extensible so that researchers can extend the simulation factor space over time.

Generating data on demand or having predefined data sets available for download is less challenging than identifying a hosting service or personnel to support the endeavor. Further, supplying data sets in lieu of code to generate data helps alleviate the potential issues of individuals generating data incorrectly, having limited access to software, or the requirement to maintain code in multiple languages. Perhaps a bigger concern is creating a collection of data sets that reasonably cover the space of common applications. There are at least a few possible approaches to this problem. First, users can suggest or contribute simulated data sets for which they understand their favorite methods to perform well. Such data sets should be vetted for validity and closeness to real-life scenarios. Over time, the collection of such data sets would at least provide benchmarks for existing methods against which new methods can be compared. Second, a design of experiments approach can be utilized to systematically choose combinations of simulation factors to effectively cover the factor space. Finally, an adaptive strategy may be appropriate to first address simulation factors where a particular class of methods excels, then examine other areas of the factor space.

24.3.3 Biomarker Subgroup Identification

The BSID component is the most flexible portion of the PBP. Here, authors are free to use their knowledge, expertise, and imagination to develop and apply any methodology of their choosing. This includes the methods described above, as well as any methods suggested by the framework outlined in (Shen et al. 2015). The benefit of the PBP web portal is that methods do not need to be published, and can provide near instant feedback on the performance of the candidate BSID method, compared to the other methods that have been contributed. General good performance against other methods, or excellent performance localized to various subspaces of simulation attributes could be key findings for publication of the method in the literature. Further, the performance of other methods tracked in the PBP web portal could suggest refinements to the candidate BSID method in situations where the performance is disappointing. Some facility for storing and sharing contributed software would be ideal to make a method generally available to the research community.

24.3.4 Performance Measures

BSID methods will ultimately be compared by a number of performance measures, and it may be likely that not all metrics will favor the same model. In these cases, the particular problem may suggest the most important metrics to consider. However, it is important that all metrics be computed so that comparisons across the BSID methods can at least be performed. At a minimum, reporting will include the identified biomarkers, the final subgroup that was selected for purposes of designing the next study, and the estimated treatment effect within this subgroup (which should at least be as high as currently available therapies).

There are a number of important and specific metrics that can be considered, and this depends on the particular objective of the subgroup identification exercise. For example, identifying important biomarkers related to the treatment response would be considered a testing problem, and the performance metrics here would be at the covariate level. Next, measuring the enhanced treatment effect is an estimation problem, with the metrics obtained at the subgroup level. Deciding which patients are ultimately treated with which medication is a prediction problem, with metrics defined at the patient level. The web portal should have some means of summarizing performance measures across simulation criteria and contributed methods so that the key attributes and scenarios under which a given method performs can be identified and described.

24.3.4.1 Testing

Testing problems are important to improve our understanding of the underlying biology and how this interacts with the treatments we hope to prescribe. Here, we compare the set of identified biomarkers with the truly predictive biomarkers for a given data set using statistics commonly used in epidemiology (Table 24.1).

1. How many true biomarkers were identified? Sensitivity $= \frac{a}{a+b}$
2. How many false biomarkers were incorrectly identified? $1 -$ specificity $= \frac{c}{c+d}$
3. Among identified biomarkers, how many are true biomarkers? Positive predictive value (PPV) $= \frac{a}{a+c}$

Table 24.1 Contingency table for true versus identified biomarkers

	Identified biomarker	
Predictive biomarker	Yes	No
True	a	b
False	c	d

4. Among biomarkers not identified, how many are true biomarkers? 1 − negative predictive value (NPV) $= \frac{b}{b+d}$

These quantities can be computed for each simulation, with the overall average, minimum, maximum, and standard deviation used as summary measures. Measures of variability are important to assess the sensitivity of the results to individual simulated data sets. Other quantities of interest include accuracy, the proportion of simulations that correctly identify each individual biomarker, as well as proportion of simulations that identify the set of biomarkers. Note, the analysis suggested above only considers whether the biomarker is identified, and not the particular cutpoints or alleles for the biomarkers. For continuous variables or categorical variables with multiple categories, there can be numerous subgroups to consider that number far beyond the total number of biomarkers. However, these varying cutpoints or groupings are often limited by the number of patients available in the resulting subgroups.

24.3.4.2 Estimation

At the subgroup level, the goal is to compare the estimated treatment effect against the truth. The true treatment effect can be calculated using the expected treatment effect from the simulation model for each patient that is a member of the identified subgroup. The accuracy of the estimated treatment effect can be compared to the truth in terms of magnitude and direction of estimation error. The example described in Sect. 24.2 illustrates the potential bias that could occur if covariate imbalance between the treatment groups is not considered.

The implications of the identified subgroup for further clinical trials can be investigated by calculating the sample size needed for a trial with a specified (for example, 90 %) power compared to the standard of care. The accuracy mentioned above is important; an overestimate of the treatment effect can result in an underpowered study or even a suboptimal decision to pursue tailoring, while an underestimated effect results in an unnecessarily large trial. Further, the cost of the trial can be estimated (largely driven by the number of enrolled patients) as well as the time needed to complete the trial (driven by the number of patients screened).

24.3.4.3 Prediction

Finally, the goal of tailored therapeutics is to understand a patient's personal and disease characteristics so they can be prescribed the most effective medication. Ultimately, it is important to ascertain how well the identified subgroup(s) classify the

Table 24.2 Comparison of simple accuracy between virtual twins and prune as you go based on 100 simulated samples

Simulation	Baseline	Virtual twins	Prune as you go
Binary, base case	0.75	0.75	0.75
Binary, base case $\times$ 2	0.75	0.88	0.79
Normal, base case	0.75	0.94	0.94
Normal, base case $\times$ 2	0.75	0.98	0.99

response to the treatment. Here, a model can be used to predict the response to the treatment (or not). The accuracy of these predictions can then be compared to the true response the patients exhibited.

24.3.5 Application to the Example

To illustrate one combination of the preceding approach, we conducted a small simulation study comparing the method described in Sect. 24.2 with virtual twins (VT) (Foster et al. 2011). The simulated data follow the "base case" described in (Foster et al. 2011). This simulates 1000 patients, half treated and half not, with predictors X_1–X_{15} iid N(0,1) and a binary response B with

$$P(B = 1) = \text{logit}^{-1}(-1 + 0.5X_1 + 0.5X_2 - 0.5X_7 + 0.1T + 0.5X_2X_7 + 0.9TA)$$

where T denotes the treatment variable coded as 0 or 1 and A indicates the subgroup $X_1 > 0$ and $X_2 < 0$, also coded as 0 or 1. We performed 100 simulations and also simulated a normal response with the same linear predictor and variance 1. The depth of the tree was set to 2 for both methods and the *p* value cutoff for PAYGO was set to 0.0005 to temper the greedy nature of the algorithm.

As a performance metric, we chose simple accuracy, which is the proportion of all patients classified into their true subgroup. Note the featured subgroup comprises 25 % of the data on average, so a baseline minimal accuracy is 0.75. Finally, to increase the power of the methods, we simulated a "base case $\times$ 2" scenario, which doubles every coefficient in the linear predictor. Results are shown in Table 24.2.

We see that virtual twins perform better with the binary response for base case $\times$ 2 and that the two methods perform almost identically for the normal response.

The preceding brief analysis represents one example thread through the simulation options discussed previously. We would envisage simulated data sets corresponding to each of the four rows of Table 24.2 being available in the repository to facilitate comparison with the two methods shown here.

24.4 Conclusions

In this chapter, we have outlined a novel approach to performing methodological research using subgroup identification methods for tailored therapeutics as a motivating example. There are many benefits to the proposed PBP web portal. First, and the most important, is the benefit of consistency in the simulated data and performance criteria for comparing BSID methodologies. This consistency allows for direct comparisons against current and future methods in order to identify the best approach to be used in practice. Further, should no single method prove optimal across all scenarios, the PBP web portal will fully characterize the study attributes for which each BSID method performs best so that an appropriate choice can be made based on the current clinical trial design. Heat maps and clustering analyses can identify methods with similar performance, which could suggest more computationally straightforward methods to apply. Finally, the PBP web portal enables the researcher in a number of important ways by simplifying their simulation studies by fully characterizing important simulation criteria and providing code and/or data for use, negating the need to locate or develop software for comparator methods to be used as a benchmark, and providing immediate feedback for performance. Though the PBP web portal is not yet generally available as described above, some efforts have been made at individual companies (such as Eli Lilly) and working groups of industry statisticians.

Given the importance of personalized medicine and considering the potential abuses and overinterpretations of subgroup analyses (Rothwell 2005; Wang et al. 2007), as well as past failures of research (Ioannidis 2005), the PBP may benefit from an industry-wide effort through the participation of the Clinical Trials Transformation Initiative (CTTI) (Clinical Trials Transformation Initiative 2013) or TransCelerate BioPharma Inc (TransCelerate BioPharma Inc 2008). Involving either or both of these organizations will make best use of the expertise across numerous pharmaceutical, regulatory, and academic institutions. Further, the PBP is no straightforward feat; the combined technical and financial resources of the member groups will be needed to develop and maintain the PBP web portal. However, once the infrastructure is developed, such collaborative efforts can be applied to other problems. For example, the simulated data sets can be easily utilized for other methodological developments, though modifications and extensions to simulated data may be needed in order to be appropriate for other applications (such as OTR).

Identifying subgroups with enhanced treatment response addresses one small part of tailored therapeutics; OTR is another. The next step is to apply the findings to the clinical program. While BSID methods often employ resampling methods to prevent overfitting, it is still possible to have identified a subgroup where the enhanced response was an artifact of the particular trial. Whenever possible, identified subgroups should be examined for scientific plausibility of the enhanced response, while independent trials should be used for enrichment and reproducibility of the result. Various strategies for enriching and analyzing trials with patients from "important" subgroups have been described elsewhere (Alosh and Huque 2009; Simon 2010).

Acknowledgments The authors thank an editor and reviewer for the constructive comments and suggestions that improved this manuscript. RCZ would like to thank LS for the invitation to speak at the 2013 ICSA Symposium. He would also like to thank Padraic Neville and Pei-Yi Tan for the example presented in Fig. 24.4. The authors thank the editors for their invitation to contribute to this collected volume. We are grateful for the support and insights of several colleagues: Chakib Battioui, Ming-Long Lam, Stephen Ruberg, and John Sall.

References

Alosh M, Huque MF (2009) A flexible strategy for testing subgroups and overall population. Stat Med 28:3–23

Baselga J, Perez EA, Pienkowski T, Bell R. (2006) Adjuvant trastuzumab: a milestone in the treatment of HER-2-positive early breast cancer. Oncologist 11(Suppl 1):4–12

Battioui C, Shen L, Ruberg SJ (2013) A resampling-based ensemble tree method to identify patient subgroups with enhanced treatment effect. Proceedings to the Joint Statistical Meetings

Benjamini Y, Hochberg Y (1995) Controlling the false discovery rate: a practical and powerful approach to multiple testing. J R Stat Soc Series B Stat Methodol 57:289–300

Bron, AJ (2001) Diagnosis of dry eye. Surv Ophthamol 45(Suppl 2):S221–S226

Clinical Trials Transformation Initiative (n.d.) http://www.ctti-clinicaltrials.org/

Dusseldorp E, Mechelen IV (2014) Qualitative interaction trees: a tool to identify qualitative treatment-subgroup interactions. Stat Med 33:219–237

Foster JC, Taylor JMG, Ruberg SJ (2011) Subgroup identification from randomized clinical trial data. Stat Med 30:2867–2880

Hochberg, Y (1988) A sharper Bonferonni procedure for multiple tests of significance. Biometrika 75:800–802

Ioannidis JPA (2005) Why most published research findings are false. PLoS Med. 2(8): e124 http://www.plosmedicine.org/article/info:doi/10.1371/journal.pmed.0020124

Lipkovich I, Dmitrienko A (2014) Strategies for identifying predictive biomarkers and subgroups with enhanced treatment effect in clinical trials using SIDES. J Biopharm Stat 24:130–153

Lipkovich I, Dmitrienko A, Denne J, Enas G (2011) Subgroup identification based on differential effect search—a recursive partitioning method for establishing response to treatment in patient subpopulations. Stat Med 30:2601–2621

Loh WY (2011) Classification and regression trees. Data Min Knowl Discov 1:14–23

Negassa A, Ciampi A, Abrahamowicz M, Shapiro S, Boivin JF (2005) Tree-structured subgroup analysis for censored survival data: validation of computationally inexpensive model selection criteria. Stat Comput 15:231–239

Radcliffe NJ, Surry PD (2011) Real-world uplift modelling with significance-based uplift trees, Portrait Technical Report TR-2011–1, Stochastic Solutions White Paper. Available at http://www.stochasticsolutions.com/pdf/sig-based-up-trees.pdf

Ramsey BW, Davies J, McElvaney NG, Tullis E, Bell SC, Dřevínek P, Griese M, McKone EF, Wainwright CE, Konstan MW, Moss R, Ratjen F, Sermet-Gaudelus I, Rowe SM, Dong Q, Rodriguez S, Yen K, Ordoez C, Elborn JS (2011) A CFTR potentiator in patients with cystic fibrosis and the G551D mutation. N Engl J Med 365:1663–1672

Rothwell PM (2005) Subgroup analysis in randomized controlled trials: importance, indications, and interpretation. Lancet 365:176–86

Ruberg SJ, Chen L, Wang Y (2010) The mean does not mean as much anymore: finding sub-groups for tailored therapeutics. Clin Trials 7:574–583

Shen L, Ding Y, Battioui C (2015) A framework for statistical methods to identify subgroups with differential treatment effects in randomized trials. Proceedings from International Chinese Statistics Association

Simon R (2010) Clinical trial designs for evaluating the medical utility of prognostic and predictive biomarkers in oncology. Pers Med 7:33–47
Su X, Zhou T, Yan X, Fan J, Yang S (2008) Interaction trees with censored survival data. Int J Biostat 4: 1–26. doi: 10.2202/1557–4679.1071
Su X, Tsai CL, Wang H, Nickerson DM, Li B (2009) Subgroup analysis via recursive partitioning. J Mach Learn Res 10:141–158
TransCelerate BioPharma Inc (n.d.) http://www.transceleratebiopharmainc.com/ Accessed Dec 2014
Wang R, Lagakos SW, Ware JH, Hunter DJ, Drazen JM (2007) Statistics in medicine—reporting of sub-group analyses in clinical trials. N Engl J Med 357:2189–2194
Xu Z, Kalbfleisch JD (2010) Propensity score matching in randomized clinical trials. Biometrics 66:813–823
Zhang B, Tsiatis AA, Davidian M, Zhang M, Laber EB (2012) Estimating optimal treatment regimes from a classification perspective. Statistics 1:103–114
Zhao Y, Zheng D, Rush AJ, Kosorok MR (2012) Estimating individualized treatment rules using outcome weighted learning. J Am Stat Assoc 107:1106–1118

Chapter 25
A Framework of Statistical Methods for Identification of Subgroups with Differential Treatment Effects in Randomized Trials

Lei Shen, Ying Ding and Chakib Battioui

Abstract The problem of identifying subgroups of patients with differential treatment effects in randomized trials plays an important role in the effort to tailor therapies to patients who are most likely to get benefit from them. It has attracted active research effort in recent years, and a growing number of statistical methods have been developed. In this chapter, after first examining the major challenges with subgroup identification that these methods are designed to address, we create a structured framework into which many of the methods can be placed. Such a framework provides insight into the subgroup identification problem and methods, and can be utilized to generate additional methods from existing ones. Using a small simulation study, we also demonstrate a recently proposed approach to systematically evaluate the performance of subgroup identification methods. Together, the methodological framework and systematic assessment of performance can help to determine the optimal analyses for various applications.

25.1 Introduction

In the drug development process, there is now an increasing amount of attention on tailoring a new therapy to those patients who are most likely to benefit from it. An important part of the effort to develop tailored therapeutics is the identification, using data from randomized clinical trials, of patient subgroups that enjoy an enhanced treatment response.

A number of statistical methods for the identification of such subgroups have been proposed (Loh 2002; Su et al. 2008; Lipkovich et al. 2011; Dusseldrop and Van

L. Shen (✉) · C. Battioui
Eli Lilly and Company, Indianapolis, USA
e-mail: Shen_Lei@Lilly.com

C. Battioui
e-mail: Battioui_Chakib@Lilly.com

Y. Ding
Department of Biostatistics, University of Pittsburgh, Pittsburgh, USA
e-mail: YingDing@Pitt.edu

Z. Chen et al. (eds.), *Applied Statistics in Biomedicine and Clinical Trials Design*,
ICSA Book Series in Statistics, DOI 10.1007/978-3-319-12694-4_25

Mechelen 2014; Foster et al. 2011; Battioui et al. 2014; Bell et al. 2012), and new ones regularly appear in the literature. With methods becoming more numerous, there comes an acute need to understand these methods and their performance in various settings. Although publications that present novel methods often contain simulation studies, the many differences in the setup of these simulation studies make it difficult to understand the relative performance of various methods. There is a strong interest in consistent and rigorous evaluation of subgroup identification methods, a topic addressed in Zink et al. (2015). In this chapter, we focus on a different question: Can we create a framework into which most of these methods would fit? Such a framework could help us gain much insight into the subgroup identification problem itself and its desirable solutions. On the surface, many of the statistical methods for subgroup identification look quite different from each other. However, in this chapter, we attempt to show that a useful framework can indeed be used to capture the key components of these methods. We will then demonstrate some important benefits of this framework and new insights gleaned from it.

In Sect. 25.2, we briefly review some of the subgroup identification methods in preparation for the discussion that follows. A methodological framework is proposed in Sect. 25.3, and we show a few important applications of this framework in Sect. 25.4 before concluding with Sect. 25.5.

25.2 Subgroup Identification Problem and Methods

25.2.1 Major Challenges

We first discuss the major challenges inherent in the problem of subgroup identification, which the various methods attempt to address in different ways. Perhaps the most often mentioned of these challenges is multiplicity, appropriately so, given the potentially severe impact it has on inflated type I error rate as well as on overly optimistic estimates of treatment effect. An analysis to identify interesting subgroups almost always includes multiple predictors—numbering in dozens for baseline pathophysiological variables and sometimes thousands for genomic or genetic variables. The number of predictors in an analysis is, however, not the only source of multiplicity, as there are at least two others. If a predictor is measured on a continuous scale—such as expression level of a gene or the amount of a protein—the same predictor can define many different patient subgroups when various cutoff values are used. In addition, when an analysis attempts to explore beyond subgroups defined by a single biomarker, the number of potential subgroups defined by the same set of predictors increases exponentially with higher complexity of the subgroups under consideration. For example, 100 binary biomarkers define 200 single-marker subgroups, but about 20,000 subgroups when two biomarkers are used jointly.

Another major challenge, also derived from the potentially large number of candidate subgroups, is computational. Not only do we need to efficiently search through a large number of subgroups in order to identify the most promising ones but we also often need to apply resampling approaches to address the aforementioned multiplicity issue. Any of the various resampling techniques require an additional computational loop around the search for subgroups. When these two factors—searching among many subgroups and repeating the search for a larger number of resampled datasets—are put together, the computational burden can be so severe as to render an otherwise reasonable method infeasible.

High degree of multiplicity is not unique to the problem of subgroup identification; rather it is prevalent in fields such as "high dimensional data analyses" or "statistical learning," of which subgroup identification can be considered a special case. It is therefore natural to assume that many of the modern statistical techniques developed for these fields can be applied to subgroup identification, and indeed many of them prove to be useful. But now we come to a third major challenge of subgroup identification. If we analyze data from patients receiving the same treatment and try to identify subgroups with higher average response, we can directly utilize methods such as classification-and-regression trees (CART) (Breiman et al. 1984). However, since we are interested in subgroups with differential *treatment effects,* with "treatment effect" defined as the difference in average responses between two treatment groups (typically a new treatment and a control, the latter often in the form of placebo or standard-of-care), the problem is one of identifying treatment-by-subgroup interactions. Many statistical learning algorithms such as CART cannot be directly applied to solve this more complex problem.

It should be noted that, while these challenges are the most important ones, there are certainly others. For example, the naïve estimate of treatment effect in the identified subgroup is known to be overly optimistic due to ascertainment bias associated with the process of searching for the best subgroups. It is therefore desirable if a subgroup identification method can provide bias-corrected estimates of treatment effect so that the clinical importance of an identified subgroup can be properly judged.

25.2.2 Subgroup Identification Methods

Having discussed three major challenges in subgroup identification, we now provide a brief survey of three methods that have been proposed for this problem.

In what is traditionally termed as "subgroup analysis," most phase 2 and phase 3 clinical trials have in their statistical analysis plans lists of prespecified subgroups to be investigated using interaction testing. In this chapter, we will refer to this method as the "traditional" method. The testing for treatment by subgroup interaction is performed one-at-a-time. Often, no formal multiplicity adjustment is made although the Bonferroni correction is sometimes used (if informally) in the interpretation of results.

Recursive partitioning techniques are utilized by many modern statistical methods for subgroup identification, including the next two methods to be reviewed in this chapter (as well as Loh 2002; Su et al. 2008; Lipkovich et al. 2011; Dusseldrop and Van Mechelen 2014; Bell et al. 2012). A detailed review of recursive partitioning can be found in the references (Breiman et al. 1984; Loh 2014). Briefly, a recursive partitioning method creates a decision tree that classifies patients into subgroups with differential treatment effects using sequential splits based on dichotomous (or dichotomized) predictors.

The second method we consider in detail is the "virtual twin" method by Foster et al. (2011). It borrows concepts from counterfactual models for causal inference. As a first step, this method applies random forest model (Breiman 2001) to impute the unobserved outcome for each patient; that is, the outcome of the patient if he or she had been randomized to the other treatment group. This allows an individualized treatment effect to be calculated for each patient since his or her responses to both treatments are now available, for example, by subtracting one treatment response from the other if the response variable is continuous. Recursive partitioning is then applied to these individualized treatment effects in order to identify subgroups with enhanced treatment effect. The authors considered a number of techniques to account for multiplicity.

The final method to be discussed here is the "treatment-specified subgroup detection tool" (TSDT) method by Battioui et al. (2014). It also utilizes recursive partitioning to identify promising subgroups, albeit in two steps. First, one of the treatment groups is selected based on practical considerations; this is often—although not always—the group receiving the new treatment, since a hypothesized subgroup effect is such that response to the new treatment is impacted much more by the group status than is response to placebo or standard-of-care. Recursive partitioning is applied to this selected treatment group to yield a list of candidate subgroups that manifest differential response (note, not differential *treatment effect,* at this point). As the second step, data from the other treatment group are utilized to ensure that a given candidate subgroup does not reflect a similar differential response in the other treatment group, which would render the subgroup uninteresting since there would be little or no differential treatment effect. This two-step analysis is performed on a number of datasets resampled from the original dataset using bootstrap or subsampling. And finally, response values are permuted within each treatment arm to allow the calculation of an adjusted p value for the best subgroup identified.

While other methods for subgroup identification have been proposed (e.g., Loh 2002; Su et al. 2008; Lipkovich et al. 2011; Dusseldrop and Van Mechelen 2014; Bell et al. 2012), the above review of three representative methods is sufficient for the introduction of a general methodological framework in the next section.

25.3 A Framework for Subgroup Identification Methods

Although the three methods reviewed above have many differences among them, a number of important components emerge when we examine how they handle the major challenges of subgroup identification presented in the previous section. We will discuss each of these components below.

25.3.1 Component "T": How to Handle Treatment-By-Subgroup Interaction

The "traditional" method deals with this directly by testing for interactions. An interesting idea used by the "virtual twin" method is to first impute unobserved outcomes, hence changing a problem of differential treatment effect (interaction) to a simpler problem of differential response (main effect). Yet another strategy is used by the "TSDT" method, where one treatment group is analyzed first, before the other group is incorporated into the analysis to ensure an interaction effect.

By reviewing these and other methods, we can see at least the following approaches:

1. "Model": Testing for treatment-by-subgroup interaction in a regression model.
2. "Transformation": Transforming the observed response, such as imputing for unobserved outcome and then calculating individualized treatment effect (Foster et al. 2011).
3. "Sequential": Analyzing one treatment group first, before incorporating the other group (Battioui et al. 2014).
4. "Direct": Directly contrasting the observed average responses to two treatments for any given subgroup (Lipkovich et al. 2011).

25.3.2 Component "S": How to Search for Candidate Subgroups, Ideally in a Computationally Efficient Manner

In this regard, the "traditional" method simply considers all possible subgroups, but in doing so, essentially limits itself to considering only single-marker subgroups, since testing treatment-by-subgroup interactions for more complex subgroups is often computationally prohibitive in practice. The other two reviewed methods both utilize recursive partitioning, which counts computational efficiency as one of its main strength. Although not all possible subgroups are considered, the recursive nature of the algorithm allows much more complex subgroups to be considered, such as those defined by two or even more predictors.

We therefore have the following options for this component:

1. "Exhaustive": Studying all possible subgroups.
2. "Recursive partitioning": Creating a decision tree that classifies patients into subgroups with differential treatment effects using sequential splits based on dichotomous (or dichotomized) predictors (Loh 2014).
3. "Stepwise modeling": We use this option to represent the various penalized regression techniques (Zou and Zhang 2012), which can also identify candidate subgroups efficiently without considering all possible subgroups, but (unlike option #2) does so in a regression setting.

25.3.3 Component "M": How to Address Multiplicity

The Bonferroni correction sometimes used in traditional subgroup analysis can be impractical and overly conservative, and most subgroup identification methods utilize one or a combination of resampling techniques. We have the following options regarding this component:

1. "Simple": Such as the Bonferroni correction.
2. "Permutation": Using permutations of the original data to generate a reference distribution of the test statistic under an appropriate null.
3. "Bootstrap": Bootstrapping the original data to estimate the sampling distribution of the test statistic and/or a bias-corrected estimates of effect sizes using out-of-bag samples.
4. "Cross-validation": Using m-fold cross-validation to estimate prediction accuracy or other key quantities associated with a particular application.
5. "Subsampling": Randomly dividing the original data into two smaller datasets with prespecified proportions, with one used as training data and the other testing data; this is often repeated a number of times with results then averaged over subsamples.
6. "Combinations": Using a combination of above approaches, such as "subsampling & permutation."

It should be noted that there are other options for each of the components above, as the lists are not intended to be comprehensive. For example, some methods utilize variable importance to further control false-positive findings. One could also say that some of the options are fairly broad. For example, "recursive partitioning" covers a wide range of actual methods, with one of the key differences being the criteria used to determine whether and how to split at each node. In this regard, the "TSDT" method uses a specific approach, while the method by Bell et al. (2012) allows any user-defined criteria to be used. In theory, the user-defined criteria can optimize the desirability of the identified subgroup according to practical considerations for the specific application, such as the proper balance between subgroup size and the magnitude of treatment effect in the subgroup. Nevertheless, we will see in the next section that such a framework, even with simplifications on the options for each component, can be quite useful.

25.4 Utilizing the Framework

An immediate application of this framework is that we can now catalogue seemingly different methods for subgroup identification. For example, the "TSDT" method can be represented by *T(sequential)* × *S(recursive partitioning)* × *M(subsampling & permutation)*. As another example, the method by Lipkovich et al. (2011) can be represented by the following entry in the framework: *T(direct)* × *S(recursive partitioning)* × *M(permutation)*. Of course, it should be stated that such representation captures the key elements of each method, but not all its details. The "TSDT" method utilizes out-of-bag samples from bootstrapping or subsampling to correct ascertainment bias in estimating the treatment effect size in the identified subgroup, and such details are not easily captured in a framework.

By considering the key components of subgroup identification methods, we are able to enumerate multiple options for each component, hence gaining valuable insight. By dissecting even a small number of methods, we now have a "toolbox" where options for each component can be combined. This leads to an even more interesting application, namely many "new" methods for subgroup identification generated by this toolbox. For example, one can naturally combine *T(transformation)* with *S(exhaustive)*. In other words, we can perform the first step of the "virtual twin" method and calculate individualized treatment effects, then perform a test for each subgroup that is simpler than interaction tests. Intuitively, in situations where the imputed outcome is of high quality, this method should outperform the "traditional" method. With the options given above for each component, we have $4 \times 3 \times 6 = 72$ combinations, each of which corresponds to a unique "method." Some of these methods, once described, are clearly impractical or inferior; but at the same time, many of these methods appear reasonable, yet are "novel" in the sense that they have not been proposed in the literature.

25.4.1 Systematic Method Evaluation

In addition to the value described above, we posit that such a framework of numerous methods for subgroup identification should work very well with a system to consistently and rigorously evaluate these methods, as proposed by Zink et al. (2015). There are three components in this evaluation system: data generation, application of analysis methods, and performance measurement. Consistency in data generation and performance measurement allows a wide array of analysis methods to be compared directly, thus leading to insight on strengths and weaknesses of each method.

Of both technical and practical importance is the proposal to evaluate the performance of a method on three levels: marker-level, subgroup-level, and subject-level. Briefly, the marker-level performance measures capture the accuracy in which the markers are correctly identified as predictive markers (or not); the subgroup-level performance measures include the average size and treatment effect of the identified subgroups, while the quality of associated treatment decisions for individual patients is measured at the subject level. Section 25.4.2 will elaborate on these measures in the context of a simulation study; additional details can be found in Zink et al. (2015).

Table 25.1 Three subgroup identification methods compared in the simulation study

Method	Component "T"	Component "S"	Component "M"
"Traditional"	Model	Exhaustive	Simple (Sidak correction)
"VT"	Transformation	Recursive partitioning	Permutation
"TSDT"	Sequential	Recursive partitioning	Subsampling + permutation

25.4.2 Simulation Study

Here, as an example to demonstrate how this system works, we present a small simulation study to compare three subgroup identification methods.

25.4.2.1 Subgroup Identification Methods

The methods have been briefly described in Sect. 25.2 and presented in Table 25.1 according to the framework we established. Here, we provide additional details of each method:

- Traditional Method: Test for treatment by subgroup interaction ("T: model") one-at-a-time for all variables ("S: exhaustive"), with multiplicity adjustment made using Sidak correction ("M: simple").
- Virtual Twin Method: First apply random forest model to impute for each patient the unobserved outcome as if he or she had been randomized to the other treatment group ("T: transformation"). Then apply recursive partitioning ("S: recursive partitioning") to the individualized treatment effects calculated by subtracting the "control outcome" from the "new treatment outcome" of the same patient. Finally, use permutations of the original data to estimate a reference null distribution of the test statistics for differential treatment effect in an identified subgroup, which in turn provides a multiplicity adjusted p value ("M: permutation").
- TSDT Method: In a subsample of the original data, construct candidate subgroups with differential response based solely on the new treatment arm, and then incorporate data from the control arm to exclude any candidate subgroup that does not show sufficient treatment-by-subgroup interaction ("T: sequential"). Candidate subgroups are constructed using recursive partitioning ("S: recursive partitioning"). Confirm the directional consistency of any remaining candidate subgroup in the corresponding out-of-bag sample. Averaging the results over all the random subsamples, for each candidate subgroup, and calculate the proportion of subsamples for which the subgroup is identified and shown to be consistent in the out-of-bag sample. Finally, apply permutation of the original data to obtain a reference null distribution of the consistency measure, which in turn provides a multiplicity adjusted p value ("M: subsampling + permutation").

For each of the subgroup identification methods, three different α levels ($\alpha = 0.1$, 0.2, 0.3) are used for controlling type I error rate.

Table 25.2 Five scenarios used in the simulation study

Scenario	Number of subjects	Number of markers	Number of predictive markers
A	240	20	1
B	240	50	2
C	240	50	1
D	240	20	0
E	240	50	0

25.4.2.2 Simulation Scenarios

We generated 200 datasets in each of five scenarios, with Table 25.2 providing a summary of these scenarios. In scenario A, each dataset contains 20 predictors, with one of them being a predictive marker and hence the target of identification. The number of predictors is increased to 50 in scenario B, with two of them being predictive markers. Scenario C is chosen to provide comparisons with the first two scenarios. It calls for generation of datasets with 50 predictors, one of which is a predictive marker. Contrasting scenarios A and C will allow us to observe the impact of the total number of predictors, while the comparison between scenarios B and C can demonstrate the impact of the number of predictive markers. Scenarios D and E are null scenarios with no predictive marker, included here for the purpose of evaluating control of type I errors.

In all scenarios, there are 240 subjects, with a 3:1 randomization ratio between the new treatment and control. For each dataset, an appropriate number (20 or 50) of genetic markers with identical distribution were generated. Specifically, each marker is a three-level ordinal variable with proportions of the three levels being 49, 42, and 9 %. According to the scenario, responses on a continuous scale were then generated with either zero, one, or two of the genetic markers being predictive. The predictive markers each confer the same magnitude of effect. When there is one predictive marker (scenario A and C), the population consists of two subpopulations that are both about 50 % in size and have average treatment effects 0.1 and 0.55, respectively. When there are two predictive markers (scenario B), the population is divided into four subpopulations that are each about 25 % in size and have average treatment effects 0.1, 0.55, 0.55, and 1.00, respectively.

25.4.2.3 Performance Measures

The aforementioned performance measures were calculated for each method across datasets. Specifically:

- Marker-level performance measures: Natural choices for presenting the accuracy with which predictive markers are correctly identified by an analysis method are sensitivity, specificity, positive predictive value, and negative predictive value.

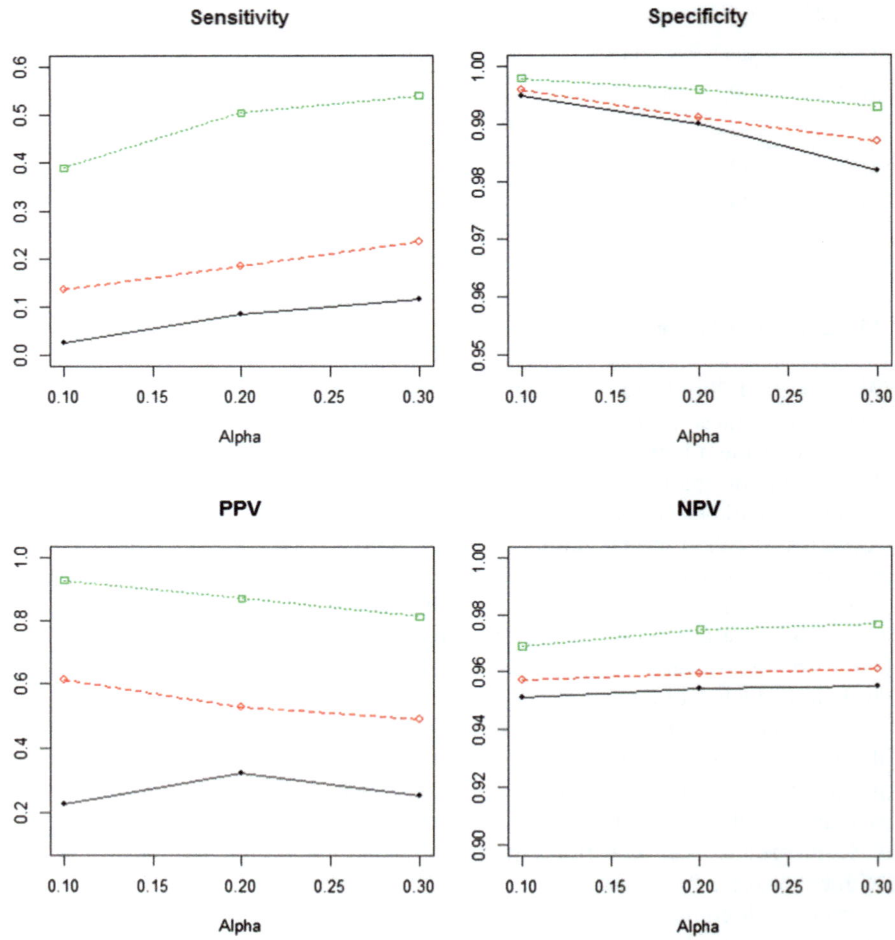

Fig. 25.1 *Marker level performance for scenario A* (solid line/solid dots = "Traditional," dashed line/hollow dots = "Virtual Twin," dotted line/square dots = "TSDT"). **a** *Sensitivity* = proportion of times that true predictive marker(s) are identified as predictive. **b** *Specificity* = proportion of times that nonpredictive markers are identified as nonpredictive. **c** *PPV* = proportion of true predictive markers among the markers identified as predictive. **d** *NPV* = proportion of nonpredictive markers among the markers identified as nonpredictive

These values for a single analysis are easily calculated from the 2 × 2 table with rows being the true status of a marker (predictive or not) and columns being the results of identification (identified as predictive or not). The proportions are then averaged across datasets.

- Subgroup-level performance measures: Toward the eventual objective of subgroup identification—to tailor a potential medicine to those patients who are more likely to respond—it is often desired that subsequent clinical trials would focus on the

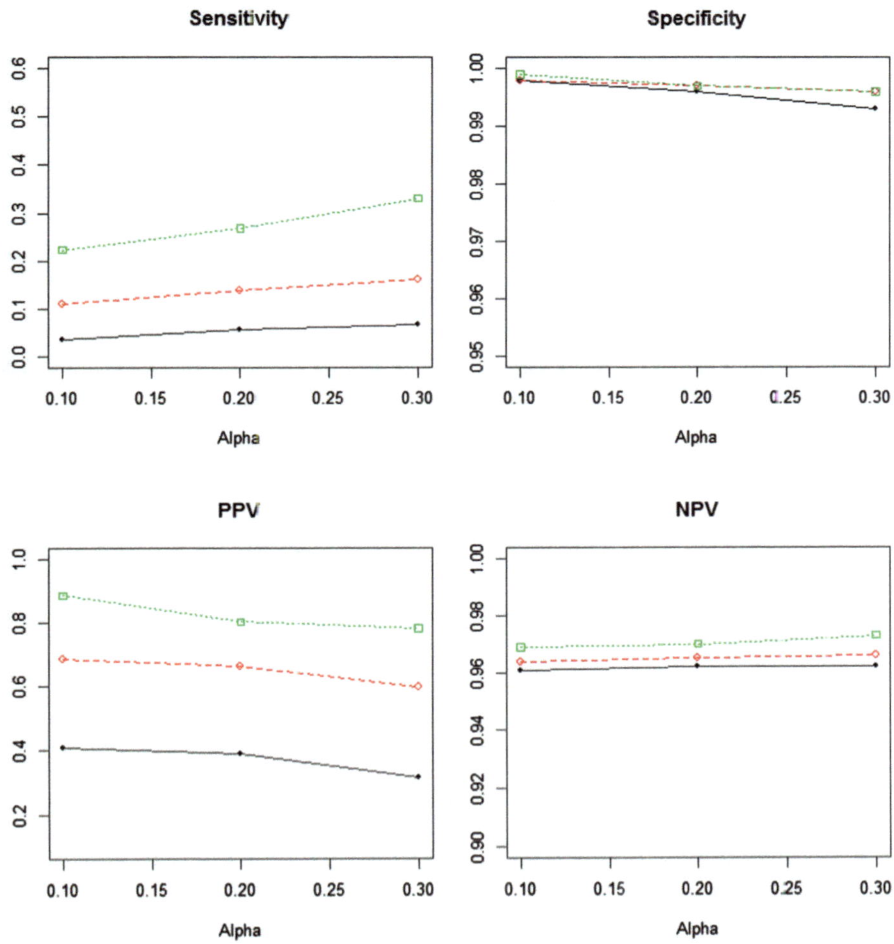

Fig. 25.2 *Marker level performance for scenario B* (solid line/solid dots = "Traditional," dashed line/hollow dots = "Virtual Twin," dotted line/square dots = "TSDT"). **a** *Sensitivity* = proportion of times that true predictive marker(s) are identified as predictive. **b** *Specificity* = proportion of times that nonpredictive markers are identified as nonpredictive. **c** *PPV* = proportion of true predictive markers among the markers identified as predictive. **d** *NPV* = proportion of nonpredictive markers among the markers identified as nonpredictive

subgroup that has been identified. Whether such a tailored drug development program is clinically and commercially prudent depends critically on the size and treatment effect associated with the subgroup. Therefore, it is important to capture these quantities (averaged over datasets) in simulation studies. While other summaries across simulated datasets can be constructed, we start with the most obvious ones by simply averaging the size and treatment effect of the identified subgroup for each dataset.

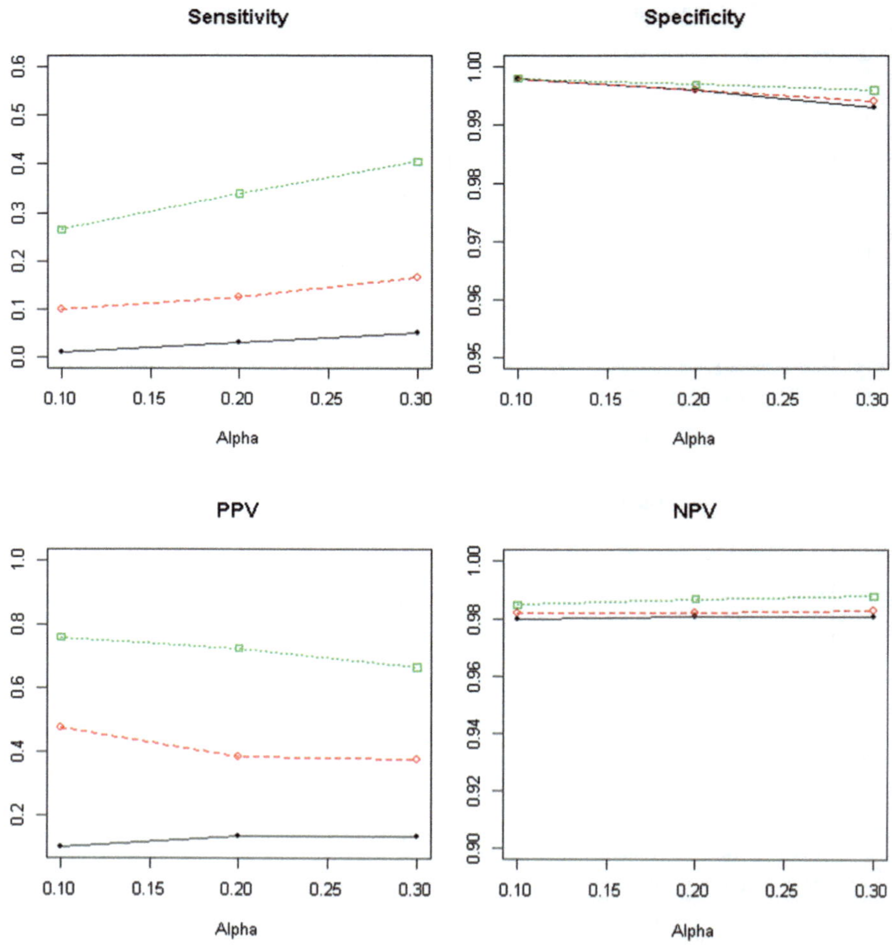

Fig. 25.3 *Marker-level performance for scenario C* (solid line/solid dots = Traditional," dashed line/hollow dots = "Virtual Twin," dotted line/square dots = "TSDT"). **a** *Sensitivity* = proportion of times that true predictive marker(s) are identified as predictive. **b** *Specificity* = proportion of times that nonpredictive markers are identified as nonpredictive. **c** *PPV* = proportion of true predictive markers among the markers identified as predictive. **d** *NPV* = proportion of nonpredictive markers among the markers identified as nonpredictive

- Subject-level performance measures: Upon approval of a potential treatment by regulatory agencies, the subgroup identified and confirmed in the drug development program will impact clinical decision making. The status of each patient—in terms of whether he or she belongs to the subgroup—can be considered as a decision rule of whether the patient should be given the new treatment. Naturally, the quality of this decision rule can be measured using sensitivity, specificity, positive

Table 25.3 Subgroup-level performance ($\alpha = 0.1$)

Scenario	Method	Subgroup identified (%)	Subgroup size (%)	Subgroup treatment effect
A	T	11	93.1	0.335
	VT	22	88.8	0.359
	TSDT	42	79.2	0.415
B	T	16	92.5	0.574
	VT	32	83.6	0.609
	TSDT	49	75.8	0.658
C	T	10	95.2	0.332
	VT	21	89.7	0.352
	TSDT	34	83.0	0.389
D	T	9	93.7	–
	VT	10	94.8	–
	TSDT	10	94.9	–
E	T	9	95.7	–
	VT	12	94.3	–
	TSDT	12	94.0	–

predictive value, and negative predictive value—this time with each subject as a unit. However, since clinical decision making does not become important until the new medicine is successfully developed, our simulation study here will not focus on these measures.

25.4.2.4 Results

Figures 25.1, 25.2, 25.3 present the marker-level performance for each non-null scenario, method, and α level. Across all scenarios and all measures, we can see that the "TSDT" method performed the best, while the "traditional" method performed the worst. The choice of α level had a moderate impact on the results. When comparing between scenarios, we can see that when the number of predictors increased (scenario C vs. A), sensitivity decreased for all three methods, as expected. On the other hand, an interesting observation is that, when the number of predictive markers increased (scenario B vs. C), sensitivity did not seem to improve.

The first column ("Subgroup identified") of Table 25.3 provides further information on how often each method identified a subgroup in these scenarios. We start with the two null scenarios D and E, where all three methods appear to do a good job of controlling the type I error rate at the stated nominal α level of 0.1. When we look at the three non-null scenarios A, B, and C, we see that in every scenario, the

"TSDT" method identified subgroups most often, whereas the "traditional" method did so the least often.

The final two columns of Table 25.3 present the subgroup-level performance measures (for $\alpha = 0.1$). It is evident that when the "TSDT" method identified subgroups in non-null scenarios, the subgroups also tended to be of the best quality in terms of having the largest treatment effect ("Subgroup Treatment Effect" column). Comparing across scenarios, it is clear that identification of subgroup, especially high-quality subgroups, is the most difficult for scenario C and easiest for scenario B, as one would expect. The average size of subgroups identified by each method is closely related to the frequency of identifying subgroups (since the size is 100 % of the population when no subgroup is identified), and in this case it is not otherwise informative given the identical distribution of all the predictors.

In summary, since all three methods control type I error rate at the same level in the null scenarios, the performance in non-null scenarios indicates that the "TSDT" is the most powerful method among the three in this simulation study.

25.5 Conclusions

In this chapter, we established a framework for statistical methods to identify patient subgroups with differential treatment effects in randomized clinical trials. By focusing on three major challenges with subgroup identification, we submit that the methods can be viewed as combinations of three key components: how treatment by subgroup interaction is handled, how candidate subgroups are searched, and how multiplicity is accounted for. This framework allows us to dissect existing methods, identify the options they utilize for each component, and then combine these options in other ways to easily generate additional methods. Such a system to catalogue and index various methods also works well with the framework proposed by Zink et al. (2015) to consistently evaluate performance of subgroup identification methods.

Acknowledgment The authors would like to sincerely thank their colleagues Hollins Showalter and Brian Denton for assistance with computation.

References

Battioui C, Shen L, Ruberg SJ (2014) A resampling-based ensemble tree method to identify patient subgroups with enhanced treatment effect. Proceedings of 2014 Joint Statistical Meetings, pp 4013–4023

Bell M, Higgs R, Lipkovich I, Lu Y, Ruberg S (2012) Flexible subgroup search tool. Presented at 2012 FDA/DIA Statistics Forum

Breiman L (2001) Random forests. Mach Learn 45:5–32

Breiman L, Friedman JH, Olshen RA, Stone CJ (1984) Classification and regression trees. Wadsworth, Belmont

Dusseldorp E, Van Mechelen I (2014) Qualitative interaction trees: a tool to identify qualitative treatment-subgroup interactions. Stat Med 33:219–217

Foster JC, Taylor JMG, Ruberg SJ (2011) Subgroup identification from randomized clinical trial data. Stat Med 30:2867–2880

Lipkovich I, Dmitrienko A, Denne J, Enas G (2011) Subgroup identification based on differential effect search—a recursive partitioning method for establishing response to treatment in patient subpopulations. Stat Med 30:2601–2621

Loh WY (2002) Regression trees with unbiased variable selection and interaction detection. Stat Sin 12:361–386

Loh WY (2014) Fifty years of classification and regression trees. International Statistics Review 82(3):329–348. doi:10.1111/insr.12016

Su X, Zhou T, Yan X, Fan J, Yang S (2008) Interaction trees with censored survival data. Int J Biostatist 4(1):1557–4679. doi:10.2202/1557–4679.1071

Zink RC, Shen L, Wiolfinge RD, Showalter HD (2015) Assessment of methods to identify patient subgroups with enhanced treatment response in randomized clinical trials. Applied Statistics in Biomedicine and Clinical Trials Design: Selected Papers from 2013 ICSA/ISBS Joint Statistical Meetings. Springer (in press)

Zou H, Zhang HH (2012) On the adaptive elastic-net with a diverging number of parameters. Ann Stat 37:1733–1751

Chapter 26
Biomarker Evaluation and Subgroup Identification in a Pneumonia Development Program Using SIDES

Alex Dmitrienko, Ilya Lipkovich, Alan Hopkins, Yu-Ping Li and Whedy Wang

Abstract This chapter discusses the general problem of exploratory subgroup analysis in the context of late-stage clinical development. In this context, exploratory subgroup analysis focuses on biomarker discovery and identification of subgroups with enhanced treatment effect in large clinical trial databases. A case study based on a Phase III development program in patients with nosocomial pneumonia is used to compare traditional approaches to subgroup search, based on univariate assessments of individual biomarkers, and a novel subgroup exploration method, which utilizes a recursive partitioning algorithm with a local treatment effect modeling approach. The SIDES (Subgroup Identification based on Differential Effect Search) method and its extensions (SIDEScreen method) have been used in multiple Phase II and Phase III programs to perform a comprehensive evaluation of candidate biomarkers and identify biomarker-based subgroup of patients with desirable characteristics (improved efficacy or acceptable safety). The chapter provides a detailed summary of key features of the SIDES method, including complexity control (subgroup pruning), biomarker screening to prevent data overfitting and application of resampling-based techniques to account for Type I error rate inflation inherent in subgroup exploration.

A. Dmitrienko (✉) · I. Lipkovich
Quintiles, Inc, 4820 Emperor Boulevard, Durham, NC 27703, USA
e-mail: alex.dmitrienko@quintiles.com

I. Lipkovich
e-mail: ilya.lipkovich@quintiles.com

A. Hopkins · Y. Li · W. Wang
Theravance, Inc, 901 Gateway Boulevard, South San Francisco, CA 94080, USA
e-mail: ahopkins@theravance.com

Y. Li
e-mail: yli@theravance.com

W. Wang
e-mail: wwang@theravance.com

Z. Chen et al. (eds.), *Applied Statistics in Biomedicine and Clinical Trials Design*,
ICSA Book Series in Statistics, DOI 10.1007/978-3-319-12694-4_26

26.1 Introduction

Assessment of treatment effect heterogeneity in clinical trials is one of the most important and challenging problems in drug development which has received much attention in both statistical and medical literature over the past 15 years. Several research groups have published extensive guidelines and detailed checklists that (if properly followed) would ensure credible subgroup analysis (Brookes et al. 2001; Rothwell 2005; Sun et al. 2010). However, these guidelines have not eliminated important concerns about validity of subgroup analysis strategies. In particular, should subgroup analysis focus on only a (small) set of predefined subpopulations while applying clearly defined multiplicity adjustment procedures, or can statistically valid data-driven strategies resulting in the identification of patient subgroups that were not prespecified (or even envisioned as likely important) be applied as well? These two approaches can be loosely labeled as "confirmatory" and "exploratory" subgroup analysis, respectively (see Varadhan et al. 2013; Lipkovich and Dmitrienko 2014a).

The need for principled data-driven approaches to evaluating treatment effects across biomarker-driven subgroups of patients is stressed by a recent paradigm shift from the idea of developing "one treatment which fits all patients" to *personalized medicine* (Ruberg et al. 2010). The recently published draft guidance documents on enrichment strategies and subgroup analysis in clinical trials (Food and Drug Administration 2012; Committee for Medicinal Products for Human Use 2014) discuss the role of subgroup search and exploration. The draft Committee for Medicinal Products for Human Use (CHMP) guidance states that ignoring possible treatment effect heterogeneity in phase III trials (with respect to both safety and efficacy) may be unacceptable as it may create a false impression of consistency of treatment effect, whereas in fact this may be not the case. At the same time, this guidance document emphasizes that data-driven subgroup analysis may result in inflated type I error rates and "discovering" spurious patient subgroups.

It has been previously accepted that the use of unconstrained ad hoc methods in subgroup analysis and biomarker evaluation is likely to lead to unreliable results. However, downplaying data-driven subgroup exploration may be in conflict with the "discovery spirit" of personalized medicine and science in general. Ones view is that exploratory subgroup analysis should be treated as a special case of model selection within the unifying statistical/machine learning framework. As with any statistical learning method, the focus is on specifying an analytic strategy with known operating characteristics rather than on prespecifying the final model.

Within this paradigm, biomarker evaluation and subgroup identification should start with the prespecification of:

- A set of clinically relevant biomarkers that will be used to form a (typically quite large) search space of candidate subgroups.
- Analysis strategy that will evaluate candidate subgroups and identify promising subgroups.

An important element of this analytic strategy is that it should protect against selection bias which may result in selecting spurious and overfit subgroups that are very unlikely to be replicated in the future trials. Another important consideration (and less common to other applications of statistical learning) is the need for controlling an appropriately defined false positive rate (overall type I error rate or false discovery rate) associated with the entire strategy, which typically can only be achieved by using resampling methods.

Several methods extending the methodologies developed within machine learning and data mining communities have been proposed recently for the selection of biomarkers in clinical trial databases and choosing biomarker cutoffs to define subgroups of patients with enhanced treatment effect. The following classification was proposed in Lipkovich and Dmitrienko (2014b):

- *Global outcome modeling* comprises strategies that first estimate the "response surface" for the clinical outcome, given a patient's biomarker values and assigned treatment arm (which typically results in a complex "black box model") and then "extract" each patient's treatment effect from that model. Examples include the virtual twins method by Foster et al. (2011) and penalized regression by Imai and Ratcovic (2013).
- *Global treatment effect modeling* includes strategies aimed at directly estimating an individual patient's treatment effect, which obviates the need to fit the main effects. This approach is used in the Interaction tree method of Su et al. (2009), modified covariate method by Tian et al. (2012), qualitative interaction trees (QUINT) by Dusseldorp and Mechelen (2014). A special case of this general approach includes strategies for estimating optimal treatment regimes that require only estimating the sign of the individual treatment effect as the basis for assigning optimal treatment for each patient, see Zhao et al. (2012) and Zhang et al. (2012).
- The last class of subgroup search methods that can be called *local treatment effect modeling* focuses on a direct search for treatment-by-covariate interactions and selecting subgroups with desirable characteristics. Examples include the adaptive signature designs by Freidlin et al. (2005, 2010) and bump hunting approach of Kehl and Ulm (2006)

This chapter focuses on a powerful biomarker evaluation and subgroup identification method known as subgroup identification based on differential effect search (SIDES). The method was developed in Lipkovich et al. (2011) and belongs to the class of local treatment effect modeling approaches. An advantage of the local approach to subgroup search is that the researchers do not need to estimate the response function over the entire covariate space. SIDES and other local treatment effect modeling approaches focus on identifying specific regions of the search space with a large differential treatment effect.

The SIDES method is based on a recursive partitioning subgroup search which uses a set of candidate biomarkers to progressively split promising subgroups into child subgroups to define groups of patients who are likely to experience significant treatment benefit. The SIDES method offers several attractive features to clinical drug developers, including complexity control (subgroup pruning) and biomarker screening to reduce the chances of data overfitting which may result in forming spurious subgroups. SIDES utilizes resampling-based techniques to efficiently account for selection bias inherent in biomarker exploration. In addition, one can construct bias-adjusted estimates of the treatment effect (honest estimates) within the selected subgroups using resampling methods such as cross-validation and bootstrap (see, for example, Foster et al. 2011 and Simon et al. 2011).

The SIDES method has been successfully applied to multiple phase II and phase III development programs to provide a comprehensive evaluation of candidate biomarkers and perform subgroup searches (see, for example, Hardin et al. 2013). Most commonly, this method is utilized to better characterize the efficacy profile of new treatments and identify the subgroups of patients who experience a highly beneficial effect. However, due to its focus on differential treatment effects, the SIDES method can be used to discover subgroups where the treatment could be harmful and thus it offers a complete platform for developing tailored therapies.

In this chapter, the SIDES methodology will be used to facilitate the process of identifying subgroups of patients who experience a strong beneficial effect in a phase III development program for the treatment of nosocomial pneumonia (the ATTAIN program).

This chapter is organized as follows. Section 26.2 provides background information on the ATTAIN development program and defines the general problem of biomarker and subgroup identification in clinical trials. Section 26.3 discusses traditional approaches to subgroup exploration and evaluation. Section 26.4 introduces the SIDES method and provides information on its use in biomarker discovery and subgroup identification problems. Section 26.5 describes applications of the SIDES method to the analysis of the ATTAIN database. Section 26.6 provides a summary of the results. Technical details, including a detailed description of the SIDES subgroup search algorithm, are provided in the Appendix.

26.2 Case Study

This section introduces a case study based on two phase III randomized, double-blind, parallel group, multinational trials of identical non-inferiority design (assessment of telavancin for treatment of hospital-acquired pneumonia (ATTAIN) trials). The studies will be referred to as studies 0015 and 0019. The studies were conducted by Theravance, Inc. to evaluate the safety and efficacy of telavancin (test antibiotic) compared to vancomycin (active control antibiotic) for the treatment of adults with nosocomial pneumonia caused by Gram-positive methicillin resistant *Staphylococcus aureus* (MRSA) bacteria. The studies were conducted using identical protocols that included a provision for a pooled analysis in those patients with MRSA. Nosocomial pneumonia encompasses hospital-acquired bacterial pneumonia (HABP) and ventilator-associated bacterial pneumonia (VABP), both of which are important causes of morbidity and mortality. A total of 1503 patients were randomized across both studies. The primary end point was clinical response at a test-of-cure visit after completion of antibiotic therapy. Both studies demonstrated non-inferiority at the prespecified 10 % level for clinical response (Rubinstein 2011).

The mortality analyses reported in this chapter are based on 1289 patients who met the criteria for American Thoracic Society/Infectious Disease Society of America (ATS/IDSA) pneumonia diagnosis (American Thoracic Society/Infectious Diseases Society of America 2005; Food and Drug Administration 2010). The ATS/IDSA analysis set included patients in the all-treated analysis set who met the ATS/IDSA pneumonia criteria. These criteria are included in the proposed inclusion criteria for clinical trials of hospital-acquired bacterial pneumonia-associated bacterial pneumonia/VABP in the 2010 Food and Drug Administration (FDA) guidance. Additionally, they are included in the ATS/IDSA consensus guidelines for the diagnosis of pneumonia to identify patients who should be treated with antibiotics, offering the optimal balance of sensitivity and specificity in making the diagnosis.

26.2.1 Mortality End Point

Subsequent to completion of the ATTAIN trials, the US FDA's focus shifted to all-cause mortality as an important end point for nosocomial pneumonia treatment assessment. In the ATTAIN studies, timing of the last study visit varied depending on the duration of treatment and the lag time between the end of treatment and the last visit (which could occur between 7 and 14 days after the end of treatment), resulting in different durations of patient follow-up. To minimize bias and increase the precision of estimates of mortality rates, vital status information (through at least day 49, i.e., up to 21 treatment days plus 28 post-treatment days) was collected post study closure for all patients who participated in studies 0015 and 0019. Follow-up queries were generated for nearly half of the study participants, and responses were obtained for nearly 90 % of the 697 queries at 175 clinical sites, resulting in about 5 % censored data at 28 days post randomization and less than 10 % censored data at 49 days (censoring refers to the number of subjects lost to follow-up at 28 and 49 days). Although collected after the studies had been completed, this additional patient follow-up for vital status provides a near complete data set for analysis of mortality.

The program's sponsor conducted a post hoc analysis of the 28-day all-cause mortality data from studies 0015 and 0019 in the ATTAIN program. The crude all-cause mortality results based on the ATS/IDSA population are shown in Table 26.1. Based on a 10 % non-inferiority margin for mortality (telavancin minus vancomycin), study 0019 showed that the treatment had a nonstatistically significant numerical advantage concluding non-inferiority based on the 10 % margin. However, study 0015 showed a numerical disadvantage for the treatment arm. Since both studies were conducted under the identical protocol, it was of interest to understand the differences between the mortality results in the two studies. The clinical trial database was utilized to perform a series of exploratory subgroup searches with the objective of identifying important predictive subgroups of patients that might explain the influential factors

Table 26.1 Crude 28-day all-cause mortality in the ATTAIN program (based on the American Thoracic Society/Infectious Disease Society of America (ATS/ITSA) population, $N = 1289$)

	Study 0015		Study 0019	
	Telavancin $N = 309$	Vancomycin $N = 316$	Telavancin $N = 325$	Vancomycin $N = 339$
Number of deaths	75	67	74	80
Crude mortality	24.3 %	21.2 %	22.8 %	23.6 %
Treatment difference	3.1		−0.8	
(95 % CI)	(−3.5, 9.6)		(−7.2, 5.6)	

Treatment difference: Telavancin−vancomycin
Confidence intervals were computed using the Agresti–Caffo adjustment

that were associated with the outcome variables. Other references which include mortality analyses for the ATTAIN studies include Torres et al. (2014) and Corey et al. (2014).

26.2.2 Key Patient Characteristics

Mortality in nosocomial pneumonia varies considerably depending on preexisting chronic health condition(s), acute comorbid disease, severity of acute illness, and type of infecting microorganism. Also relevant is whether a patient is hospitalized in a medical, surgical, neurosurgical, or other type of specialized unit, each of which is associated with risk factors that have a bearing on mortality. This diversity of risk factors in nosocomial pneumonia contributes to the wide variability in reported mortality. Mortality rate is also significantly influenced by early, appropriate antibiotic and supportive therapy, with inappropriate therapy contributing considerably to higher rates of mortality (Sorbello et al. 2010). Interpretation of a mortality end point in nosocomial pneumonia studies is confounded by the contribution of non-attributable mortality, particularly due to factors described above, many of which are unrelated to the pneumonia and are preexisting conditions that are the cause for hospitalization.

Baseline patient characteristics (covariates) selected for the exploratory analysis of mortality in the ATTAIN program are defined in Table 26.2. The covariates were not prespecified but represented a set of baseline characteristics potentially related to mortality. As we have done in other publications, in order to simplify the terminology, we will refer to the covariates as *biomarkers*.

26.2.3 Differences Between Studies 0015 and 0019

To understand the differences between studies 0015 and 0019 in the ATTAIN program, the 27 patient baseline characteristics listed in Table 26.2 were compared between the treatment arms from study 0015 and from study 0019. The same

Table 26.2 Candidate biomarkers in the ATTAIN program

Biomarker	Description	Values
X_1	Age (years)	Continuous
X_2	APACHE II score	Continuous
X_3	Acute respiratory distress syndrome/acute lung injury status	No, yes
X_4	Bacteremia status	No, yes
X_5	Intensive care unit status	No, yes
X_6	Body mass index (kg/m^2)	Continuous
X_7	Cerebrovascular accident	No, yes
X_8	Renal risk (diabetes)	No, yes
X_9	Presence of cardiovascular disease	No, yes
X_{10}	Two or more chronic illnesses	No, yes
X_{11}	Serum creatinine clearance (mL/min)	Continuous
X_{12}	Adequacy of Gram-negative HAP treatment	No, yes
X_{13}	Immunocompromised status	No, yes
X_{14}	Mixed infection (Gram-positive or -negative)	No, yes
X_{15}	MRSA infection at baseline	No, yes
X_{16}	Multilobe pneumonia	No, yes
X_{17}	Nephrotoxic medication use	No, yes
X_{18}	Prior treatment failure	No, yes
X_{19}	AN/PS/SMAL infection	No, yes
X_{20}	Presence of any pulmonary comorbidity	No, yes
X_{21}	Race	White, other
X_{22}	Sex	Male, female
X_{23}	Sepsis, septic shock, multiple organ failure at any time	No, yes
X_{24}	Total Glasgow coma score	Continuous
X_{25}	Ventilator status	No, yes
X_{26}	Use of vasopressors	No, yes
X_{27}	Geographical region	North America; Latin America; Asia; Middle East; Europe, Australia and South Africa

HAP hospital-acquired bacterial pneumonia, *MRSA* methicillin-resistant Gram-positive bacteria, *AN/PS/SMAL Acinetobacter/Pseudomonas/Stenotrophomonas maltophilia* infection

comparisons were performed for the control arms between the two studies. In addition, the two studies were combined and differences among the 27 covariates were examined between the treatment and control arms. Based on unadjusted p values, differences between the treatment arms in the two studies were found on 16 covariates and differences between the control arms were found on 9 covariates. However, when the studies were pooled, a difference was discovered only for biomarker X_{26} (use of vasopressors).

Justifications for combining evidence from the two telavancin studies include the following:

- The study protocols were identical in all respects.
- The studies were conducted concurrently.
- The statistical analysis plan called for combining the studies for the analysis of an efficacy endpoint (clinical response in patients with MRSA).
- There was no difference between the treatment arms for 26 out of 27 baseline covariates.
- Confidence intervals for the all-cause mortality rates overlap between the studies (see Table 26.1).

The consistency between the treatment arms on baseline characteristics is remarkable, and the diversity is representative of the intended population. Based on this information, it was felt that pooling the two studies was appropriate. The biomarker evaluation presented in Sects. 26.3 and 26.5 is based on the pooled analysis of the data collected in studies 0015 and 0019.

26.2.4 Predictive and Prognostic Biomarkers

Predictive biomarkers play a central role in evaluating subgroup effects in large clinical trial databases such as the combined ATTAIN database. Predictive biomarkers are defined as treatment-specific patient characteristics that help identify patients who are more likely to respond to a particular treatment (Food and Drug Administration 2012). It is instructive to contrast predictive biomarkers with prognostic biomarkers, i.e., patient characteristics that help predict disease-related outcomes independently of the assigned treatment. Biomarker X_2 (APACHE II score) defined in Table 26.2 serves as an example of a prognostic covariate. A higher APACHE II score is associated with a higher risk of death for an individual patient (Knaus et al. 1985) but it is not clear if the APACHE II score can be used for predictive purposes, i.e., if this score may help identify patients who are most likely to benefit from telavancin.

Predictive biomarkers provide a foundation for developing individualized/tailored therapies. A well-known example is the use of a protein expression-based classifier in the trastuzumab (Herceptin) development program in metastatic breast cancer. Based on the data collected earlier in the program, the program's sponsor concluded that patients whose tumors demonstrated high levels of human epidermal growth factor receptor 2 (HER-2) expression would be most likely to benefit from the new treatment. Patients in the phase III program were classified as biomarker-positive if their tumors tested positive for HER-2 and biomarker-negative otherwise. Only biomarker-positive patients were enrolled in the phase III trials and a positive effect of trastuzumab was confirmed in this subpopulation of patients (Romond et al. 2005). However, further investigation of the treatment effect trastuzumab on breast cancer indicated that the HER-2 status might not be a strong predictive biomarker and biomarker-negative patients could also benefit from this treatment (Paik et al. 2008; Hayes 2011). This example highlights the importance of a comprehensive assessment of the predictive value of candidate biomarkers before launching a large development program.

As shown above, the main purpose of studying predictive biomarkers in clinical development programs is to help identify the subpopulations of patients with a modified (enhanced or reduced) treatment effect. The subpopulations are constructed by dichotomizing one or more selected biomarkers. Any biomarker with more than two levels, including continuous variables, needs to be converted to a simple binary classifier which defines biomarker-negative and biomarker-positive patients. For example, with a continuous variable, values below a certain threshold correspond to a biomarker-negative status and values above the threshold define a biomarker-positive status. The thresholds may be chosen based on clinically relevant cutoffs or based on statistical criteria, e.g., criteria that are aimed at maximizing the differential treatment effect between the subsets of biomarker-negative and biomarker-positive patients. Patient subgroups are then formed based on a single classifier or by combining several classifiers.

26.3 Initial Biomarker Evaluation in ATTAIN Trials

We first describe a series of preliminary analyses aimed at characterizing the effect of the candidate biomarkers listed in Table 26.2 on the outcome variable in the ATTAIN program. The analyses were driven by the divergent results from the two randomized phase III studies (studies 0015 and 0019) on the post hoc efficacy end point (mortality).

The preliminary analyses rely on traditional "univariate" approaches to subgroup exploration. Limitations of the traditional approaches are discussed in Sect. 26.3.2. Advanced approaches to biomarker evaluation and identification of patient subgroups with an enhanced treatment effect are defined in Sects. 26.4 and 26.5. These approaches are based on the SIDES method, which employs a "multivariate" approach to evaluating sets of candidate biomarkers and features multiplicity adjustment and complexity control tools.

26.3.1 Model-Based Biomarker Assessment

As explained in Sect. 26.2, the primary end point defined in the protocol was clinical response at a test-of-cure visit approximately a week after completion of antibiotic therapy. The clinical response results were shown to be non-inferior to the active control in both phase III studies. The main objective of the exploratory biomarker evaluation was to identify potential predictive biomarkers while minimizing bias in the process of analyzing the individual covariates. Proportional hazards regression models were applied to compare the two treatment groups in each study adjusted for important prognostic covariates related to mortality. The prespecified biomarkers were further tested for treatment interactions to check for differential subgroup effects. This general methodology is similar to approaches to biomarker evaluation that are often used in exploratory sections of statistical analysis plans.

The following five-step algorithm was used to develop a common proportional hazards regression model based on studies 0015 and 0019 using the all-treated population. A single regression model for analyzing the combined ATTAIN database resulted from the evaluation algorithm. PROC PHREG in SAS version 9.2 was used to implement the algorithm.

Step 1. Screen potential prognostic biomarkers with univariate proportional hazards regression

Each candidate biomarker was separately screened for its association with mortality. The screen was conducted (1) on all patients in the database, combined across treatment arms, (2) on all patients in study 0015, combined across treatment arms, (3) on all patients in study 0019 combined across treatment arms, and (4) on each treatment arm separately, combined across studies. Covariates with $p \leq 0.1$ were considered as candidate variables in further steps. At this step the candidate biomarkers were not selected based upon their impact on any treatment group comparison.

Step 2. Use screened biomarkers in a stepwise proportional hazards regression ignoring treatment

Stepwise proportional hazards regression was applied to identify the biomarkers associated with outcome in each of the data groups defined in step 1. In each data group, only the biomarkers found significant in step 1 in that data group were used for the stepwise regression. The entry and removal criteria were both based on $p \leq 0.1$. The study and treatment terms were ignored in these models.

Step 3. Check for interactions among selected variables with study

All biomarkers from the models in step 2 were evaluated in a stepwise regression model that included all patients. In addition, the study term and interactions with study for each of these biomarkers were included in the model. The entry and removal criteria were both based on $p \leq 0.1$. If any covariate-by-study interactions are identified, proportional hazards regression models in subsequent steps was to be stratified by study.

Step 4. Check for interactions among selected biomarkers with treatment to identify potential predictive biomarkers

The same process as in step 3 was repeated for treatment interactions. Treatment interactions were included for all biomarkers. If any study-by-biomarker interaction was significant in step 3, the models were stratified by study. A hierarchical model fitting procedure with treatment in the first hierarchy was used. The entry and removal criteria were both based on $p \leq 0.1$. After step 5 below, a test for the study-by-treatment interaction term in the model was assessed.

Step 5. Final model: Force treatment into the model and check for treatment interactions with $p \leq 0.1$

All the main effects and the significant interaction terms from steps 3 and 4 were included in step 5. At this step, the treatment term was included in the model. Treatment was forced to stay in the model and stepwise proportional hazards regression was used to identify a final set of significant biomarkers. The entry and removal criteria were both set to $p \leq 0.1$. An interaction and its component could be entered or be eliminated in a single step using the HIERARCHY option in PROC PHREG.

To summarize the results from the univariate analysis, there were 17 statistically significant biomarkers identified from the combined ATTAIN database. The resulting unadjusted hazard ratio and 95 % confidence intervals for levels of each biomarker are shown in Table 26.3 under "univariate assessment." Most of the biomarkers were related to severity of disease or other preexisting conditions. The sole exception is biomarker X_{27} (geographic region), where mortality rates were higher in Latin America and Middle East than in North America, although the confidence interval of the unadjusted hazard ratio included 1 for Middle East.

The results of the final model identified in step 5 are reported in Table 26.3 under "model-based assessment." This table lists the ten biomarkers plus an interaction between treatment and X_{11} (creatinine clearance) that were included in the final model.

In Table 26.3, several prognostic covariates associated with the outcome of mortality were identified in the ATTAIN program. These covariates were each evaluated for treatment interactions. Only one covariate (biomarker X_{11}, serum creatinine clearance) showed a strong differential mortality response. It is natural to hypothesize that creatinine clearance is a predictive biomarker. A higher creatinine clearance rate (>80 mL/min and above) demonstrated a trend toward lower mortality in the telavancin arm compared to vancomycin. This predictive biomarker illustrated a qualitative interaction between the level of creatinine clearance and treatment. Proportional hazards regression models showed how effects of the prognostic factors and the predictive biomarker can be quantitatively expressed in terms of hazard ratios.

The conclusion is an important one, but how robust is the result? A lot of variable screening of the covariate space was conducted using univariate regressions with a prespecified cutoff point $p \leq 0.10$ and a stepwise regression was then used to develop a final model. p values in the stepwise model development did not have real probability interpretations but were simply measures of the strength of evidence upon which decisions were made in the model development process. The final model p values were not adjusted for multiplicity, which is a particularly important deficiency for regulatory decision making. Note also that several continuous biomarkers were categorized and one clearly runs the risk of using incorrect cutoff points and losing precision in the model without the continuous representation. In addition, the classifications used for biomarker X_{11} were based on the levels generally considered normal versus mild, moderate or severe renal deficiency.

Table 26.3 Summary of hazard ratios based on univariate assessment and final model

Biomarker	Subgroup	Hazard ratio (95 % confidence interval)	
		Univariate assessment	Model-based assessment
X_1	≤65		
	>65	2.35 (1.84, 3.01)	1.46 (1.09, 1.95)
X_2	0 − 14		
	15 − 20	2.58 (1.93, 3.46)	1.85 (1.37, 2.51)
	>20	3.91 (2.90, 5.28)	2.06 (1.49, 2.84)
X_3	No		
	Yes	1.92 (1.41, 2.62)	
X_4	No		
	Yes	2.26 (1.58, 3.21)	1.74 (1.21, 2.51)
X_5	No		
	Yes	1.32 (1.04, 1.67)	
X_7	No		
	Yes	1.30 (0.98, 1.71)	
X_8	No		
	Yes	1.35 (1.05, 1.73)	
X_9	No		
	Yes	2.11 (1.64, 2.73)	1.33 (1.00, 1.77)
X_{10}	No		
	Yes	2.07 (1.62, 2.64)	
X_{11}	>80		0.69 (0.44, 1.08) [>80: T–V]
	50 − 80	1.76 (1.28, 2.42)	0.92 (0.57, 1.47) [50 − 80: T–V]
	30 − 50	2.23 (1.61, 3.07)	1.30 (0.81, 2.11) [30 − 50: T–V]
	≤30	4.17 (3.05, 5.70)	1.81(1.13, 2.89) [≤ 30: T–V]
X_{15}	No		
	Yes	1.60 (1.27, 2.02)	1.35 (1.08, 1.69)
X_{16}	No		
	Yes	1.73 (1.34, 2.24)	1.50 (1.15, 1.96)
X_{23}	No		
	Yes	4.16 (3.29, 5.27)	2.83 (2.19, 3.64)
X_{24}	>6		
	≤6	1.42 (1.02, 1.98)	
X_{25}	No		
	Yes	1.26 (0.99, 1.60)	

Table 26.3 (continued)

Biomarker	Subgroup	Hazard ratio (95 % confidence interval)	
		Univariate assessment	Model-based assessment
X_{26}	No		
	Yes	2.36 (1.74, 3.20)	
X_{27}	North America		
	Latin America	1.63 (1.15, 2.30)	1.39 (0.96, 2.01)
	Asia	0.98 (0.69, 1.39)	0.82 (0.57, 1.19)
	Middle East	1.26 (0.82, 1.94)	1.33 (0.84, 2.09)
	Europe, Australia, and South Africa	0.87 (0.62, 1.22)	0.97 (0.68, 1.37)

T–Vis telavancin versus vancomycin

26.3.2 Limitations of the Traditional Approach

As illustrated earlier in this section, simple biomarker evaluation approaches are commonly used in clinical drug development. In the context of time-to-event analysis, proportional hazards regression models including the terms for treatment, single biomarker, and treatment-by-biomarker interaction may be applied to a set of candidate biomarkers. Biomarkers with interaction effects that are significant at a prepecified level are retained for further examination. For selected continuous/ordinal biomarkers, such examination would typically involve evaluating all possible cutoffs using multiplicity adjusted p values. This approach to biomarker evaluation can be referred to as a "univariate" approach. An important feature of this approach is that it can only identify patient subgroups defined by a single biomarker. In addition, the approach does not control the overall alpha level or false discovery rate and at the same time suffers from low power.

As an alternative to simplistic univariate approaches, multiple candidate biomarkers and their higher-order interactions with treatment may be evaluated in a single regression model. Subgroups are identified based on the significance of specific interaction terms. However, this analytic strategy is similar to the univariate approach in that it also suffers from low power and arbitrary choice of the significance levels used in the interaction tests. Besides, the alternative approach requires the prespecification of interaction terms and covariate cutoffs to form the individual subgroups.

Regression with stepwise selection of the main and interactions effects may also be employed to help select important biomarkers; however, the stepwise selection methods are notoriously unstable and their operating characteristics are not well understood. There are other problems common to fitting parametric models with a large number of interaction terms. Hence, methods of penalized regression and their extensions, as well as other methods adopted from statistical/machine learning, have been proposed that may mitigate some of these issues. These complex methods are rarely employed in evaluating biomarkers in clinical trials and may require very careful tuning. For example, penalized regression may fail to detect important interactions since they may be obscured by much stronger main effects, i.e., effects of prognostic biomarkers, compared to the predictive biomarker effects, which would require using different penalties for the main and interaction terms (Imai and Ratkovic 2013).

One of the main drawbacks of the biomarker evaluation approaches described above is that they do not fully explore the relationships among the individual biomarkers and their synergistic effect on the outcome variable. As a consequence, these approaches do not fully assess the predictive value of individual biomarkers which often manifests itself through their relationships with other covariates. Also, univariate and stepwise selection methods overlook an inherent multiplicity problem. Without a proper adjustment for the multiplicity and selection bias arising in the analysis of multiple covariate and subgroups based on these covariates, one cannot perform reliable inferences and is bound to face a highly inflated probability of incorrect conclusions. Basic biomarker evaluation approaches often suggest patterns that are not confirmed by more advanced approaches that rely on a joint assessment of candidate biomarkers. Advanced approaches to biomarker evaluation are presented in Sects. 26.4 and 26.5.

26.4 SIDES Method

The SIDES method is a novel subgroup identification/biomarker discovery method which offers a viable alternative to traditional biomarker exploration methods described in Sect. 26.3. This method is based on key principles of data mining and machine learning and utilizes recent advances in this expanding area of research.

The general SIDES methodology was introduced in Lipkovich et al. (2011) and an extended version of the SIDES subgroup identification procedure which utilizes biomarker screening was proposed in Lipkovich and Dmitrienko (2014a). Comprehensive simulation-based assessments of the operating characteristics of the standard and enhanced SIDES methods are presented in Lipkovich and Dmitrienko (2014a, 2014b). For a detailed overview of the SIDES method as well as other approaches aimed at efficient subgroup identification and biomarker evaluation, see Lipkovich and Dmitrienko (2014b).

Note that for the simplification of the presentation, the analyses presented in this section focus on superiority p values to compare the mortality rates between the treatment and control arms. A similar approach can be used to investigate non-inferiority of the treatment compared to the control arm.

26.4.1 Key Components of SIDES Method

We will begin with a high-level summary of the key components of the SIDES method, including:

- Component I. Subgroup generation algorithm (subgroup partitioning rules).
- Component II. Subgroup pruning tools (growth and treatment effect restrictions, biomarker screening).
- Component III. Subgroup interpretation tools (multiplicity adjustment, subgroup proximity assessment, and reproducibility assessment).

A detailed description of the general SIDES subgroup search algorithm is given in the Appendix.

26.4.2 Component I. Subgroup Generation

To define the main building blocks of the SIDES method, the subgroup generation component includes an efficient algorithm aimed at the identification of covariates with treatment modification properties (predictive covariates) and promising subgroups of patients. This is a *recursive partitioning algorithm* which relies on the local treatment effect modeling approach defined in the Introduction. Beginning with the overall population, the algorithm generates subgroups by finding an optimal split of each *parent group* into two complementary *child subgroups* for each candidate biomarker. The optimality criterion used in the algorithm is known as the *partitioning criterion* and is based on evaluating the treatment-by-split interaction. The resulting set of subgroups forms a forest with a large number of subgroup trees.

26.4.3 Component II. Subgroup Pruning

If subgroup generation is performed in an unconstrained manner, the number of subgroups grows at an exponential rate and the final set of subgroups is quite difficult to manage and interpret. It is therefore natural to consider ways to efficiently select the most relevant subgroups from the extremely large *search space* (set of all subgroups produced by the subgroup generation algorithm). Subgroup selection utilizes a number of subgroup pruning tools that help control the complexity of the subgroup identification problem and reduce the size of the search space. This includes *growth restrictions* and treatment effect restrictions in child subgroups. Setting a limit on the absolute number of children or a fraction of the total number of children for any parent group keeps the subgroups trees from growing at an unacceptably high rate. Most commonly, growth restrictions are defined using the "rule of three children" or "rule of five children," e.g., only three or five subgroups are retained for any parent.

In addition, restrictions on the magnitude of the treatment effect in child subgroups are commonly applied (*treatment effect restrictions*). A child subgroup is retained only if it provides a certain amount of improvement over the parent group. The improvement is typically measured on a p value scale; however, other measures of treatment effect such as the effect size can be utilized as well.

A closely related tool is *biomarker screening* based on the concept of *variable importance* (VI). A VI score provides a quantitative estimate of a biomarkers ability to modify treatment effect. This approach enables clinical trial researchers to assess the relative effects of candidate biomarkers on the treatment response and build a biomarker screen which filters out covariates with weak predictive properties. This screen can be used as part of a two-stage procedure which first selects the strongest predictors of treatment benefit and then applies the standard SIDES subgroup search algorithm to the small subset of most promising biomarkers. The resulting procedures (known as *SIDEScreen procedures*) help reduce the impact of nuisance covariates, which results in improved performance of the subgroup identification method.

26.4.4 Component III. Subgroup Interpretation

The last component of the SIDES method is a set of tools that facilitate the interpretation of the patient subgroups in the final set. This includes *multiplicity adjustment*, *subgroup proximity assessment,* and *reproducibility assessment*. As was pointed out in Sect. 26.3, traditional subgroup search methods are likely to produce spurious results due to an inherent but commonly overlooked problem of testing a very large number of null hypotheses. This multiplicity problem is directly related to the "curse of dimensionality." SIDES relies on resampling-based multiplicity adjustments that account for subgroup selection bias, which leads to a considerable overstatement of the treatment effect within individual subgroups. Properly adjusted p values provide a foundation for reliable inferences in the subgroups identified using the SIDES method.

Subgroup proximity assessment provides tools for measuring the overlap between individual subgroups. It is not unusual to discover that two or more subgroups based on different sets of biomarkers in fact define virtually identical sets of patients. The Jaccard index is utilized to measure the pairwise similarities (or proximities) between subgroups in the final set. The proximities can be converted to distances and analyzed further using hierarchical clustering methods to find families of subgroups that are quite similar to each other. The resulting assessment plays an important role in facilitating the clinical interpretation of patient subpopulations generated by the SIDES subgroup search algorithm.

Another important consideration in subgroup exploration is reproducibility assessment. The assessment is performed by splitting the original clinical trial database into training and test subsets (learn and confirm approach) using the balanced allocation procedure (Lipkovich et al. 2011). A set of most promising subgroups is constructed based on the training subset and the probability of confirming these subgroups in the test subset is then estimated.

26.4.5 *Application of Key SIDES Components*

It is important to point out that the components defined in Sect. 26.4.1, i.e., subgroup generation, subgroup pruning, and subgroup interpretation, serve as building blocks of the general SIDES method and should not be viewed as sequential steps of a subgroup search algorithm. In fact, within the SIDES method, subgroup pruning can be either integrated into subgroup generation or performed as the second step following subgroup generation (harvesting).

In the former case, the search space is restricted by imposing constraints as part of the recursive partitioning process, e.g., requiring that the treatment effect in a subgroup exceeds that in the parent group by some margin (treatment effect restrictions).

In the latter case, a large number of subgroups is first formed with a few or no restrictions and then the biomarkers are scored by averaging their contributions to each subgroup, which is conceptually similar to ensemble procedures, e.g., bagging, random forest, boosting (an important difference is that SIDES does not use random components in generating subgroups). As a result, the search space can be restricted by selecting only the biomarkers with top scores; the ensemble of subgroups can be pruned by identifying subgroups based on the selected biomarkers. Two-stage SIDEScreen procedures with VI assessment utilize this algorithm.

These two approaches correspond to two philosophies in model selection: the first one indexes models by some free parameter(s) describing the complexity of the model. The model is selected by fixing complexity parameters at some levels, which is often done via cross-validation, external data, or expert knowledge. The second approach relies on first harvesting a large ensemble of models that likely overfit the data and contain many irrelevant covariates; however, it then takes advantage of the fact that noise variables contribute sparsely to the ensemble and are suppressed by averaging their contributions over the entire ensemble.

26.5 Biomarker Evaluation and Subgroup Identification in ATTAIN Trials Using SIDES Method

A SIDES-based subgroup search method with a biomarker screening stage, known as the SIDEScreen method (Lipkovich and Dmitrienko 2014a), was applied to the analysis of the combined ATTAIN database, which includes studies 0015 and 0019. The candidate set in this analysis included biomarkers X_1 through X_{26} defined in Table 26.2 (the geographic region was excluded). The main objective of this exercise was to characterize the predictive ability of the 26 biomarkers and select subgroups of patients who are most likely to experience beneficial therapeutic effect.

To facilitate the presentation of the material, we will focus on the three main components of the SIDES method introduced in Sect. 26.4.1, namely, component I (subgroup generation), component II (subgroup pruning), and component III (subgroup interpretation).

An Excel add-in package (SIDESxl package) developed by Ilya Lipkovich and Alex Dmitrienko was used to perform subgroup search in the ATTAIN database. This package can be downloaded from the Biopharmaceutical Network website at `http://biopharmnet.com/wiki/Software`.

26.5.1 Component I. Subgroup Generation

As explained in Sect. 26.4, the first step in the general SIDES method deals with the generation of promising subgroups that are later examined and compared to identify the final set of subgroups with enhanced treatment effect. The subgroup generation algorithm was applied recursively to the combined data set from the two ATTAIN trials beginning with the overall population of patients (1289 patients). In the first step of the algorithm, the overall population served as the parent group and a family of child subgroups based on each biomarker in the candidate set was found. The overall population was optimally partitioned using two splitting criteria:

- Criterion 1: Differential effect criterion.
- Criterion 2: Maximum effect criterion.

To define the splitting criteria, consider a continuous biomarker X (splitting criteria for categorical biomarkers are constructed in a similar manner). For a given cut-off point c, the biomarker-low and biomarker-high child subgroups are defined as follows:

$$L(c) = \{X \leq c\},\ H(c) = \{X > c\}.$$

Further, $Z_L(c)$ and $Z_H(c)$ denote the log-rank test statistics for comparing the mortality rates between the treatment and control arms in the biomarker-low and biomarker-high subgroups. Criterion 1 (differential effect criterion) is based on a standardized absolute difference between the two test statistics, i.e.,

$$D(c) = 2\left[1 - \Phi\left(\frac{|Z_H(c) - Z_L(c)|}{\sqrt{2}}\right)\right],$$

where $\Phi(x)$ is the cumulative distribution function of the standard normal distribution. By contrast, criterion 2 (maximum effect criterion) focuses on the more significant of the test statistics in the two child groups:

$$D(c) = 2\min[1 - \Phi(Z_H(c)), 1 - \Phi(Z_L(c))].$$

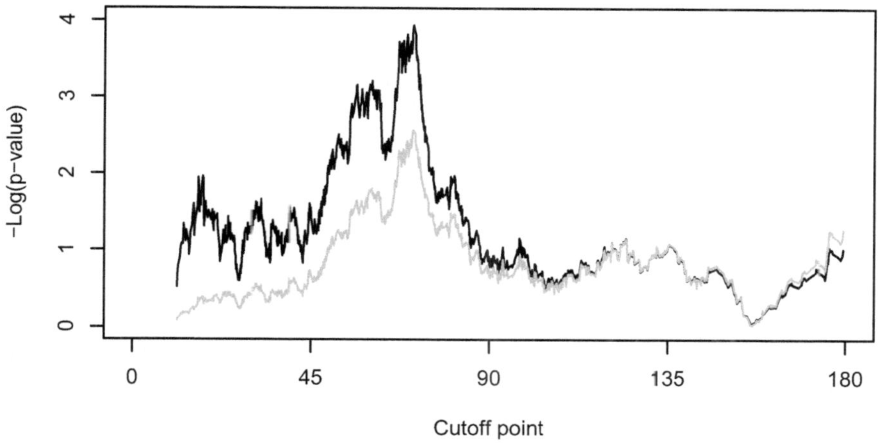

Fig. 26.1 Comparison of two splitting criteria for determining an optimal split of the overall population on biomarker X_{11} (creatinine clearance). *Black curve*, differential effect criterion; *gray curve*, maximum effect criterion

Note that splitting criteria are typically defined on a p value scale and therefore they are optimized by finding the lowest/most significant value. Alternatively, a log scale can be utilized, i.e., $-\log(D)$ can be used instead of D. This scale helps highlight the more subtle yet important differences between very small values of a criterion. For example, it is very difficult to detect the difference between $D = 0.001$ and $D = 0.0001$ on a regular scale but, with the log scale, this difference becomes much more prominent.

Each splitting criterion was applied to partition the parent group into two mutually exclusive child subgroups for each biomarker. The optimal cutoff c was defined as the value which maximized the criterion on the log scale (or minimized the criterion on the regular p value scale). To compare the two approaches to defining optimal subgroups, Fig. 26.1 plots the splitting criteria as a function of the cutoff point for biomarker X_{11} (creatinine clearance). Even though there was a fair amount of variation across the criterion functions, the general pattern was quite similar and the two criteria resulted in the same optimal cutoff point ($c = 67$).

A more detailed comparison of criteria 1 and 2 as well as other splitting criteria is provided in Lipkovich and Dmitrienko (2014b). In general, criteria 1 and 2 produce very similar results and, for this reason, we will focus on criterion 1 (differential effect criterion) in this section. In addition, to speed up the subgroup generation algorithm, all continuous biomarkers were converted to categorical covariates with 20 levels. This transformation had trivial impact on the final subgroups.

The differential effect criterion was applied to define promising subgroups based on all biomarkers in candidate set 1. These subgroups will be referred to the level 1 subgroups. The SIDES subgroup generation algorithm was applied recursively up to level 2, i.e., in the next step of the algorithm, each level 1 subgroup was treated as a parent subgroup and additional child subgroups were found. The level 2 subgroups were based on two biomarkers.

A simple sample size restriction is typically applied in each step of the SIDES subgroup generation algorithm, e.g., subgroups with less than a predefined number of patients per treatment arm are discarded. The smallest sample size per arm was set to 30 in the analysis of the ATTAIN database.

26.5.2 Component II. Subgroup Pruning

Due to its recursive nature, the subgroup generation algorithm tends to create a vast search space with an exponentially growing set of promising subgroups. It is critical to apply efficient subgroup pruning tools to reduce the number of subgroups to help facilitate their analysis and interpretation.

The following two subgroup pruning tools were initially considered to reduce the complexity of subgroup exploration in the ATTAIN program. Growth restrictions based on the rule of five children were applied and thus up to five children subgroups were retained for each parent group. In general, focusing on a single best child subgroup for a parent subgroup may be misleading. Selecting several subgroups better reflects the uncertainty around the choice of the most promising subgroup. To make an analogy with model selection problems, reliance on a single best model is known to be one of the key weaknesses of stepwise multiple regression. Treatment effect restrictions were formulated in terms of the treatment effect p value (log-rank p value for the difference in survival rates between the control and treatment arms). Given a prespecified constant γ ($0 < \gamma \leq 1$), a child subgroup was kept only if

$$p_C \leq \gamma p_P,$$

where p_C and p_P are the treatment effect p-values in the child and parent subgroups, respectively, and γ is termed the child-to-parent ratio. Several child-to-parent ratio values were considered to help control the size of the search space and choose the most relevant subgroups. A lower value of γ resulted in more aggressive pruning. Since the subgroup selection criterion was formulated in terms of the strength of the treatment effect, this pruning tool focused on identifying the best subgroups for a given parent.

The effect of the commonly used subgroup pruning tools is illustrated in Fig. 26.2. This figure displays the relationship between the treatment effect and subgroup size in the final set of subgroups identified using four different approaches:

- Approach 1: Unconstrained subgroup generation without pruning. The final set contained 390 subgroups.
- Approach 2: Subgroup pruning with growth restrictions (up to five children subgroups were retained for each parent group). The final set contained 15 subgroups.

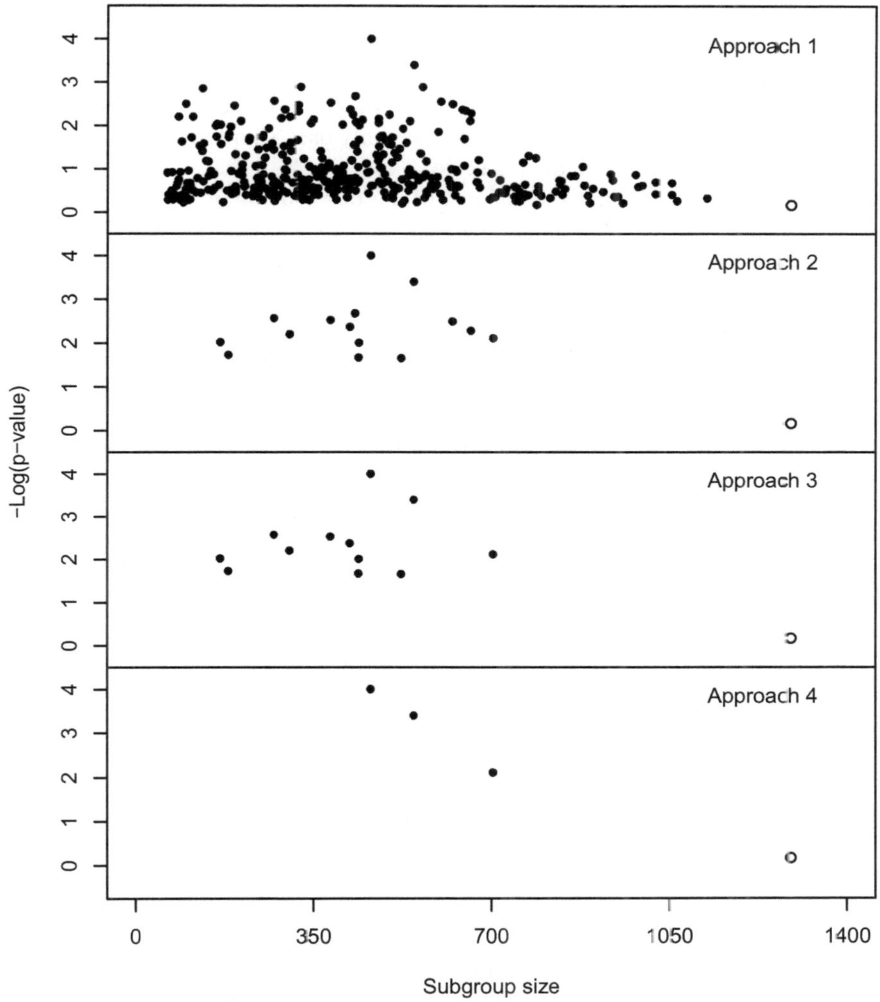

Fig. 26.2 Effect of subgroup pruning on the number of subgroups (*closed circles*, patient subgroups in the final set; *open circle*, overall population of patients)

- Approach 3: Subgroup pruning with growth restrictions (up to five children subgroups were retained for each parent group) and treatment effect restrictions (child-to-parent ratio $\gamma = 0.5$). The final set contained 12 subgroups.
- Approach 4: Subgroup pruning with growth restrictions (up to five children subgroups were retained for each parent group) and treatment effect restrictions (child-to-parent ratio $\gamma = 0.25$). The final set contained three subgroups.

Each dot in Fig. 26.2 represents a subgroup produced by the SIDES subgroup generation algorithm and the overall population of patients is provided as a reference point. As in Fig. 26.1, the treatment effect p values within the subgroups and overall population are presented on a log scale. The value of zero corresponds to an infinitely negative treatment difference. A commonly used significance level of 0.025 (one-sided) is equal to 1.6 on the log scale.

It is instructive to examine the impact of subgroup pruning on the size of the final subgroup set in Fig. 26.2. Beginning with approaches 1 and 2, it is clear that the rule of five children helps reduce the search space to a much more manageable size (from 390 subgroups down to 15 subgroups). Further improvement in the size of the final set is achieved by applying treatment effect restrictions. The set tends to shrink quite rapidly with the increasing child-to-parent ratio γ since child subgroups are pruned more aggressively. In this particular setting, the size of the final set was reduced from 15 subgroups in approach 2 (no treatment effect restrictions) to 12 subgroups in approach 3 (treatment effect restriction with $\gamma = 0.5$), and only 3 subgroups in approach 4 (treatment effect restriction with $\gamma = 0.25$).

An important feature of subgroup pruning is that it provides complexity control by discarding the less relevant subgroups. The clinical relevance of a subgroup of patients is usually defined as a composite measure of the treatment difference within this subgroup and the subgroup's size. Even though different measures can be considered, a more "attractive" patient subgroup has a larger size and a more significant treatment effect. Figure 26.2 shows that the subgroup pruning methods defined above retain about 4 % of the final subgroups obtained using approach 1 and the selected subgroups are generally larger or exhibit a more significant treatment effect than the discarded subgroups. This is accomplished by creating an efficient sieving mechanism which helps identify the most promising subgroups from an expanding set of eligible subgroups in each step of the algorithm.

An additional advantage of stricter subgroup pruning is that it reduces the burden of multiplicity in complex subgroup search problems. It was explained in Sect. 26.4 that an unadjusted analysis of treatment differences across multiple subgroups of patients is highly unreliable due to selection bias. SIDES utilizes a resampling-based method to perform multiplicity adjustments within each final subgroup and compute a properly adjusted treatment effect p value (for more information on multiplicity adjustments, see Dmitrienko and D'Agostino 2013). To briefly introduce the key idea, consider a subgroup identified by the SIDES method and let p denote the raw treatment effect p value within this subgroup, which is computed directly from the log-rank test. Using a resampling method, a large number of null data sets (e.g., $m = 10,000$ data sets) are generated from the original database by removing the treatment effect across all possible subsets. The SIDES method is applied to each null data set and the best subgroup is chosen. Let q_j denote the treatment effect p value in the best subgroup identified from the jth null data set, $j = 1, \dots, m$. A multiplicity-adjusted treatment effect p value within the selected subgroup, denoted by $\widetilde{p}$, is defined as the proportion of the null data sets such that the p value in the

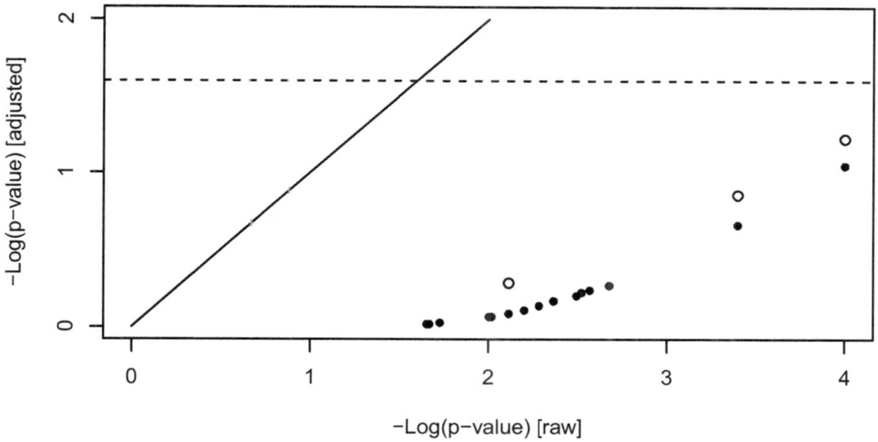

Fig. 26.3 Relationship between the raw and multiplicity-adjusted treatment effect p values in the final subgroup sets based on approach 2 (*closed circles*) and approach 4 (*open circles*). The *dotted line* is drawn at the standard significance level (one-sided 0.025). The *solid line* is an equality line (adjusted p value is equal to raw p value)

best subgroup is less than or equal to the raw p value for the selected subgroup, i.e.,

$$\widetilde{p} = \frac{1}{m} \sum_{j=1}^{m} I\{q_j \leq p\}.$$

Due to strong selection bias, multiplicity-adjusted p values tend to be much less significant than raw p values. Adjusted treatment effect p values that are significant at a 0.025 level (based on a one-sided test) are very rare in subgroup identification problems.

To illustrate multiplicity adjustments in subgroup search, Fig. 26.3 displays the raw and adjusted one-sided treatment effect p values using approaches 2 and 4 defined above (as before, the p values are displayed on the log scale). The figure shows that the raw treatment effect p values identified using either approaches were highly significant and ranged between 1.66 and 4 on the log scale (i.e., between 0.0001 and 0.0221 on the regular scale). When the less aggressive pruning approach (approach 2 with the child-to-parent ratio $\gamma = 0.75$) was applied and resampling-based multiplicity-adjusted p values were computed in the resulting 15 subgroups, the most significant adjusted p value was greater than 0.09. Recall that, due to the treatment effect restrictions, the subgroup search algorithm systematically chose the subsets with the most significant results. The apparent significance of the treatment effect in the resulting subgroups of patients before the multiplicity adjustment is a direct effect of selection bias.

When the more stringent pruning rules with a treatment effect restriction based on $\gamma = 0.25$ were considered (approach 4), only three subgroups were discovered. The burden of multiplicity was reduced in this setting due to a smaller search space, which led to a smaller multiplicity penalty. Indeed, Fig. 26.3 demonstrates that the adjusted p values obtained under approach 4 were uniformly more significant compared to approach 2 (even though the difference was generally small). To see this more concretely, consider one of the subgroups identified under approach 4, i.e.,

$$S_{11} = \{X_{11} > 67\}.$$

A naive analysis based on the raw one-sided log-rank p-value suggested a strong treatment effect within this subgroup ($p = 0.0077$). Under approach 2, the adjusted treatment effect p value was 0.82. When approach 4 was applied, the adjusted p value was reduced to 0.52. Thus, the use of a more efficient subgroup search provided a somewhat stronger evidence of significance.

26.5.3 Component II. Biomarker Screening

It was demonstrated earlier in this section that standard subgroup pruning provides efficient tools aimed at slowing the growth of subgroup trees. This helps control the complexity of the subgroup identification problem. However, subgroup pruning based on growth and treatment effect restrictions does not address the fundamental problem of nuisance/noise covariates. Most biomarkers are either non-informative or may be valuable mostly from a prognostic perspective. Very few biomarkers are reliable predictors of treatment response. Non-informative and prognostic biomarkers lower the signal-to-noise ratio in subgroup search problems and it is highly desirable to find tools that help screen out the noise biomarkers. This approach is consistent with the general scientific principle of parsimony.

In order to develop an effective screening method, we need to find a way to quantitatively assess the predictive ability of a given biomarker. As proposed in Lipkovich and Dmitrienko (2014a), clinical trial researchers can take advantage of the concept of *VI* which has been successfully used in machine learning methods. The VI index is defined as the impact of a biomarker on treatment response which is averaged over the final set of subgroups. More formally, consider the final set identified by the SIDES procedure and let

$$F_1, \ldots, F_m$$

denote the subgroups included in this set. Further, for a given biomarker, let d_i denote the value of the partitioning criterion on the log scale (i.e., criterion 1 defined in Sect. 26.5.1) associated with this biomarker in subgroup F_i, $i = 1, \ldots, m$. Note that $d_i = 0$ if the biomarker is not used in subgroup F_i. The VI index is then computed as the average of $d_1, \ldots, d_m$. The resulting VI index will be larger for the biomarkers that are included in multiple subgroups and, in addition, demonstrate a stronger differentiating effect within these subgroups as measured by the partitioning criterion. For a thorough discussion of VI, see Lipkovich and Dmitrienko (2014a).

A key feature of VI scores is that they explicitly account for (potentially complex) interactions among the candidate covariates. For example, a simplistic version of the VI score could have been obtained by using the partitioning criterion in the level 1 subgroups only. This score provides an initial estimate of VI since this approach focuses on a "univariate" effect of each biomarker on the outcome variable (all-cause mortality). Higher-order interactions are not taken into account even though they may be quite valuable in assessing the predictive strength of a biomarker. As explained in Lipkovich and Dmitrienko (2014a), a biomarker may not be strongly associated with a differential treatment effect compared to the other biomarkers in the very first step of the algorithm (i.e., when the level 1 subgroups are examined). However, a careful review of all subgroups in the final set may reveal that this biomarker modifies the treatment effect within the level 2 subgroups based on two covariates. In this case, a biomarkers treatment modification effect may be conditional upon another biomarker.

To illustrate the importance of accounting for higher-order interactions when computing the VI score, consider biomarker X_{14} (presence of mixed infection). This biomarker was included in the following four subgroups in the final set:

$$
\begin{aligned}
S_{2,14} &= \{X_2 \leq 10,\ X_{14} = \text{`No'}\}, \\
S_{14,5} &= \{X_{14} = \text{`No'},\ X_5 = \text{`No'}\}, \\
S_{17,14} &= \{X_{17} = \text{`No'},\ X_{14} = \text{`No'}\}, \\
S_{11,14} &= \{X_{11} > 67,\ X_{14} = \text{`No'}\}.
\end{aligned}
$$

Figure 26.4 displays the values of the partitioning criterion for these subgroups along with the value of the partitioning criterion in the level 1 subgroup based on biomarker X_{14}, i.e., $\{X_{14} = \text{`No'}\}$. The latter is equal to 3.3 and is represented by the horizontal line. It is clear that the partitioning criterion for subgroups $S_{2,14}$, $S_{17,14}$, and $S_{11,14}$ was much different from 3.3. For example, consider first subgroup $S_{2,14}$. This subgroup was formed by splitting a level 1 subgroup based on X_2 by X_{14}. The associated partitioning criterion equaled 2.2 and thus it was lower than 3.3. This indicates that, after accounting for the impact of biomarker X_2 on the survival rate, biomarker X_{14} exhibited a more "modest" differential effect. On the other hand, when subgroup $S_{11,14}$ was examined, the partitioning criterion increased to 5. This implies that a synergistic effect of biomarkers X_{11} and X_{14} considerably improved the latter's ability to predict the treatments effect on survival. Higher-order interactions turn out to be quite important for assessing the predictive value of biomarker X_{14} and clearly need to be incorporated into the VI score.

Figure 26.5 shows the final VI scores for the top four biomarkers (the scores for the remaining biomarkers were less than 0.5 and they were treated as noise covariates). It follows from this figure that the VI score can be used as an effective biomarker screening tool. For example, biomarker X_{11} (creatinine clearance) had a high VI score compared to the other biomarkers, which indicates that baseline creatinine clearance is a strong predictor of telavancin-related survival benefit.

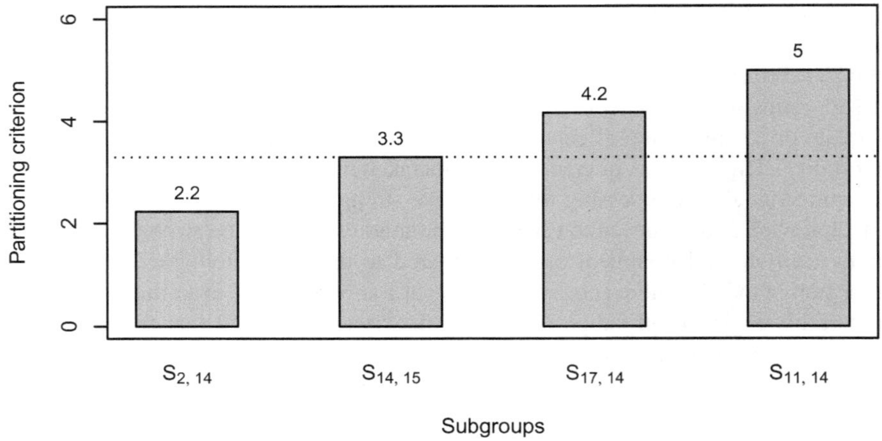

Fig. 26.4 Values of the partitioning criterion for the four subgroups based on biomarker X_{14} (creatinine clearance). The *horizontal line* is drawn at the value of the partitioning criterion in the level 1 subgroup based on biomarker X_{14} (3.3)

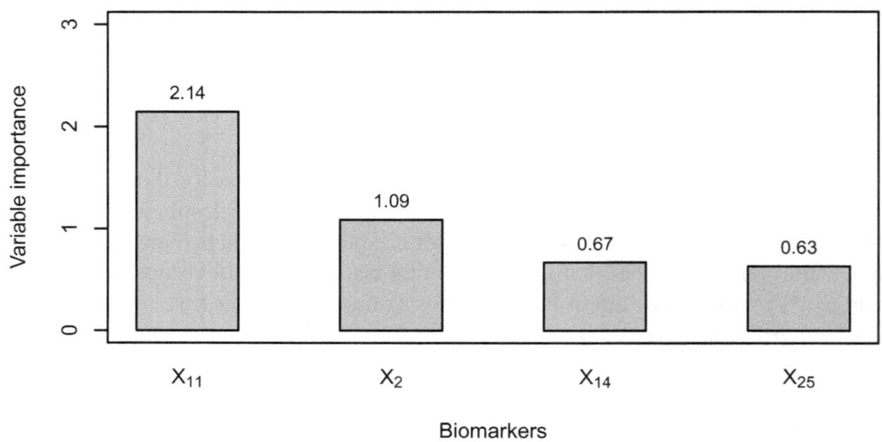

Fig. 26.5 Variable importance scores for the top four biomarkers (biomarker X_{11}, creatinine clearance; biomarker X_2, APACHE II score; biomarker X_{14}, presence of mixed infection; biomarker X_{25}, ventilator status)

A biomarker screening rule can be constructed either by choosing a fixed number of biomarkers with the highest VI scores, e.g., $k = 3$ biomarkers, or by applying an adaptive approach which identifies a variable number of biomarkers in order to protect an appropriately defined selection error rate. The fixed biomarker screening rule is easy to implement. For example, based on the results presented in Fig. 26.5, the fixed rule with $k = 3$ selected the following biomarkers:

- Biomarker X_{11} (creatinine clearance).
- Biomarker X_2 (APACHE II score).
- Biomarker X_{14} (presence of mixed infection).

This screening rule is somewhat simplistic and an adaptive approach with built-in error rate control provides a useful alternative. The error rate is defined in this case as the probability of incorrectly selecting at least one biomarker when all biomarkers are in fact non-informative. The selection error rate is computed from the null distribution of the maximum VI score. To apply the adaptive biomarker screening rule to the 26 biomarkers in candidate set 1, the null distribution was computed based on 1000 permutations. This distribution was approximately normal with mean $\mu = 0.85$ and standard deviation $\sigma = 0.32$. Using this reference distribution, we can compute normalized VI scores using the same principle which is used in the definition of a p value:

$$v^* = 1 - \Phi\left(\frac{v - \mu}{\sigma}\right),$$

where v and v^* are the regular and normalized VI scores, respectively, and $\Phi(x)$ is the cumulative distribution function of the normal distribution. The normalized VI scores have a simple interpretation. A lower score indicates that the associated biomarker is important. In particular, if the normalized VI score for a biomarker is equal to v^*, this biomarker will be chosen by the adaptive rule based on the selection error rate of $100v^*$ %.

It is easy to see that the normalized VI scores for the most important four biomarkers were given by

- Biomarker X_{11}: $v^* = 0.00002$.
- Biomarker X_2: $v^* = 0.228$.
- Biomarker X_{14}: $v^* = 0.717$.
- Biomarker X_{25}: $v^* = 0.756$.

If a restrictive adaptive biomarker selection rule based on the selection error rate of 10 % was applied, only one biomarker would be chosen for the second stage of the procedure (normalized VI score for biomarker X_{11} was less than 0.1). If the selection error rate was increased to 30 %, two biomarkers would be selected (normalized VI scores for biomarkers X_{11} and X_2 were less than 0.3).

Using the fixed and adaptive biomarker screening rules, a two-stage subgroup identification procedure (SIDEScreen procedure) can be built as follows:

- Step 1. Apply the SIDES subgroup search algorithm with liberal subgroup pruning rules to a set of biomarkers. Compute the VI score for all candidate biomarkers and select the most promising biomarkers.
- Step 2. Apply the SIDES subgroup search algorithm to the biomarkers identified in step 1.

Fixed and adaptive SIDEScreen procedures were applied to the combined ATTAIN database to perform biomarker assessment.

Table 26.4 Final sets of subgroups identified by the the fixed and adaptive SIDEScreen procedures in the ATTAIN program

Subgroup	Subgroup size	One-sided p values	
		Raw p value	Adjusted p value
Overall patient population			
All patients	1289	0.6894	NA
Fixed SIDEScreen procedure			
$S_{11,14} = \{X_{11} > 67 \text{ and } X_{14} = \text{'No'}\}$	547	0.0004	0.0990
$S_{11,2} = \{X_{11} > 67 \text{ and } X_2 \leq 15\}$	426	0.0056	0.4530
$S_{11} = \{X_{11} > 67\}$	703	0.0077	0.5160
$S_{2,11} = \{X_2 \leq 13 \text{ and } X_{11} > 49\}$	432	0.0083	0.5310
$S_{14,2} = \{X_{14} = \text{'No' and } X_2 \leq 13\}$	439	0.0099	0.5650
$S_2 = \{X_2 \leq 13\}$	522	0.0221	0.7430
Adaptive SIDEScreen procedure			
$S_{11} = \{X_{11} > 67\}$	703	0.0077	0.0680

26.5.4 Component II. Two-Stage Subgroup Search

To illustrate the two-stage approach to subgroup identification based on SIDEScreen procedures with biomarker screening, we applied the fixed and adaptive procedures to the combined ATTAIN database. Both procedures utilized the SIDES subgroup search algorithm with the following parameters in the first step:

- No treatment effect restrictions.
- Up to five children subgroups selected for each parent.
- Two-level subgroup search with subgroups defined using one or two biomarkers.

The fixed SIDEScreen procedure then applied the SIDES algorithm to the three biomarkers with the largest VI indices (X_{11}, X_2, and X_{14}). The adaptive SIDEScreen procedure only selected the biomarkers with VI exceeding a prespecified threshold, which was computed using the "rule of one standard deviation." In particular, as discussed in Sect. 26.5.3, the null distribution of the maximum VI score was computed. This distribution was approximately normal with mean $\mu = 0.85$ and standard deviation $\sigma = 0.32$ and the threshold was defined as

$$\mu + \sigma = 1.17.$$

This biomarker screening rule corresponded to a 16 % selection error rate. The adaptive approach resulted in selection of only one biomarker (X_{11}). The resulting sets of subgroups are summarized in Table 26.4.

Table 26.4 presents key characteristics of the subgroups identified by the fixed and adaptive SIDEScreen procedures and compares them to the overall patient population. The relative size of the subgroups identified by the fixed procedure ranged

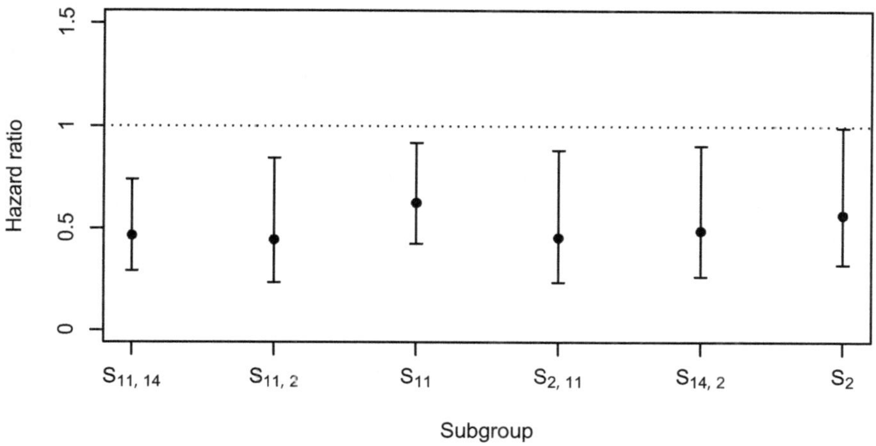

Fig. 26.6 Hazard ratios and 95 % confidence intervals in the subgroups identified by the the fixed and adaptive SIDEScreen procedures in the ATTAIN program

from 33 to 55 % (from 426 to 703 patients) and all subgroups provided a substantial improvement over the general population in terms of survival benefit. The raw one-sided p values within the six subgroups ranged from 0.0004 to 0.0221 but, after the resampling-based multiplicity adjustment, none of the p values were even remotely significant. Consider, for example, subgroup $S_{11,14}$. The raw p value computed from the log-rank test in this subgroup was highly significant (one-sided $p = 0.0004$). However, when the null data sets without treatment effect across all possible subgroups were generated, it turned out that a subgroup with a one-sided treatment effect p value of 0.0004 or smaller was found in 9.9 % of the null sets. As a consequence, the multiplicity-adjusted p value in subgroup $S_{11,14}$ was set to 0.0990.

As explained in Sect. 26.5.2, the multiplicity penalty in subgroup identification problems is greatly affected by the size of the search space. With stricter biomarker screening rules, the search space is often substantially shrunk, which reduces the degree of multiplicity adjustment. Indeed, as shown in Table 26.4, the multiplicity-adjusted p value in subgroup S_{11} was considerably smaller when the adaptive SIDEScreen procedure was applied. With the fixed procedure, the adjusted treatment effect p value in this subgroup was very large ($p = 0.516$) whereas the adjusted p value associated with the adaptive procedure was $p = 0.068$, which may be viewed as marginally significant.

Figure 26.6 provides a summary of the treatment effects (estimated hazard ratios and 95 % confidence intervals) in the subgroups listed in Table 26.4. It is worth noting that the estimated hazard ratios are obviously biased estimates of the true treatment differences in the individual subgroups and are used here mostly as benchmarks. Secondly, no adjustment for multiplicity was performed across the subgroups and marginal 95 % confidence intervals are presented in Fig. 26.6 to describe the variability of the treatment effect estimates.

Figure 26.6 shows that a highly beneficial effect was observed in most subgroups with the hazard ratios ranging between 0.44 and 0.63. With the exception of S_2, the upper confidence limits were well below the horizontal line drawn at 1. For comparison, the hazard ratio in the overall patient populations was 1.059. Also, since the biomarker screening rule used in the fixed SIDEScreen procedure was more liberal than the adaptive screening rule, the apparent effect size in the top subgroup selected by the fixed procedure ($S_{11,14}$) was much larger (and the corresponding hazard ratio was lower) than in the subgroup identified by the adaptive procedure (S_{11}):

- Hazard ratio of 0.46 in the best subgroup identified by the fixed SIDEScreen procedure.
- Hazard ratio of 0.63 in the best subgroup identified by the adaptive SIDEScreen procedure.

The results presented in Table 26.4 and Fig. 26.6 suggest that biomarker X_{11} (creatinine clearance) is a reliable predictor of treatment benefit in the combined ATTAIN database and subgroup S_{11} is worth investigating further in future trials as the best candidate for developing a tailored strategy. For comparison, a negative treatment effect was observed in the complementary subgroup $\{X_{11} \leq 67\}$. The hazard ratio in this subgroup was 1.4 with a significant treatment effect in favor of the control group (one-sided $p = 0.008$).

Considering subgroup S_{11}, it is helpful to assess the balance of key patient characteristics between the two treatment arms within this subgroup. In general, a positive treatment effect within a particular subset of the overall patient population may be induced by imbalance with respect to important prognostic covariates (note that covariates with a weak prognostic ability have virtually no impact on the outcome variable). To rule out such an explanation of the observed beneficial effect in subgroup S_{11}, treatment imbalance was examined across the 26 covariates listed in Table 26.2. Since the candidate set of biomarkers included a mix of continuous and binary covariates, the standardized treatment difference between the treatment arms (effect size) was computed for the 26 biomarkers. The standardized treatment difference was defined as the difference in sample means or proportions divided by the pooled sample standard deviation. In addition, the prognostic strength of each individual biomarker was assessed using a Cox proportional hazards model for 28-day all-cause mortality with the biomarker as the only independent variable. A p value computed from this model was used to quantify the impact of the biomarker on the outcome variable. As in Sect. 26.5.2, a log transformation was applied to each p value to compute a measure of prognostic effect.

Figure 26.7 plots the measures of treatment imbalance (standardized treatment differences) as a function of the prognostic effect for the 26 biomarkers included in the candidate set. The standardized treatment differences are quite small (most of the differences lie between -0.1 and 0.1), which demonstrates that the treatment arms were balanced with respect to the most important patient characteristics within subgroup S_{11}. It is also worth noting that the magnitude of treatment imbalance is independent of the prognostic ability of the individual biomarkers.

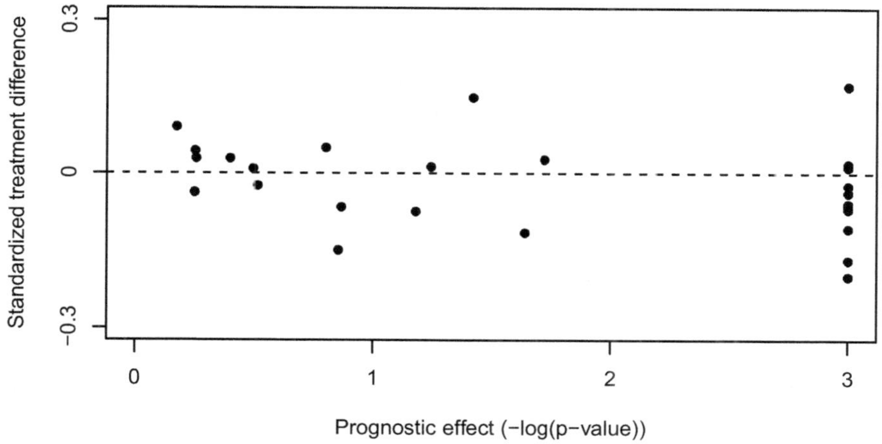

Fig. 26.7 Assessment of treatment imbalance within subgroup $S_{11} = \{X_{11} > 67\}$. The standardized treatment difference is plotted as a function of the prognostic strength (on a log scale) for the 26 biomarkers in the candidate set

26.5.5 Component III. Proximity Assessment

The output of the SIDES procedures (both single-stage and two-stage procedures) is a collection of subgroups that would typically require further examination. Some of the groups may substantially overlap and essentially represent the same type of patients. This would obviously happen because of using common biomarkers in defining subgroups; however, subgroups defined by different markers are also likely to overlap because they are based on correlated covariates. As an extreme case, if two copies of the same covariate were accidentally included in the set of candidate biomarkers, e.g., X_1 and X_2, the SIDES method would report two identical subgroups $\{X_1 \leq c\}$ and $\{X_2 \leq c\}$.

In general, it is always beneficial to assess the "amount of overlap" among the subgroups, based on the actual group memberships rather than on the labels of the biomarkers that define subgroups. Since a subgroup can be thought of as a binary variable assuming values $Z = 1$ for the patients who are included in the subgroup and $Z = 0$ for those who are not, the similarity between two subgroups can be measured by any of the variety of similarity (proximity) measures for binary variables. One popular measure is the Jaccard index which measures the overlap between subgroups S_i and S_j. This index is defined as the ratio of the number of patients included in both subgroups to the number of patients included in either subgroup, i.e.,

$$J(S_i, S_j) = \frac{|S_i \cap S_i|}{|S_i \cup S_i|},$$

where $|S|$ is the size of subgroup S. The Jaccard index equals 0 if the two subgroups do not overlap and 1 if the two subgroups are identical to each other. A dissimilarity measure or, in other words, "distance" between subgroups S_i and S_j, is defined simply as $1 - J(S_i, S_j)$.

The matrix of pairwise subgroup similarities can be analyzed using cluster analysis methods (e.g., hierarchical cluster analysis) or multidimensional scaling (e.g., principal coordinate plots based on singular value decomposition of the dissimilarity matrix).

The results of proximity assessment can be graphically presented using:

- Heatmaps with rows and columns arranged according to their order in a dendrogram produced by a hierarchical clustering method.
- Low-dimensional plots using coordinates from (metric or nonmetric) multidimensional scaling methods.

As an illustration, Fig. 26.8 presents a heatmap based on hierarchical clustering of dissimilarities among the six subgroups generated by the SIDEScreen procedure with a fixed biomarker screening rule (three most important biomarkers were taken forward to the second stage of the subgroup search algorithm, see Table 26.4). Lighter cells in this figure correspond to dissimilar subgroups and darker cells help identify subgroups with a considerable overlap. In addition, a dendrogram shows the groups of clusters defined by combining the individual subgroups. Due to a strong correlation between biomarkers X_2 (APACHE II score) and X_{14} (presence of mixed infection), subgroups S_2 and $S_{14,2}$ are fairly close to each other with the Jaccard index of 0.84. Indeed, it can be seen from Table 26.4 that most patients at a lower risk of death based on the APACHE II score ($X_2 \leq 13$) do not present with mixed infections (X_{14} = 'No'). Further, Biomarkers X_{11} (creatinine clearance) and X_{14} are also strongly correlated. As a result, two other pairs of subgroups, namely, subgroups S_{11} and $S_{11,14}$, and subgroups S_2 and $S_{2,11}$, exhibit a considerable overlap.

Based on the results presented in Figure 26.8, the six subgroups identified by the SIDEScreen procedure can be grouped as follows:

- Cluster 1: Subgroups $S_{2,11}$, S_2 and $S_{14,2}$ are similar to each other.
- Cluster 2: Subgroups S_{11} and $S_{11,14}$ are similar to each other.
- Cluster 3: Subgroup $S_{11,2}$ is dissimilar to the other groups of patients.

26.5.6 Component III. Reproducibility Assessment

As was pointed out in Sect. 26.4, an important goal of subgroup analysis is to support reliable predictive inferences by selecting the subgroups that are likely to be reproduced in subsequent trials. Lipkovich et al. (2011) described the use of a *learn-and-confirm* approach to performing reproducibility assessments. This approach relies on splitting the original data set into two random subsets that are balanced with respect to the key patient characteristics (the two subsets are created using the *balanced allocation procedure*). A single-stage or two-stage SIDES procedure is applied to the first subset (known as the *training set*) and the confirmation rate is estimated by examining the subgroups in the other subset (known as the *test set*). The

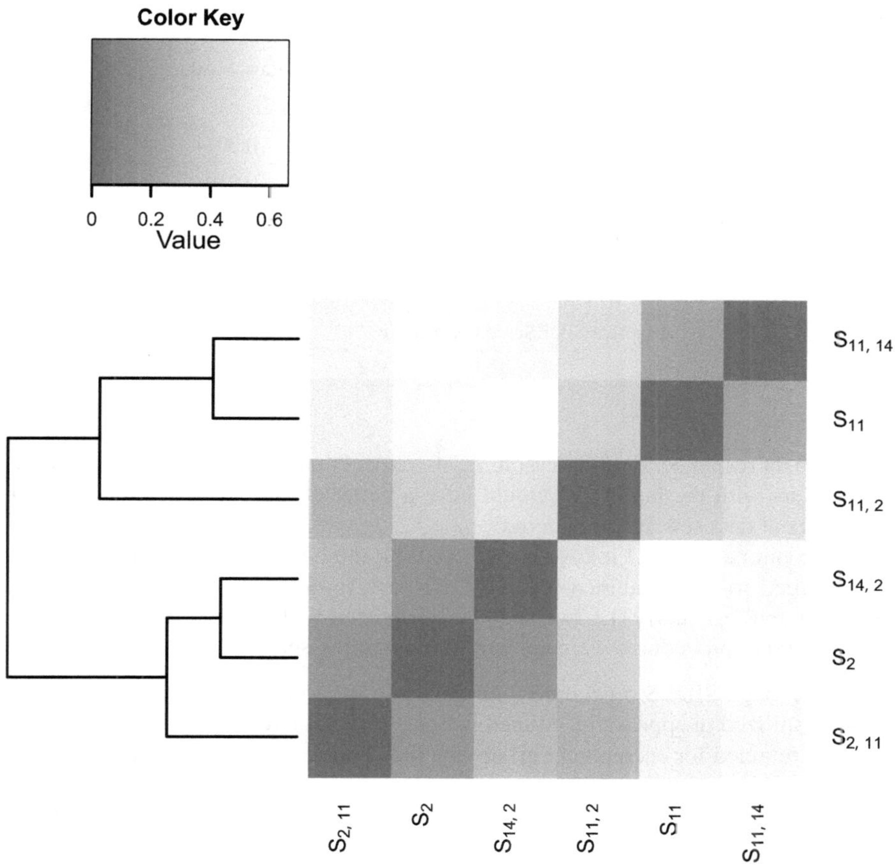

Fig. 26.8 Heatmap-based proximity assessment in the six subgroups produced by the SIDEScreen procedure with a fixed biomarker screening rule

confirmation rate is defined as the probability that the beneficial effect in a subgroup identified in the training set is confirmed in the test set.

As we would expect, subgroups identified by SIDES in the training set may be quite different from those found in the analysis of the full data set. Recursive partitioning methods are known to be unstable and the results often change across multiple replicates from the same data set. The main reason for that is that most of the candidate biomarkers are noise covariates and some of them are likely to be incorrectly "identified" as significant predictors of treatment response in a greedy search process. By creating random subpopulations, we may redistribute the "contributions" of the noise biomarkers in the ensemble of subgroups. However, as discussed in Sect. 26.5.3, when averaged over a collection of subgroups, the contribution of the noise biomarkers tends to shrink toward zero, which helps reveal the true predictors

Table 26.5 Subgroup sets identified by the the fixed and adaptive SIDEScreen procedures in the training set

Subgroup	Subgroup size	Raw p value
Fixed SIDEScreen procedure		
$S_{11} = \{X_{11} > 67\}$	352	0.0044
$S_{11,1} = \{X_{11} > 67 \text{ and } X_1 > 50\}$	211	0.0108
$S_{16,1} = \{X_{16} = \text{'No' and } X_1 \leq 60\}$	98	0.0162
$S_{1,11} = \{X_1 \leq 60 \text{ and } X_{11} > 57\}$	236	0.0167
$S_{11,16} = \{X_{11} > 67 \text{ and } X_{16} = \text{'No'}\}$	132	0.0206
Adaptive SIDEScreen procedure		
$S_{11} = \{X_{11} > 67\}$	352	0.0044

of treatment response. By this reasoning, we expect that the subgroups based on the biomarkers with the largest VI would have a better chance to be replicated when independent data sets are considered.

As recommended in Lipkovich et al. (2011), the balanced allocation procedure was applied to the combined ATTAIN database to define two sets of equal size (training and test sets). The two sets were balanced with respect to all covariates. The following procedures were applied to the training set:

- Single-stage SIDES procedure with the same subgroup pruning parameters that were utilized in approach 3 defined in Sect. 26.5.2 (up to five children subgroups were retained for each parent group and the child-to-parent ratio was set to $\gamma = 0.5$).
- Fixed SIDEScreen procedure (three biomarkers with the highest VI were selected for the second stage).
- Adaptive SIDEScreen procedure (biomarkers with high VI were selected using the rule of one standard deviation defined in Sect. 26.5.4).

The single-stage SIDES procedure selected 9 subgroups in the training set that were quite different from the 12 subgroups that were identified on the full data set (see Sect. 26.5.2). The results produced by the fixed and adaptive SIDEScreen procedures were generally more consistent with those presented in the analysis of the full ATTAIN database (see Table 26.4). The three biomarkers chosen by the fixed screening rule were X_{11} (creatinine clearance), X_1 (age) and X_{16} (multilobe pneumonia) with biomarker X_{11} exhibiting a much higher VI score compared to the other two covariates. The adaptive screening rule selected only one biomarker (X_{11}).

The final subgroups identified by the two SIDEScreen procedures are listed in Table 26.5. It can be seen from this table that the fixed SIDEScreen procedure selected fewer subgroups compared to the full database and there was a fair amount of variability across the subgroups. By contrast, the adaptive SIDEScreen procedure returned the same subgroup on the training data as it did on the full data, i.e., $S_{11} = \{X_{11} > 67\}$.

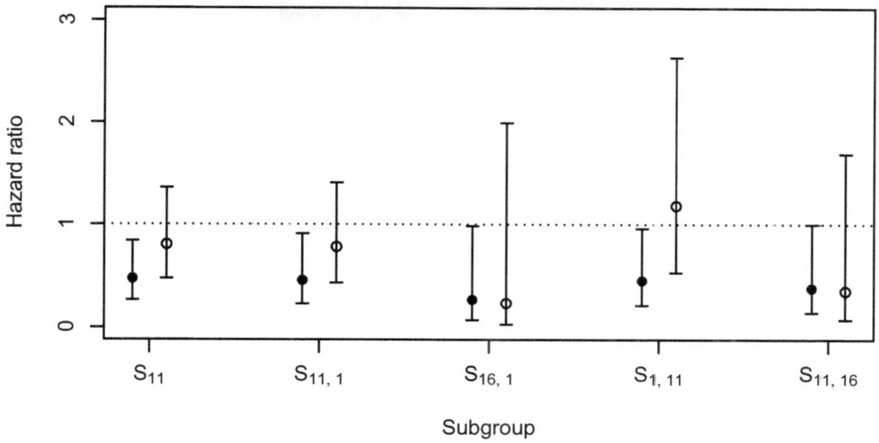

Fig. 26.9 Hazard ratios and 95 % confidence intervals in the subgroups identified by the the fixed and adaptive SIDEScreen procedures in the ATTAIN program. Training set, *closed circles*; test set, *open circles*

To evaluate the extent to which the subgroups identified on the training set are likely to be confirmed in an independent data set, Figure 26.9 displays the hazard ratios estimated in the training and test sets. It was emphasized in Sect. 26.5.4 that, due to selection bias, the observed hazard ratios overstate the magnitude of the treatment difference. The treatment effects within the individual subgroups are expected to attenuate in the test set and thus the hazard ratios will most likely shrink towards 1 (or, in other words, the effect sizes measured on a log-hazard ratio scale will shrink towards 0). In fact, with ad hoc subgroup search methods, the reproducibility rate is typically quite low. Even though a strong beneficial effect may be found within a subgroup based on one data set, a confirmation exercise on another data set often reveals no evidence of a positive effect or a negative treatment difference may be observed. This phenomenon is a simple example of regression to the mean.

In this setting, Fig. 26.9 demonstrates that a negative treatment effect with the hazard ratio of 1.18 was detected in subgroup $S_{1,11}$. However, the hazard ratios were comparable between the two data sets in subgroups $S_{16,1}$ and $S_{11,16}$ and a meaningful fraction of the effect size was retained in subgroups S_{11} and $S_{11,1}$. However, even if the effect sizes were generally similar between the training and test data sets in selected subgroups, the confidence intervals were clearly wider when the treatment differences were estimated in the test set.

This simple example illustrates the importance of reproducibility assessment based on cross-validation. In general, "repeated cross-validation" can be applied to better characterize the magnitude of selection bias in the subgroups discovered by SIDEScreen procedures. This can be accomplished by randomly generating a larger number of complementary training and test sets and evaluating an appropriate measure of discordance between each pair of sets. For example, one could compute the average difference between the effect size in the top subgroup identified in each training set and the effect size in the corresponding subgroup in the test set. Another approach to assessing the "optimism bias" could focus on computing the rate at which the top subgroup was confirmed on the test data using the treatment effect p value < 0.05 or 0.1.

To summarize, the reproducibility assessment strengthened an earlier conclusion that biomarker X_{11} (creatinine clearance) is a strong predictor of telavancin's effect on survival. The survival benefit observed in patients with higher rates of creatinine clearance and related subgroups of patients is likely to be confirmed in future clinical trials.

26.6 Discussion

The general topic of personalized medicine and tailored therapeutics has attracted much attention in the clinical trial literature. Clinical trial sponsors are increasingly interested in the evaluation of treatment effects within specific subsets of the overall patient population that are defined using biomarkers. However, the use of basic approaches to biomarker exploration and subgroup identification remains widespread in clinical trials. In this chapter, we outlined the main weaknesses of the traditional methods that rely mainly on univariate assessments of the individual biomarkers. Recent developments in subgroup identification methodology provide viable alternatives to traditional approaches. This chapter describes an application of a novel subgroup identification method (SIDES) to a large clinical trial database with the goal of selecting most promising predictors of treatment response and associated subgroups of patients who are most likely to experience a beneficial effect.

The SIDES method overcomes important limitations of simplistic biomarker exploration methods. The proposed method emphasizes a multivariate treatment of the general problem of biomarker discovery and characterization, and explicitly accounts for the multiplicity induced by the analysis of a massive number of subgroups. It was shown in recent publications (see, for example, Lipkovich and Dmitrienko 2014b) that the SIDES methodology, including extended SIDES procedures that utilize biomarker screening, performs well in a broad class of realistic settings with up to a 100 candidate biomarkers.

Both the regression- and SIDES-based approaches to biomarker evaluation identified baseline creatinine clearance as a predictive biomarker. The traditional regression-based method showed the interaction favoring telavancin for patients with baseline creatinine clearance > 50 mL/min and the opposite for baseline creatinine clearance ≤ 50 mL/min. The SIDES method found the optimal baseline creatinine clearance cutoff point at >67 mL/min for telavancin benefit associated with the multiplicity adjusted treatment effect p value of 0.068. This predictor may be a potential candidate for developing a tailored treatment strategy.

To provide relevant background information, the phase III ATTAIN trials provided the basis for the 2013 FDA approval of telavancin for HABP/VABP caused by susceptible isolates of *Staphylococcus aureus* when other alternatives are not suitable. The label contains a black box warning concerning treatment of patients with decreased renal function:

> Patients with pre-existing moderate/severe renal impairment (CrCl $\leq$ 50 mL/min) who were treated with VIBATIV for hospital-acquired bacterial pneumonia/ventilator-associated bacterial pneumonia had increased mortality observed versus vancomycin. Use of VIBATIV in patients with pre-existing moderate/severe renal impairment (CrCl $\leq$ 50 mL/min) should be considered only when the anticipated benefit to the patient outweighs the potential risk.

The SIDES method offers several attractive features that help clinical drug developers address challenging problems in biomarker evaluation, e.g., efficient subgroup search strategies and selection bias control. The method provides multiplicity-adjusted p values for statistical comparisons. We hope that the adjusted probabilities can be evaluated by regulators as evidence of superiority or inferiority to help better establish a risk/benefit profile for future drug reviews.

26.7 Appendix

The Appendix defines the subgroup search algorithm used in the SIDES method.

26.7.1 Algorithm Parameters

The following parameters need to be specified before the algorithm is applied to a clinical trial database:

- D: Partitioning criterion.
- L: Depth (maximum number of levels in subgroup).
- M: Width (maximum number of child subgroups for a parent group used in subgroup pruning).
- γ: Child-to-parent ratio used in subgroup pruning (degree of improvement in the treatment effect p-value).
- $n_{\min}$: Lower bound for the sample size per treatment arm in a subgroup.
- $p_{\max}$: Upper bound on the treatment effect p in a subgroup.

26.7.2 Description

The subgroup search algorithm includes the three main steps:

Initialization

A single level 0 parent group is formed of all patients in the data set. Initialize the set of promising subgroups as an empty set, $\mathcal{P} = \emptyset$.

Iteration

Partition the current level l parent group, $0 \leq l \leq L$. If $l = L$, the current parent group is included in the final set and is not partitioned further. Otherwise perform the following steps:

- Form the ordered list of biomarkers from the "best" to "worst" in terms of the optimal value of the partitioning criterion, i.e., $\widetilde{D}_{(1)}, \ldots, \widetilde{D}_{(k)}$. Here, D_j is the value of the partitioning criterion for the best split on biomarker X_j for all allowable partitions. If biomarker X_j is ordinal, the allowable partitions include all binary splits into sets $\{X_j \leq c\}$ and $\{X_j > c\}$, where c ranges over the values of X_j. If X_j is nominal, the binary splits are formed as all possible partitions of the values of X_j into two nontrivial sets, e.g.,. $\{X_j =$ 'No'$\}$ and $\{X_j =$ 'Yes'$\}$. The restriction on the minimum sample size is imposed at this step. Further, $\widetilde{D}_j$ is the adjusted value of the partitioning criterion based on local multiplicity adjustment.
- For each of the top M biomarkers, say, X_j, based on the above criterion, form two children subgroups L_j and H_j and select the subgroup with the larger treatment effect (this promising subgroup is denoted by S_j and included in $\mathcal{P}$). Retain this subgroup if it meets the treatment effect restrictions, i.e., $p_j \leq \gamma p_0$, where p_j is the treatment effect p value in subgroup S_j and p_0 is the treatment effect p value in the parent subgroup.
- For each promising subgroup S_j, set S_j as the current parent group, let $l = l + 1$ and repeat the iteration step.
- If none of the biomarkers has allowable splits resulting in a promising child subgroup, the current parent group is included in the final set and is not considered for further partitioning.

Selection

Define the final set of subgroups as the subset of $\mathcal{P}$ with the treatment effect p values $\leq p_{\max}$. Compute multiplicity-adjusted p values for the subgroups in the final set using resampling-based techniques.

References

American Thoracic Society/Infectious Diseases Society of America (2005) Guidelines for the management of adults with hospital-acquired, ventilator-associated, and healthcare-associated pneumonia. Am J Respir Crit Care Med 171:388–416

Brookes ST, Whitley E, Peters TJ, Mulheran PA, Egger M, Davey Smith G (2001) Subgroup analyses in randomised controlled trials: quantifying the risks of false-positives and false-negatives. Health Technol Assess 5:1–56

Committee for Medicinal Products for Human Use (2014) Guideline on the investigation of subgroups in confirmatory clinical trials. EMA/CHMP/539146/2013

Corey GR, Kollef MH, Shorr AF, Rubinstein E, Stryjewski ME, Hopkins A, Barriere SL (2014) Telavancin for hospital-acquired pneumonia: clinical response and 28-day survival. Antimicrob Agents Chemother 58:2030–2037

Dmitrienko A, D'Agostino RB (2013) Tutorial in biostatistics: traditional multiplicity adjustment methods in clinical trials. Stat Med 32:5172–5218

Dusseldorp E, Van Mechelen I (2014) Qualitative interaction trees: a tool to identify qualitative treatment subgroup interactions. Stat Med 33:219–237

Food and Drug Administration (2010) Guidance for industry: hospital-acquired bacterial pneumonia and ventilator-associated bacterial pneumonia: developing drugs for treatment

Food and Drug Administration (2012) Guidance for industry: enrichment strategies for clinical trials to support approval of human drugs and biological products

Foster JC, Taylor JMC, Ruberg SJ (2011) Subgroup identification from randomized clinical trial data. Stat Med 30:2867–2880

Freidlin B, Simon R (2005) Adaptive signature design: an adaptive clinical trial design for generating and prospectively testing a gene expression signature for sensitive subjects. Clin Cancer Res 11:7872–7878

Freidlin B, Jiang W, Simon R (2010) Adaptive signature design: the cross-validated adaptive signature design. Clin Cancer Res 16:691–698

Hardin DS, Rohwer RD, Curtis BH, Zagar A, Chen L, Boye KS, Jiang HH, Lipkovich IA (2013) Understanding heterogeneity in response to antidiabetes treatment: a post hoc analysis using SIDES, a subgroup identification algorithm. J Diabetes Sci Technol 7:420–429

Hayes DF (2011) Steady progress against HER2-positive breast cancer. New Engl J Med 365:1336–1338

Imai K, Ratkovic M (2013) Estimating treatment effect heterogeneity in randomized program evaluation. Ann Appl Stat 7:443–470

Kehl V, Ulm K (2006) Responder identification in clinical trials with censored data. Comput Stat Data Anal 50:1338–1355

Knaus WA, Draper EA, Wagner DP, Zimmerman JE (1985) APACHE II: a severity of disease classification system. Crit Care Med 13:818–829

Lipkovich I, Dmitrienko A (2014a) Strategies for identifying predictive biomarkers and subgroups with enhanced treatment effect in clinical trials using SIDES. J Biopharm Stat 24:130–153

Lipkovich I, Dmitrienko A (2014b) Biomarker identification in clinical trials. In: Carini C, Menon S, Chang M (eds) Clinical and statistical considerations in personalized medicine. Chapman and Hall/CRC, New York

Lipkovich I, Dmitrienko A, Denne J, Enas G (2011) Subgroup identification based on differential effect search (SIDES): a recursive partitioning method for establishing response to treatment in patient subpopulations. Stat Med 30:2601–2621

Paik S, Kim C, Wolmark N (2008) HER-2 status and benefit from adjuvant trastuzumab in breast cancer. New Engl J Med 358:1409–1411

Romond EH, Perez EA, Bryant J (2005) Trastuzumab plus adjuvant chemotherapy for operable HER2-positive breast cancer. New Engl J Med 353:1673–1684

Rothwell PM (2005) Subgroup analysis in randomized controlled trials: importance, indications, and interpretation. Lancet 365:176–186

Ruberg SJ, Chen L, Wang Y (2010) The mean does not mean as much anymore: finding sub-groups for tailored therapeutics. Clin Trials 7:574–583

Rubinstein E, Lalani T, Corey GR, et al (2011). Telavancin versus vancomycin for hospital-acquired pneumonia due to gram-positive pathogens. Clin Infect Dis 52:31–40

Simon RM, Subramanian J, Li M-C, Menezes S (2011) Using cross validation to evaluate the predictive accuracy of survival risk classifiers based on high dimensional data. Brief Bioinform 12:203–214

Sorbello A, Komo S, Valappil T (2010) Noninferiority margin for clinical trials of antibacterial drugs for nosocomial pneumonia. Drug Inf J 44:165–176

Su X, Tsai CL, Wang H, Nickerson DM, Li B (2009) Subgroup analysis via recursive partitioning. J Mach Learn Res 10:141–158

Sun X, Briel M, Walter SD, Guyatt GH (2010) Is a subgroup effect believable? Updating criteria to evaluate the credibility of subgroup analyses. Br Med J 340:c117 (850–854)

Tian L, Alizaden AA, Gentles AJ, Tibshirani R (2012) A simple method for detecting interactions between a treatment and a large number of covariates. http://arxiv.org/abs/1212.2995
Torres A, Rubinstein E, Core GR, Stryjewski ME, Barriere SL (2014) Analysis of Phase 3 telavancin nosocomial pneumonia data excluding patients with severe renal impairment and acute renal failure. J Antimicrob Chemother 69:1119–1126
Varadhan R, Segal JB, Boyd CM, Wu AW, Weiss CO (2013) A framework for the analysis of heterogeneity of treatment effect in patient-centered outcomes research. J Clin Epidemiol 66:818–825
Zhao Y, Zheng D, Rush AJ, Kosorok MR (2012) Estimating individualized treatment rules using outcome weighted learning. J Am Stat Assoc 107:1106–1118
Zhang B, Tsiatis AA, Davidian M, Zhang M, Laber E (2012) Estimating optimal treatment regimes from a classification perspective. Statistics 1:103–114

Part VI
Statistical Genomics and High-Dimensional Data Analysis

Chapter 27
A Stochastic Segmentation Model for the Indentification of Histone Modification and DNase I Hypersensitive Sites in Chromatin

Haipeng Xing, Yifan Mo, Will Liao, Ying Cai and Michael Zhang

Abstract Focal alterations in chromatin structure are essential for the proper functioning of various classes of transcriptional regulatory elements in the human genome. These changes can be detected through an increased sensitivity to DNase I and other nucleases due to an open and accessible chromatin conformation. Currently, quantitative analysis approaches use heuristic procedures to identify regions enriched for histone modifications and DNase I hypersensitivity. We here develop a stochastic segmentation model and associate inference framework to characterize the categorical and continuous features of hierarchical structures hidden in sequences. The proposed model has attractive statistical and computational properties and yields explicit formulas for posterior distribution of hidden states with a hierarchical structure. We propose an approximation method whose computational complexity is only linear in sequence length. We demonstrate the performance of the model via extensive simulations. We further use our model to identify DNase I sensitivity and DNase I hypersentitive sites over the Encyclopedia of DNA Elements (ENCODE) regions in human lymphoblastoid cells.

H. Xing (✉) · Y. Cai
Department of Applied Mathematics and Statistics, State University of New York,
Stony Brook, NY 11794, USA
e-mail: xing@ams.sunysb.edu

Y. Cai
e-mail: ying.cai@stonybrook.edu

Y. Mo
Mount Sinai Hospital, New York, NY 10029, USA
e-mail: jasonmo2006@gmail.com

W. Liao
New York Genome Center, New York, NY 10013, USA
e-mail: wliao@nygenome.org

M. Q. Zhang
Department of Molecular & Cell Biology, Center for Systems Biology,
The University of Texas at Dallas, Richardson, TX 75080, USA
e-mail: michael.zhang@utdallas.edu

MOE Key Laboratory of Bioinformatics and Bioinformatics Division,
Center for Synthetic and System Biology, TNLIST, Department of Automation,
Tsinghua University, 100084 Beijing, P. R. China

Z. Chen et al. (eds.), *Applied Statistics in Biomedicine and Clinical Trials Design*,
ICSA Book Series in Statistics, DOI 10.1007/978-3-319-12694-4_27

27.1 Introduction

Recent advances in sequencing technologies have led to a vast leap in our understanding of the genome. It is now well accepted that genomic features beyond simple protein-coding sequence are of significant import. The extent of functional relevance of this noncoding DNA has been the topic of much debate of late. A hotly discussed study by the Encyclopedia of DNA Elements (ENCODE) Project Consortium postulated that as much as 80 % of these regions have some functional roles clear departure from the days where this so-called junk DNA was largely overlooked (Consortium TEP et al. 2012). Whether or not this figure proves true or not, their main point—that deciphering the regulatory role of noncoding DNA is critical to understanding the complexity of the genome—clearly has taken hold. Now, significant work is being undertaken to make sense of how DNA outside of protein-coding regions might participate in gene regulation in a cell- and tissue-specific manner.

No area of research has contributed more to this understanding than that of epigenomics comprised primarily DNA methylation, posttranslational histone modifications, noncoding RNA species, and chromatin structure. These features, as the name suggests, sit "upon" or "outside" the genome and may provide key distinctions between functional and nonfunctional DNA that cannot be discerned from the primary sequence. Already, ENCODE and other collectives like the Roadmap Epigenomics Mapping Consortium (Bernstein et al. 2010) have invested considerable effort into characterizing epigenomic profiles in various cellular contexts. Their work has validated many previously described correlative, and putatively causal, relationships with function, e.g., enrichment of the posttranslational histone modifications H3K4me3 at active promoters, and H3K4me1 and H3K27ac at distal enhancers (Barski et al. 2007; Mikkelsen et al. 2007).

Many of their findings were based on enrichment assays designed to isolate fragments of chromatin DNA, by way of specific antibodies, which are complexed with posttranslationally modified histone protein of interest an assay termed chromatin immunoprecipitation. Similar efforts employed an assay that selects for fragments more easily digested by an enzyme, DNase I, which preferentially cuts at open, accessible DNA. Regions that are "hotspots" for DNase I cleavage are thought to pinpoint areas of active transcription or targeting by regulatory DNA-binding proteins (Sabo et al. 2006). Given this, improving methods to reliably and accurately identify regions of enrichment, by chromatin immunoprecipitation or DNase I digestion, have been the subject of great interest to computational biologists.

Analyses of these types of enrichment assays have largely been described as a peak detection problem, where the main goal is segmenting the genome into regions that are absent of and those that are overrepresented by observed sequence. The abundance of fragments at genomic locations is usually quantified using either tiling arrays or next-generation sequencing. Several successful solutions have been introduced to address this problem (Zhang et al. 2008; Rozowsky et al. 2009; Qin et al. 2010). The model-based analysis for chromatin immunoprecipitation sequencing (ChIP-Seq; MACS) is one of the most popular methods. This method uses a window-based approach to solve the peak-calling problem. MACS slides twice of preset bandwidth windows across the genome to search the locations with very enriched signals of the Watson strand and Crick strand, where they estimate the mean distance between the summit of these two strand as d. Then the reads will be moved to the middle of these two strands by $d/2$ base pairs. They model the tag distribution along the genome by a Poisson distribution and use one parameter, λ, to capture both the mean and the variance. Then, $2d$ windows are slid across the genome to find candidate peaks. MACS uses a dynamic parameter λ_{local} defined as $\lambda_{\text{local}} = \max(\lambda_{\text{background}}, \lambda_{1k}, \lambda_{5k}, \lambda_{10k})$, where $\lambda_{1k}, \lambda_{5k}, \lambda_{10k}$ are estimated around each candidate peak region in the control data. MACS uses local to calculate the p value and smooth out the potential false positives.

Heuristic solutions like MACS are quite common and perform reasonably well for identifying regions enriched for histone modifications and DNase I hypersensitivity, but they do not make full use of the pertinent characteristics of the data. One notable feature of these assays is that the fragment size often exceeds the maximum resolution of tiling arrays or sequencing. Consequently, if signal is observed at a particular position, it is far more likely to be observed at adjacent positions, as well. Given this longitudinal nature of the data and a dependency of the signal on neighboring positions, a more sophisticated hidden Markov model could provide a much more refined solution. Furthermore, these methods produce a binary classification for a region—as either enriched or not. Due to the stochasticity inherent to enrichment assays, it would be particularly useful to have a sort of "smoothed" estimate of the true signal as an intermediate output, in addition to the simple call on enrichment. This could provide additional insights into the actual physical characteristics of the region.

Furthermore, enrichment assays produce data with features that are not entirely unique from other tailing array and sequencing platforms and as a result we imagine models could easily be modified to address other similar issues. For example, there is a similar spatial relationship in DNA methylation levels from array hybridization or sequencing of bisulfite-treated DNA as well as in copy number detection from genome sequencing. A Markov chain-based approach would also be well suited for these problems.

To address the above issues, we propose in this chapter a stochastic segmentation model and associated inference framework. The proposed model has a hierarchical hidden Markov structure that yields attractive statistical and computational properties. In particular, our model assumes a latent finite state Markov chain for categorical features of a region, and then conditional on the latent finite-state Markov chain, the true signal levels on the region follow a continuous state hidden Markov chain. As a working model, such assumptions give us more flexibility to capture the categorical and continuous features of signals with hierarchical structures simultaneously. Although these assumptions seem to lead to complicated or computationally intensive inference procedures, it turns out that the proposed model yields explicit recursive formulas for the posterior distributions of latent finite state and continuous states of Markov chains. To make implement the inference procedure more efficiently, we further develop a bounded complexity mixture (BCMIX) approximation scheme to reduce the computational complexity of the algorithm to linear order. We also develop an expectation-maximization (EM) algorithm to estimate the model hyperparameters for practical applications. The proposed model and developed inference methods are closely related to the ones in Xing et al. (2014), which characterizes the categorical and continuous features of the means and variances of observed data in the recurrent copy number alteration analysis.

The rest of the chapter is organized as follows. Section 27.2 presents the model assumptions and develops an inference procedure. It also discusses some computational issues of the model and propose a BCMIX approximation scheme and an EM estimation procedure for model hyperparameters. Section 27.3 demonstrate the performance of the model and associated inference procedure through extensive simulation studies. Section 27.4 applies our model to identify the DNase I sensitivity and DNase I hypersensitive sites (DHS) over the ENCODE regions in human lymphoblastoid cells. Section 27.5 concludes the chapter.

27.2 A Stochastic Segmentation Model

27.2.1 Model Specification

We assume the following stochastic segmentation model for observations y_t:

$$y_t = \mu_t + \sigma_t \varepsilon_t, \qquad t = 1, \ldots, n, \tag{27.1}$$

where ε_t are independent normal random variables with mean 0 and variance 1. The latent states $\theta_t := (\mu_t, \sigma_t)$ take continuous values; however, they are governed by a K-state irreducible hidden Markov chain $\{s_t\}$ with transition probability matrix $Q = (q_{ij})$ and a stationary distribution π. Note that such specification corresponds to the qualitative description of the hidden states. For example, $K = 3$ could represent the three states (major DHS, minor DHS, and insensitive) discussed in Sect. 27.4. As θ_t are continuous state variables, we assume that the dynamics of θ_t is given by

$$\theta_t = 1_{\{s_t = s_{t-1}\}} \theta_{t-1} + 1_{\{s_t \neq s_{t-1}\}} (z_t, \nu_t^2), \tag{27.2}$$

where

$$z_t | \nu_t \sim N(z^{(k)}, \nu_t^2 \kappa^{(k)}), \quad (2\nu_t^2)^{-1} \sim \text{gamma}\,(g^{(k)}, \lambda^{(k)}),$$

and $z^{(k)}, \kappa^{(k)}, \lambda^{(k)}$, and $g^{(k)}$ $(k = 1, \ldots, K)$ are hyperparameters. This indicates that if the categorical state s_t undergoes a transition, the continuous variable θ_t will jump to another level, and the new level can be sampled from a normal-inverted gamma prior distribution.

In the above specification, the existence of stationary distribution of Markov chain $\{s_t\}$ could define as a reversed chain for $\{s_t\}$. This further implies that the Markov chain $\{\theta_t\}$ has a stationary distribution. Moreover, if we assume that θ_0 is initialized at the stationary distribution, $\{\theta_t\}$ becomes a reversible Markov chain, which provides substantial simplification for computing the posterior distributions of θ_t and s_t.

27.2.2 Forward Filters

Let $J_t^{(k)} = \max\{i \leq t : s_{i-1} \neq s_i = \cdots = s_t = k\}$ be the most recent location prior or equal to t on which s_t switches to state K from another state. Denote $\xi_t^{(k)} = P(s_t = k|\mathcal{F}_t)$ and $\xi_{i,t}^{(k)} = P(J_t^{(k)} = i|\mathcal{F}_t)$ for $1 \leq i \leq t$ and $1 \leq k \leq K$, in which $\mathcal{F}_{i,j}$ and $\mathcal{F}_t$ are defined as follows: $\mathcal{F}_{i,j} := \{y_i, \ldots, y_j\}$, and $\mathcal{F}_t := \mathcal{F}_{1t}$. Then by definition, $\xi_t^{(k)} = \sum_{i=1}^t \xi_{i,t}^{(k)}$. We then note that, given $\mathcal{F}_t$ and $J_t^{(z)} = i$, the conditional distribution of θ_t is given by

$$\mu_t|(\sigma_t, \mathcal{F}_{it}) \sim N\left(z_{it}^{(s_t)}, \sigma_t^2 \kappa_{it}^{(s_t)}\right), \qquad \left(2\sigma_t^2\right)^{-1}|\mathcal{F}_{it} \sim \text{gamma}\left(g_{it}^{(k)}, \lambda_{it}^{(k)}\right). \quad (27.3)$$

in which

$$\kappa_{it}^{(k)} = \left(\frac{1}{\kappa^{(k)}} + t - i + 1\right)^{-1}, \qquad z_{it}^{(k)} = \kappa_{it}^{(k)}\left(\frac{z^{(k)}}{\kappa^{(k)}} + \sum_{j=i}^t y_j\right).$$

$$g_{it}^{(k)} = g^{(k)} + (t - i + 1)/2, \qquad \frac{1}{\lambda_{it}^{(k)}} = \frac{1}{\lambda^{(k)}} + \frac{(z^{(k)})^2}{\kappa^{(k)}} + \sum_{j=i}^t y_j^2 - \frac{(z_{it}^{(k)})^2}{\kappa_{it}^{(k)}}.$$

Based on the above conditional distribution, the posterior distribution of θ_t given $\mathcal{F}_t$ become mixtured normal-inverted gamma distributions:

$$\theta_t|\mathcal{F}_t \sim \sum_{k=1}^K \sum_{i=1}^t \xi_{i,t}^{(k)}\left[\theta_t|\mathcal{F}_{it}, J_t^{(k)} = i\right]. \quad (27.4)$$

Making use of $\sum_{k=1}^K \sum_{i=1}^t \xi_{i,t}^{(k)} = 1$, we show in appendix that the conditional probabilities $\xi_{i,t}^{(k)}$ can be determined by the following recursions:

$$\xi_{i,t}^{(k)*} := \begin{cases} \left(\sum_{l \neq k} \xi_{t-1}^{(l)} q_{lk}\right) \psi_{0,0}^{(k)} / \psi_{t,t}^{(k)} & i = t, \\ q_{kk} \xi_{i,t-1}^{(k)} \psi_{i,t-1}^{(k)} / \psi_{i,t}^{(k)} & i < t, \end{cases} \quad (27.5)$$

and the conditional probabilities $\xi_{i,t}^{(k)}$ can be computed by

$$\xi_{i,t}^{(k)} = \xi_{i,t}^{(k)*} \Bigg/ \left[\sum_{h=1}^K \sum_{j=1}^t \xi_{j,t}^{(h)*}\right],$$

in which

$$\psi_{0,0}^{(k)} = (\kappa^{(k)})^{-\frac{1}{2}} \frac{(\lambda^{(k)})^{-g^{(k)}}}{\Gamma(g^{(k)})}, \qquad \psi_{i,j}^{(k)} = \frac{1}{\sqrt{\kappa_{ij}^{(k)}}} \frac{1}{\Gamma(g_{ij}^{(k)})} \left[\lambda_{ij}^{(k)}\right]^{-g_{ij}^{(k)}}.$$

Therefore, making use of (27.4) yields:

$$P(s_t = k|\mathcal{F}_t) = \sum_{i=1}^t \xi_{i,t}^{(k)}, \qquad E(\theta_t|\mathcal{F}_t) = \sum_{k=1}^K \sum_{i=1}^t \xi_{i,t}^{(k)} E(\theta_t|\mathcal{F}_{it}). \quad (27.6)$$

27.2.3 Backward Filters

The model assumption implies that a stationary distribution of θ_t exists and can be expressed as

$$\sum_{k=1}^{K} \pi_k \text{ normal } (z^{(k)}, V^{(k)}). \tag{27.7}$$

As mentioned in Sect. 27.2.1, this allows us defining a reversed chain for θ_t, and such reversed chain has the same structure as the one in the forward filter. In particular, we define $R_t^{(k)} = \min\{j \geq t : k = s_t \cdots = s_{j-1} \neq s_j\}$ as the closest switching positions larger than or equal to t on which s_t switches from state k to another state. Let $\eta_t^{(k)} = P(s_t = k|\mathcal{F}_{t,T})$ and $\eta_{j,t}^{(k)} = P(R_t^{(k)} = j|\mathcal{F}_{t,T})$ for $t \leq j \leq T$ and $1 \leq k \leq K$. The quantity $\eta_t^{(k)}$ is the conditional probability that the current state is k given information $\mathcal{F}_{t,T}$, and $\eta_{i,t}^{(k)}$ is the conditional probability that the current state is k and the next transition occurs at location j given $\mathcal{F}_{t,T}$. Thus, $\eta_t^{(k)} = \sum_{j=t}^{T} \eta_{t,j}^{(k)}$. If we know all the information from time t to T and that the next transition occurs at location j, we only need to use the information before the change to estimate the current value of θ_t.

We then use the time-reversed chain of θ_t to obtain a backward analog of (27.4):

$$\theta_{t+1}|\mathcal{F}_{t+1,T} \sim \sum_{k=1}^{K} \sum_{j=t+1}^{T} \eta_{t+1,j}^{(k)} \left[\theta_{t+1}|\mathcal{F}_{t+1,j}\right], \tag{27.8}$$

in which the weights $\eta_{t+1,j}^{(k)}$ can be obtained by backward induction using the time-reversed counterpart of (27.5):

$$\eta_{t+1,j}^{(k)} \propto \eta_{t+1,j}^{(k)*} := \begin{cases} \left(\sum_{l\neq k} \eta_{t+2}^{(l)} \widetilde{q}_{lk}\right) \psi_{0,0}^{(k)}/\psi_{t+1,t+1}^{(k)} & j = t+1, \\ \widetilde{q}_{kk} \eta_{t+2,j}^{(k)} \psi_{t+2,j}^{(k)}/\psi_{t+1,j}^{(k)} & j > t+1, \end{cases} \tag{27.9}$$

where $\widetilde{Q} = (\widetilde{q}_{lk})$ is the transition matrix of the reversed chain of $\{s_t\}$, and $\widetilde{q}_{lk} = P(s_t = k|s_{t+1} = l)$. Since for $B \subset \mathbb{R}^d$, $P(\beta_t \in B|\mathcal{F}_{t,T}) = \int P(\beta_t \in B|\beta_{t+1}) dP(\beta_{t+1}|\mathcal{F}_{t,T})$, it follows from (27.8) that

$$\theta_t|\mathcal{F}_{t+1,T} \sim \sum_{k=1}^{K} \left\{ \widetilde{q}_{kk} \sum_{j=t+1}^{T} \eta_{t+1,j}^{(k)} \left[\theta_t|\mathcal{F}_{t+1,j}\right] + \left(\sum_{l\neq k} \widetilde{q}_{lk} \eta_{t+1}^{(l)}\right) [\theta_t|\mathcal{F}_0] \right\}. \tag{27.10}$$

27.2.4 Smoothing Estimates of Hidden States

We now use Bayes' theorem to combine the forward filter (27.4) with its backward variant (27.10) to estimate θ_t and s_t given $\mathcal{F}_T$. Note that the posterior distribution of

θ_t given $\mathcal{F}_T$ can also be expressed as the following mixture:

$$\theta_t|\mathcal{F}_T \sim \sum_{k=1}^{K} \sum_{1\leq i\leq t\leq j\leq T} \alpha_{ij,t}^{(k)} \left[\theta_t|\mathcal{F}_{i,j}\right], \tag{27.11}$$

in which the mixture weights $\alpha_{ij,t}^{(k)}$ are posterior probabilities explained below. Consider the event

$$C_{ij}^{(k)} = \{s_i = \cdots = s_j = k, s_i \neq s_{i-1}, s_j \neq s_{j-1}\},$$

i.e., $C_{ij}^{(k)}$ represents the event that the categorical state s_t is k from location $t = i$ to $t = j$, but not before or afterward. We can see that, for $i \leq t \leq j$, $\alpha_{ijt}^{(k)} = P(C_{ij}^{(k)}|\mathcal{F}_n)$. We then show in Appendix that $\alpha_{ij,t}^{(k)}$ can be calculated recursively as follows:

$$\alpha_{ijt}^{(k)} = \alpha_{ijt}^{(k)*}/D_t, \qquad D_t = \sum_{k=1}^{K} \sum_{1\leq i\leq t\leq j\leq T} \alpha_{ijt}^{(k)*},$$

$$\alpha_{ijt}^{(k)*} = \begin{cases} \xi_{i,t}^{(k)} \left(\sum_{l\neq k} \eta_{t+1}^{(l)} q_{kl}/\pi_l\right) & i \leq t = j, \\ q_{kk}\xi_{i,t}^{(k)} \eta_{t+1,j}^{(k)} \psi_{i,t}^{(k)} \psi_{t+1,j}^{(k)} / (\pi_k \psi_{i,j}^{(k)} \psi_{0,0}^{(k)}) & i \leq t < j. \end{cases} \tag{27.12}$$

Therefore, the smoothing estimates of θ_t and s_t given $\mathcal{F}_T$ are given by

$$E(\mu_t|\mathcal{F}_T) = \sum_{k=1}^{K} \sum_{1\leq i\leq t\leq j\leq T} \alpha_{ijt}^{(k)} z_{i,j}^{(k)}, \tag{27.13}$$

$$E(\sigma_t^2|\mathcal{F}_T) = \sum_{k=1}^{K} \sum_{1\leq i\leq t\leq j\leq T} \frac{1}{2}(g_{ij}^k - 1)^{-1}(\lambda_{ij}^k)^{-1}, \tag{27.14}$$

$$P(s_t = k|\mathcal{F}_T) = \sum_{1\leq i\leq t\leq j\leq T} \alpha_{ijt}^{(k)}. \tag{27.15}$$

27.2.5 *BCMIX Approximation*

Although the Bayes filter (27.4) uses a recursive updating formula (27.5) for the weights $\xi_{i,t}^{(k)}$ $(1 \leq i \leq t, 1 \leq k \leq K)$, the number of weights increases dramatically with t, resulting in rapidly increasing computational complexity and memory requirements in estimating θ_t as t keeps increasing. To address the issue of computational efficiency, we follow (Xing et al. 2006) and consider a *BCMIX* approximation procedure with much lower computational complexity yet comparable to the Bayes estimates in statistical efficiency. The idea of BCMIX approximation is to keep only a fixed number M of weights at every stage t, in particular, the most recent m $(1 \leq m < M)$ weights $\xi_{i,t}^{(k)}$ (with $t - m < i \leq t$) and the largest $M - m$ of the remaining weights.

Denote $\mathcal{K}_{t-1}^{(k)}$ the set of induces i for which $\xi_{i,t-1}^{(k)}$ in (27.5) is kept at stage $t-1$ for regime k. Note that there are at most M induces in $\mathcal{K}_{t-1}^{(k)}$ and $\mathcal{K}_{t-1}^{(k)} \supset \{t-1, \cdots, t-m\}$. When a new observation arrives at time t, we still define $\xi_{i,t}^{(k)*}$ by (27.5) for $i \in \{t\} \cup \mathcal{K}_{t-1}^{(k)}$ and denote i_t the index not belonging to the most recent m stages, $\{t, t-1, \ldots, t-m+1\}$, such that

$$\xi_{i_t,t}^{(k)*} = \min\{\xi_{i,t}^{(k)*} : i \in \mathcal{K}_{t-1}^{(k)} \quad \text{and} \quad i \leq t - m\}, \tag{27.16}$$

choosing $i_t^{(k)}$ to be the one farthest from t if the minimizing set in (27.16) has more than one element. Define $\mathcal{K}_t^{(k)} = \{t\} \cup (\mathcal{K}_{t-1}^{(k)} - \{i_t^{(k)}\})$, and then

$$\xi_{i,t}^{(k)} = \left(\xi_{i,t}^{(k)*} \Big/ \sum_{j \in \mathcal{K}_t^{(k)}} \xi_{j,t}^{(k)*} \right), \qquad i \in \mathcal{K}_t^{(k)}, \tag{27.17}$$

yields a BCMIX approximation to the forward filter.

Similarly, to obtain a BCMIX approximation to the backward filter (27.9), let $\widetilde{\mathcal{K}}_{t+1}^{(k)}$ denote the set of indices j for which $\eta_{j,t+1}^{(k)}$ in (27.9) is kept at stage $t+1$ for regime k; thus, $\widetilde{\mathcal{K}}_{t+1}^{(k)} \supset \{t+1, \cdots, t+m\}$. At time t, define $\eta_{j,t}^{(k)}$ by (27.9) for $j \in \{t\} \cup \mathcal{K}_{t+1}^{(k)}$ and let j_t be the index not belonging to the most recent m stages, $\{t, t+1, \cdots, t+m-1\}$ such that

$$\eta_{j_t,t}^{(k)*} = \min\{\eta_{j,t}^{(k)*} : j \in \widetilde{\mathcal{K}}_{t+1}^{(k)} \quad \text{and} \quad j \geq t + m\}, \tag{27.18}$$

choosing $j_t^{(k)}$ to be the one farthest from t if the minimizing set in (27.18) has more than one element. Define $\widetilde{\mathcal{K}}_t^{(k)} = \{t\} \cup (\mathcal{K}_{t+1}^{(k)} - \{i_t^{(k)}\})$, and then

$$\eta_{j,t}^{(k)} = \left(\eta_{j,t}^{(k)*} \Big/ \sum_{j \in \widetilde{\mathcal{K}}_t^{(k)}} \eta_{j,t}^{(k)*} \right), \qquad j \in \widetilde{\mathcal{K}}_t^{(k)}, \tag{27.19}$$

yields a BCMIX approximation to the backward filter.

For the smoothing estimate $E(\theta_t|\mathcal{F}_T)$ and its associated posterior distribution, we construct BCMIX approximations by combining the preceding forward and backward BCMIX filters with index sets $\mathcal{K}_t^{(k)}$ and $\widetilde{\mathcal{K}}_{t+1}^{(k)}$, respectively, at time t. Then the BCMIX approximations to (27.12) are given as

$$\widetilde{\alpha}_{ijt} = \alpha_{ijt}^* / \widetilde{D}_t, \qquad \widetilde{D}_t = \sum_{i \in \mathcal{K}_t^{(k)}, j \in \{t\} \cup \widetilde{\mathcal{K}}_{t+1}^{(k)}} \alpha_{ijt}^*,$$

$$\alpha_{ijt}^{(k)*} = \begin{cases} \xi_{i,t}^{(k)} \left(\sum_{l \neq k} \eta_{t+1}^{(l)} q_{kl} / \pi_l \right) & i \in \mathcal{K}_t^{(k)}, \\ q_{kk} \xi_{i,t}^{(k)} \eta_{t+1,j}^{(k)} \psi_{i,t}^{(k)} \psi_{t+1,j}^{(k)} / (\pi_k \psi_{i,j}^{(k)} \psi_{0,0}^{(k)}) & i \in \mathcal{K}_t^{(k)}, j \in \{t\} \cup \widetilde{\mathcal{K}}_{t+1}^{(k)}. \end{cases}$$

Therefore, the BCMIX smoother for θ_t and s_t given $\mathcal{F}_T$ are expressed as

$$E(\theta_t|\mathcal{F}_T) \approx \sum_{k=1}^{K} \sum_{i \in \mathcal{K}_t^{(k)}, j \in \{t\} \cup \widetilde{\mathcal{K}}_{t+1}^{(k)}} \widetilde{\alpha}_{ijt}^{(k)} \left[\theta_t | \mathcal{F}_{ij}\right], \tag{27.20}$$

$$P(s_t = k|\mathcal{F}_T) \approx \sum_{k=1}^{K} \sum_{i \in \mathcal{K}_t^{(k)}, j \in \{t\} \cup \widetilde{\mathcal{K}}_{t+1}^{(k)}} \widetilde{\alpha}_{ijt}^{(k)}. \tag{27.21}$$

The BCMIX approximation fixes the number of filters as M at each time, and keeps the m closest weights and the other $M - m$ largest weights. This reduces the computational complexity, $O(T^2)$ of the filter in Sects. 27.2.1 and 27.2.2 and $O(T^3)$ of the smoother in Sect. 27.2.3, to $O(T)$. The specification of M and m are discussed in Sect. 27.3.

27.3 Simulation Studies

In this section, we access the performance of the proposed inference procedure via extensive simulation studies. Since our estimates deal with means and variables of continuous state variables and finite state variables, we use the following three measures to access the performance. We define the mean squared error (MSE) between true and estimated means:

$$\text{SSE} = \frac{1}{T}\sum_{t=1}^{T} (\mu_t - \widehat{\mu}_t)^2.$$

To measure the divergence between the true and estimated (μ_t, σ_t), we consider the Kullback–Leibler (KL) divergence:

$$2\text{KL}(\theta_t, \widehat{\theta}_t) = \frac{(\mu_t - \widehat{\mu}_t)^2}{\widehat{\sigma}_t^2} + \frac{\sigma_t^2}{\widehat{\sigma}_t^2} - 1 - \log\left(\frac{\sigma_t^2}{\widehat{\sigma}_t^2}\right).$$

We use κ to represent the average of KL for the whole sample

$$\kappa := \frac{2}{T}\sum_{t=1}^{T} \text{KL}(\theta_t, \widehat{\theta}_t).$$

To evaluate the estimates $\widehat{r}_{t|T}^{(k)} = P(s_t = k|\mathcal{F}_t)$ for s_t, we first estimate s_t by k such that the computed probability $\widehat{r}_{t|T}^{(k)}$ for k is larger than 0.5. We then define the identification ratio (IR) as

$$\text{IR} := \frac{1}{T}\sum_{t=1}^{T}\sum_{k=1}^{K} \mathbf{1}_{(\widehat{r}_{t|T}^{(k)} > 0.5) \cap (s_t = k)},$$

27.3.1 Comparison of Bayes and BCMIX Estimates in Frequentist Setting

We first evaluate the performance of Bayes and BCMIX estimates and see if the BCMIX approximation is close enough to Bayes estimates. We consider four cases of the hidden state $\{s_t\}$ with $K = 2$ and $T = 1000$.

Case 1. $s_t = 1 \cdot 1_{\{1 \le t \le 200\}} + 2 \cdot 1_{\{201 \le t \le 1000\}}$.
Case 2. $s_t = 1 \cdot 1_{\{1 \le t \le 800\}} + 2 \cdot 1_{\{801 \le t \le 1000\}}$.
Case 3. $s_t = 1 \cdot 1_{\{1 \le t \le 350, 701 \le t \le 1000\}} + 2 \cdot 1_{\{351 \le t \le 700\}}$.
Case 4. $s_t = 1 \cdot 1_{\{1 \le t \le 200, 401 \le t \le 600\}} + 2 \cdot 1_{\{201 \le t \le 400, 601 \le t \le 1000\}}$.

Given $\{s_t\}$, the signals θ_t are generated by (27.2) with following hyperparameters, $z^{(1)} = 2.0, \kappa^{(1)} = 0.8, \lambda^{(1)} = 0.8, g^{(1)} = 2.5$; $z^{(2)} = 4.0, \kappa^{(2)} = 1.0, \lambda^{(2)} = 0.5, g^{(2)} = 1.8$ and transition probability matrix Q such that $q_{11} = 0.99$, $q_{22} = 0.9$.

We then compute the Bayes and BCMIX estimates using the procedure in Sect. 27.3. For BCMIX estimates, we consider four settings of (M, m), which includes $(10, 5), (20, 10), (30, 15)$, and $(40, 20)$. To evaluate the performance of our estimates, we also consider an oracle estimate that assumes the hidden state of each position is known, so that the Bayes estimates of θ_t between two transitions can be computed via standard Bayes formulas (Sect. 2.7 of Box and Tiao 1973). We then run such simulation 500 times for each case, and summarize the results in Table 27.1 (the standard errors are given in parentheses).

We find that, in terms of the estimates of μ_t, the oracle estimate has the smallest MSE while the performance of BCMIX estimates are comparable to the Bayes estimates. The relative differences between the BCMIX(10,5) and oracle estimates is less than 2 % in all cases, suggesting the BCMIX estimate is also comparable to the oracle estimate. In terms of the estimated μ_t and σ_t, the KL divergence in Table 27.1 has the similar pattern to the MSE measure in all cases. For categorical states s_t, the IRs of Bayes and BCMIX estimates in Table 27.1 are very high, and the BCMIX estimates performs even slighly better than the Bayes estimates. Actually, the standard errors of the IRs estimated by BCMIX methods are smaller than that of Bayes methods, indicating that BCMIX has less variations or better stability. We further notice that the difference of MSE among four settings of (M, m) in BCMIX estimates is very small, so we focus on the performance of BCMIX estimates in the sequel for $(M, m) = (20, 10)$.

27.3.2 Performance of BCMIX Estimates Under Model Assumptions

We then evaluate the performance of the BCMIX estimate when s_t is indeed a hidden Markov chain. In this study, we only consider the BCMIX estimate with $(M, m) = (20, 10)$ for different types of transition probabilities. Specifically, we assume $K = 2$,

Table 27.1 Performance of the oracle, Bayes and BCMIX estimates

				BCMIX(M, m)			
	Case	Oracle	Bayes	(10, 5)	(20, 10)	(30, 15)	(40, 20)
MSE	*1*	0.0023 (1.3e-4)	0.0031 (1.6e-4)	0.0025 (1.6e-4)	0.0025 (1.6e-4)	0.0025 (1.6e-4)	0.0025 (1.6e-4)
	2	0.0024 (1.3e-4)	0.0031 (1.5e-4)	0.0024 (1.4e-4)	0.0024 (1.4e-4)	0.0025 (1.4e-4)	0.0025 (1.4e-4)
	3	0.0027 (1.3e-4)	0.0035 (1.7e-4)	0.0030 (1.6e-4)	0.0030 (1.6e-4)	0.0030 (1.6e-4)	0.0030 (1.6e-4)
	4	0.0027 (1.3e-4)	0.0051 (2.3e-4)	0.0045 (2.2e-4)	0.0045 (2.2e-4)	0.0045 (2.2e-4)	0.0045 (2.2e-4)
$10^3\kappa$	*1*	3.973 (1.2e-4)	5.461 (2.1e-4)	4.269 (2.0e-4)	4.268 (2.0e-4)	4.268 (2.0e-4)	4.268 (2.0e-4)
	2	4.027 (1.3e-4)	5.394 (1.8e-4)	4.200 (1.7e-4)	4.199 (1.7e-4)	4.198 (1.7e-4)	4.198 (1.7e-4)
	3	5.882 (1.4e-4)	7.434 (2.8e-4)	6.245 (2.8e-4)	6.244 (2.8e-4)	6.244 (2.8e-4)	6.242 (2.8e-4)
	4	7.883 (1.4e-4)	9.557 (2.8e-4)	8.365 (2.7e-4)	8.365 (2.7e-4)	8.364 (2.7e-4)	8.362 (2.7e-4)
IR×100 %	*1*		99.9892 (2.0e-5)	99.9992 (4.0e-6)	99.9992 (4.0e-6)	99.9992 (4.0e-6)	99.9992 (4.0e-6)
	2		99.9898 (1.9e-5)	99.9994 (4.5e-6)	99.9994 (4.5e-6)	99.9994 (4.5e-6)	99.9994 (4.5e-6)
	3		99.9894 (2.0e-5)	99.9999 (4.5e-6)	99.9999 (4.5e-6)	99.9999 (4.5e-6)	99.9999 (4.5e-6)
	4		99.9884 (2.1e-5)	99.9984 (5.6e-6)	99.9984 (5.6e-6)	99.9984 (5.6e-6)	99.9984 (5.6e-6)

BCMIX bounded complexity mixture, *IR* identification ratio, *MSE* mean squared error

$z^{(1)} = 2.0, \kappa^{(1)} = 0.8, \lambda^{(1)} = 0.8, g^{(1)} = 2.5, z^{(2)} = 4.0, \kappa^{(2)} = 1.0, \lambda^{(2)} = 0.5,$ $g^{(2)} = 1.8$. The 2×2 transition matrix Q has the following nine scenarios:

Scenario S1. $(q_{11}, q_{22}) = (0.001, 0.001)$.
Scenario S2. $(q_{11}, q_{22}) = (0.002, 0.001)$.
Scenario S3. $(q_{11}, q_{22}) = (0.002, 0.002)$.
Scenario S4. $(q_{11}, q_{22}) = (0.004, 0.001)$.
Scenario S5. $(q_{11}, q_{22}) = (0.004, 0.002)$.
Scenario S6. $(q_{11}, q_{22}) = (0.008, 0.004)$.
Scenario S7. $(q_{11}, q_{22}) = (0.008, 0.008)$.
Scenario S8. $(q_{11}, q_{22}) = (0.016, 0.008)$.
Scenario S9. $(q_{11}, q_{22}) = (0.016, 0.016)$.

For each scenarios, we first simulate observations $\{y_t\}$ based on our model assumption for $T = 3000, 4000, 5000, 6000$, and 7000, then use the EM algorithm to estimate the hyperparameters, and compute the BCMIX (20, 10) estimates. We then run 500

Table 27.2 Performance of BCMIX(20, 10) estimate under model assumption

	T	S1	S2	S3	S4	S5	S6	S7	S8	S9
MSE	3000	1.79e-3 (7.1e-5)	2.23e-3 (9.1e-5)	2.63e-3 (9.9e-5)	2.42e-3 (9.5e-5)	3.01e-3 (1.1e-4)	4.10e-3 (1.4e-4)	4.78e-3 (1.5e-4)	5.21e-3 (1.6e-4)	5.67e-3 (1.7e-4)
	4000	1.67e-3 (6.6e-5)	2.12e-3 (7.6e-5)	2.55e-3 (8.4e-5)	2.30e-3 (7.9e-5)	2.89e-3 (9.2e-5)	3.96e-3 (1.2e-4)	4.60e-3 (1.3e-4)	4.90e-3 (1.4e-4)	5.19e03 (1.4e-4)
	5000	1.60e-3 (5.9e-5)	1.95e-3 (6.5e-5)	1.44e-3 (5.3e-5)	2.17e-3 (7.0e-5)	2.86e-3 (8.8e-5)	3.87e-3 (1.1e-4)	4.54e-3 (1.3e-4)	4.83e-3 (1.4e-4)	5.18e-3 (1.5e-4)
	6000	1.66e-3 (6.5e-5)	1.98e-3 (7.0e-5)	2.40e-3 (7.9e-5)	2.22e-3 (8.0e-5)	2.72e-3 (8.4e-5)	3.76e-3 (1.2e-4)	4.28e-3 (1.3e-4)	4.57e-3 (1.3e-4)	4.96e-3 (1.5e-4)
	7000	1.50e-3 (5.3e-5)	1.79e-3 (6.3e-5)	2.20e-3 (7.0e-5)	2.02e-3 (6.9e-5)	2.62e-3 (8.6e-5)	3.55e-3 (1.1e-4)	4.03e-3 (1.3e-4)	4.31e-3 (1.3e-4)	4.76e-3 (1.6e-4)
$10^3\kappa$	3000	3.829 (1.5e-4)	4.517 (1.6e-4)	5.555 (1.8e-4)	4.890 (1.7e-4)	6.434 (1.9e-4)	8.810 (2.1e-4)	10.246 (2.1e-4)	11.122 (2.2e-4)	12.439 (2.5e-4)
	4000	3.541 (1.2e-4)	4.377 (1.4e-4)	5.459 (1.5e-4)	4.973 (1.6e-4)	6.344 (1.7e-4)	8.772 (1.9e-4)	10.324 (2.2e-4)	11.297 (2.5e-4)	12.144 (2.2e-4)
	5000	3.372 (1.1e-4)	4.138 (1.2e-4)	4.358 (7.8e-5)	4.715 (1.3e-4)	6.323 (1.6e-4)	8.728 (1.6e-4)	10.333 (1.8e-4)	11.309 (1.9e-4)	12.217 (2.1e-4)
	6000	3.441 (1.1e-4)	4.177 (1.2e-4)	5.161 (1.2e-5)	4.668 (1.2e-4)	6.043 (1.3e-4)	8.645 (1.6e-4)	9.979 (1.7e-4)	10.848 (1.7e-4)	12.005 (1.8e-4)
	7000	3.191 (8.9e-5)	3.817 (9.6e-5)	4.813 (9.8e-5)	4.346 (9.9e-5)	5.727 (1.1e-4)	8.239 (1.4e-4)	9.708 (1.6e-4)	10.551 (1.7e-4)	11.859 (1.8e-4)

Table 27.2 (continued)

	T	S1	S2	S3	S4	S5	S6	S7	S8	S9
IR×100%	3000	0.932 (9.0e-3)	0.932 (7.0e-3)	0.944 (6.5e-3)	0.961 (5.2e-3)	0.976 (3.6e-3)	0.984 (3.2e-3)	0.983 (3.5e-3)	0.986 (2.8e-3)	0.987 (2.9e-3)
	4000	0.932 (7.8e-3)	0.949 (5.5e-3)	0.955 (5.5e-3)	0.970 (3.7e-3)	0.977 (3.8e-3)	0.987 (2.6e-3)	0.986 (2.9e-3)	0.989 (2.3e-3)	0.989 (2.4e-3)
	5000	0.932 (7.8e-3)	0.937 (6.0e-3)	0.959 (5.8e-3)	0.962 (3.7e-3)	0.980 (3.2e-3)	0.990 (2.1e-3)	0.991 (2.0e-3)	0.995 (1.3e-3)	0.993 (1.7e-3)
	6000	0.933 (7.6e-3)	0.940 (5.5e-3)	0.961 (5.0e-3)	0.962 (4.4e-3)	0.982 (3.4e-3)	0.991 (1.9e-3)	0.991 (1.8e-3)	0.994 (1.4e-3)	0.993 (1.5e-3)
	7000	0.935 (7.2e-3)	0.953 (4.9e-3)	0.962 (4.5e-3)	0.966 (4.0e-3)	0.983 (3.0e-3)	0.991 (2.0e-3)	0.992 (2.0e-3)	0.993 (1.5e-3)	0.994 (1.3e-3)

BCMIX bounded complexity mixture, *IR* identification ratio, *MSE* mean squared error simulation for each specific setting. Table 27.2 summarizes the simulation result, and also provided the corresponding standard errors based on 500 simulations in parentheses of each cell. We can see that the MSE is very small and keeps almost constant when T increases. κ has a tendency of decreasing when T increases. When T changes from 3000 to 4000, there is a significant decrease in κ. Furthermore, the IRs in all scenarios are larger than 95 %. The above observations suggest the BCMIX estimates show good performance in identifying the hidden categorical states s_t and continuous states θ_t.

27.4 A Real Data Analysis

We applied the stochastic segmentation model to a real dataset: Nimblegen ENCODE Arrays for identifying DNase I sensitivity and *DHS* over the ENCODE regions in human lymphoblastoid cells (GSE4334). We display some characteristic results of our model such as posterior means, variance, and state probabilities. Genome browser screenshots are also used to demonstrate the biological relevance of the results.

This data were published on July 27, 2006, with the series number GSE4334 in the Gene Expression Omnibus (GEO) database. The goal of this study was to map DNase I sensitive and DHS over the covered ENCODE regions in human lymphoblastoid cells (GM06990, Coriell). The assay protocol used by (Sabo et al. 2006) is a "quantitative chromatin profiling" method previously introduced by (Dorschner et al. 2004). In brief, intact nuclei were first isolated and divided into two fractions, one treated with DNase I, another which was not. In a departure from the (Dorschner et al. 2004) method that utilized a single enzymatic cut, (Sabo et al. 2006) further size-selected for small fragments by cutting a second time with DNase I in close proximity. Then, using a custom-designed Nimblegen array which employed around 39,000 50-mer probes tiled with 12-mer overlaps and falling within 44 genomic ENCODE segments, signal-to-noise ratios were calculated from the observed intensities at each probe position by comparing DNase-I-treated versus untreated samples. It was these signal-to-noise ratios that served as the input for our algorithm.

Since the study involves three states (major DHS, minor DHS, and insensitive sites), we label those states as state 1, 2, and 3, respectively, in the model and perform the analysis for each of 23 chromosomes. Due to the page limit, we only show numerical results of six randomly selected chromosomes (chromosomes 1, 5, 7, 8, 9, and 12) and provide graphical interpretation for two chromosomes (chromosomes 1 and 6). In particular, for each chromosome, we first use the EM algorithm to estimate the hyperparameters of the model. Tables 27.3 and 27.4 show the estimated parameters in hyper priors and transition probabilties of the model for each chromosome. We can see that the patterns of estimated transition probabilities for each chromosome are quite similar. We then use the estimated parameters to compute the postier distribution of continuous and categorical states via BCMIX(20, 10) algorithm. Table 27.5 summarizes some relevant statistics of the results. For example, major and minor hypersensitive sites comprise only a small fraction of the genome

Table 27.3 Estimated parameters in hyperpriors of the model for six chromosomes

	Chr 1	Chr 5	Chr 7	Chr 8	Chr 9	Chr 12
z_1	1.6287	1.4385	1.3999	1.3320	1.6070	1.4157
z_2	0.3614	0.3387	0.3102	0.2784	0.2162	0.3038
z_3	−0.0166	−0.0339	−0.0238	−0.0442	−0.0174	−0.0204
κ_1	0.9716	1.4020	1.4041	1.0464	0.9235	1.2234
κ_2	2.0104	2.0329	2.1900	2.5055	2.4176	2.2494
κ_3	1.3335	1.0567	1.0551	0.8612	1.2474	1.0216
λ_1	1.3860	1.4965	1.7600	1.9908	1.2697	1.8861
λ_2	4.4515	4.5131	5.2046	5.3476	4.3205	5.3941
λ_3	10.2532	7.9558	8.5532	8.1350	8.2500	8.6679

Table 27.4 Estimated transition probabilities for six chromosomes

		Major DHS (State 1)	Minor DHS (State 2)	Insensitive (State 3)		Major DHS (State 1)	Minor DHS (State 2)	Insensitive (State 3)
Chr1	State 1	0.8637	0.1001	0.0362	Chr5	0.8104	0.1430	0.0466
	State 2	0.0325	0.7985	0.1690		0.0234	0.8118	0.1648
	State 3	0.0048	0.0250	0.9702		0.0025	0.0214	0.9761
Chr7	State 1	0.8162	0.1293	0.0545	Chr8	0.8272	0.1200	0.0528
	State 2	0.0162	0.8220	0.1618		0.0108	0.8025	0.1867
	State 3	0.0020	0.0203	0.9777		0.0017	0.0128	0.9855
Chr9	State 1	0.8253	0.1133	0.0614	Chr12	0.8170	0.1215	0.0615
	State 2	0.0128	0.7741	0.2131		0.0204	0.8343	0.1453
	State 3	0.0021	0.0313	0.9666		0.0020	0.0173	0.9807

DHS DNase I hypersensitive sites

Table 27.5 Base level coverage and segment lengths for three states

	Major DHS (State 1)	Minor DHS (State 2)	Insensitive (State 3)
Number of segments	815	5127	31,104
Number of bases	234 kb	802 kb	13,325 kb
Percent of bases	1.60 %	5.60 %	92.80 %
Mean of segment length	287	156	428

DHS DNase I hypersensitive sites

(7.2 %) as compared to insensitive regions (92.8 %). This suggests that the majority of the genome exists in a more compact, less accessible state and only a fraction is openly accessible, a state more amenable to regulation or transcription, at any given moment.

We then chose chromosomes 1 and 6 to visualize the posterior means, variance and state probabilities that are estimated by our model. Figure 27.1 displays the observed

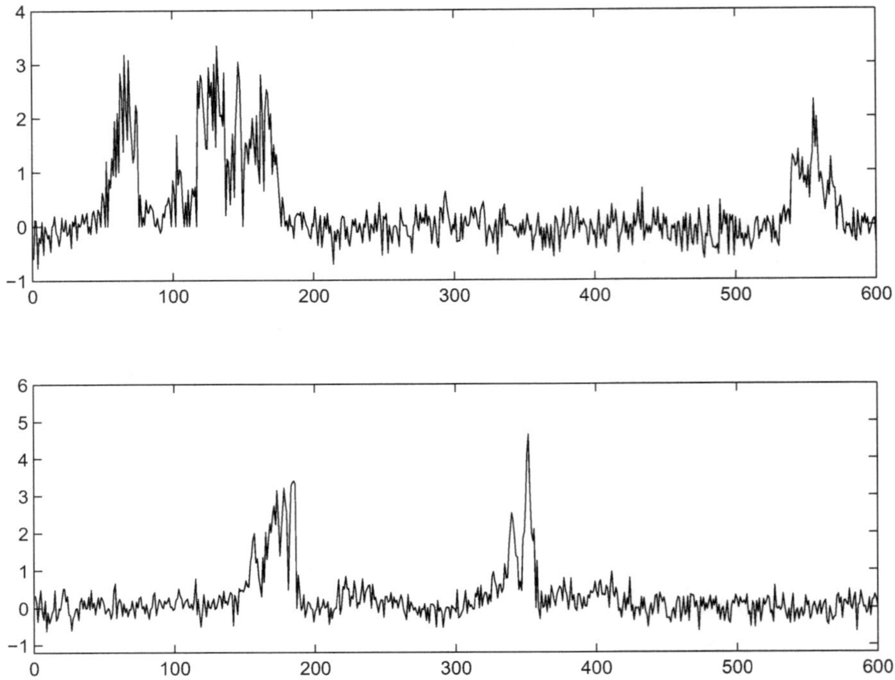

Fig. 27.1 The observation of 600 probes in chromosomes 1 (*upper panel*) and 6 (*lower panel*)

signal-to-noise ratios across the first 600 probes on chromosome 1 which cover 55024 basepairs (chr1:148374643-148429666) and another 600 probes on chromosome 6 which cover 37164 basepairs (chr6:41537432-41574595). The presence of clear peaks on both chromosomes demarcate the regions of increased coverage due to DNase I hypersensitivity that we are trying to capture. We then show the posterior estimates of chromosomes 1 and 6 in Figs. 27.2 and 27.3, respectively. These two figures demonstrate that our model performs well at smoothing the highly variable signals and generates reasonable state calls. Based on estimated state probabilities, we can identify the categorical states by using a threshold line of 0.5, as the way suggested in the beginning of Sect. 27.3. Shown in Fig. 27.4 is a genome browser screenshot for the series from chromosome 1, in which some of the major and minor hypersensitive sites called by our model are annotated. Notably, there is a distinct hypersensitive region in the upstream promoter of *PLEKH01* gene and extending across its transcription start site (TSS) into its gene body. This is consistent with the expectation for highly accessible chromatin, which would be extremely susceptible to DNase I, within cis-regulatory regions that are commonly associated with gene promoters and enhancers.

To assess DNase I hypersensitive (DHS) island accuracy, we operated on the assumption that high signal-to-noise ratios falling within DHS islands would be

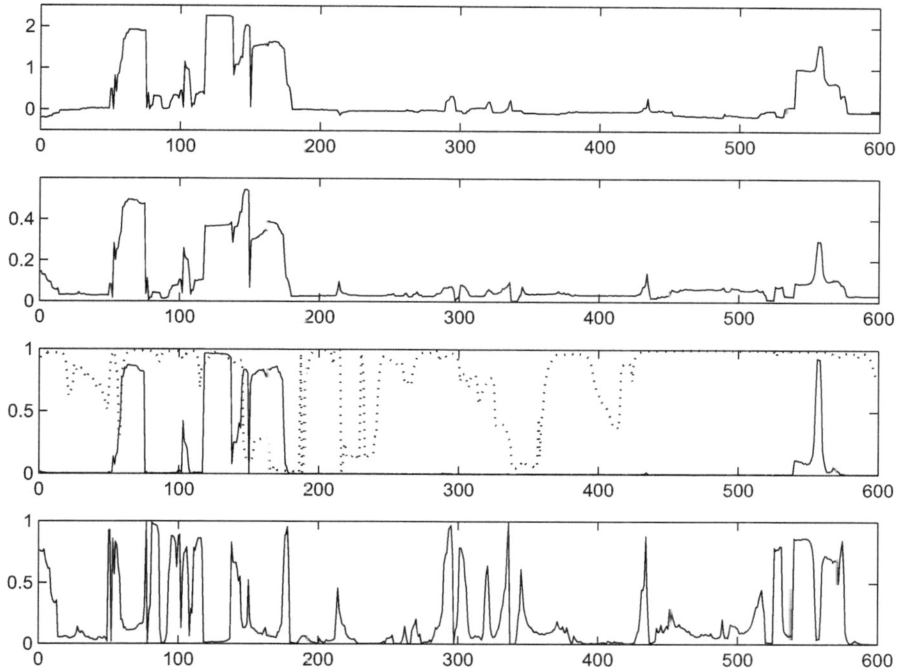

Fig. 27.2 The posterior estimation of mean (the *first panel*), variance (the *second panel*) and state probabilities (*bottom two panels*) for chromosome 1

enriched and flanked by significantly reduced ratios outside of the island boundaries thereby forming a plateau-shaped profile. Given this, we examined the profiles of our call and the DHS island calls in Sabo et al. (2006), including flanking regions up- and downstream half the island length. We divided the islands, plus flanks, into 100 equal-sized bins and calculated average read densities within each bin. Our method showed a much more pronounced plateau (Figure 27.5), which implies our DHS islands more accurately defined island boundaries dividing regions of higher and lower DNase I accessibility.

As mentioned, common wisdom suggests that functionally relevant regions of DNA are more susceptible to enzymatic digestion by DNase treatment due to increased accessibility at cis-regulatory elements. We assessed the degree of enrichment of our DHS islands within regions of known functional importance, including CpG islands, known genes, mRNA transcripts, spliced expressed sequence tags (ESTs), and regions enriched for histone modification marks. We adopted the same enrichment calculation as Lian et al. (2008). Compared to the DHS called by Sabo et al. (2006), our results exhibit better enrichment at major DHS and similar enrichment on the union of major and minor DHS (Fig. 27.6). The method of calculation of enrichment is same as in Lian et al. (2008). These results suggest our model is capable of more accurately capturing regions hypersensitive for DNase I cleavage.

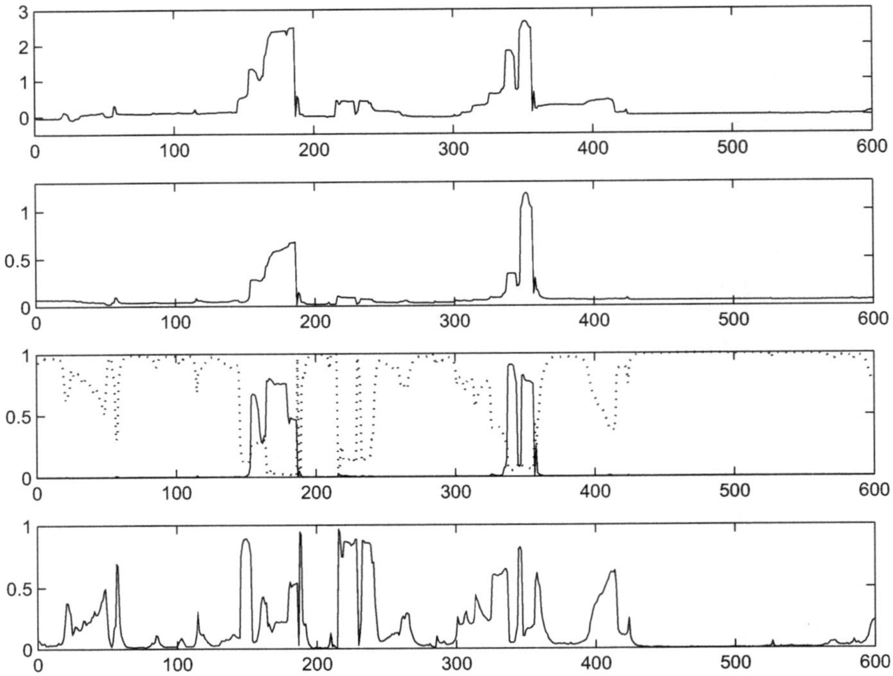

Fig. 27.3 The posterior estimation of mean (the *first panel*), variance (the *second panel*) and state probabilities (*bottom two panels*) for chromosome 6

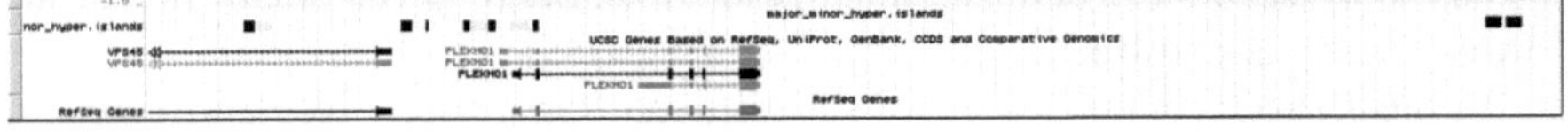

Fig. 27.4 A screenshot corresponding to the selected series of chromosome 1 from UCSC genome browser. *UCSC* University of California Santa Cruz

The boundaries of such regions are more clearly and accurately defined which minimizes the amount of false positive signal and search space propagated to downstream analysis. For example, one consequence of accurately identifying DHS is the identification of more concise regions of possible transcription factor binding. Therefore, analysis for enrichment of motif recognition sites within these DHS regions would

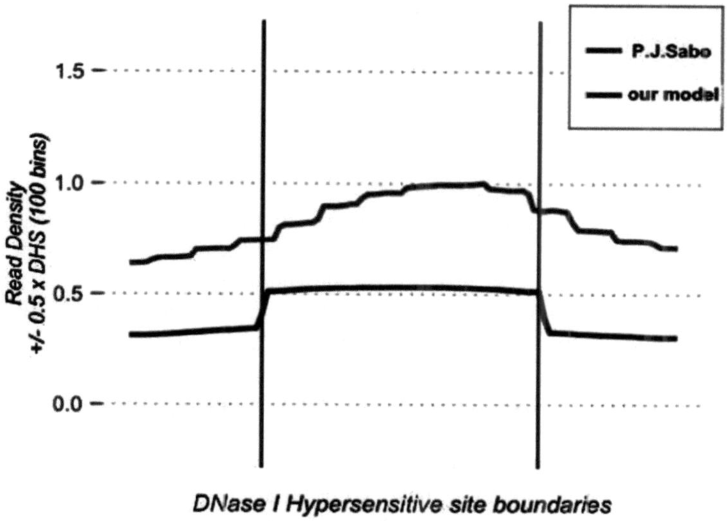

Fig. 27.5 The assessment of DHS island accuracy. *DHS* DNase I hypersensitive sites

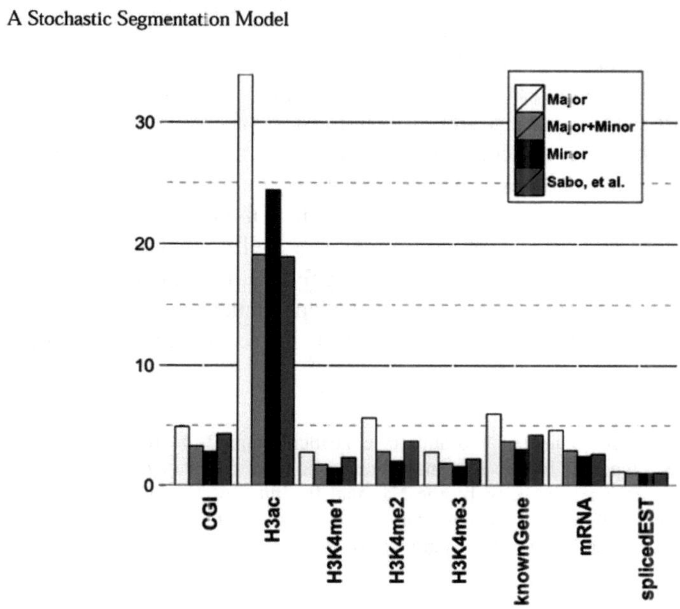

Fig. 27.6 Enrichment of annctation functional elements

be simplified. All in all, our model provides a sound statistical basis for improved analysis of enrichment assays like DNase I hypersensitivity.

27.5 Conclusion

We have developed a stochastic segmentation model and an associated inference framework to identify DNase I sensitivity and DHS over the ENCODE regions in human lymphoblastoid cells. The proposed model yields explicit recursive formulas for posterior distributions of both categorical and continuous states. To reduce the computational comlexity to linear order, an approximation to the exact explicit formulas is also developed. These make the model more attractive statistically and computationally. To estimate the hyperparameters for the practical purpose, an explicit EM algorithm is also developed and described in the appendix.

As demonstrated by application to the Nimblegen ENCODE Array dataset, our model makes important advances to existing heuristic algorithms used to identify regions of DNase I hypersensitivity. The explicitly determined posterior means of signal-to-noise ratios can be viewed as a more representative smoothed estimate of the true underlying signal and should more accurately pinpoint regions of increased DNA accessbility. This estimate leverages the known correlation of nearby genomic positions through a Markov chain, thus providing a sound statistical underpinning. As has been pointed out previously, our model is able to more accurately identify regions hypersensitive to DNase I digestion at higher resolution, with segmentation points more clearly distinguishing enriched and unenriched genomic regions. This type of sequential data structure is actually quite common in genomics research. Many other assays share a similar relationship where local genomic regions are expected to have highly correlated signals. Two immediately obvious data types, DNA methylation and copy number variation, are areas of intense research and it is clear that the principles of the model we describe here can easily be modified to address the peculiarities of these problems as well. Notably, methods in common usage for analyzing these datasets are largely heuristic or make use of finite state Hidden Markov models with significant dependency on simulations. As was the case with DNase I hypersensitivity detection, we see notable room for improvement through implementation of our work.

Acknowledgement The first two authors contributed equally to the chapter. Haipeng Xing's research was supported by the National Science Foundation grant DMS-1206321. Michael Q. Zhang's research was supported by the National Institutes of Health grant HG001696 and ES-17166, the National Basic Research Program of China grant 2012CB316503, and the National Natural Science Foundation of China grant 91019016.

Appendix A. Proof of 27.5 and 27.12

Proof of 27.5: To derive the mixture weight $\xi_{i,t}^{(k)}$, we first note that

$$f(\theta_t, y_t, s_{t-1} = k|\mathcal{F}_{t-1}) = \sum_{l=1}^{K} f(\theta_t, y_t, s_{t-1} = k, s_t = l|\mathcal{F}_{t-1}).$$

When $l \neq k$,

$$\begin{aligned} & f(\theta_t, y_t, s_{t-1} = k, s_t = l|\mathcal{F}_{t-1}) \\ =& f(\theta_t, y_t|\mathcal{F}_{t-1}, s_{t-1} = k, s_t = l)P(s_{t-1} = k, s_t = l|\mathcal{F}_{t-1}) \\ =& f(y_t|\mathcal{F}_{t-1}, J_t^{(l)} = t)f(\theta_t|\mathcal{F}_t, J_t^{(l)} = t)P(s_t = l|s_{t-1} = k)P(s_{t-1} = k|\mathcal{F}_{t-1}) \\ =& f(y_t|\mathcal{F}_{t-1}, J_t^{(l)} = t)f(\theta_t|\mathcal{F}_t, J_t^{(l)} = t)p_{k,l}\xi_{t-1}^{(k)}. \end{aligned}$$

When $l = k$,

$$f(\theta_t, y_t, s_{t-1} = k, s_t = k|\mathcal{F}_{t-1}) = \sum_{i=1}^{t-1} f(J_t^{(k)} = i, \theta_t, y_t|\mathcal{F}_{t-1})$$

$$= \sum_{i=1}^{t-1} f(\theta_t, y_t|\mathcal{F}_{t-1}, J_t^{(k)} = i)P(s_{t-1} = k, s_t = k|\mathcal{F}_{t-1})$$

$$= \sum_{i=1}^{t-1} f(y_t|\mathcal{F}_{t-1}, J_t^{(k)} = i)f(\theta_t|\mathcal{F}_t, J_t^{(k)} = i)P(s_t = k|s_{t-1} = k)P(s_{t-1} = k|\mathcal{F}_{t-1})$$

$$= \sum_{i=1}^{t-1} f(y_t|\mathcal{F}_{t-1}, J_t^{(l)} = t)f(\theta_t|\mathcal{F}_t, J_t^{(k)} = i)p_{k,k}\xi_{i,t-1}^{(k)}.$$

Let

$$\xi_{i,t}^{(k)*} = \begin{cases} \left(\sum_{l\neq k} \xi_{t-1}^{(l)} p_{lk}\right) f(y_t|J_t^{(k)} = t) & i = t, \\ p_{kk}\xi_{i,t-1}^{(k)} f(y_t|\mathcal{F}_{t-1}, J_t^{(k)} = i) & i < t. \end{cases}$$

We then have

$$f(\beta_t|\mathcal{F}_t) \propto \sum_{k=1}^{K} \xi_{t,t}^{(k)*} f(\theta_t|\mathcal{F}_t, J_t^{(l)} = t) + \sum_{k=1}^{K}\sum_{i=1}^{t-1} \xi_{i,t}^{(k)*} f(\theta_t|\mathcal{F}_t, J_t^{(k)} = i).$$

Hence, the mixture weight $\xi_{i,t}^{(k)}$ is the conditional probability which can be determined via normalization of $\xi_{i,t}^{(k*)}$. Furthermore, simple algebra shows that

$$f(y_t|J_t^{(k)} = t) = \psi_{0,0}^{(k)}/\psi_{t,t}^{(k)}, \qquad f(y_t|\mathcal{F}_{t-1}, J_t^{(k)} = i) = \psi_{i,t-1}^{(k)}/\psi_{i,t}^{(k)},$$

where

$$\psi_{0,0}^{(k)} = (\kappa^{(k)})^{-\frac{1}{2}} \frac{(\lambda^{(k)})^{-g^{(k)}}}{\Gamma(g^{(k)})}, \qquad \psi_{ij}^{(k)} = (\kappa_{ij}^{(k)})^{-\frac{1}{2}} \frac{(\lambda_{ij}^{k})^{-g_{ij}^{(k)}}}{\Gamma(g_{ij}^{(k)})},$$

for $i \leq j$. This proves (27.5).

Proof of (27.12): We use Bayes' theorem to combine the forward filter (27.4) with its backward variant (27.10) to derive the posterior distribution of θ_t given $\mathcal{F}_T$ $(1 \leq t < T)$

$$f(\theta_t|\mathcal{F}_T) = \sum_{k=1}^{K} f(\theta_t, s_t = k|\mathcal{F}_T) \propto \sum_{k=1}^{K} f(\theta_t, s_t = k|\mathcal{F}_t) \frac{f(\theta_t, s_t = k|\mathcal{F}_{t+1,T})}{f(\theta, s_t = k)}. \tag{27.22}$$

We first consider the following:

$$\begin{aligned}
&f(\theta_t, s_t = k|\mathcal{F}_t) f(\theta_t, s_t = k|\mathcal{F}_{t+1,T}) \big/ f(\theta, s_t = k) \\
&= \frac{\sum_{i=1}^{t} \xi_{i,t}^{(k)} f(\theta_t|\mathcal{F}_{i,t}) \cdot \{\widetilde{q}_{kk} \sum_{j=t+1}^{T} \eta_{t+1,j}^{(k)} f(\theta_t|\mathcal{F}_{t+1,j}) + \sum_{l \neq k} \widetilde{q}_{lk} \eta_{t+1}^{(l)} f(\theta_t|s_t = k)\}}{P(s_t = k) f(\theta_t|s_t = k)} \\
&= \frac{\sum_{i=1}^{t} \xi_{i,t}^{(k)} f(\theta_t|\mathcal{F}_{i,t}) \cdot \widetilde{q}_{kk} \sum_{j=t+1}^{T} \eta_{t+1,j}^{(k)} f(\theta_t|\mathcal{F}_{t+1,j})}{\pi_k f(\theta_t|s_t = k)} \\
&\quad + \frac{\sum_{i=1}^{t} \xi_{i,t}^{(k)} f(\theta_t|\mathcal{F}_{i,t}) \cdot \sum_{l \neq k} \widetilde{q}_{lk} \eta_{t+1}^{(l)} f(\theta_t|s_t = k)}{\pi_k f(\theta_t|s_t = k)} \\
&= \sum_{i}^{t} \xi_{i,t}^{(k)} \sum_{l \neq k} \frac{\widetilde{q}_{lk}}{\pi_k} \eta_{t+1}^{(l)} f(\theta_t|\mathcal{F}_{i,t}) + \frac{\widetilde{q}_{kk}}{\pi_k} \sum_{1 \leq i \leq t \leq j \leq T} \xi_{i,t}^{(k)} \eta_{t+1,j}^{(k)} \frac{f(\theta_t|\mathcal{F}_{i,t}) f(\theta_t|\mathcal{F}_{t+1,j})}{f(\theta_t|s_t = k)}.
\end{aligned}$$

Note that

$$\frac{f(\theta_t|\mathcal{F}_{i,t}) f(\theta_t|\mathcal{F}_{t+1,j})}{f(\theta_t|s_t = k)} = \frac{\psi_{i,t}^{(k)} \psi_{t+1,j}^{(k)}}{\psi_{i,j}^{(k)} \psi_{0,0}^{(k)}} f(\theta_t|\mathcal{F}_{i,j}),$$

we then obtain

$$\begin{aligned}
f(\theta_t|\mathcal{F}_T) = \sum_{k=1}^{K} \Bigg(&\sum_{i}^{t} \xi_{i,t}^{(k)} \sum_{l \neq k} \frac{\widetilde{q}_{lk}}{\pi_k} \eta_{t+1}^{(l)} f(\theta_t|\mathcal{F}_{i,t}) \\
&+ \frac{\widetilde{q}_{kk}}{\pi_k} \sum_{1 \leq i \leq t \leq j \leq T} \xi_{i,t}^{(k)} \eta_{t+1,j}^{(k)} \frac{\psi_{i,t}^{(k)} \psi_{t+1,j}^{(k)}}{\psi_{i,j}^{(k)} \psi_{0,0}^{(k)}} f(\theta_t|\mathcal{F}_{i,j}) \Bigg).
\end{aligned}$$

Hence, (27.12) is proved.

Appendix B. EM Algorithm for Hyperparameter Estimation

The inference procedure in the above sections involve the hyperparameters $\Phi = \{Q, z^{(k)}, \kappa^{(k)}, \lambda^{(k)}, g^{(k)}; k = 1, \ldots, \}$, is a $[4K + K(K-1)]$-dimensional vector. We can use the EM algorithm to exploit the much simpler structure of the log likelihood $l_c(\Phi)$ of the complete data $\{(y_t, s_t, \theta_t), 1 \le t \le T\}$, which is expressed as

$$
\begin{aligned}
l_c(\Phi) &= \sum_{t=1}^{T} \log f(\{y_t, s_t, \theta_t\}) \\
&= \sum_{t=1}^{T} \Big\{ \log f(y_t|\theta_t) + \sum_{k=1}^{K} f(\theta_t|s_t = k)\mathbf{1}_{\{s_t=k\}} + \sum_{k,l=1}^{K} \log(p_{kl})\mathbf{1}_{\{s_{t-1}=k, s_t=l\}} \Big\} \\
&= -\sum_{t=1}^{T} \Big\{ \frac{(y_t - \mu_t)^2}{2\sigma_t^2} + \frac{1}{2}\log(2\sigma_t^2) \Big\} - \sum_{t=1}^{T}\sum_{k=1}^{K} \Big\{ \frac{(\mu_t - z^{(k)})^2}{2\sigma_t^2 \kappa^{(k)}} + \frac{1}{2}\log(2\sigma_t^2 \kappa^{(k)}) \Big\} \\
&\quad - \sum_{t=1}^{T}\sum_{k=1}^{K} \Big\{ g^{(k)}\log(\lambda^{(k)}) - \log(\Gamma(g^{(k)})) - (g^{(k)} - 1)\log(2\sigma_t^2) + \frac{1}{2\sigma_t^2 \lambda^{(k)}} \Big\} \mathbf{1}_{\{s_t=k\}} \\
&\quad + \sum_{t=1}^{T}\sum_{k,l=1}^{K} \log(p_{kl})\mathbf{1}_{\{s_{t-1}=k, s_t=l\}}. \qquad (27.23)
\end{aligned}
$$

The E-step of the EM algorithm calculates $E[l_c(\Phi)|\mathcal{F}_t]$, which involves the computation of the conditional expectations:

$$
E\left[\frac{(y_t - \mu_t)^2}{2\sigma_2^2}|\mathcal{F}_T\right], \qquad E[\log(2\sigma_t^2)|\mathcal{F}_T], \qquad E\left(\frac{(\mu_t - z^{(k)})^2}{2\sigma_t^2 \kappa^{(k)}}\mathbf{1}_{\{s_t=k\}}|\mathcal{F}_T\right),
$$

$$
E[\log(2\sigma_t^2 \kappa^{(k)})\mathbf{1}_{\{s_t=k\}}|\mathcal{F}_T], \quad E[\log(2\sigma_t^2)\mathbf{1}_{\{s_t=k\}}|\mathcal{F}_T], \quad E\left(\frac{1}{2\sigma_t^2 \lambda^{(k)}}\mathbf{1}_{\{s_t=k\}}|\mathcal{F}_T\right),
$$

and the conditional probability:

$$
P(s_t = k|\mathcal{F}_T), \qquad P(s_{t-1} = k, s_t = l|\mathcal{F}_T).
$$

The M-step of the EM algorithm involves calculating the partial derivatives of $E[l_c(\Phi)|\mathcal{F}_t]$ with respect to Φ. Simple algebra yields the following updating formulas for Φ:

$$
\widehat{q}_{kl,\text{new}} = \frac{\sum_{t=2}^{T} P(s_{t-1} = k, s_t = l|\mathcal{F}_T, \widehat{\Phi}_{\text{old}})}{\sum_{t=2}^{T} P(s_{t-1} = k|\mathcal{F}_T, \widehat{\Phi}_{\text{old}})},
$$

$$
\widehat{z}^{(k)}_{\text{new}} = \frac{\sum_{t=1}^{T} E[\mu_t/(2\sigma_t^2)\mathbf{1}_{\{s_t=k\}}|\mathcal{F}_T, \widehat{\Phi}_{\text{old}}]}{\sum_{t=1}^{T} E[P_t \mathbf{1}_{\{s_t=k\}}|\mathcal{F}_T, \widehat{\Phi}_{\text{old}}]},
$$

$$\widehat{\kappa}^{(k)}_{\text{new}} = \frac{2\sum_{t=1}^{T} E[(\mu_t - \widehat{z}^{(k)}_{\text{old}})^2/(2\sigma_t^2)\mathbf{1}_{\{s_t=k\}}|\mathcal{F}_T, \widehat{\Phi}_{\text{old}}]}{\sum_{t=1}^{T} E[\mathbf{1}_{\{s_t=k\}}|\mathcal{F}_T, \widehat{\Phi}_{\text{old}}]},$$

$$\widehat{\lambda}^{(k)}_{\text{new}} = \frac{\sum_{t=1}^{T} E[(2\sigma_t)^{-1}\mathbf{1}_{\{s_t=k\}}|\mathcal{F}_T, \widehat{\Phi}_{\text{old}}]}{\sum_{t=1}^{T} g^{(k)}_{\text{old}} E[\mathbf{1}_{\{s_t=k\}}|\mathcal{F}_T, \widehat{\Phi}_{\text{old}}].} \tag{27.24}$$

I-terms in (27.24) can be obtained as follows:

$$E\left(\frac{\mu_t}{2\sigma_t^2}\mathbf{1}_{\{s_t=k\}}\middle|\mathcal{F}_T, \widehat{\Phi}_{\text{old}}\right) = \sum_{t=1}^{T} \alpha^{(k)}_{ijt} E\left(\frac{\mu_t}{2\sigma_t^2}\middle|C^{(k)}_{ij}, \mathcal{F}_T, \widehat{\Phi}_{\text{old}}\right), \tag{27.25}$$

$$E\left(\frac{\mu_t}{2\sigma_t^2}\middle|C^{(k)}_{ij}\mathcal{F}_T, \widehat{\Phi}_{\text{old}}\right) = \lambda^{(k)}_{ij} g^{(k)}_{ij} z^{(k)}_{ij}, \tag{27.26}$$

$$E\left(\frac{1}{2\sigma_t^2}\mathbf{1}_{\{s_t=k\}}\middle|\mathcal{F}_T, \widehat{\Phi}_{\text{old}}\right) = \sum_{1\le i\le t\le j\le T} \alpha^{(k)}_{ijt} g^{(k)}_{ijt} \lambda^{(k)}_{ijt}. \tag{27.27}$$

$$E\Big(\frac{\mu_t - z^{(k)}_{\text{old}})^2}{2\sigma_t^2}\mathbf{1}_{\{s_t=k\}}\Big|\mathcal{F}_T, \widehat{\Phi}_{\text{old}}\Big) = \sum_{1\le i\le t\le j\le T} \alpha^{(k)}_{ijt}\Big\{E\left(\frac{\mu_t^2}{2\sigma_t^2}\middle|C^{(k)}_{ij}, \mathcal{F}_T, \widehat{\Phi}_{\text{old}}\right)$$
$$- 2z^{(k)}_{\text{old}} E\left(\frac{\mu_t}{2\sigma_t^2}\middle|C^{(k)}_{ij}, \mathcal{F}_T, \widehat{\Phi}_{\text{old}}\right) + (z^{(k)}_{\text{old}})^2) E\left(\frac{1}{2\sigma_t^2}\middle|C^{(k)}_{ij}, \mathcal{F}_T, \widehat{\Phi}_{\text{old}}\right)\Big\}, \tag{27.28}$$

in which

$$E\left(\frac{\mu_t^2}{2\sigma_t^2}\middle|C^{(k)}_{ij}, \mathcal{F}_T, \widehat{\Phi}_{\text{old}}\right) = \frac{\kappa^{(k)}_{ij}}{2} + \lambda^{(k)}_{ij} g^{(k)}_{ij}\left(z^{(k)}_{ij}\right)^2. \tag{27.29}$$

We can use the BCMIX approximations instead of the full recursions to determine the items (27.25)–(27.29) in order to speed up computation. The iteration scheme (27.24) is carried out until convergence to estimate hyperparameters.

References

Barski A, Cuddapah S, Cui K, Roh Tae-Y, Schones DE, Wang Z, Wei G, Chepelev I, Zhao, K (2007) Highresolution profiling of histone methylations in the human genome. Cell 129:823–837

Bernstein BE, Stamatoyannopoulos JA, Costello JF, Ren B, Milosavljevic A, Meissner A, Kellis M, Marra MA, Beaudet, AL, Ecker JR et al (2010) The NIH roadmap epigenomics mapping consortium. Nat Biotechnol 28:1045–1048

Consortium TEP, data analysis coordination OC, data production DPL, data analysis LA, group W, scientific management NPM, steering committee PI, Boise State University and University of North Carolina at Chapel Hill Proteomics groups (data production and analysis), Broad Institute Group (data production and analysis), Cold Spring Harbor, University of Geneva, Center for Genomic Regulation, Barcelona, RIKEN, Sanger Institute, University of Lausanne, Genome Institute of Singapore group (data production and analysis), Data coordination center at UC

Santa Cruz (production data coordination), Duke University, EBI, University of Texas, Austin, University of North Carolina-Chapel Hill group (data production and analysis), Genome Institute of Singapore group (data production and analysis), HudsonAlpha Institute, Caltech, UC Irvine, Stanford group (data production and analysis), targeted experimental validation LBNLG, data production and analysis NG, Sanger Institute, Washington University, Yale University, Center for Genomic Regulation, Barcelona, UCSC, MIT, University of Lausanne, CNIO group (data production and analysis), Stanford-Yale, Harvard, University of Massachusetts Medical School, University of Southern California/UC Davis group (data production and analysis), University of Albany SUNY group (data production and analysis) (2012) An integrated encyclopedia of DNA elements in the human genome. Nature 488:57–74

Dorschner MO, Hawrylycz M, Humbert R, Wallace JC, Shafer A, Kawamoto, J, Mack J, Hall R, Goldy J, Sabo PJ et al (2004) High-throughput localization of functional elements by quantitative chromatin profiling. Nat Methods 1:219–225

Lian H, Thompson WA, Thurman R, Stamatoyannopoulos JA, Noble WS, Lawrence CE (2008) Automated mapping of large-scale chromatin structure in ENCODE. Bioinformatics 24:1911–1916

Sabo PJ, Kuehn MS, Thurman R, Johnson BE, Johnson EM, Cao H, Yu M, Rosenzweig E, Goldy J, Haydock A et al (2006) Genome-scale mapping of DNase I sensitivity in vivo using tiling DNA microarrays. Nat Methods 3:511–518

Xing H, Mo Y, Liao W, Zhang MQ (2006) Genome-wide localization of protein-DNA binding and histone modification by a Bayesian change-point method with ChIP-seq data. PLoS Comput Biol 8:e1002613

Xing H, Ying C (2014) A stochastic segmentation model for recurrent copy number alteration analysis. Technical Report, Department of Applied Mathematics and Statistics, State University of New York at Stony Brook

Mikkelsen TS, and Ku M, Jaffe DB, Issac B, Lieberman E, Giannoukos G, Alvarez P, Brockman W, Kim T-K, Koche RP et al (2007) Genome-wide maps of chromatin state in pluripotent and lineage-committed cells. Nature 448:553–560

Qin ZS, Yu J, Shen J, Maher CA, Hu M, Kalyana-Sundaram S, Yu J, Chinnaiyan AM (2010) HPeak: an HMM-based algorithm for defining read-enriched regions in ChIP-Seq data. BMC bioinformatics 11:369

Rozowsky J, Euskirchen G, Auerbach RK, Zhang ZD, Gibson T, Bjornson R, Carriero N, Snyder M, Gerstein MB (2009) PeakSeq enables systematic scoring of ChIP-seq experiments relative to controls. Nat Biotechnol 27:66–75

Zhang Y, Liu T, Meyer CA, Eeckhoute J, Johnson DS, Bernstein BE, Nusbaum C, Myers RM, Brown M, Li W (2008) Model-based analysis of ChIP-Seq (MACS) . Genome Biol 9:R1375

Chapter 28
Combining *p* Values for Gene Set Analysis

Ziwen Wei and Lynn Kuo

Abstract In detecting genes which are significantly associated with a treatment, a clinical outcome, or an experimental design variable from high-throughput gene expression data, it is common to examine genes individually. However, it would be advantageous to analyze them at the level of gene sets where the sets are predefined, for example, as the genes belong to the same biological pathway, chromosomal location, or regulation. Gene set analysis (GSA) will ease the interpretation of a large-scale experiment by identifying important pathways and processes. An increasing number of GSA methods are being proposed.

In this chapter, we propose another method based on aggregating individual *p* values within the set. We evaluate the proposed approach along with six other gene set methods including gene set enrichment analysis (GSEA), GSA by Efron and Tibshirani (GSA-ET), random set, significance analysis of microarray for gene sets (SAM-GS), global test, and global analysis of covariance (ANCOVA) by a simulation experiment, where we compare them in terms of the false positive rate (FPR), false negative rate (FNR), false discovery rate (FDR), false non-discovery rate (FNDR), and receiver operating characteristic (ROC) curve.

28.1 Introduction

When microarray technology was first developed, a large number of statistical methods were developed to screen for differentially expressed (DE) genes between two groups of samples. They are mostly individual gene analysis (IGA) consisting of two steps: first, we select a set of significant genes based on individual gene scores and a threshold, and second, we seek a biological interpretation of this selected set. The IGA is sensitive to the noise in the microarray data and thresholds that are selected

Z. Wei (✉)
Merck & Co., Inc., 126 E Lincoln Ave, Rahway, NJ 07065, USA
e-mail: ziwen.wei@merck.com

L. Kuo
Departement of Statistics, University of Connecticut, 215 Glenbrook Road, U-4120, Storrs, CT 06029, USA
e-mail: lynn.kuo@uconn.edu

Z. Chen et al. (eds.), *Applied Statistics in Biomedicine and Clinical Trials Design*, ICSA Book Series in Statistics, DOI 10.1007/978-3-319-12694-4_28

(Pan et al. 2005). Hence, we saw gradual interests in the development of gene set analysis (GSA) to identify DE sets across different conditions, where the sets are predefined, for example, consisting of genes in a pathway. The null hypothesis of GSA can be summarized into two types (Nam and Kim 2008): (1) The level of the association of a gene set with the phenotype is the same as the complement of the gene set with the phenotype; (2) consider only genes within the set, in which no gene is associated with the phenotype. Consequently, the methods developed accordingly were termed competitive and self-contained tests, respectively. As opposed to IGA, GSA is a single-step process to infer the biological meaning of the set by either applying a sampling or a gene randomization test. It is more appealing than IGA in understanding the cellular process, because weak expression changes in individual genes gathered together may show a significant effect.

In this chapter, we propose a new gene set method which summarizes a gene set using individual p values in the set instead of individual gene scores, for example, the t-statistic. It relies on the fact that the individual p values tend to be small for both upregulated genes and downregulated genes. Let us consider a gene set denoted by S. We start with individual p values from t-statistics for genes in set S, denoted by p_i, $i \in S$. Next, let $s_i = -2\log(p_i)$, and summarize them by the total sum score $TS_{obs} = \sum_{i \in S} s_i$. Then we evaluate the p value of the total sum score by the permutation method. Fisher (1932) first develops the combined p value approach which is also known as the Fisher's combined probability test to combine the results from several independent tests having the same null hypothesis. It has been used routinely in meta-analysis (Hedges and Olkin 1985). It has also been extended to combine dependent p values with either known covariance by Brown (1975) or unknown covariance by Kost and McDermott (2002). Although we use the same combined probability test (essentially a product of p values) proposed by Fisher, our hypothesis is very different from that in the meta-analysis. In meta-analysis, the null hypothesis is that all of the separate null hypotheses are true. The alternative hypothesis is that at least one of the separate alternative hypotheses is true. When we apply the same Fisher's combined p value test statistics to the GSA, our null hypothesis is that the set is not particularly enriched by significant genes associated with the clinical outcome. To test this null hypothesis, Fisher's exact test is often used. Z-test, t test, Kolmogorove–Smirnov test, and unpaired Wilcoxon's test have also been developed for GSA. All these procedures evaluate the proportion of DE genes in the set to a reference. As far as we know, our method of aggregating p values within the set has not been applied to GSA. Our method not only takes into account the number of DE genes in the set but also incorporates the strength of DE evidence for individual genes. So we would like to examine it in the perspective of testing sets of DE genes and argue that it is desirable to apply this test to GSA by the following simulation study.

We conduct a simulation study to compare our method to six other GSA methods in terms of false positive rate (FPR), false negative rate (FNR), false discovery rate (FDR), false non-discovery rate (FNDR), and receiver operating characteristic (ROC) curve. These six methods are: gene set enrichment analysis (GSEA) by Subramanian et al. (2005), GSA by Efron and Tibshirani (2007; GSA-ET), random set (RS) method by Newton et al. (2007), significance analysis of microarray for gene sets (SAM-GS) by Dinu et al. (2007), global test by Goeman et al. (2004), and global analyis of covariance (ANCOVA) test by Mansmann and Meister (2005).

Our simulation study demonstrates that the proposed method has more power in detecting DE gene sets than several other commonly used methods, especially when sets contain a lot of DE genes in both directions, up- and downregulated.

There are other studies to evaluate GSA methods. For example, Liu et al. (2007) conduct a comparative study on global test, global ANCOVA test, and SAM-GS test; Dinu et al. (2008) evaluate the biological performance of six GSA: SAM-GS, global test, global ANCOVA test, the method of Tian et al. (2005), the method of Tomfohr et al. (2005), and GSEA; and Abatangelo et al. (2009) compare four methods: Fisher's exact test, GSEA, RS, and gene list analysis with prediction accuracy (GLAPA). An even broader range of 16 approaches are compared in Tarca et al. (2013).

A brief summary of the six GSA methods that were used for comparison to our method is provided in Sect. 28.2. Our proposed approach based on aggregating individual p values within each gene set is discussed in Sect. 28.3. In Sect. 28.4, we evaluate these seven methods by a simulation experiment in which five scenarios with different number of DE sets and different magnitude of differentiation are considered. Section 28.4.1 describes the simulated data, and Sect. 28.4.2 presents and discusses the simulation results, including a comparison among the seven methods in terms of the accuracy and the receiver operating characteristic (ROC) curve. Section 28.5 is devoted to a real data analysis using preferred methods. At the end, discussions are given in Sect. 28.6.

28.2 Review of Existing Methods

28.2.1 GSEA

GSEA was initially proposed by Mootha et al. (2003) to provide a set enrichment score for assessing its association with a phenotype, say D for example, using the Kolmogorov–Smirnov running sum statistic. The method is then improved by Subramanian et al. (2005) in which the components of the original Kolmogorov–Smirnov statistic are weighted by the strength of associations between the genes and the phenotype.

GSEA Procedure

Step 1: For gene i, $i = 1, \ldots, N$, compute a Pearson correlation r_i (or other metrics) between gene i and phenotype D.

Step 2: Establish a gene list L by sorting N genes according to r_i from maximum to minimum.

Step 3: Let ES be the running sum score for gene set S. Start with $ES = 0$, walking down the list L, add ES by $\frac{|r_i|}{\sum_{l \in S} |r_l|}$ if $i \in S$; decrease ES by $\frac{1}{N-M}$ if $i \notin S$.

Step 4: Let $ES(S)$ be the enrichment score of gene set S, where $ES(S)$ =maximum deviation of ES from 0.

Step 5: Permute labels of phenotype D and repeat steps 1–4 a large number of times to obtain the permutation distribution of $ES(S)$.

Step 6: Statistical significance for the association between the gene set S and the phenotype D is obtained by the proportion of permutations with $ES(S)$ larger than the observed $ES(S)$ which is positive, or proportion of permutations with $ES(S)$ smaller than the observed $ES(S)$ which is negative.

28.2.2 GSA-ET

GSA-ET is introduced by Efron and Tibshirani (2007) improving upon GSEA by using a more robust statistics called maxmean and a permutation test that employs both subject resampling and gene resampling. The maxmean statistics would prevent a few large positive or negative scores in the gene set dominating the whole set. Efron and Tibshirani (2007) call their procedure GSA. Given we have used GSA for the gene set analysis in general, we just use GSA-ET for this procedure, where ET are the first letters of the two authors.

GSA-ET Procedure

Step 1: Start with a gene-level t-statistic t_i for gene i, and convert it to a z value by

$$z_i = \Phi^{-1}(F_{n-2}(t_i)), \tag{28.1}$$

where F_{n-2} is cdf of the t distribution with $df = n - 2$, Φ^{-1} is the inverse cdf of a standard normal random variable, and z_i follows $N(0, 1)$ under the null hypothesis.

Step 2: Define $s(z) = (s^{(+)}(z), s^{(-)}(z))$, where $s^{(+)}(z) = \max(z, 0)$ and $s^{(-)}(z) = -\min(z, 0)$. And define $(\overline{s_S^{(+)}}, \overline{s_S^{(-)}})$ to be the average of $s(z)$. Then the proposed maxmean statistic for set S, is defined as

$$S_{maxmean} = \max\left(\overline{s_S^{(+)}}, \overline{s_S^{(-)}}\right). \tag{28.2}$$

Step 3: Randomly shuffle the gene labels and repeat step 2 for a large number of times to get the mean denoted by $\text{mean}_{S_{maxmean}}$ and the standard deviation $\text{SD}_{S_{maxmean}}$. Standardize $S_{maxmean}$ by

$$S'_{maxmean} = \frac{S_{maxmean} - \text{mean}_{S_{maxmean}}}{\text{stdev}_{S_{maxmean}}}. \tag{28.3}$$

Step 4: Repeat steps 1–3 for B times (B is large) by column permuted bootstrap data sets, yielding $S'^{*1}_{maxmean}, S'^{*2}_{maxmean}, \ldots, S'^{*B}_{maxmean}$.

Step 5: Statistical significance for association between gene set S and phenotype D is obtained by the proportion of permutations with $S'^{*}_{maxmean}$ from step 4 greater than $S'_{maxmean}$ observed from the data.

28.2.3 Random Set

RS method is proposed by Newton et al. (2007) in which the set-level score is defined as the average of the gene-level scores in this set. RS method treats the unstandardized enrichment score of the gene set as a random variable as in the simple random sampling without replacement. With the first two moments of this random variable given analytically, RS method is one of the computationally most efficient methods.

RS Procedure

Step 1: Starting with a gene-level score d_i for gene i, for example, log(fold change) or t-statistic, obtain a set-level score as the average of d_i's in gene set S of size M:

$$\overline{X} = \frac{1}{M}\sum_{i \in S} d_i. \tag{28.4}$$

Step 2: Consider $\overline{X}$ as a random variable. It is claimed that the distribution of $\overline{X}$ is approximately Gaussian, with mean and variance given by:

$$\mu = E(\overline{X}) = \frac{\sum_{i=1}^{N} d_i}{N} \tag{28.5}$$

and

$$\sigma^2 = Var(\overline{X}) = \frac{1}{M}\left(\frac{N-M}{N-1}\right)\left\{\left(\frac{\sum_{i=1}^{N} d_i^2}{N}\right) - \left(\frac{\sum_{i=1}^{N} d_i}{N}\right)^2\right\}. \tag{28.6}$$

Step 3: Standardize $\overline{X}$ by $Z = \frac{\overline{X}-\mu}{\sigma}$, which is $N(0,1)$ under the null hypothesis.

Step 4: Statistical significance for association between the gene set S and the phenotype D is obtained by p value $= 1 - \Phi(Z)$ for positive Z or p value $= \Phi(Z)$ for negative Z.

28.2.4 SAM-GS

SAM-GS is introduced by Dinu et al. (2007). It is based on the individual t-like statistic from the SAM proposed in Tusher et al. (2001). It calculates the observed gene set score as the sum of squares of the SAM statistic scores of all genes in that set, and conducts a permutation test to obtain the statistical significance of the association between the gene set and phenotype D. Assume we have N genes, and n samples in the gene expression data set. We are interested in the gene set S which contains M genes. Let d_i denote the gene-level score for gene i. We summarize the SAM-GS procedure as below.

SAM-GS Procedure

Step 1: As in SAM, calculate the gene-level statistic d_i for gene i,

$$d_i = \frac{\overline{x}_1(i) - \overline{x}_2(i)}{S(i) + S_0}, \tag{28.7}$$

where $\overline{x}_1(i)$ is the average gene intensity over the samples of phenotype 1, $\overline{x}_2(i)$ is the average gene intensity over the samples of phenotype 2, $S(i)$ is the pooled standard deviation over all samples of both phenotype 1 and 2, and S_0 is a small positive constant that adjusts for the small variability encountered for some genes in the data, so the method would not be biased toward genes with small intensity.

Step 2: For set S, calculate the observed set score as

$$SAMGS = \sum_{i \in S} d_i^2. \tag{28.8}$$

Step 3: Permute labels of phenotype D (i.e., shuffle 1's and 2's) and repeat steps 1 and 2 to obtain the permutation distribution of *SAMGS*.

Step 4: The statistical significance for association between set S and phenotype D is obtained by comparing the observed *SAMGS* from step 2 and its permutation distribution from step 3.

28.2.5 Global Test

Global test is proposed by Goeman et al. (2004) to test whether the global expression pattern of a gene set is significantly related to some clinical outcome of interest using a random-effect logistic model. Let $X_{M \times n}$ be the data matrix that contains expression data of set S with M genes and n samples, and let $Y_{1 \times n}$ be a 0-1 vector indicating clinical outcome, where 0 is for the control group and 1 is for the treatment group. The procedure of global test is summarized as below.

Global Test Procedure

Step 1: Fit a logistic regression model,

$$E(Y_j|\boldsymbol{\beta}) = h^{-1}\left(\alpha + \sum_{i=1}^{M} x_{ij}\beta_i\right), i = 1, 2, ..., M; j = 1, 2, .., n. \tag{28.9}$$

where h^{-1} is the link function (e.g., logit link), α is the intercept, and $\beta_i' s$ are regression coefficients, which are random. The null hypothesis of interest is

$$H_0 : \beta_1 = \beta_2 = ... = \beta_M = 0. \tag{28.10}$$

Assume $\beta_1, \beta_2, ..., \beta_M$ come from a distribution with mean 0 and variance τ^2, then (28.10) is equivalent as:

$$H_0 : \tau^2 = 0. \tag{28.11}$$

Table 28.1 Data set for global ANCOVA

	Genes	$j = 1$	...	$j = n_1$	...	$j = n_2$
	g_1	x_{111}	...	x_{11n_1}		
$k = 1$	...	...	...	...		
	g_N	x_{1N1}	...	x_{1Nn_1}		
	g_1	x_{211}	...	...	...	x_{21n_2}
$k = 2$	...	...	...	...		
	g_N	x_{2N1}	...	...	...	x_{2Nn_2}

ANCOVA analysis of covariance

Step 2: Let $\zeta_j = \sum_i x_{ij}\beta_i$, then $\boldsymbol{\zeta} = (\zeta_1, ..., \zeta_n)$, $E(\boldsymbol{\zeta}) = 0$, and $cov(\boldsymbol{\zeta}) = \tau^2 XX'$. Hence, the model (28.9) can be simplified into a simple random effects model,

$$E(Y_j|\zeta_j) = h^{-1}(\alpha + \zeta_j), j = 1, 2, ..., n. \tag{28.12}$$

Step 3: The score test (Le Cessie and Van Houwelingen 1995) uses complicated test statistic T or a simpler statistic Q,

$$Q = \frac{(Y - \mu)R(Y - \mu)'}{\mu_2} \tag{28.13}$$

where $R = \frac{1}{M}X'X$, $\mu = h^{-1}(\alpha) = E(Y)$, and μ_2 is the second central moment of Y under H_0.

Step 4: Permute the labels of all samples and recalculate Q value. Repeat above steps for a large number of times.

Step 5: The empirical p value is computed as a proportion of permutations with Q values greater than the observed Q value from the data.

28.2.6 Global ANCOVA

Global ANCOVA test is derived by Mansmann and Meister (2005) to compete with the global test. It tests the same hypothesis in the global test, but applies an ANCOVA approach and exchanges the roles of genes and phenotype in the regression modeling framework of the global test. Note that for all methods mentioned here, genes in the same set are assumed to contribute equally to the set.

In this method, it is further assumed that the n samples consists of n_1 samples from group 1 and n_2 samples from group 2. The data can be organized as in Table 28.1 (as an example, we assume $n_1 < n_2$), where x_{kij} is the gene intensity of the jth sample in group k for gene i, $k = 1, 2$, $i = 1, 2, ..., N$, and $j = 1, 2, ..., n_k$.

Global ANCOVA Procedure

Step 1: Consider the saturated (full) model given by

$$x_{kij} = \mu_{ki} + e_{kij}, \tag{28.14}$$

with $E(e_{kij}) = 0$, and μ_{ki}, the mean expression for gene i in group k, can be split up into a two-way ANOVA layout as

$$\mu_{ki} = \mu + \alpha_k + \beta_i + \gamma_{ki}, \tag{28.15}$$

where α_k is the group effect, β_i is the gene effect, γ_{ki} is the interaction, and $\sum_k \alpha_k = \sum_i \beta_i = \sum_k \gamma_{ki} = \sum_i \gamma_{ki} = 0$.

Step 2: Consider the null hypothesis of interest $H_0 : \mu_{1i} = \mu_{2i}$, $i = 1, \ldots, N$ which is equivalent to $H_0 : \alpha_k = \gamma_{ki} = 0, k = 1, 2$. So under H_0, $\mu_{ki} = \mu + \beta_i$. If we only only test for interaction $\gamma_{ki} = 0, k = 1, 2; i = 1, \ldots N$, then under H_0, $\mu_{ki} = \mu + \alpha_k + \beta_i$.

Step 3: Providing the residual sums of squares for full model and reduced model, the F-statistic is derived as

$$F = \frac{[SSE_{reduced} - SSE_{full}]/df_1}{SSE_{full}/df_2}, \tag{28.16}$$

where $df_1 = N$, $df_2 = N(n_1 + n_2 - 2)$. If test interaction only, $df_1 = N - 1$.

Step 4: Permute the labels of all samples and recalculate the F value. Repeat the above step for a large number of times.

Step 5: The empirical p value is computed as a proportion of permutations with F values greater than the observed F value from the data.

28.3 Proposed Approach

The performance of GSA methods, to a large extent, depends on how one summarizes the gene-level scores of a set. Therefore, whether the summary score of the gene set is representative becomes an important concern. We propose a combined p score, which aggregates p values for each gene in the set instead of individual gene scores (the t-statistic, d-statistics, etc.).

28.3.1 Combined p Score

The p value of a simple hypothesis testing framework is uniformly distributed under the null hypothesis and all other assumptions are met (Tippett 1931). The validity of this statement can be verified in a one-step derivation as below. Under the null hypothesis, the test statistic, denoted by T, has the null distribution $F(t)$ (e.g., standard normal). The p value, denoted by $P = F(T)$, has a probability distribution

$$\begin{aligned} Pr(P < p) &= Pr(F^{-1}(P) < F^{-1}(p)) \\ &= Pr(T < t) \\ &\equiv p. \end{aligned}$$

In other words, P is uniformly distributed. An explicit explanation is given in Murdock et al. (2008).

If we assume that a set of M hypotheses are independent, with p value for the ith hypothesis denoted by p_i, $i = 1, ..., M$, and let

$$s_i = -2\log(p_i),$$

then

$$s_i \sim \chi_2^2, \text{ for all } i, \tag{28.17}$$

and the sum of s_i, $\sum_{i=1}^{M} s_i$, yields a chi-square distribution with degree of freedom $2M$. That is,

$$\sum_{i=1}^{M} s_i \sim \chi_{2M}^2. \tag{28.18}$$

Such way of combing p values is known as Fisher's method, or Fisher's combined probability test. Fisher's method of combining the probabilities is asymptotically optimal among essentially all methods of combining independent tests (Littell and Folks 1971, 1973) according to Bahadur relative efficiency (Bahadur 1967). In meta-analysis, this technique is known as the inverse chi-square method. It is one of the combined test procedures for testing the significance of combined results (Hedges and Olkin 1985). Here, we propose to apply the same technique in summarizing the set scores.

While combining p values, one needs to assume all individual tests are independent in order to apply the chi-square distribution. When the individual statistical tests are not independent, one can approximate the null distribution of s_i with a scaled chi-square distribution. Brown's method (Brown 1975) or Kost's method (Kost and McDermott 2002) can be used depending on whether or not the covariance between the p values is known. More sophisticated methods can be developed. But this is beyond the scope of this chapter.

In addition to the Fisher's method, Owen (2009) describes Pearson's method for meta-analysis that also has potential to be applied to GSA. That is to be investigated in the future.

28.3.2 Combined p Procedure

The test procedure proposed is listed as below:

Step 1: Let us consider set S which contains M genes. We start with individual p values from t-statistic for genes in the set, denoted by p_i, $i \in S$.

Step 2: For each p_i, let

$$s_i = -2\log(p_i), \tag{28.19}$$

and summarize s_i's, $i \in S$ by

$$TS_{obs} = \sum_{i \in S} s_i. \tag{28.20}$$

Step 3: Permute labels of phenotype D and repeat steps 1 and 2 for a large number of times. Each time we obtain a summarized set score, TS, from the permuted data, hence it yields a permutation distribution.

Step 4: The p value representing the significance of the gene set S is estimated by the proportion of TS that is larger than TS_{obs}.

The combined p method relies on the fact that the individual p value tends to be small for both upregulated genes and downregulated genes. Therefore, it avoids canceling out the upregulation and downregulation effects in one set. It is an effective way to test the significance of gene sets, especially for the gene set containing both up- and downregulated genes.

28.4 Simulation Study

28.4.1 Simulated Data

We focus on two-condition situations along our study, similar to the simulation scheme of Efron and Tibshirani (2007), we generated a larger data set with more variation. Assume that we have $N = 5000$ genes, coming from 200 disjoint gene sets of size 25 each. We also assume there are two conditions, A and B, each of which has 50 replicated samples. First, we generated a 5000×100 matrix with each entry from the standard normal distribution. Then, we prepared gene expression data sets for five different scenarios by adding effect to the first 30 gene sets. Specifically:

Scenario 1: For all 25 genes of the first 30 gene sets, add 0.2 units for condition B.

Scenario 2: For the first 15 genes of the first 30 gene sets, add 0.3 units for condition B.

Scenario 3: For the first 10 genes of the first 30 gene sets, add 0.4 units for condition B.

Scenario 4: For the first 5 genes of the first 30 gene sets, add 0.6 units for condition B.

Scenario 5: For the first 10 genes of the first 30 gene sets, add 0.6 units for condition B; and for second 10 genes of the first 30 gene sets, subtract 0.4 units for condition B.

Table 28.2 provides a summary on how we simulated the data for different scenarios.

The first 30 gene sets in all scenarios were constructed as DE sets. Specifically, scenarios 1–4 set the first 30 gene sets to be upregulated to different extents. In scenario 1, all members in the first 30 sets have a 0.2 higher average expression in condition B. In scenarios 2, 3/5 of genes in the first 30 sets have a 0.3 higher average expression in condition B. In scenarios 3, 2/5 of genes in the first 30 sets

Table 28.2 Simulated data summary

	Genes that are manually altered in the first 30 sets	Condition A	Condition B
Scenario 1	$\{g1, ..., g25\}$	$N(0, 1)$	$N(0, 1) + 0.2$
Scenario 2	$\{g1, ..., g15\}$	$N(0, 1)$	$N(0, 1) + 0.3$
Scenario 3	$\{g1, ..., g10\}$	$N(0, 1)$	$N(0, 1) + 0.4$
Scenario 4	$\{g1, ..., g5\}$	$N(0, 1)$	$N(0, 1) + 0.6$
Scenario 5	$\{g1, ..., g10\}$	$N(0, 1)$	$N(0, 1) + 0.6$
	$\{g11, ..., g20\}$	$N(0, 1)$	$N(0, 1) - 0.4$

have a 0.4 higher average expression in condition B. In scenario 4, 1/5 of genes in the first 30 sets have a 0.6 higher average expression in condition B. In scenario 5, 2/5 of genes in the first 30 sets have a 0.6 higher average expression in condition B, another 2/5 of genes in the first 30 sets have a 0.4 lower average expression in condition B, and the remaining 1/5 have no average difference in the two conditions. Scenarios 5 represents the situation that the set contains genes having higher average expressions in both conditions. This is commonly seen and can be difficult to detect if the summary statistics allow the cancellation of upregulated and downregulated effects.

We evaluate all seven methods in terms of FPR, FNR, FDR, FNDR. In this study, we set 0.05 as the cutoff p value for significance gene sets for each method. We estimate FPR as the fraction of false positives out of negatives, FNR as the fraction of false negatives out of positives, FDR as the fraction of negatives out of claimed positives, and FNDR as the fraction of positives out of claimed negatives. Note that positives (or negatives) in the GSA setting means the set is DE (or EE, equivalently expressed). Methods with small values in all four metrics, FPR, FNR, FDR, and FNDR, are considered to be superior. In addition, all methods are also compared via the ROC curve, which is created by plotting TPR versus FPR, at various threshold settings. TPR stands for true positive rates, which is estimated by the fraction of true positives out of the positives. In terms of the ROC plot, the closer the ROC curve is to the upper left corner, the higher the overall accuracy of the test is. The simulation results are discussed in detail in the next section.

28.4.2 Simulation Results

In this section, we present the results of the FPR, FNR, FDR, and FNDR first, followed by a discussion on ROC curves. All values in Tables 28.3–28.7 are calculated based on 100 simulations, so are the rate values used to plot ROC curves.

Table 28.3 FPR, FNR, FDR, and FNDR for scenario 1

Methods	**FPR** Mean (SE)	**FNR** Mean (SE)	**FDR** Mean (SE)	**FNDR** Mean (SE)
GSEA	0.0065 (0.0006)	0.0173 (0.0022)	0.0350 (0.0031)	0.0031 (0.0004)
GSA-ET	0.0049 (0.0006)	0.0200 (0.0024)	0.0270 (0.0031)	0.0035 (0.0004)
RS	0.1625 (0.0024)	0.0060 (0.0013)	0.4784 (0.0036)	0.0012 (0.0003)
SAM-GS	0.0068 (0.0006)	0.4213 (0.0110)	0.0583 (0.0051)	0.0693 (0.0017)
Global test	0.0356 (0.0014)	0.1967 (0.0077)	0.1969 (0.0066)	0.0346 (0.0013)
Global ANCOVA	0.0471 (0.0017)	0.1683 (0.0062)	0.2380 (0.0066)	0.0301 (0.0011)
Combined p	0.0506 (0.0017)	0.1493 (0.0062)	0.2477 (0.0066)	0.0269 (0.0011)

FPR false positive rate, *FNR* false negative rate, *FDR* false discovery rate, *FNDR* false non-discovery rate, *GSEA* gene set enrichment analysis, *GSA-ET* gene set analysis by Efron and Tibshirani, *RS* random set, *SAM-GS* significance analysis of microarray for gene sets, *ANCOVA* analysis of covariance

28.4.2.1 FPR, FNR, FDR, and FNDR

FPR, FNR, FDR, and FNDR are used to assess the accuracy of the seven methods. Mean and standard error for each metric are computed based on 100 simulations. Methods with small values in all four metrics are considered to be superior.

Table 28.3 presents the FPR, FNR, FDR, and FNDR from seven GSA methods for simulation scenario 1. From this table, we see GSEA and GSA-ET have smaller rates in FPR, FNR, FDR, and FNDR, while others have at least one rate appearing to be high, which suggests that GSEA and GSA-ET perform better than others in cases that all genes in the set have 0.2 higher average expression in condition B. Between GSEA and GSA-ET, GSA-ET is slightly better.

The results for other simulated scenarios are presented in Tables 28.4–28.7. From these tables, we notice that none of the methods beats others in all four rates. SAM-GS has large FNR in scenario 1. Global test consistently has large FDR. It also has large FNR in scenario 1. The rates of global ANCOVA are comparable to global test. It has relatively larger FDR but smaller FNR than global test. For scenarios 1–4, the rates for GSEA and GSA-ET are relatively low, but not always the lowest. For example, in scenario 1, RS achieves smaller FNR and FNDR than both GSA-ET and GSEA. Also, in scenario 4, the FNR for all other methods except RS are smaller than the FNR for GSA-ET and GSEA. These two methods also have large FNR in scenario 5. On the other hand, SAM-GS turns out to be the optimal in this case. RS method has highest FDR in general, and its FNR in scenario 5 goes as high as 0.6710. However, it can achieve very small FNR and FNDR in the first two scenarios. Our proposed combined p method performs satisfactorily in terms of FPR, FNR, FNDR. Its FDR is never the highest. Moreover, it has a smaller FNDR comparing to most of the other methods, especially in scenarios 3, 4, and 5.

Table 28.4 FPR, FNR, FDR, and FNDR for scenario 2

Methods	FPR Mean (SE)	FNR Mean (SE)	FDR Mean (SE)	FNDR Mean (SE)
GSEA	0.0071 (0.0006)	0.0387 (0.0031)	0.0393 (0.0031)	0.0068 (0.0005)
GSA-ET	0.0039 (0.0005)	0.0227 (0.0025)	0.0216 (0.0028)	0.0040 (0.0004)
RS	0.1362 (0.0023)	0.0203 (0.0023)	0.4377 (0.0042)	0.0041 (0.0005)
SAM-GS	0.0094 (0.0008)	0.1667 (0.0076)	0.0580 (0.0044)	0.0287 (0.0013)
Global test	0.0356 (0.0014)	0.0610 (0.0045)	0.1730 (0.0058)	0.0110 (0.0008)
Global ANCOVA	0.0470 (0.0016)	0.0497 (0.0041)	0.2152 (0.0058)	0.0091 (0.0007)
Combined *p*	0.0508 (0.0017)	0.0467 (0.0036)	0.2277 (0.0059)	0.0086 (0.0007)

FPR false positive rate, *FNR* false negative rate, *FDR* false discovery rate, *FNDR* false non-discovery rate, *GSEA* gene set enrichment analysis, *GSA-ET* gene set analysis by Efron and Tibshirani, *RS* random set, *SAM-GS* significance analysis of microarray for gene sets, *ANCOVA* analysis of covariance

Table 28.5 FPR, FNR, FDR, and FNDR for scenario 3

Methods	FPR Mean (SE)	FNR Mean (SE)	FDR Mean (SE)	FNDR Mean (SE)
GSEA	0.0089 (0.0007)	0.0590 (0.0040)	0.0500 (0.0036)	0.0104 (0.0007)
GSA-ET	0.0041 (0.0005)	0.0250 (0.0027)	0.0225 (0.0025)	0.0044 (0.0005)
RS	0.1145 (0.0022)	0.0527 (0.0036)	0.4031 (0.0046)	0.0103 (0.0007)
SAM-GS	0.0094 (0.0007)	0.0733 (0.0059)	0.0528 (0.0039)	0.0128 (0.0010)
Global test	0.0356 (0.0014)	0.0227 (0.0027)	0.1674 (0.0056)	0.0041 (0.0005)
Global ANCOVA	0.0474 (0.0016)	0.0177 (0.0024)	0.2105 (0.0058)	0.0032 (0.0004)
Combined *p*	0.0508 (0.0017)	0.0173 (0.0024)	0.2224 (0.0058)	0.0032 (0.0004)

FPR false positive rate, *FNR* false negative rate, *FDR* false discovery rate, *FNDR* false non-discovery rate, *GSEA* gene set enrichment analysis, *GSA-ET* gene set analysis by Efron and Tibshirani, *RS* random set, *SAM-GS* significance analysis of microarray for gene sets, *ANCOVA* analysis of covariance

28.4.2.2 ROC Curve

On the ROC curve, each point represents a (TPR, FPR) pair corresponding to a particular decision threshold. To establish (TPR, FPR) pairs, we first sort all the gene sets according to increasing p values, yielding a top-ranked set list. Then cut the DE set at different places in the top-ranked set list. A perfect test should have an ROC plot that passes through the upper left corner. Therefore, the closer the ROC curve is to the upper left corner, the higher the overall accuracy of the test is (Zweig and Campbell 1993).

The plots of TPR versus FPR for all scenarios are shown in Fig. 28.1. For scenario 1, where all members in the sets of interest have 0.2 higher average expression in condition B, we see from these plots that, GSA-ET and GSEA perform best, much

Table 28.6 FPR, FNR, FDR, and FNDR for scenario 4

Methods	**FPR** Mean (SE)	**FNR** Mean (SE)	**FDR** Mean (SE)	**FNDR** Mean (SE)
GSEA	0.0134 (0.0009)	0.1430 (0.0061)	0.0787 (0.0048)	0.0248 (0.0010)
GSA-ET	0.0048 (0.0005)	0.1030 (0.0058)	0.0287 (0.0031)	0.0178 (0.0010)
RS	0.0885 (0.0020)	0.2420 (0.0066)	0.3942 (0.0058)	0.0446 (0.0012)
SAM-GS	0.0104 (0.0007)	0.0360 (0.0037)	0.0562 (0.0038)	0.0063 (0.0006)
Global test	0.0356 (0.0014)	0.0103 (0.0019)	0.1656 (0.0056)	0.0019 (0.0003)
Global ANCOVA	0.0474 (0.0016)	0.0083 (0.0017)	0.2091 (0.0057)	0.0015 (0.0003)
Combined *p*	0.0509 (0.0017)	0.0103 (0.0019)	0.2215 (0.0057)	0.0019 (0.0003)

FPR false positive rate, *FNR* false negative rate, *FDR* false discovery rate, *FNDR* false non-discovery rate, *GSEA* gene set enrichment analysis, *GSA-ET* gene set analysis by Efron and Tibshirani, *RS* random set, *SAM-GS* significance analysis of microarray for gene sets, *ANCOVA* analysis of covariance

Table 28.7 FPR, FNR, FDR, and FNDR for scenario 5

Methods	**FPR** Mean (SE)	**FNR** Mean (SE)	**FDR** Mean (SE)	**FNDR** Mean (SE)
GSEA	0.0102 (0.0007)	0.2460 (0.0084)	0.0689 (0.0046)	0.0418 (0.0014)
GSA-ET	0.0012 (0.0003)	0.1300 (0.0057)	0.0075 (0.0017)	0.0224 (0.0010)
RS	0.0346 (0.0014)	0.6710 (0.0087)	0.3670 (0.0103)	0.1091 (0.0012)
SAM-GS	0.0108 (0.0008)	0.0000 (0.0000)	0.0562 (0.0039)	0.0000 (0.0000)
Global test	0.0356 (0.0014)	0.0000 (0.0000)	0.1642 (0.0055)	0.0000 (0.0000)
Global ANCOVA	0.0468 (0.0016)	0.0000 (0.0000)	0.2059 (0.0055)	0.0000 (0.0000)
Combined *p*	0.0531 (0.0018)	0.0000 (0.0000)	0.2268 (0.0059)	0.0000 (0.0000)

FPR false positive rate, *FNR* false negative rate, *FDR* false discovery rate, *FNDR* false non-discovery rate, *GSEA* gene set enrichment analysis, *GSA-ET* gene set analysis by Efron and Tibshirani, *RS* random set, *SAM-GS* significance analysis of microarray for gene sets, *ANCOVA* analysis of covariance

better than other methods. The next best is RS. The performance of SAM-GS, global test, global ANCOVA, and the proposed combined p method are quite similar but not as good as GSA-ET, GSEA, and RS. As less genes in the sets of interest have larger average expression in condition B, GSEA and RS start working not as good, but GSA-ET still works well. Also, SAM-GS, global test, global ANCOVA, and combined p all show improved performance. This can be seen from Fig. 28.1, scenario 4, in which these four methods are superior to others. It indicates that SAM-GS, global test, global ANCOVA, and combined p are capable of detecting the gene sets with only 1/5 of the genes having 0.6 higher average expression in condition B. In the last scenario, SAM-GS, global test, global ANCOVA, and combined p show better performance than GSA-ET, GSEA, and RS. It is worth mentioning that our proposed combined p method is one of the best approaches in this particular case.

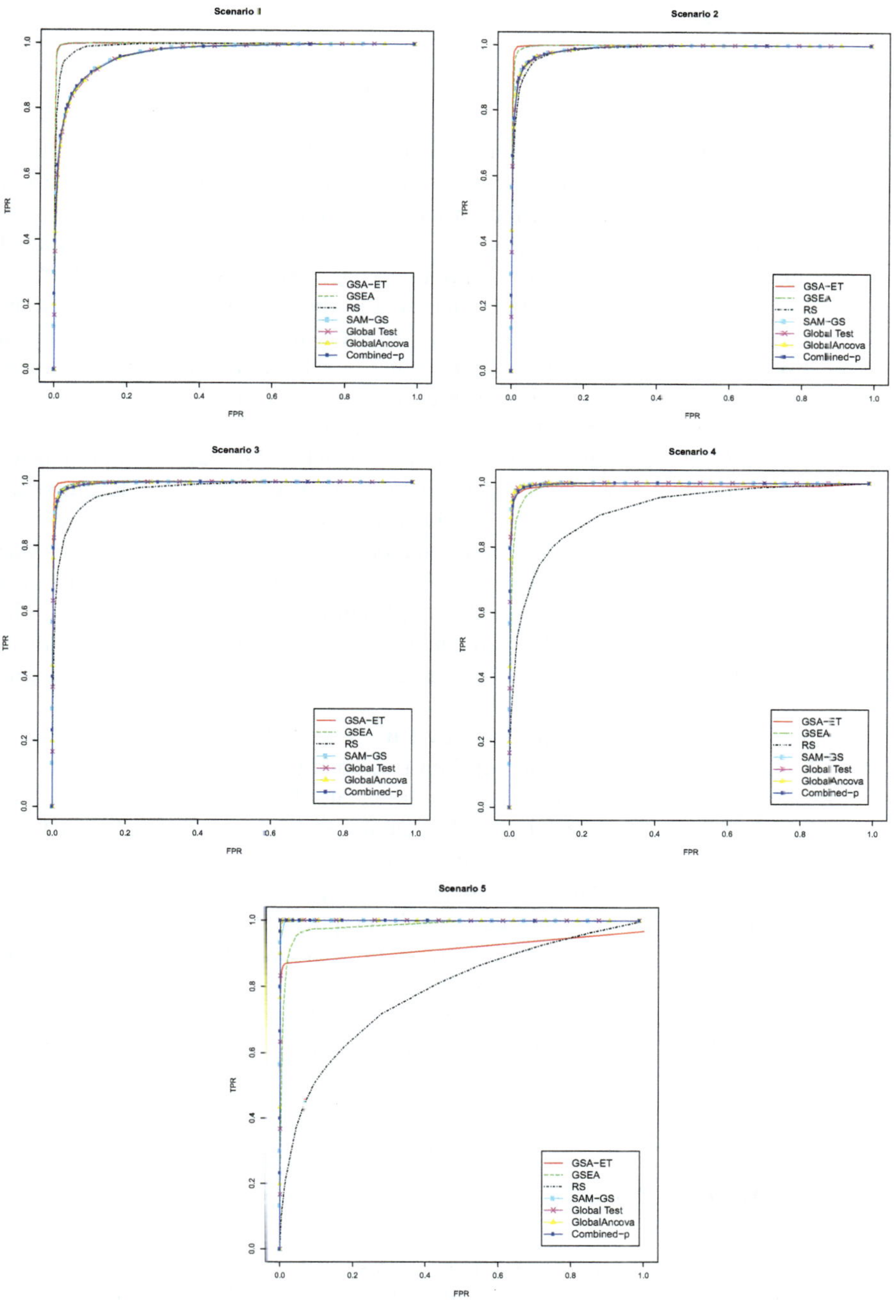

Fig. 28.1 Receiver operating characteristic (*ROC*) curves for scenarios 1–5

28.5 Real Data Analysis

28.5.1 Bone Data

Bone is a multifunctional, highly dynamic mineralized connective tissue that undergoes significant turnover. Osteoprogenitor lineage differentiation is one of the key processes responsible for bone formation and remodeling. During this process, a subpopulation of mesenchymal progenitors undergoes osteoblast lineage commitment and matures through a series of differentiation steps. Osteocytes represent the most abundant cellular component of mature mammalian bones with important functions in bone mass maintenance and remodeling. In order to selectively isolate defined populations of cells uncontaminated with other cell fractions, dual green fluorescent protein (GFP) reporter mice are utilized in which osteocytes are expressing GFP (topaz) directed by the DMP1 promoter, while osteoblasts are identified by expression of GFP (cyan) driven by 2.3 kb of the Col1a1 promoter. Comprehensive analysis of gene profiles and regulatory networks involved in skeletal development and remodeling is a prerequisite to elucidate the differential gene expression between osteoblasts and osteocytes, and completely understand physiological bone structure, function, and homeostasis. In Paic et al. (2009), the cRNA preparation and array hybridization are performed using Illumina microarray technology. The presence/absence call is determined and intensity values derived from the hybridization signals of each gene (i.e., Illumina source IDs) to represent their raw expression level.

We use the same data set considered by Paic et al. (2009) for our real data analysis. We consider the comparison between two conditions, cyan (osteoblasts) and topaz (osteocytes). There are four biological replicates for each condition and a total number of 45,856 genes in the data set. The scanned data are normalized before GSA using the R Bioconductor package "lumi" (Du et al. 2008) to rescale gene expression intensities across all Mouse-WG6 v1 BeadChip arrays used for hybridization of cRNA samples from four analyzed biological replicas. The annotations of the Illumina probe sets (source IDs) and corresponding genes are derived using the nuID part of the lumi software package (Du et al. 2007).

We use the 127 Kyoto Encyclopedia of Genes and Genomes (KEGG) pathways from the KEGG pathway database (*http://www. genome.jp/kegg*) as the gene sets for our GSA.

28.5.2 Analysis Results

Considering each KEGG pathway as a gene set, we are interested in those DE between osteoblasts and osteocytes. To achieve this goal, we apply GSA-ET, SAM-GS, and combined p method on the bone data introduced above, focusing on investigating DE KEGG pathways. For each method, we use 1000 as the number of permutations

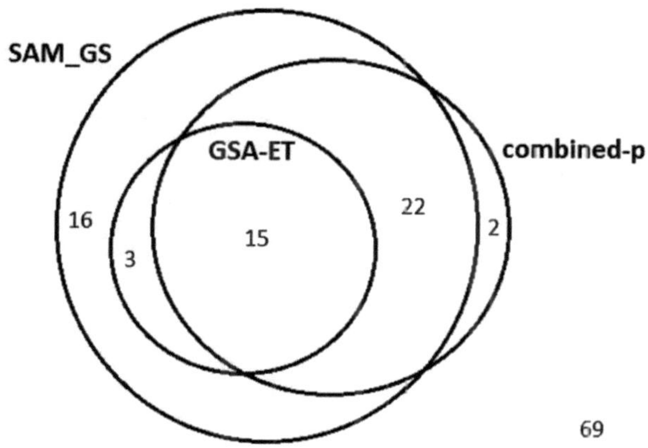

Fig. 28.2 Venn diagram of Kyoto Encyclopedia of Genes and Genomes (*KEGG*) pathway analysis

for the permutation test, and we use 0.1 as a cutoff of p value for each method to select pathways of interest.

We have summarized the number of pathways selected by each method from the 127 KEGG pathways in a Venn diagram as in Fig. 28.2. Out of 18 KEGG pathways selected by GSA-ET, 15 are also selected by SAM-GS and combined p, indicating a high likelihood of differential expression for these 15 pathways. There are a total of 25 pathways selected by two methods, where 22 of them are selected by SAM-GS and combined p, and the other three pathways are selected by only GSA-ET and SAM-GS. They should still be of interest. Additionally, there are 18 pathways selected only by one method, hence further investigations are needed to determine their regulation.

Note that two pathways, *glycosphingolipid (GSL) biosynthesis—globo series* and *sphingolipid metabolism* pathways, are selected by our proposed combined p method, but not by any of the other two methods. This finding that these two pathways are involved in the differentiation between osteoblasts and osteocytes is further supported by the following literature search. GSLs are a subtype of glycolipids containing the amino alcohol sphingosine. They are cell type-specific markers that change dramatically during ontogenesis and oncogenesis. Hakomori and Igarashi (1995) partially clarify the functional roles of GSLs in cellular interactions and control of cell proliferations in multicellular organisms. In addition, GSLs of the globo series are found to be associated with the monocytic lineage of human myeloid cells in Kniep et al. (1985). Sphingolipids are important for cell growth and differentiation (Wells and Lester 1983, Hanada et al. 1992), and they play major roles in cell recognition and adhesion (Hakomori and Igarashi 1995). Sphingolipids and their degradation products are claimed to be involved in signal transduction (Hannun 1996), and the formation of lipid rafts (Simons and Ikonen 1997). Spiegel and Merril (1996) point out that sphingolipid metabolites appear to serve as second messengers for growth factors, cytokines, and other "physiological" agonists. Tables 28.8 and 28.9 in Appendix illustrate the detailed information for these two pathways.

Table 28.8 Kyoto Encyclopedia of Genes and Genomes (*KEGG*) pathway: *Glycosphingolipid biosynthesis—globo series*

Gene symbol	Gene name	t_i	d_i	p_i
St6galnac2	ST6 (alpha-*N*-acetyl-neuraminyl-2,3-beta-galactosyl-1,3)-*N*-acetylgalactosaminide alpha-2,6-sialyltransferase 2	0.384	0.419	0.640
B4galt1	UDP-Gal:betaGlcNAc beta 1,4- galactosyltransferase, polypeptide 1	−0.100	−0.136	0.885
St8sia3	ST8 alpha-*N*-acetyl-neuraminide alpha-2,8-sialyltransferase 3	−1.220	−1.721	0.105
St8sia5	ST8 alpha-*N*-acetyl-neuraminide alpha-2,8-sialyltransferase 5	−1.116	−1.525	0.135
St3gal2	ST3 beta-galactoside alpha-2,3-sialyltransferase 2	1.196	1.416	0.139
St3gal2	ST3 beta-galactoside alpha-2,3-sialyltransferase 2	0.300	0.325	0.715
St8sia4	ST8 alpha-*N*-acetyl-neuraminide alpha-2,8-sialyltransferase 4	0.077	0.087	0.922
Gla	Galactosidase, alpha	−0.573	−0.656	0.467
St8sia1	ST8 alpha-*N*-acetyl-neuraminide alpha-2,8-sialyltransferase 1	−0.154	−0.223	0.822
Hexa	Hexosaminidase A	1.721	2.006	0.048
Hexb	Hexosaminidase B	2.429	2.643	0.016
St8sia3	ST8 alpha-*N*-acetyl-neuraminide alpha-2,8-sialyltransferase 3	0.855	1.368	0.239
St8sia2	ST8 alpha-*N*-acetyl-neuraminide alpha-2,8-sialyltransferase 2	−0.082	−0.092	0.917
Fut2	Fucosyltransferase 2	0.978	1.582	0.185
St6galnac2	ST6 (alpha-*N*-acetyl-neuraminyl-2,3-beta-galactosyl-1,3)-*N*-acetylgalactosaminide alpha-2,6-sialyltransferase 2	−0.401	−0.674	0.572
Naga	N-acetyl galactosaminidase, alpha	2.053	2.521	0.020
B4galnt2	Beta-1,4-*N*-acetyl-galactosaminyl transferase 2	−0.509	−0.831	0.472
St3gal2	ST3 beta-galactoside alpha-2,3-sialyltransferase 2	0.216	0.271	0.765
B3galt5	UDP-Gal:betaGlcNAc beta 1,3-galactosyltransferase, polypeptide 5	−0.050	−0.075	0.942

Table 28.8 (continued)

Gene symbol	Gene name	t_i	d_i	p_i
Fut7	Fucosyltransferase 7	0.775	1.037	0.285
B3galnt1	UDP-GalNAc:betaGlcNAc beta 1,3-galactosaminyltransferase, polypeptide 1	1.905	2.302	0.029
B4galt1	UDP-Gal:betaGlcNAc beta 1,4- galactosyltransferase, polypeptide 1	1.109	1.480	0.140
St8sia4	ST8 alpha-*N*-acetyl-neuraminide alpha-2,8-sialyltransferase 4	−0.728	−0.983	0.312
B4galt5	UDP-Gal:betaGlcNAc beta 1,4-galactosyltransferase, polypeptide 5	−0.424	−0.654	0.543
B4galt5	UDP-Gal:betaGlcNAc beta 1,4-galactosyltransferase, polypeptide 5	0.015	0.017	0.985
St8sia1	ST8 alpha-*N*-acetyl-neuraminide alpha-2,8-sialyltransferase 1	−0.620	−1.048	0.390
Fut4	Fucosyltransferase 4	0.073	0.089	0.921
Gla	Galactosidase, alpha	−2.497	−3.135	0.007
Summary Statistic		$S'_{maxmean} = 0.070$	$\overline{SAMGS} = \frac{\sum_{i=1}^{28} d_i^2}{28} = 1.855$	$\overline{TS_{obs}} = \frac{-2\sum_{i=1}^{28} \log(s_i)}{28} = 2.755$

UDP uridine diphosphate galactose

Table 28.9 Kyoto Encyclopedia of Genes and Genomes (*KEGG*) pathway: *Sphingolipid metabolism*

Gene symbol	Gene name	t_i	d_i	p_i
B4galt1	UDP-Gal:betaGlcNAc beta 1,4- galactosyltransferase, polypeptide 1	−0.100	−0.136	0.885
Glb1	Galactosidase, beta 1	−0.231	−0.259	0.770
Galc	Galactosylceramidase	−0.159	−0.228	0.817
Glb1	Galactosidase, beta 1	0.339	0.462	0.627
Glb1	Galactosidase, beta 1	0.764	1.062	0.286
Smpd2	Sphingomyelin phosphodiesterase 2, neutral	0.547	0.719	0.445
Sphk1	Sphingosine kinase 1	0.343	0.400	0.654
Gba	Glucosidase, beta, acid	−0.895	−1.058	0.255
Galc	Galactosylceramidase	−0.587	−0.736	0.425
Sphk2	Sphingosine kinase 2	0.173	0.233	0.804
Sphk2	Sphingosine kinase 2	0.908	1.264	0.212
Sphk1	Sphingosine kinase 1	−0.209	−0.275	0.766
Smpd1	Sphingomyelin phosphodiesterase 1, acid lysosomal	0.470	0.488	0.589
Smpd3	Sphingomyelin phosphodiesterase 3, neutral	−0.546	−0.573	0.527
Asah1	*N*-acylsphingosine amidohydrolase 1	0.004	0.004	0.997
Asah1	*N*-acylsphingosine amidohydrolase 1	−0.953	−1.463	0.191
Sptlc1	Serine palmitoyltransferase, long chain base subunit 1	0.613	0.792	0.398
Smpd2	Sphingomyelin phosphodiesterase 2, neutral	−0.309	−0.387	0.670
Sphk1	Sphingosine kinase 1	1.781	2.075	0.043
Sptlc2	Serine palmitoyltransferase, long chain base subunit 2	−0.383	−0.523	0.584
Gla	Galactosidase, alpha	−0.573	−0.656	0.467
Glb1	Galactosidase, beta 1	2.425	3.428	0.007
Galc	Galactosylceramidase	0.082	0.101	0.910
Neu1	Neuraminidase 1	2.291	3.019	0.010
Gal3st1	Galactose-3-*O*-sulfotransferase 1	−0.201	−0.229	0.797
Galc	Galactosylceramidase	0.741	0.959	0.311
Sptlc2	Serine palmitoyltransferase, long chain base subunit 2	0.560	0.805	0.424
Sgpp1	Sphingosine-1-phosphate phosphatase 1	0.805	0.900	0.325
Glb1	Galactosidase, beta 1	−0.564	−0.866	0.422
Neu1	Neuraminidase 1	0.358	0.428	0.633
Neu3	Neuraminidase 3	1.115	1.440	0.143

Table 28.9 (continued)

Gene symbol	Gene name	t_i	d_i	p_i
Sgpl1	Sphingosine phosphate lyase 1	1.203	1.382	0.147
Smpd1	Sphingomyelin phosphodiesterase 1, acid lysosomal	−0.036	−0.041	0.963
Sphk1	Sphingosine kinase 1	1.648	2.257	0.040
Ugcg	UDP-glucose ceramide glucosyltransferase	−1.489	−1.719	0.081
B4galnt2	Beta-1,4-*N*-acetyl-galactosaminyl transferase 2	−0.509	−0.831	0.472
Smpd3	Sphingomyelin phosphodiesterase 3, neutral	−0.575	−0.651	0.470
Fut7	Fucosyltransferase 7	0.775	1.037	0.285
Sgms2	Sphingomyelin synthase 2	−0.155	−0.174	0.844
B4galt1	UDP-Gal:betaGlcNAc beta 1,4-galactosyltransferase, polypeptide 1	1.109	1.480	0.140
Neu2	Neuraminidase 2	−0.456	−0.545	0.545
Sphk2	Sphingosine kinase 2	0.181	0.191	0.830
Phca	Phytoceramidase, alkaline	3.087	3.778	0.003
Phca	Phytoceramidase, alkaline	2.730	3.448	0.005
B4galt5	UDP-Gal:betaGlcNAc beta 1,4-galactosyltransferase, polypeptide 5	−0.424	−0.654	0.543
B4galt5	UDP-Gal:betaGlcNAc beta 1,4-galactosyltransferase, polypeptide 5	0.015	0.017	0.935
Degs2	Degenerative spermatocyte homolog 2 (Drosophila), lipid desaturase	0.288	0.442	0.677
Asah1	*N*-acylsphingosine amidohydrolase 1	3.219	4.609	0.001
Degs1	Degenerative spermatocyte homolog 1 (Drosophila)	−0.691	−0.943	0.334
Fut4	Fucosyltransferase 4	0.073	0.089	0.921
Gla	Galactosidase, alpha	−2.497	−3.135	0.007
Summary Statistic		$S'_{maxmean} =$ 0.145	$\overline{SAMGS} = \frac{\sum_{i=1}^{51} d_i^2}{51} = 2.231$	$\overline{TS_{cbs}} = \frac{-2\sum_{i=1}^{51} \log(s_i)}{51} = 2.790$

UDP uridine diphosphate galactose

We have also used 0.05 as the cutoff of *p* value for each of the three methods. Only one pathway is in common among all three methods and ten pathways are selected by the combined *p* method only and missed by both GSA-ET and SAM-GS. However, eight out of the ten pathways are not "real" miss because they have relatively small *p* values (between 0.05 and 0.1) by other methods. If we eliminate these eight pathways which are in the borderline, the remaining two pathways are exactly the same as what we have obtained before by using the *p* value = 0.1 as the cutoff. Therefore, this reduces to our previous gene ontology (GO) findings.

28.6 Discussions

We have reviewed six different methods on the analysis of the high-throughput microarray gene expression data at the level of groups of genes rather than individual genes. A new gene set method based on combining individual *p* values for genes in the set is proposed. All seven methods, including the proposed one, are compared via simulation studies. Based on our simulation results, we cannot say any single method is superior to others all the time, or any one is the weakest among all. As we have discussed in Sect. 28.4.2, GSEA and GSA-ET outperform others in the case that all genes in the set have 0.2 higher average expression or 3/5 of genes in the set have 0.3 higher average expression in condition B. Nevertheless, in cases that only 1/5 of genes in the set have 0.6 higher average expression in condition B or there are genes with higher average expression in both conditions, SAM-GS works relatively better. Furthermore, our proposed combined *p* approach performs satisfactorily. It maintains low FNR and low FNDR all the time. One advantage of combined *p* method worthy mentioning is that when data are confidential and only *p* values are available, one can still implement GSA. Therefore, we suggest including it in the data analysis to complement with other methods. For the real data analysis, we apply GSA-ET, SAM-GS, and combined *p* method on the bone data set and search for the DE pathways between osteoblasts and osteocytes. Fifteen pathways are commonly selected by all three methods. In particular, we note that the proposed combined *p* method selects *GSL biosynthesis—globo series* and *sphingolipid metabolism* pathways. The importance of these two pathways in osteoblast lineage differentiation are further supported by our literature search. We suggest further study to be conducted to confirm this finding.

Acknowledgements The authors would like to thank Dr. David Rowe and Dr. Dong-Guk Shin for sharing the data set used in the real data analysis. They further acknowledge a stem cell grant 06SCC04 from Connecticut Innovations, Connecticut, that provided partial support for the early phase of the first author's graduate study.

Appendix

Tables 28.8 and 28.9 illustrate the information of *GSL biosynthesis—globo series* and *sphingolipid metabolism* pathways in detail. This information includes gene source IDs in the particular pathway (meaning the overlap of mouse Illumina source IDs from the KEGG pathway database and our data set), corresponding gene symbols and gene names, individual gene-level scores used for GSA-ET, SAM-GS, and combined p method. Summary statistics indicating the observed set scores for these three methods are $S'_{maxmean}$ (28.2), $SAMGS$ (28.8), and TS_{obs} (28.20), respectively. Note that $S'_{maxmean}$ is an average, while $SAMGS$ and TS_{obs} are summations, so we divided $SAMGS$ and TS_{obs} by the set size (denoted by $\overline{SAMGS}$ and $\overline{TS_{obs}}$) to make them more comparable to $S'_{maxmean}$. These three summary statistics are also listed at the bottom in the tables.

References

Abatangelo L, Maglietta R, Distaso A, D'Addabbo A, Creanza TM, Mukherjee S, Ancona N (2009) Comparative study of gene set enrichment methods. BMC Bioinform 10:275–286

Bahadur RR (1967) Rates of convergence of estimates and tests statistics. Ann Math Stat 38:303–324

Brown M (1975) A method for combining non-independent, one-sided tests of significance. Biometrics 31(4):987–992

Dinu I, Potter JD, Mueller T, Liu Q, Adewale AJ, Jhangri GS, Einecke G, Famulski KS, Halloran P, Yasui Y (2007) Improving gene set analysis of mocroarray data by SAM-GS. BMC Bioinform 8:242

Dinu I, Liu Q, Potter JD, Adewale AJ, Jhangri GS, Mueller T, Einecke G, Famulsky K, Halloran P, Yasui Y (2008) A biological evaluation of six gene set analysis methods for identification of differentially expressed pathways in microarray data. Cancer Bioinform 6:357–368

Du P, Kibbe WA, Lin SM (2007) Nuid: a universal naming schema of oligonucleotides for Illumina, Affymetrix, and other microarrays. Biol Direct 2:16

Du P, Kibbe WA, Lin SM (2008) Lumi: A pipeline for processing Illumina microarray. Bioinformatics 24(13):1547–1554

Efron B, Tibshirani R (2007) On testing the significance of a set of genes. Ann Appl Stat 1(1):107–129

Fisher RA (1932) Statistical methods for research workers, 4th edn. Oliver and Boyd, Edinburgh

Goeman JJ, Van de Geer SA, De Kort F, Van Houwelingen HC (2004) A global test for groups of genes: testing association with a clinical outcome. Bioinformatics 20(1):93–99

Hakomori S, Igarashi Y (1995) Functional role of glycosphingolipids in cell recognition and signaling. J Biochem 118(6):1091–1103

Hanada K, Nishijima M, Kiso M, Hasegawa A, Fujita S, Ogawa T, Akamatsu Y (1992) Sphingolipids are essential for the growth of Chinese hamster ovary cells. restoration of the growth of a mutant defective in sphingoid base biosynthesis by exogenous sphingolipids. J Bio Chem 267:23527–23533

Hannun YA (1996) Functions of ceramide in coordinating cellular responses to stress. Science 274:1855–1859

Hedges LV, Olkin I (1985) Statistical methods for meta-analysis. Academic, Orlando

Kniep B, Monner DA, Schwulléra U, Mühlradt PF (1985) Glycosphingolipids of the globo-series are associated with the monocytic lineage of human myeloid cells. Eur J Biochem 149:187–191

Kost J, McDermott M (2002) Combining dependent p-values. Stat Probab Lett 60(2):183–190

Le Cessie S, Van Houwelingen HC (1995) Testing the fit of a regression model via score tests in random effects models. Biometrics 61(2):600–614
Littell RC, Folks JL (1971) Asymptotic optimal of Fisher's method of combining independent tests. J Am Stat Assoc 66:802–807
Littell RC, Folks JL (1973) Asymptotic optimal of Fisher's method of combining independent tests. II. J Am Stat Assoc 68:193–196
Liu Q, Dinu I, Adewale AJ, Potter JD, Yasui Y (2007) Comparative evaluation of gene-set analysis methods. BMC Bioinform 8:431–445
Mansmann U, Meister R (2005) Testing differential gene expression in functional groups. Methods Inf Med 44:449–453
Mootha VK, Lindgren CM, Eriksson KF, Subramanian A, Sihag S, Lehar J, Puigserver P, Carlsson E, Ridderstrale M, Laurila E (2003) PGC-1alpha-responsive genes involved in oxidative phosphorylation are coordinately downregulated in human diabetes. Nat Genet 34:267–273
Murdock D, Tsai Y, Adcock J (2008) P-values are random variables. Am Stat 62:242–245
Nam D, Kim SY (2008) Gene-set approach for expression pattern analysis. Brief Bioinform 9:189–197
Newton MA, Quintana FA, Boon JA, Sengupta S, Ahlquist P (2007) Random-set methods identify distinct aspect of the enrichment signal in gene-set analysis. Ann Appl Stat 1(1):85–106
Owen AB (2009) Karl Pearson's meta-analysis revisited. Ann Stat 37(6B):3867–3892
Paic F, Igwe JC, Nori R, Kronenberg MS, Franceschetti T, Harrington P, Kuo L, Shin DG, Rowe DW, Harris SE, Kalajzic I (2009) Identification of differentially expressed genes between osteoblasts and osteocytes. Bone 45(4):682–692
Pan KH, Lih CJ, Cohen SN (2005) Effects of threshold choice on biological conclusions reached during analysis of gene expression by DNA microarrays. Proc Natl Acad Sci U S A 102:8961–8965
Simons K, Ikonen E (1997) Functional rafts in cell membranes. Nature 387:569–572
Spiegel S, Merril AJ (1996) Sphingolipid metabolism and cell growth regulation. FASEB J 10:1388–1397
Subramanian A, Tamayo P, Mootha VK, Mukherjee S, Ebert BL, Gillette MA, Paulovich A, Pomeroy SL, Golub TR, Lander ES, Mesirov JP (2005) Gene set enrichment analysis: a knowledge-based approach for interpreting genome-wide expression profiles. Proc Natl Acad Sci U S A 102:15545–15550
Tarca AL, Bhatti G, Romero R (2013) A comparison of gene set analysis methods in terms of sensitivity, prioritization and specificity. PLoS ONE 8(11):e79217
Tian L, Greenberg SA, Kong SW, Altschuler J, Kohane IS, Park PJ (2005) Discovering statistically significant pathways in expression profiling studies. Proc Natl Acad Sci U S A 102:13544–13549
Tippett LH (1931) The methods of statistics. Williams and Norgate, London
Tomfohr J, Lu J, Kepler TB (2005) Pathway level analysis of gene expression using singular value decomposition. BMC Bioinform 6:225
Tusher V, Tibshirani R, Chu G (2001) Significance analysis of microarrays applied to the ionizing radiation response. Proc Natl Acad Sci U S A 98:5116–5121
Wells GB, Lester RL (1983) The isolation and characterization of a mutant strain of *Saccharomyces cerevisiae* that requires a long chain base for growth and for synthesis of phosphosphingolipids. J Bio Chem 258:10200–10203
Zweig MH, Campbell G (1993) Receiver-operating characteristic (ROC) plots: a fundamental evaluation tool in clinical medicine. Clin Chem 39:561–577

Chapter 29
A Simple Method for Testing Global and Individual Hypotheses Involving a Limited Number of Possibly Correlated Outcomes

A. Lawrence Gould

Abstract Tests for the presence of a global treatment effect expressed by possibly correlated "primary" outcome variables taken together frequently use Bonferroni-type adjustments. These procedures accommodate an arbitrary number of comparisons, but can be conservative if the outcome variables are highly correlated. This conservatism can be ameliorated by a simple rule requiring essentially no calculation (and therefore convenient to apply when exact calculation is impractical) that is relatively robust to the correlation structure of the responses when the number of comparisons is not large (16 or less for 5 % level tests). The recommended global testing rule is: For a type 1 error rate of α and up to $K(\alpha)$ "primary" response variables, reject the global null hypothesis if (a) the smallest marginal p value is slightly less than $\alpha_1 = \alpha/K$, (b) the second smallest marginal p value is $\leq 2\alpha_1$, or (c) the third smallest marginal p value is $\leq \alpha$. Analytic expressions that do not assume independence or any particular distribution for the responses are provided for the probability of rejecting the global null hypothesis. The type 1 error rates and power generally are preserved regardless of the correlation structure. Individual comparisons can be tested if the global null hypothesis is rejected, with reasonable preservation of comparison-wise type 1 error rates and of the false discovery rates (FDRs).

29.1 Introduction

Effects of treatments or interventions often are expressed by several prespecified outcome variables instead of a single "primary" variable in, for example, the clinical evaluation of psychotherapeutic and antiarthritic agents, treatments of asthma and gastroesophageal reflux disease, and nondrug interventions. When inferences regarding the existence of a treatment effect are based on tests of hypotheses about the effect of treatment on each individual outcome variable, multiplicity adjustments to the individual critical values generally are necessary to control at a specified level α, the probability of concluding that there is a treatment effect overall or for the

---

A. L. Gould (✉)
Merck Research Laboratories, UG1D-88, North Wales, PA 19454, USA
Tel.: (267) 305-6888
e-mail: goulda@merck.com

Z. Chen et al. (eds.), *Applied Statistics in Biomedicine and Clinical Trials Design*,
ICSA Book Series in Statistics, DOI 10.1007/978-3-319-12694-4_29

individual outcome variables when there truly is none. These usually require calculations that may not be convenient in some circumstances, such as when listening to a presentation or when evaluations need to be done quickly or manually. The prespecification of the outcome variables means that the individual hypotheses are identified at the outset.

Many recent articles describe methods for controlling type 1 error rates of various kinds in the evaluation of the outcomes of genotyping experiments based on micorarrays when there are hundreds or thousands of individual comparisons to identify enhanced or suppressed gene expression. Farcomeni (2008) and Storey et al. (2004) provide reviews of current methods. When the number of component hypotheses is relatively small (≤ 16, say), which typically happens in large scale clinical trials when there are multiple primary outcomes, a suggestion by Sen (1999) can be exploited to yield a testing procedure that requires no calculation.

Testing strategies using individual comparisons for multiple outcome variables generally proceed as follows. Let p_i denote the conventional p value computed for testing the i-th of K individual null hypothesis $H_{0i}, i = 1, \ldots, K$, and let $p_{(1)} \leq . p_{(2)} \leq \cdots \leq p_{(K)}$ denote the ordered p values. If $\alpha_K = \{\alpha_{K1}, \alpha_{K2}, \ldots, \alpha_{KK}\}$ with $\alpha_{K1} \leq \alpha_{K2,} \leq \ldots \leq \alpha_{KK}$ denotes a set of adjusted type 1 error rates, then the i-th null hypothesis H_{0i} (and the global null hypothesis H_0) could be rejected if $p_{(i)} < \alpha_{Ki}$ for some i. Different tests arise from different choices for α_K, e.g., (Sen 1999; Benjamini and Stark 1996; Bonferroni 1936; Farcomeni and Pacillo 2011; Farcomeni and Finos 2013; Finner and Roters 2002; Finner and Gontscharuk 2009; Finos and Farcomeni 2011; Hochberg 1988; Hochberg and Rom 1995; Hochberg and Benjamini 1990; Holland and Copenhaver 1987; Holland and Copenhaver 1988; Holm 1979; Hommel 1988; James 1991; Liu 1996; Rom 1990; Rom and Connell 1994; Sarkar and Chang 1997; Sarkar 1998; Sarkar 2008; Simes 1986; van der Laan M et al. 2004). Classical testing method set $\alpha_{K1} = \alpha_{K2,} = \ldots = \alpha_{KK} = \alpha^*$, e.g., the Bonferroni procedure (1936) that sets $\alpha^* = \alpha_B = \alpha/K$. These methods can be very conservative, especially if the outcome variables are positively correlated. This chapter addresses a particularly interesting choice for α_K that does not seem to have been considered in detail. The method sets $\alpha_{K3} = \ldots = \alpha_{KK}$ (Sen 1999) and rejects the global null hypothesis if $p_{(1)} < \alpha_{K1}$ or if $p_{(2)} < \alpha_{K2}$ or if $p_{(3)} < \alpha_{K3}$, where α_{K1}, α_{K2}, and α_{K3} are chosen to control the global type 1 error rate at α. This rule is not the same as any of the conventional step-up or step-down rules. Recent reviews of methods for testing multiple hypotheses based on ordered p values do not address this testing strategy (Farcomeni 2008; Storey et al. 2004; Sarkar 2008; Hommel et al. 2011; Sarkar et al. 2012).

The elements of the procedure are described in Sect. 2, including guidance on sample size determination. Power comparisons over a variety of correlation patterns are provided in Sect. 3 when K = 5. Section 4 addresses tests of the individual members of the collection of outcomes. A number of examples are presented in Sect. 5, and some concluding remarks are given in Sect. 6. Technical details and derivations are provided in Appendix 1. Appendix 2 provides R code for carrying out the simulations discussed in Sects. 3 and 4.

29.2 Elements of the Method

Suppose that a collection Ω of prespecified null hypotheses $\{H_{0i}\}$ to be tested using the outcomes of an experiment or trial is minimal (Gabriel 1969) or "free-combination" (Grechanovsky and Pinsker 1999) in the sense that the component hypotheses are not functionally related. Suppose further that there are at most $K(\alpha)$ such null hypotheses, where α is the nominal type 1 error rate.

A global null hypothesis that all of the component null hypotheses are true is tested using the following simple strategy: Reject the global null hypothesis if $p_{(1)} \le \alpha_{K1}$, or if $p_{(2)} \le \alpha_{K2}$, or if $p_{(3)} \le \alpha$. The critical values α_{K1} and α_{K2} must satisfy $\alpha_{K1} = \alpha/K - \varepsilon$ and $\alpha_{K2} = 2\alpha_{K1}$, where ε is a small, analytically determined, positive number, $\varepsilon \ll \alpha/K$, so that α_{K1} and α_{K2} are slightly less than the corresponding bounds for Simes's test (1986) when $K > 3$ (they are the same when $K \le 3$). The ability to reach a decision using the first three ordered p values more than compensates for the slight diminution of the first two bounds, and the proposed procedure has power no less than that of Simes's test. Slightly decreasing the value of α_{K1} below α_3 provides an opportunity to increase α_{K3} to α when the number of component tests is bounded.

Table 29.1 provides the maximum values that can be taken by α_{K1} (see Appendix 1). These values are for all practical purposes negligibly less than the values used for Simes's test, especially when fewer than ten comparisons are to be made. The values are scaled for readability, e.g., the upper leftmost entry (167) means that the value of α_{1max} is 0.0167. If $K = 8$, then both α/K and α_{1max} are approximately equal to 0.006 (actually, 0.00625 and 0.0058, respectively).

The power and, therefore, the sample size needed, for rejecting a global null hypothesis depends on the joint distribution of the outcomes under an alternative hypothesis. An alternative hypothesis could specify a constant shift for each component outcome such as $H_{1i} : \theta_i = \theta^* \ne \theta_{i0}$ for all i, or a shift with respect to some, but not all, of the component outcome distributions, so that the alternative hypothesis would be defined by $H_{1i} : \theta_i = \theta_{i1} \ne \theta_{i0}$ for $i \in \{i_1, \ldots, i_m\} \subset \{1, \ldots, K\}$, and $\theta_i = \theta_{i0}$ otherwise. Section A1.5 of Appendix 1 describes the computation of noncentrality parameter and sample size values. Noncentrality parameter values commonly are expressed as a ratio such as $\theta = \mu\sqrt{n}/\sigma$, where μ denotes a shift, n denotes a sample size, and σ is a measure of variability such as the standard deviation. Table 29.2 provides noncentrality parameter values calculated assuming normality for $K = 3$ (1) 16 and when $m = 1$ (1) min (5,K) of the K means are positive.

29.3 Computational Results

The statistical properties of the proposed method relative to the methods described by Benjamini and Hochberg (1995) and by Benjamini and Liu (1999) are addressed in Tables 29.3, 29.4, 29.5, 29.6, and 29.7 of this section and the following section for various correlation structures and patterns of nonzero means assuming a common

Table 29.1 Values of α_{1max}, α/K, and their difference ($\times\ 10^{-4}$)

	$\alpha = 0.05$			$\alpha = 0.025$			$\alpha = 0.05$			$\alpha = 0.025$			
K	α_{1max}	α_B	ε	α_{1max}	α_B	ε	K	α_{1max}	α_B	ε	α_{1max}	α_B	ε
3	167	167	0	83	83	< 1	10	41	5	09	24	25	1
4	125	125	0	63	63	< 1	11	35	45	11	21	23	2
5	99	100	1	50	50	< 1	12	28	42	13	19	21	2
6	81	83	2	41	42	< 1	13	22	38	16	17	19	2
7	68	71	3	35	36	< 1	14	16	36	19	15	18	3
8	58	62	5	31	31	1	15	11	33	22	14	17	3
9	49	56	6	27	28	1	16	05	31	26	12	16	4

Table 29.2 Noncentrality parameter values $\theta\ (= \mu\sqrt{n}/\sigma)$ yielding 90 % power for rejecting at the 5 % level H_0: "all K independent responses have zero mean" using the rule based on $S_1 \cup S_2 \cup S_3$, when m of the K means are positive

m	K = 3	4	5	6	7	8	9
1	3.65	3.75	3.83	3.89	3.95	4.00	4.04
2	2.83	2.93	3.00	3.05	3.10	3.15	3.18
3	2.43	2.52	2.58	2.62	2.66	2.69	2.72
4		2.26	2.31	2.35	2.38	2.41	2.43
5			2.12	2.16	2.18	2.20	2.22
m	K = 10	11	12	13	14	15	16
1	4.09	4.14	4.20	4.26	4.34	4.45	4.63
2	3.22	3.26	3.30	3.35	3.41	3.49	3.65
3	2.74	2.77	2.79	2.82	2.86	2.91	2.99
4	2.45	2.46	2.48	2.51	2.53	2.56	2.61
5	2.24	2.25	2.27	2.28	2.30	2.32	2.36

variance via simulations consisting of 10,000 random observations from (K =) 5-dimensional multivariate normal distributions. A set of 286 correlation patterns were considered initially, consisting of ordered combinations of some or all of 0, 0.1, 0.5, and 0.9. Not all of the corresponding correlation patterns turned out to be positive definite. The calculations used the 141 correlation patterns corresponding to the positive definite correlation matrices. The determinants of the correlation matrices (det(R)) ranged from 0.0005 to 1. The variable least correlated with the other variables has a nonzero mean in case 2, while the variable most correlated with the other variables has a nonzero mean in case 3. A similar comment applies for case 5 as opposed to case 6.

29.3.1 *Type 1 Error Rate*

The top row of Table 29.3 presents the type 1 error rates for the $S_1 \cup S_2 \cup S_3$ rule calculated directly from expression (A4) in Appendix 1. The simulated type 1 error rates for all of the cases were (mean, min, max) = (4.9, 4.5, 5.5), suggesting good type 1 error control. For comparison, the corresponding (mean, min, max) values for the Benjamini–Hochberg and Benjamini–Liu procedures based on all of the cases were (B–H: 4.6, 3.6, 5.4; B–L: 4.4, 3.1, 5.4).

29.3.2 *Power*

The power of the $S_1 \cup S_2 \cup S_3$ rule for rejecting the global null hypothesis depends on the pattern of the nonzero noncentrality parameters when the outcomes are not independent. Table 29.3 summarizes the power values corresponding to 15 configurations of the nonzero means (noncentrality parameters). The noncentrality parameter values were drawn from Table 29.2.

The power was 89–90 % when the variables were uncorrelated [det(R) = 1] for all cases. The effect of intercorrelations among the variables on the power depended on the number of nonzero means and the degree of correlation. In general, the average power was less for cases when det(R) < 0.4. The range of achieved power was much smaller for cases when det(R) > 0.4. The power tended to be less when the nonzero means were among the most highly correlated variables, as in cases 6 and 10, for example. This was especially pronounced when the correlation matrices were nearly singular. Table 29.4 compares the average power for rejecting a false global null hypothesis of the $S_1 \cup S_2 \cup S_3$ hypothesis-testing rule with the average power for the Benjamini–Hochberg and Benjamini–Liu rules. The power is about the same for all of the approaches in all of the cases.

29.4 Individual Comparisons

Comparison-wise testing procedures often are evaluated using the "false discovery rate" (FDR) = Pr(H_{0i} true | H_{0i} rejected) (Benjamini Hochberg 1995), as opposed to the Type 1 error rate = Pr(H_{0i} rejected | H_{0i} true). The type 1 error rate does not depend on how many individual H_{0i} are true. However, the FDR increases when few of the individual null hypotheses are false because it is the same as 1—positive predictive value used to evaluate diagnostic procedures, which does depend on the prevalence of true negatives (true H_{0i}). The strategy for testing individual comparisons therefore depends on how many null hypotheses are tested and how many are likely to be false.

The following variation of the Benjamini and Hochberg (1995) approach for individual comparisons is proposed. First, carry out individual comparisons only if the global null hypothesis is rejected. If half or more of the comparison-wise *p* values

Table 29.3 Size and power properties of the $S_1 \cup S_2 \cup S_3$ rule for testing the global null hypothesis as a function of the degree of correlation among the outcome variables and the pattern of true nonzero means (denoted by "X" in the pattern) when there are five outcome variables, except for case 1 which corresponds to the null hypothesis that all means equal to zero. The target power is 90 %. det(R) is the determinant of the correlation matrix

		All ($n = 141$)			det(R) ≥ 0.4 (38)			det(R) < 0.4 (103)		
Case	Pattern	Mean	Min.	Max.	Mean	Min.	Max.	Mean	Min.	Max.
1	00000	4.9	4.5	5.5	5.0	4.5	5.5	4.8	4.5	5.3
2	X0000	90.1	89.5	91.2	90.1	89.5	90.7	90.1	89.5	91.7
3	0000X	90.7	89.6	91.9	90.4	89.6	91.1	90.9	90.1	91.9
4	X000X	88.5	82.8	90.9	89.6	88.3	90.7	88.0	75.8	90.9
5	XX000	89.8	83.3	91.1	90.0	88.6	90.8	89.6	76.7	91.1
6	000XX	80.3	75.4	90.7	85.1	82.7	90.7	78.5	75.4	84.6
7	00XX0	84.4	75.5	90.6	88.1	83.3	90.6	83.0	75.5	90.0
8	0XX00	87.4	76.0	90.9	89.5	88.5	90.6	86.5	76.0	90.9
9	XXX00	87.8	74.7	90.7	89.5	87.7	90.7	87.0	68.4	90.5
10	00XXX	78.0	68.5	89.9	83.8	77.9	89.9	75.7	68.5	83.3
11	XX00X	86.6	74.4	90.8	89.2	87.7	90.8	85.5	68.2	90.4
12	X00XX	83.1	74.4	90.0	86.7	84.5	90.0	81.7	68.5	86.8
13	0XXX0	83.4	68.5	90.8	88.0	84.5	90.8	81.5	68.5	90.3
14	XXXX0	84.4	68.5	90.1	88.1	84.9	90.1	82.9	62.3	90.0
15	0XXXX	78.0	61.9	90.2	84.8	80.5	90.2	75.4	61.9	85.1
16	XXXXX	80.0	62.7	89.6	85.7	81.4	89.6	77.8	57.9	86.0

are less than α, then reject the individual null hypotheses whose *p* values are less than α. If fewer than half are less than α, then calculate adjusted *p* values as described by Benjamini and Hochberg (1995):

$$p_{adj(K)} = p_{(K)} \tag{29.1}$$

$$p_{adj(i)} = \min(p_{adj(i+1)},\ (K/i) \times p_{(i)}, i = K-1,\ \ldots,\ 1$$

and reject the individual null hypotheses whose adjusted *p* values are $< \alpha$. A simpler way to state (29.1) when using the procedure described here is to reject H_{0i} if $p_{(i)} < i\alpha/K$.

Table 29.5 summarizes the FDR for the proposed procedure and the Benjamini and Hochberg, and Benjamini and Liu procedures for the same correlation patterns used to construct Tables 29.3 and 29.4, and for a variety of patterns of nonzero means whose values were drawn from Table 29.2.

Cases 1 and 16 are omitted because their corresponding FDRs are fixed by definition (FDR ≡ 100 % in case 1 and FDR = 0 in case 16). All of the procedures controlled the FDR reasonably well when the outcomes were not highly correlated

Table 29.4 Average percent power of the $S_1 \cup S_2 \cup S_3$ ("Rule 3") rule for testing the global null hypothesis relative to the Benjamini–Hochberg and Benjamini–Liu approaches. Case 1 corresponds to the global null hypothesis (pattern = 00000); "X" denotes a positive mean

		All			det(R) ≥ 0.4			det(R) < 0.4		
Case	Pattern	Rule3	B–H	B–L	Rule3	B–H	B–L	Rule3	B–H	B–L
1	00000	4.9	4.6	4.4	5.0	5.0	5.0	4.8	4.5	4.2
2	X0000	90	90	90	90	90	90	90	90	90
3	0000X	91	91	91	90	90	90	91	91	91
4	X000X	89	88	88	90	89	89	88	88	87
5	XX000	90	90	89	90	90	89	90	89	89
6	000XX	80	80	79	85	85	84	78	78	77
7	00XX0	84	84	83	88	88	87	83	83	82
8	0XX00	87	87	86	89	89	89	87	86	86
9	XXX00	88	87	86	90	89	88	87	86	85
10	00XXX	78	76	74	84	83	82	76	74	72
11	XX00X	87	86	85	89	88	87	86	85	83
12	X00XX	83	82	80	87	86	85	82	80	79
13	0XXX0	83	82	81	88	87	86	82	80	79
14	XXXX0	84	83	81	88	87	85	83	81	80
15	0XXXX	78	76	74	85	83	82	75	73	71
16	XXXXX	80	78	76	86	84	82	78	75	73

(det(R) > 0.4). The FDR values for the Benjamini–Hochberg and Benjamini–Liu procedures generally were less than a nominal 5 % error rate. The FDR values for all of the procedures tended to decrease substantially when many of the component null hypotheses were false.

The FDR is not the only metric that can be used to assess misclassification. It also is possible to fail to identify true differences, that is, the probability that a particular hypothesis H_{0i} is false given that it was not rejected, which we term the "missed discovery rate" or MDR (See also Hwang et al. 2011, where it is called the "false non-discovery rate."). Table 29.6 displays MDR values for the "Rule of 3," Benjamini–Hochberg, and Benjamini–Liu procedures for the cases considered in Table 29.5.

The MDRs are slightly lower for the Rule of 3 procedure than for the other two procedures. They do not depend greatly on the correlation structure but, as expected, do depend on how many of the component null hypotheses are false.

Another desirable property of multiple comparison procedures is control of the family-wise error rate (FWER), that is, the probability of rejecting a true null hypothesis. In the context of diagnostic testing, the probability of rejecting any true null hypothesis is the complement of the specificity, which here is the probability of not

Table 29.5 False discovery rates (FDR) of tests for individual comparisons for various mean vector patterns (X denotes a nonzero component obtained from Table 29.3) and high or low intercorrelation as measured by the determinant of the correlation matrix

Case	All			det(R) > 0.4			det(R) < 0.4		
	Rule 3	B–H	B–L	Rule 3	B–H	B–L	Rule 3	B–H	B–L
2	4.7	3.9	2.6	4.6	4.1	2.7	4.7	3.9	2.5
3	4.6	4.2	2.9	4.6	4.2	2.8	4.7	4.1	2.9
4	4.2	2.9	1.9	4.3	2.8	1.8	4.2	2.9	1.9
5	4.0	2.6	1.8	4.2	2.7	1.7	3.9	2.6	1.8
6	5.1	3.3	2.3	4.6	3.0	1.9	5.2	3.5	2.5
7	4.6	3.1	2.2	4.4	2.9	1.9	4.7	3.2	2.3
8	4.3	2.9	2.0	4.3	2.8	1.8	4.3	3.0	2.0
9	2.3	1.8	1.3	2.3	1.7	1.2	2.3	1.8	1.4
10	2.7	2.1	1.6	2.5	1.8	1.3	2.7	2.2	1.8
11	2.5	1.8	1.3	2.4	1.7	1.2	2.5	1.9	1.4
12	2.5	1.9	1.4	2.3	1.7	1.2	2.6	2.0	1.5
13	2.6	2.0	1.5	2.4	1.8	1.2	2.6	2.1	1.6
14	1.2	1.0	0.9	1.1	0.8	0.7	1.2	1.1	1.0
15	1.1	0.9	0.9	1.0	0.8	0.7	1.1	1.0	1.0

rejecting any true null hypothesis. Table 29.7 provides values of 1—the specificity for the various cases. Procedures providing strong control of the FWER guarantee that the probability of rejecting any true null hypothesis is less than the type 1 error rate regardless of the correlation structure and of how many of the null hypotheses are true. Although the proposed procedure probably does not provide strong control of the FWER, the simulation results presented in Table 29.7 suggest that the level of control it does provide may be acceptable in practice.

The power for rejecting an individual null hypothesis depends only on the true mean for that outcome variable, and may be appreciably less than the power for rejecting the global null hypothesis. In fact, the global null hypothesis can be rejected without rejecting any individual null hypothesis when most or all of the outcome variables provide modest evidence against the null hypothesis. For example, if there were $K = 5$ individual hypotheses with p values equal to 0.045, 0.045, 0.045, 0.045, and 0.06, then the global null hypothesis would be rejected by the "Rule of 3" procedure (but not by any of the conventional procedures) even though none of the individual null hypotheses would be rejected. This is the circumstance in which composite testing strategies (Tang et al. 1993) are most effective (O'Brien 1984).

Table 29.6 Missed discovery rates (MDR) of tests for individual comparisons when $K = 5$ based on 10,000 simulated draws from multivariate normal distributions with the indicated mean vectors (X denotes a nonzero component obtained from Table 29.3) and high or low intercorrelation as measured by the determinant of the correlation matrix

	All			det(R) > 0.4			det(R) < 0.4		
Case	Rule 3	B–H	B–L	Rule 3	B–H	B–L	Rule 3	B–H	B–L
2	2.0	2.1	2.1	2.0	2.0	2.1	2.1	2.1	2.1
3	2.1	2.1	2.1	2.0	2.0	2.1	2.1	2.1	2.1
4	12	13	15	12	13	15	12	13	15
5	12	13	15	12	13	15	13	13	15
6	11	12	14	12	12	14	11	12	13
7	12	12	14	12	12	14	12	12	14
8	12	12	14	12	12	15	12	12	14
9	27	31	35	27	31	36	27	31	35
10	24	28	32	26	30	34	23	27	32
11	27	30	35	27	31	36	26	30	35
12	25	29	34	26	30	35	25	29	33
13	26	29	34	27	31	35	25	29	33
14	51	55	61	53	57	62	50	54	60
15	48	51	57	51	55	61	46	50	55

29.5 Examples

29.5.1 Exercise for the Elderly

Lazowski et al. (1999) studied the effect of two exercise programs for elderly residents of long-term care institutions on the participants' strength and functional ability. The two exercise programs were functional fitness for long-term care (FFLTC) and range of motion (ROM). Ninety-six residents of five long-term care facilities who satisfied mild inclusion criteria were recruited for the study. The participants were stratified according to their degree of mobility using a standardized test as low or high mobility (LM or HM). The participants were assigned to the two exercise programs at random within each facility and each stratum. Fifty-five residents were assigned to the FFLTC program and 41 to the ROM program.

The assessments of strength and functional capacity were carried out by observers who were blinded to the participants' program assignments. Sixty-eight of the enrollees completed the study, 36 on FFLTC, and 32 on ROM. Table 29.8 summarizes the findings for functional ability. Stair-climbing ability could be assessed in only 20 participants because two of the facilities had no stairs.

Table 29.7 Family-wise error rates (FWER) of tests for individual comparisons when K = 5 based on 10,000 simulated draws from multivariate normal distributions with the indicated mean vectors (X denotes a nonzero component obtained from Table 29.3) and high or low intercorrelation as measured by the determinant of the correlation matrix

	All			det(R) > 0.4			det(R) < 0.4		
Case	Rule 3	B–H	B–L	Rule 3	B–H	B–L	Rule 3	B–H	B–L
1	1.6	1.4	1.1	1.3	1.2	1.1	1.8	1.4	1.1
2	3.0	2.3	1.5	2.5	2.1	1.3	3.2	2.4	1.5
3	2.5	2.0	1.3	2.4	2.0	1.3	2.5	2.0	1.3
4	4.0	2.6	1.6	4.1	2.6	1.5	4.0	2.6	1.6
5	4.3	2.9	1.8	4.3	2.7	1.6	4.3	2.9	1.9
6	4.0	2.5	1.5	4.1	2.6	1.5	4.0	2.5	1.5
7	3.9	2.5	1.5	4.1	2.6	1.5	3.9	2.5	1.5
8	4.1	2.7	1.6	4.2	2.6	1.5	4.1	2.7	1.6
9	4.3	3.2	2.1	4.5	3.1	1.9	4.2	3.2	2.2
10	4.0	3.0	1.9	4.3	3.1	1.8	3.9	2.9	1.9
11	4.1	3.0	1.9	4.3	3.0	1.8	4.1	3.0	2.0
12	4.0	2.9	1.8	4.3	3.0	1.8	3.9	2.9	1.9
13	4.0	2.9	1.8	4.3	3.0	1.8	3.9	2.9	1.9
14	3.9	3.2	2.5	4.3	3.3	2.3	3.7	3.2	2.6
15	4.1	3.3	2.6	4.3	3.3	2.4	4.0	3.3	2.7

It is clear from Table 29.8 that from a global perspective, participants in the FFLTC program had substantially greater improvements in functional capacity than participants in the ROM program. Where the material improvements actually occurred can be determined by evaluating the individual assessments. Applying the conventional Benjamini–Hochberg adjustments (1) causes all but one of the individual comparisons to lose significance. However, the individual assessments need no adjustment with the method described here because at least half of them were significant at the 5 % level. Consequently, one can conclude that the participants in the FFLTC program had better results than the participants in the ROM program with respect to all components of functional capacity except possibly gait and stair-climbing ability. Similar conclusions were reached by Lazowski et al. (1999).

29.5.2 Uterine Weights from Estrogen Assay

Table 29.9 illustrates the comparisons of k treatments against a control using the findings of an estrogen assay (Steel and Torrie 1980). The six differences between the activated solutions and the control solution clearly are not independent. The

Table 29.8 Significance levels from two-sided comparisons of the effect on functional capacity of two group exercise programs for elderly residents in long-term care institutions Lazowski et al. (1999). p values adjusted using (29.1)

	Mobility	Balance	Sit and reach	Shoulder flexibility	Gait (normal)	Gait (fast)	Stair climb	Function capacity
	(s)	(score)	(cm)	(degrees)	(m/s)		(watts)	(score)
n_{FFLTC}/n_{ROM}	36/30	36/32	25/19	36/29	35/29	35/30	11/9	34/31
Mean chg FFLTC	−3.7	3.9	4.7	16	0.04	0.03	−1.7	0.1
Mean chg ROM	6.2	−0.5	0.4	4.3	0.04	0.03	−1.1	−5.4
p	0.044	0.0014	0.0403	0.016	1	0.82	0.16	0.046
p_{adj}	0.074	0.0112	0.074	0.064	1	0.94	0.21	0.074

Table 29.9 One-tail p values corresponding to comparisons of effects of six in vitro-activated test solutions against a control on uterine weights (mg) of mice from an estrogen assay (Steel and Torrie 1980). p_{adj} from (29.1)

	Solutions						
	1	2	3	4	5	6	Control
Mean	88.25	75.4	68.45	84.9	78.9	70.2	96.15
1-tail p	0.183	0.012	0.002	0.101	0.028	0.003	
p_{adj}	0.183	0.024	0.012	0.112	0.042	0.009	

global null hypothesis that the mean weights for none of the solution groups differs from the mean weight for the control solution would be rejected at the (1-tailed) 5 % level. Furthermore, the mean weights for solutions 2, 3, 5, and 6 are significantly lower than the control weight. Hochberg and Tamhane (1987) and Westfall and Young (1993) reached the same conclusion from their analyses of these data.

29.5.3 Anesthesiology

Läuter (1996) presented an example in which 30 patients undergoing surgery were randomly assigned to one of two procedures for administering anesthesia. Seven correlated measurements were made on each patient. If the two procedures can be distinguished globally, what is the pattern of difference between the two procedures? The information presented by Läuter permits t-tests to be carried out for each of the measurements, although this is not how the analysis was done in the paper. The results are presented in Table 29.10. The outcomes are sorted in descending order of naïve significance level. The global null hypothesis of no difference between the procedures is rejected because $p_{(1)} < 0.05/7 = 0.0071$. Adjusted p values must be used to evaluate

Table 29.10 Two-tail significance levels for individual outcome measures comparing two procedures for surgical anesthesia (Läuter 1996). p_{adj} from (29.1)

	v1	v2	v3	v4	v5	v6	v7
Procedure 1 mean	1.44	45.7	26.6	3.28	53.7	37.7	76.2
Procedure 2 mean	1.19	33.5	15.1	1.57	33.6	19.2	33.6
p	0.752	0.393	0.112	0.100	0.060	0.025	0.006
p_{adj}	0.752	0.458	0.157	0.157	0.139	0.087	0.042

the individual outcomes because fewer than half of them were significant at the 5 % level. Only the seventh outcome measure remains significant after the adjustment. This is not surprising because Läuter's example illustrates a situation in which all (except the 7th) of the outcomes demonstrated a modest advantage for procedure 1.

29.5.4 Post-Thrombolytic Treatment

Benjamini and Hochberg (1995) presented an example of treatment differences with respect to the occurrence of cardiac and other events following the start of thrombolytic treatment. There were 15 treatment comparisons, for which the ordered p values were 0.0001, 0.0004, 0.0019, 0.0095, 0.0201, 0.0278, 0.0298, 0.0344, 0.0459, 0.3240, 0.4262, 0.5719, 0.6528, 0.7590, and 1.0; the value corresponding to 0.0095 corresponds to mortality. There are fewer than 16 comparisons, so the rule described here can be used when the type 1 error rate is 5 %. Since more than three of the comparisons had p values less than 0.05, the global null hypothesis of no treatment effect with respect to any of the comparisons can be rejected. Given that at least some of these differences are "real," the question is, "which ones?" The FDR controlling procedure (29.1) described by Benjamini and Hochberg supports rejecting only the hypotheses corresponding to the four smallest p values. The rule described here would support rejecting the nine hypotheses with p values less than 0.05 because more than half of the p values were less than 0.05.

29.6 Discussion

This chapter describes a method for carrying out multiple comparisons that controls the type 1 error rate for global null hypotheses and requires almost no computation beyond that used to produce conventional summary tables with naive p values. Although the method does not necessarily provide strong control of the FWER, it did control the FDR at a nominal 5 % level less conservatively than the Benjamini–Hochberg procedure, and showed similar power properties in a simulation study. Since basing a decision on a combination of persistence and strength of positive findings is consistent with how clinicians intuitively interpret study findings, interpreting and communicating the findings to clinicians should be relatively simple.

Moreover, it is easy to explain the need to adjust *p* values when few of the unadjusted individual comparisons reach significance, but difficult when most of them do.

Sample sizes can be kept relatively small by selecting uncorrelated outcome variables that demonstrate a treatment effect (have a positive mean). For example, the ratio of the sample sizes required when two of four instead of three of four variables have a positive mean is 1.35, which means that a trial in which two of four variables are expected to show a treatment effect would require 35 % ($(2.926/2.518)^2 - 1$) more patients than one in which three of four variables were expected to show the same treatment effect, and would require 68 % more patients than a trial in which all four variables were expected to show the effect. However, variables that demonstrate a treatment effect also may be highly correlated, so that the power may be much less than if the variables were independent. As an extreme case, if all four of the variables were perfectly correlated, then the test would amount to a test on just one variable, for which the noncentrality parameter for 90 % power with a 5 % level two-sided test would have to be 3.242 ($= 1.96 + 1.282$) instead of 2.259. The more variables that are chosen, i.e., the greater the value of K, the more serious this problem will become. Hence, K should be no larger than necessary and the outcome variables should not be highly correlated with each other as well as presumably reflecting a treatment effect (Capizzi and Zhang 1996).

In some applications, especially those involving subjective or functional evaluations such as trials of antiarthritic agents, efficacy is evaluated in terms of a number of "domains," which are sets of individual measurements. "Activities of daily living," which includes a number of questions about a patient's ability to function from day to day, is an example of one such domain. The domains occupy the roles of primary response variables. The findings from the individual responses comprising a domain provide a basis for determining whether the domain finding is "significant" at a specified level. The significance level is determined separately for each domain. This process protects the domain-wise type 1 error rate. Combining the domain findings across domains in the same manner preserves the experiment-wise error rate.

Most clinical trials have more than one relevant "primary hypothesis" because more than one issue usually needs to be addressed in reaching conclusions about the clinical utility of a drug, for example, safety or tolerability and efficacy, or whether a drug shrinks tumors *and* improves survival, or does one but not both. These marginal issues need to be addressed separately, and may not be subject to the multiplicity adjustment paradigm (Cook and Farewell 1996).

Appendix 1 Technical Details

A1.1 Acceptance Sets

Let X_i denote the i-th of K measures of the effect of an intervention obtained from a trial, with marginal cumulative distribution function (cdf) $F_i\,(x;\theta_i)$, where θ_i characterizes the intervention effect. The null hypothesis of no intervention effect with respect to the i-th measure X_i is H_{0i}: $\theta_i = \theta_{i0}$ and the alternative is H_{1i}: $\theta_i \neq \theta_{i0}$. These could be expressed as one-sided hypotheses H_{1i}: $\theta_i > \theta_{i0}$. The global null hypothesis of no overall intervention effect, $H_0 = \bigcap_{i=1}^{K} H_{0i}$ is false if any individual null hypothesis is false. Let p_i denote the usual *p* value (unadjusted for multiplicity) calculated for testing H_{0i}, i=1, ..., K so that H_{0i} would be rejected at the $100\alpha\%$ level of significance if $p_i < \alpha$ when multiplicity is ignored. Denote the ordered values of $p_1, \ldots, p_K$ by $p_{(1)} \leq p_{(2)} \leq \cdots \leq p_{(K)}$

Let $\alpha_1 \leq \alpha_2 \leq \ldots \alpha_K$ denote a set of adjusted Type 1 error rates for the ordered *p* values, and let $A_i^{(h)}$ denote the set of realizations of X_i for which H_{0i}: $\theta_i = \theta_i^{(0)}$ would *not* be rejected at the $100\alpha_h\%$ level of significance, that is, for which $p_i > \alpha_h$, i=1, ..., K. $A_i^{(h)}$ is the "acceptance set" for measure X_i when the null hypothesis H_{0i} is tested at level α_h. For positive integers h and h′ between 1 and K,

$$
\begin{aligned}
h < h' \Rightarrow\ & \text{(i) } \alpha_h \leq \alpha_{h'} \\
& \text{(ii) } A_i^{(h')} \subset A_i^{(h)} \\
& \text{(iii) } A_i^{(h)} A_i^{(h')} = A_i^{(h)} \cap A_i^{(h')} = A_i^{(h')} \\
& \text{(iv) } A_i^{(h)} \cup A_i^{(h')} = A_i^{(h)}
\end{aligned}
\tag{A1}
$$

For notational convenience,

$$
\begin{aligned}
A^{(h)} &\equiv \cap_{i=1}^{K} A_i^{(h)} \\
A_{-j}^{(h)} &\equiv \cup_{\substack{i=1, \\ i \neq j}}^{K} A_i^{(h)}
\end{aligned}
$$

and, in general,

$$
A_{-j_1 j_2 \cdots}^{(h)} \equiv \bigcap_{\substack{i = 1, \\ i \neq j_1 j_2 \cdots}}^{K} A_i^{(h)}
$$

$A^{(h)}$ is the set of outcomes such that all of the *p* values exceed α_h and $\sim A^{(h)}$ denotes its complement.

A1.2 Rejection Regions

Denote by

$$
S_1 = \sim A^{(1)}
$$

the set of outcomes for which $p_{(1)} \leq \alpha_1$. S_1 is the set of outcomes among $X_1, \ldots, X_K$ for which at least one of the component hypotheses $H_{01}, \ldots, H_{0K}$ would be rejected at the $100\alpha_1\%$ level. If $\alpha_1 = \alpha$, the nominal type 1 error rate, then controlling the

FWER at α requires $P(S_1 \mid H_0) \le \alpha$, which implies that $\alpha_1 \le 1-(1-\alpha)^{1/K} = \alpha_S$ if the outcomes are independent. The Bonferroni approach replaces α_S with $\alpha_B = \alpha/K < \alpha_S$.

Let

$$S_2 = \sim \bigcup_{i=1}^{K} A_{-i}^{(2)}$$

denote the set of outcomes $X_1, \ldots, X_K$ for which $p_{(2)} \le \alpha_2$, and let

$$S_3 = \sim \bigcup\bigcup_{i_1<i_2} A_{-i_1 i_2}^{(3)}$$

denote the set of outcomes for which $p_{(3)} < \alpha_3$. S_3 is the set of outcomes for which at least three of the component null hypotheses are rejected at the $100\alpha_3\%$ level.

Lemma: The set of outcomes for which the global null hypothesis will be rejected if $p_{(1)} < \alpha_1$ or $p_{(2)} < \alpha_2$ or $p_{(3)} < \alpha_3$ is defined in terms of the acceptance sets by

$$S_1 \cup S_2 \cup S_3 = \sim \bigcup\bigcup_{i_1<i_2} \left\{A_{i_1}^{(1)} A_{i_2}^{(2)} \cup A_{i_1}^{(2)} A_{i_2}^{(1)}\right\} A_{-i_1 i_2}^{(3)} = \sim \bigcup_{i=1}^{C_{K,2}} E_i \quad \text{(A2)}$$

where $C_{K,2} = K(K-1)/2$.

Proof:

Repeated application of relationship (iii) of (A1) yields:

$$\begin{aligned}
\sim (S_1 \cup S_2) = \sim S_1 \cap \sim S_2 &= \bigcup_{i=1}^{K} \left(\bigcap_{i=1}^{K} A_i^{(1)}\right) \cap \left(\bigcap_{j\neq i} A_j^{(2)}\right) \\
&= \bigcup_{i=1}^{K} \left(A_i^{(1)} \cap \left(\bigcap_{j\neq i} A_j^{(1)} A_j^{(2)}\right)\right) \\
&= \bigcup_{i=1}^{K} \left(A_i^{(1)} \cap \left(\bigcap_{j\neq i} A_j^{(2)}\right)\right) = \bigcup_{i=1}^{K} A_i^{(1)} A_{-i}^{(2)}
\end{aligned}$$

Expression (A2) follows from

$$\begin{aligned}
&\sim \left(S_1 \bigcup S_2 \bigcup S_3\right) = \sim S_1 \bigcap \sim S_2 \bigcap \sim S_3 \\
&= \left(\bigcup_{i=1}^{K} A_i^{(1)} A_{-i}^{(2)}\right) \bigcap \left(\bigcup\bigcup_{i_1<i_2} A_{-i_1 i_2}^{(3)}\right) \\
&= \left(A_{i_1}^{(1)} A_{-i_1}^{(2)} \cup A_{i_2}^{(1)} A_{-i_2}^{(2)} \cup \left(\bigcup_{i\neq i_1,i_2} A_i^{(1)} A_{-i}^{(2)}\right)\right) \bigcap \left(\bigcup\bigcup_{i_1<i_2} A_{-i_1 i_2}^{(3)}\right) \\
&= \bigcup\bigcup_{i_1<i_2} \left(A_{i_1}^{(1)} A_{-i_1}^{(2)} \cup A_{i_2}^{(1)} A_{-i_2}^{(2)} \cup \left(\bigcup_{i\neq i_1,i_2} A_i^{(1)} A_{-i}^{(2)}\right)\right) \cap A_{-i_1 i_2}^{(3)} \\
&= \bigcup\bigcup_{i_1<i_2} \left(A_{i_1}^{(1)} A_{i_2}^{(2)} \cup A_{i_1}^{(2)} A_{i_2}^{(1)} \cup A_{i_1}^{(2)} A_{i_2}^{(2)}\right) \cap A_{-i_1 i_2}^{(3)}
\end{aligned}$$

from relationship (iii) of (A1)

$$\bigcup\bigcup_{i_1<i_2} \left(A_{i_1}^{(1)} A_{i_2}^{(2)} \cup A_{i_1}^{(2)} A_{i_2}^{(1)}\right) \cap A_{-i_1 i_2}^{(3)}$$

from relationship (iv) of (A1) QED

A1.3 Probabilities Associated with Rejection Regions

In general (Feller 1957, p. 89), the probability associated with the events E_i in (A2) is given by

$$P(S_1 \cup S_2 \cup S_3) = 1 - P\left(\bigcup_{i=1}^{C_{K,2}} E_i\right) \tag{A3}$$

$$= 1 - \left\{\sum_{i=1}^{C_{K,2}} P(E_i) - \sum_{h=2}^{C_{K,2}} (-1)^h \sum_{i_1<} \sum_{i_2<} \cdots \sum_{i_h} P(E_{i_1} E_{i_2} \cdots E_{i_h})\right\}$$

Expressions for the joint probabilities in (A3) simplify appreciably because of the relationships among the acceptance sets. The general result is given in the following.

Theorem:

$$P(S_1 \cup S_2 \cup S_3) \tag{A4}$$

$$= 1 - \left\{\sum_{i=1}^{C_{K,2}} P(E_i) - (K-2) \sum_{j=1}^{K} P\left(A_j^{(1)} A_{-j}^{(3)}\right) + C_{K-1,2} P\left(A^{(3)}\right)\right\}$$

where the E_i are defined by (A2).

Proof:

From the Lemma, and the fact that $P(A \cup B) = P(A) + P(B) - P(AB)$,

$$P(E_i) = P\left(A_{i_1}^{(1)} A_{i_2}^{(2)} A_{-i_1 i_2}^{(3)}\right) + P\left(A_{i_1}^{(2)} A_{i_2}^{(1)} A_{-i_1 i_2}^{(3)}\right) - P\left(A_{i_1}^{(2)} A_{i_2}^{(2)} A_{-i_1 i_2}^{(3)}\right)$$

A typical product $E_i E_j$ can be written as

$$E_i E_j = \left(A_{i_1}^{(1)} A_{i_2}^{(2)} \cup A_{i_1}^{(2)} A_{i_2}^{(1)}\right)\left(A_{i_3}^{(1)} A_{i_4}^{(2)} \cup A_{i_3}^{(2)} A_{i_4}^{(1)}\right) A_{-i_1 i_2}^{(3)} A_{-i_3 i_4}^{(3)}$$

The pairs (i_1, i_2) and (i_3, i_4) are the index pairs of E_i and E_j, respectively. If i_1, i_2, i_3, and i_4 are four distinct integers, then $E_i E_j = A^{(3)}$. Otherwise, if $i_1 = i_3 = K$ or $i_2 = i_4 = K$, then $E_i E_j = A_k^{(1)} A_{-k}^{(3)}$ Hence, $P(E_i E_j) = Pr(A^{(3)})$ or $P(A_k^{(1)} A_{-k}^{(3)})$ depending on whether E_i and E_j do not or do share a common index value. The product $E_{i_1} \cdots E_{i_h} = A^{(3)}$ if the indices of the A sets for any two E factors consist of four distinct integers. Also, if k is one of the members of the index pair corresponding to each E_i of the product $E_{i_1} \cdots E_{i_h}$, then the product is equal to $A_k^{(1)} A_{-k}^{(3)}$. Consequently, $P(E_{i_1} \cdots E_{i_h}) = P(A^{(3)})$ or $P(A_k^{(1)} A_{-k}^{(3)})$ accordingly as the factors of the product $E_{i_1} \cdots E_{i_h}$ do not or do share a common index value. All told, there are $\binom{C_{K,2}}{h}$ distinct h-tuples $E_{i_1} \cdots E_{i_h}$. As long as $h < K$, there are $\binom{K-1}{h}$ ways to choose h additional distinct indices to pair with any index value i to form $E_{i_1} \cdots E_{i_h}$ products whose members' index pairs all contain i. Consequently, the term $P(A_i^{(1)} A_{-i}^{(3)})$ occurs $\binom{K-1}{h}$ times in the sum $\sum_{i_1<} \sum_{i_2<} \cdots \sum_{<i_h} P(E_{i_1} E_{i_2} \cdots E_{i_h})$ and this is true for each value of i, so there are $K\binom{K-1}{h}$ such terms. The remaining $\binom{C_{K,2}}{h} - K\binom{K-1}{h}$ terms

of the sum all equal $P(A^{(3)})$. If $h \geq K$, then all of the products $E_{i_1} \cdots E_{i_h}$ must equal $A^{(3)}$ and so $P(A^{(3)})$ must occur $\binom{C_{K,2}}{h}$ times in the sum $\sum_{i_1<} \sum_{i_2<} \cdots \sum_{<i_h} P(E_{i_1} E_{i_2} \cdots E_{i_h})$. This completes the proof.

Expression (A4) does not require independence or continuity of the outcome variables. Computationally useful forms can be obtained by assuming independence, as in the following corollaries.

Corollary 1 If the outcome variables are independent and $P\left(A_i^{(h)}\right) = p_i^{(h)}$, then

$$P(S_1 \cup S_2 \cup S_3)$$

$$= 1 - \left\{ \begin{array}{l} \sum_{i_1<i_2} \left(p_{i_1}^{(1)} p_{i_2}^{(2)} + p_{i_1}^{(2)} p_{i_2}^{(1)} - p_{i_1}^{(2)} p_{i_2}^{(2)}\right) \prod_{j \neq i_1, i_2} p_j^{(3)} \\ -(K-2) \sum_{i=1}^{K} p_i^{(1)} \prod_{j \neq i} p_j^{(3)} + C_{K-1,2} \prod_{i=1}^{K} p_i^{(3)} \end{array} \right\} \quad \text{(A5)}$$

Corollary 2 If the outcome variables are independent and continuous, and all of the component null hypotheses are true, so that $p_i^{(h)} = 1 - \alpha_h$, then the probability of rejecting the global null hypothesis is

$$P(S_1 \cup S_2 \cup S_3)$$

$$= 1 - \{C_{K,2}(1-\alpha_3)^{K-2}(1-\alpha_2)(1-2\alpha_1+\alpha_2) - K(K-2)(1-\alpha_1)(1-\alpha_3)^{K-1} + C_{K-1,2}(1-\alpha_3)^K\}$$

This is the same as expression (3.3) of Sen (1999), when $r = 3$.

A1.4 Critical Values

Corollary 2 implies that the global null hypothesis test will have level at most α under independence and continuity if and only if

$$f(\alpha_1, \alpha_2, \alpha_3) = C_{K,2}(1-\alpha_3)^{K-2}(1-\alpha_2)(1-2\alpha_1+\alpha_2) - K(K-2)(1-\alpha_1)(1-\alpha_3)^{K-1} + C_{K-1,2}(1-\alpha_3)^K \geq 1-\alpha \quad \text{(A6)}$$

Given α_1, the maximum value of f in (A6) occurs when $\alpha_2 = \alpha_3 = \alpha_1$ (the derivative of f with respect to α_2 is zero when $\alpha_2 = \alpha_1$; the derivative of f with respect to α_3 is zero when $\alpha_3 = \alpha_1$ if $\alpha_2 = \alpha_1$). Inequality (A6) is satisfied if and only if $\alpha_1 \leq \alpha_S$. If $\alpha_1 = \alpha_S$, then $f(\alpha_1, \alpha_2, \alpha_3) = 1 - \alpha$ so that neither α_2 nor α_3 can exceed α_S (Berger 1982). If $\alpha_1 < \alpha_S$, which would be true if $\alpha_1 < \alpha_B$, then α_2 and α_3 both can exceed α_1. This is the key point. In particular, (A6) can be satisfied for $\alpha_3 = \alpha$ and $\alpha_2 = 2\alpha_1$ as long as $\alpha_1 \leq \alpha_{1max}$, where

$$\alpha_{1max} =$$

$$\frac{C_{K,2} - K(K-2)(1-\alpha) + C_{K-1,2}(1-\alpha)^2 - (1-\alpha)^{3-K}}{K(K-1-(K-2)(1-\alpha))}$$

It is easy to verify that $\alpha_{1max} > 0$ when $\alpha = 0.05$ as long as $K \le K(0.05) = 16$. Smaller values of α allow for greater values of K (α): K(0.025) = 25 and K(0.01) = 44. The value of α_{1max} is not much smaller than α/K when $K \le 10$. Table 29.1 in Sect. 2 displays the values of $\alpha_{1max}, \alpha/K$, and their difference for $\alpha = 0.05$ and 0.25, and K = 3(1)16. The quantity ε mentioned in the introduction is the difference between α_{1max} and $\alpha_B = \alpha/K$.

A1.5 Power

The power and, therefore, the sample size needed, for rejecting a global null hypothesis will depend on the joint distribution of the outcomes under an alternative hypothesis. An alternative hypothesis could specify a constant shift for each component outcome such as $H_{1i} : \theta_i = \theta_{i0}$ for all *i*. Or, the alternative hypothesis could specify a shift with respect to some, but not all, of the component outcome distributions, so that the alternative hypothesis would be defined by $H_{1i} : \theta_i = \theta_{i1} \ne \theta_{i0}$ for $i \in \{i_1, \ldots, i_m\} \subset \{1, \ldots, K\}$, and $\theta_i = \theta_{i0}$ otherwise.

If the outcomes are independent, then the probability of rejecting the global null hypothesis when there is a shift in m ($1 \le m \le K$) of the component distributions, is, from (A5)

$$P(S_1 \cup S_2 \cup S_3) = 1 - \tag{A7}$$

$$\left\{\begin{array}{ll} \left[C_{K-1,2}\gamma_3 - m(K-2)\gamma_1\right]\gamma_3^{m-1}(1-\alpha_3)^{K-m} & \\ +C_{m,2}(2\gamma_1-\gamma_2)\gamma_2\gamma_3^{m-2}(1-\alpha_3)^{K-m} & m > 1 \\ +(K-m)\left[\begin{array}{r}(m-1)\left[(\gamma_1-\gamma_2)(1-\alpha_2)+\gamma_2(1-\alpha_1)\right] \\ -(K-2)(1-\alpha_1)\gamma_3\end{array}\right]\gamma_3^{m-1}(1-\alpha_3)^{K-m-1} & \\ & m < K \\ +C_{K-m,2}(1-2\alpha_1+\alpha_2)(1-\alpha_2)\gamma_3^{m}(1-\alpha_3)^{K-m-2} & m < K-1 \end{array}\right\}$$

where γ_K denotes the probability of a component event falling inside its level α_K acceptance set when H_{1i} is true. If H_{0i} is true, then $\gamma_K = 1 - \alpha_K$; if H_{1i} is true, then γ_K denotes the corresponding type 2 error rate (assumed same for all components).

The functional form of F, the distribution generating the observations, is needed to calculate the type 2 error rates γ_i in (A7) corresponding to the type 1 error rates $\alpha_i, i = 1,2,3$. Suppose the probabilities $p_i^{(h)}$ in (A5) can be calculated from

$$p_i^{(h)} = pr(A_i^{(h)}) = F(\theta_i + \zeta_{1-\alpha_h/2}; \xi) - F(\theta_i + \zeta_{\alpha_h/2}; \xi) \tag{A8}$$

for two-sided tests of H_{0i}: $\theta_i = 0$ vs $H_{1i} : |\theta_i| > 0$, where F denotes an appropriate cumulative distribution function such as the standard normal, Student *t*, etc., ξ denotes parameters with known values such as the degrees of freedom, θ_i (≥ 0) denotes the expectation of the i-th component outcome under the alternative hypothesis, and the ζ are percentiles of the null distribution of the appropriate test statistic. For power calculations under independence, we want $p_i^{(h)} \leq \gamma_h$ if $\theta_i = \theta_{i1} > 0$ and $p_i^{(h)} \geq 1 - \alpha_h$ if $\theta_i = 0$. The first term on the right-hand side of (A8) will be only slightly less than 1 when $\Delta_i > 0$, so that the requirement $p_i^{(h)} \leq \gamma_h$ if $\theta_i = \theta_{i1} > 0$ implies that a slightly conservative estimate of θ_{i1} is

$$\theta_i \cong \zeta_{1-\gamma_h} - \zeta_{\alpha_h/2} \tag{A9}$$

The value of θ_i must be the same for all h. Consequently, if θ_i is determined by α_1 and γ_1 in (A9), then γ_2 and γ_3 must be determined from

$$\zeta_{1-\gamma_h} = \zeta_{1-\gamma_1} - \zeta_{\alpha_1/2} + \zeta_{\alpha_h/2}$$

i.e.,

$$\gamma_h = 1 - F(\zeta_{1-\gamma_1} - \zeta_{\alpha_1/2} + \zeta_{\alpha_h/2}; \epsilon).$$

The quantity θ_{i1} is the value of the noncentrality parameter that gives power 1-γ_1 for rejecting the i-th individual null hypothesis H_{0i} when $\theta_i = \theta_{i1}$. It determines the required sample size through expressions such as $\theta_i = \mu_i\sqrt{n}/\sigma$ when the values of μ and σ are specified. Table 29.2 in Sect. 2 above provides noncentrality parameters values calculated assuming normality using (A9) for K = 3 (1) 16 and when m = 1 (1) min(5,K) = number of positive means.

A1.6 Confidence Sets

Let θ denote the parameters of the joint distribution of the K outcomes addressed by the null hypothesis H_0: $\theta = \theta_0$. H_0 is rejected at the 100α% level when Pr $(S_1 \cup S_2 \cup S_3 | \theta = \theta_0) \leq \alpha$. A 100(1 − α)% joint confidence region for θ consists of the parameter values for which H_0 would not be rejected, i.e., $\{\theta^* | P(S_1 \cup S_2 \cup S_3 | \theta^*) \geq \alpha\}$(Lehmann 1959, Theorem 4, p. 79). The region resembles a notched hyper-rectangle when the outcomes are independent (Benjamini and Stark 1996).

Appendix 2 R Code for Simulations

```
# THIS IS THE DRIVER ROUTINE FOR SimRunX

run.SimRunX.fn <- function(nreps,means,corrvecs,
                           alpha=0.05,eps=0.0001)
#
#  Driver routine for SimRunX.
#  INPUT:
#    nreps = number of simulation repetitions per case
#    means = matrix whose rows are mean vectors.  The
#            number of columns of 'means' determines
#            the number of null hypotheses (K)
# corrvecs = matrix of correlations (r12, r12, …, r1K,
#            r23, …) among the K outcomes corresponding
#            to the null hypotheses.
#    alpha = nominal Type 1 error rate (and FDR target)
#      eps = lower bound for determinant of positive
#            definite matrix.
#
#  The number of rows of the 'means' matrix does not
#  have to be the same as the number of rows of the
#  'corrvecs' matrix.  The 'means' and 'corrvecs'
#  arrays could be vectors (just one case for each),
#  the program will convert  them to matrices.
#
#  OUTPUT: (For the Benjamini-Hochberg, Rule of 3, and
#           Benjamini-Liu methods)
#      GR = percent of runs rejecting the global null
#           hypothesis for each case
#     FDR = FDR as percent across the runs for each case
#     MDR = MDR as percent across the runs for each case
#     EER = percentage of rejections across the
#           hypotheses and runs (see Finner & Roters)
#    Sens = sensitivity = P(Reject H0 | H0 false)
#    Spec = specificity = P(Not Reject H0 | H0 true)
#
#  Also,
#    call = calling sequence
```

```
#    Date = date of run
#    Elapsed.time = time run took
{
  tt <- proc.time()[3]
  if (length(dim(means))==0)
    means <- matrix(means,nrow=1,ncol=length(means))
  if (length(dim(corrvecs))==0)
    corrvecs <- matrix(corrvecs,nrow=1,
                       ncol=length(corrvecs))
  case <- 0
  nm <- dim(means)[1]       # No. of mean vectors
  nc <- dim(corrvecs)[1]    # No. of correlation vectors
  K <- dim(means)[2]    # Dimension of each mean vector
  results <- NULL
  x1 <- paste0("mu",1:K)
  x2 <-NULL;
  for (i in 1:(K-1))
    for (j in (i+1):K)  x2 <- c(x2,paste0("r",i,j))
  x3 <- c("Case",x1,x2,"det","BHGR","R3GR","BLGR",
          "BHFDR","R3FDR","BLFDR","BHMDR","R3MDR",
          "BLMDR","BHEER","R3EER","BLEER","BHSens",
          "R3Sens","BLSens","BHSpec","R3Spec","BLSpec")
  corrs <- NULL
  for (im in 1:nm)
    for (ic in 1:nc)
    {
      ww <- corvec2sigma.fn(K,corrvecs[ic,],eps=eps)
      if (ww$detsig > eps) # Do calculation only if cov
      {                    # matrix is positive definite
        case <- case + 1
        if (im==1) corrs <-
       rbind(corrs,c(corrvecs[ic,],
                  round(ww$detsig,4)))
        v <- c(case,means[im,],corrvecs[ic,],
              round(ww$detsig,4))
        z <- SimRunX.fn(nreps, means[im,],
```

```
                    corrvecs[ic,], alpha=alpha, eps=eps)
        attach(z)
        vv <- round(100*c(mean(BHGR),mean(GouldGR),
              mean(BLGR), mean(mean(BHFDR,na.rm=T),
              GouldFDR,na.rm=T), mean(BLFDR,na.rm=T),
              mean(BHFDR,na.rm=T),
              mean(GouldMDR,na.rm=T),
              mean(BLMDR,na.rm=T), mean(BHEER),
              mean(GouldEER),mean(BLEER),
              mean(BHSens,na.rm=T),
              mean(GouldSens,na.rm=T),
              mean(BLSens,na.rm=T),
              mean(BHSpec,na.rm=T),
              mean(GouldSpec,na.rm=T),
              mean(BLSpec,na.rm=T)),1)
        detach(z)
        results <- rbind(results,c(v,vv))
      }
    }
  dimnames(means)[[2]] <- x1
  corrs <- as.matrix(corrs)
  dimnames(corrs)[[2]]<-c(x2,"det")
  dimnames(results)[[2]] <- x3
  hdr <- 'Comparison-wise error rates following a ')
  hdr <- c(hdr,'test of the global null hypothesis ')
  hdr <- c(hdr,'that all means are zero, as a')
  hdr <- c(hdr,' function of the correlation structure
  hdr <- c(hdr,' and the true mean vector when ')
  hdr <- c(hdr,paste0('there are', K,' endpoints,'))
  hdr <- c(hdr,paste0('based on ',nreps))
  hdr <- c(hdr, 'replications.')
  hdr  <-c(hdr,'Reject null hypothesis of zero mean ')
  hdr <- c(hdr,'for individual variables according to')
  hdr <- c(hdr,'the following adaptive rule:')
  hdr <- c(hdr,'(a) If the global null is not')
  hdr <- c(hdr,'    rejected, then test none of')
  hdr <- c(hdr,'    the individual null hypotheses')
  hdr <- c(hdr,'    (i.e., reject none);')
  hdr <- c(hdr,'(b) If the global null is rejected,')
```

```
  hdr <- c(hdr,'    then first count how many ')
  hdr <- c(hdr,'    variables have p[i] <= alpha.  If')
  hdr <- c(hdr,'    p[i] < alpha for fewer than half ')
  hdr <- c(hdr,'    the variables, then adjust the ')
  hdr <- c(hdr,'    individual p[i] values using the')
  hdr <- c(hdr,'    BH procedure and reject the i-th')
  hdr <- c(hdr,'    null hypothesis Hoi if ')
  hdr <- c(hdr,'    p_adj[i] < alpha; otherwise,')
  hdr <- c(hdr,'    reject the i-th null hypothesis')
  hdr <- c(hdr,'    if p[i] < alpha ')
  hdr <- c(hdr,'The results of using decision rules')
  hdr <- c(hdr,'due to Benjamini &  Hochberg (JRSSB)'
  hdr <- c(hdr,'and Benjamini & Liu also are included')
  hdr <- c(hdr,' for comparison.')

  return(list(call=sys.call(),Date=date(),
        Elapsed.time=Elapsed.time.fn(tt), Header=hdr,
        x1=x1,x2=x2,x3=x3,means=means,
        correlations=corrs, Results=results))
}

# THIS IS THE ROUTINE THAT CARRIES OUT THE SIMULATIONS

SimRunX.fn <- function(nreps,amean,corvec,alpha=0.05,
                       eps=1E-4)
{
#
       SUBROUTINES
  alpha1Max <- function(K,alpha)
  {
    eta <- 1 - alpha
    cc <- 0.5*(K-1)
    alpha1max <- (K*cc-(K-2)*eta*(K - cc*eta)
                 - 1/eta^(K-3))/(K*(K-1-(K-2)*eta))
    return(alpha1max)
  }
```

```
DrawSamples.fn <- function(nreps,amean,sigma)
{
  X <- rmvnorm(nreps,amean,sigma)
  p <- 2*pnorm(-abs(X))
  r <- t(apply(-abs(X),1,"rank"))
  return(list(X=X,p=p,r=r))
}

BndsFns.fn <- function(bndopt,r,p,nreps,K,amean)
{
  amean0 <- t(matrix(1*(amean<1e-6),nrow=K,
                     ncol=nreps))
  amean1 <- t(matrix(1*(amean>0),nrow=K,ncol=nreps))
  nH1 <- sum(1*(amean > 0)) # No. of true alt hypoth.
  nH0 <- K - nH1           # No. of true null hypoth.
  if (bndopt==1) bnds <- (1:K)*alpha/K   # Benj-Hoch
  if (bndopt==2)
    bnds <- 1-(1-min(1,K*alpha/(K+1-1:K)))
                            ^(1/(K+1-1:K))
                                 # Benjamini-Liu
  if (bndopt < 3)
  {
    Bnds <- matrix(bnds[r],dim(r))
    Hits <- 1*(p < Bnds)
    GR <- apply(Hits,1,"max")
  }
  else                                     # Rule of 3
  {
    bnds <- c(c(1,2)*alpha1,rep(alpha,K-2))
    Bnds <- matrix(bnds[r],nrow=nreps,ncol=K)
    Hits <- 1*(p < Bnds)
    GR <- apply(Hits,1,"max")   # P(Reject Global H0)
    ii <- (1:nreps)[apply(1*(p < alpha),1,sum)
                      <= K/2]
                # Rows with no.(p < alpha) <= K/2
    if (length(ii) > 0)          # There are some
    {
      bnds <- (1:K)*alpha/K      # Get BH bounds
      nb1 <- matrix(bnds[r[ii,]],c(length(ii),K))
```

```
        Bnds[ii,] <- nb1  # Put these into rows of Bnds
      }
      Hits <- 1*(p < Bnds)
    }
    rHits <- Hits*r
    HypRejTot <- apply(rHits,1,"max")
    HypNRejTot <- K - HypRejTot
    HypRejAlt <- apply(rHits*amean1,1,"max")
    rr <- matrix(HypRejTot,nrow=nreps,ncol=K)
    HypNRejNull <- apply((1*(r > rr))*amean0,1,sum)
    if (nH1 > 0) Sens <- HypRejAlt/nH1
    else  Sens <- NA
    if (nH0 > 0) Spec <- HypNRejNull/nH0
    else  Spec <- NA
    PPV <- rep(NA,nreps)
    NPV <- rep(NA,nreps)
    ii <- (1:nreps)[HypRejTot > 0]
    jj <- (1:nreps)[HypRejTot < K]
    PPV[ii] <- HypRejAlt[ii]/HypRejTot[ii]
    NPV[jj] <- HypNRejNull[jj]/HypNRejTot[jj]
    FDR <- 1 - PPV
    MDR <- 1 - NPV
    EER <- HypRejAlt/K    # Finner & Roters EER = PCER
    return(list(Bnds=Bnds, Hits=Hits, GR=GR,
        HypRejTot=HypRejTot, HypRejAlt=HypRejAlt,
        HypNRejTot=HypNRejTot, HypNRejNull=HypNRejNull,
      FDR=FDR, MDR=MDR, EER=EER, Sens=Sens, Spec=Spec))
  }
#                         PROCESSING STARTS HERE
  options(warn=-1)
  loadlib.fn("mvtnorm")
  K <- length(amean)
  alpha1 <- alpha1Max(K,alpha)

  sig <- corvec2sigma.fn(K,corvec)
  if (sig$detsig < eps) return(sig$detsig)
```

```
            # Skip if correlation matrix is not pos def
  else
  {
    samples <- DrawSamples.fn(nreps,amean,sig$sigma)
                         # Draw samples from normal distn
    BHRes<-
       BndsFns.fn(1,samples$r,samples$p,nreps,K,amean)
    BLRes<-
       BndsFns.fn(2,samples$r,samples$p,nreps,K,amean)
    GouldRes<-
       BndsFns.fn(3,samples$r,samples$p,nreps,K,amean)
    return(list(amean=amean, corvec=corvec,
       alpha=alpha, p=samples$p, r=samples$r,
       detsig=sig$detsig, BHGR=BHRes$GR,
       BHSens=BHRes$Sens, BHSpec=BHRes$Spec,
       BHHypRejTot=BHRes$HypRejTot,
       BHHypNRejTot=BHRes$HypNRejTot,
       BHHypRejAlt=BHRes$HypRejAlt,
       BHHypNRejNull=BHRes$HypNRejNull,
       BHFDR=BHRes$FDR, BHMDR=BHRes$MDR,
       BHEER=BHRes$EER, BLGR=BLRes$GR,
       BLSens=BLRes$Sens, BLSpec=BLRes$Spec,
       BLHypRejTot=BLRes$HypRejTot,
       BLHypNRejTot=BLRes$HypNRejTot,
       BLHypRejAlt=BLRes$HypRejAlt,
       BLHypNRejNull=BLRes$HypNRejNull,
       BLFDR=BLRes$FDR, BLMDR=BLRes$MDR,
       BLEER=BLRes$EER, GouldGR=GouldRes$GR,
       GouldSens=GouldRes$Sens,
       GouldSpec=GouldRes$Spec,
       GouldHypRejTot=GouldRes$HypRejTot,
       GouldHypNRejTot=GouldRes$HypNRejTot,
       GouldHypRejAlt=GouldRes$HypRejAlt,
       GouldHypNRejNull=GouldRes$HypNRejNull,
       GouldFDR=GouldRes$FDR, GouldMDR=GouldRes$MDR,
       GouldEER=GouldRes$EER))
  }
}
```

References

Benjamini Y, Hochberg Y (1995) Controlling the false discovery rate: A practical and powerful approach to multiple testing. J R Stat Soc Series B Methodol 57:289–300
Benjamini Y, Stark PB (1996) Nonequivariant simultaneous confidence intervals less likely to contain zero. J Am Stat Assoc 91:329–337
Benjamini Y, Liu W (1999) A step-down multiple hypotheses testing procedure that controls the false discovery rate under independence. J Stat Plan Inference 82:163–170
Berger RL (1982) Multiparameter hypothesis testing and acceptance sampling. Technometrics 24:295–300
Bonferroni CE (1936) Teoria statistica della classi e calcolo delle probabilità. Pubbl del R Ist Super di Sci Econ e Commer di Firenze 8:3–62
Capizzi T, Zhang J (1996) Testing the hypothesis that matters for multiple primary endpoints. Drug Inf J 30:949–956
Cook RJ, Farewell VT (1996) Multiplicity considerations in the design and analysis of clinical trials. J R Stat Soc Series A 159:93–110
Farcomeni A (2008) A review of modern multiple hypothesis testing, with particular attention to the false discovery proportion. Stat Methods Med Res 17:347–388
Farcomeni A, Pacillo S (2011) A conservative estimator for the proportion of false nulls based on Dvoretzky, Kiefer and Wolfowitz inequality. Stat Probab Lett 81:1867–1870
Farcomeni A, Finos L (2013) FDR control with pseudo-gatekeeping based on a possibly data driven order of the hypotheses. Biometrics 69:606–613
Feller W (1957) An Introduction to Probability Theory and Its Applications. Wiley, New York.
Finner H, Roters M (2002) Multiple hypotheses testing and expected number of type I errors. Ann Stat 30:220–238
Finner H, Gontscharuk V (2009) Controlling the familywise error rate with plug-in estimator for the proportion of true null hypotheses. J R Stat Soc Series B Stat Methodol 71:1031–1048
Finos L, Farcomeni A (2011) k-FWER control without p-value adjustment, with Application to Detection of Genetic Determinants of Multiple Sclerosis in Italian Twins. Biometrics 67:174–181
Gabriel KR (1969) Simultaneous test procedures—some theory of multiple comparisons. Ann Of Math Stat 40:224–250
Grechanovsky E, Pinsker I (1999) A general approach to stepup multiple test procedures for free-combinations families. J Stat Plan Inference 82:35–54
Hochberg Y (1988) A sharper bonferroni procedure for multiple tests of significance. Biometrika 75:800–802
Hochberg Y, Tamhane AC (1987) Multiple comparison procedures. Wiley, New York
Hochberg Y, Benjamini Y (1990) More powerful procedures for multiple significance testing. Stat Med 9:811–818
Hochberg Y, Rom DM (1995) Extensions of multiple testing procedures based on Simes's test. J Stat Plan Inference 48:141–152
Holland B, Copenhaver MD (1987) An improved sequentially rejective bonferroni test procedure (corr: v43 p 737). Biometrics 43:417–423
Holland B, Copenhaver MD (1988) Improved bonferroni-type multiple testing procedures. Psychol Bull 104:145–149
Holm S (1979) A simple sequentially rejective multiple test procedure. Scand J Stat 6:65–70
Hommel G (1988) A stagewise rejective multiple test procedure based on a modified Bonferroni test. Biometrika 75:383–386
Hommel G, Bretz F, Maurer W (2011) Multiple hypotheses testing based on ordered p values—a historical survey with applications to medical research. J Biopharm Stat 21:595–609
Hwang YT, Chu SK, Ou ST (2011) Evaluations of FDR-controlling procedures in multiple hypothesis testing. Stat Comput 21:569–583

James S (1991) Approximate multinormal probabilities applied to correlated multiple endpoints in clinical trials. Stat Med 10:1123–1135

Lazowski DA, Ecclestone NA, Myers AM, Paterson DH, Tudor LC, Fitzgerald C, et al (1999) A randomized outcome evaluation of group exercise programs in long-term care institutions. J of Gerontol A Biol Sci 54:M621–M628

Läuter J (1996) Exact t and F tests for analyzing studies with multiple endpoints. Biometrics 52:964–970

Lehmann E (1959) Testing statistical hypotheses. Wiley, New York

Liu W (1996) Mulitple tests of a non-hierarchical finite family of hypotheses. J R Stat Soc Series B Methodol 58:455–461

O'Brien PC (1984) Procedures for comparing samples with multiple endpoints. Biometrics 40:1079–1087

Rom DM (1990) A sequentially rejective test procedure based on a modified Bonferroni inequality. Biometrika 77:663–665

Rom DM, Connell L (1994) A generalized family of multiple test procedures. Commun Stat Theory Methods 23:3171–3187

Sarkar SK (1998) Some probability inequalities for ordered MTP2 random variables: a proof of the Simes conjecture. Ann Of Stat 26:494–504

Sarkar SK (2008) On the Simes inequality and its generalization. In: Balakrkshnan N, Pea EA, Silvapulla MJ (eds) Beyond parametrics in interdisciplinary research: festschrift in honor of Professor Pranab K. Sen. Institute of Mathematical Statistics, Beachwood, p 231–242

Sarkar SK, Chang C-K (1997) The Simes method for multiple hypothesis testing with positively dependent test statistics. J Am Stat Assoc 92:1601–1608

Sarkar SK, Guo W, Finner H (2012) On adaptive procedures controlling the familywise error rate. J Stat Plan Inference 142:65–78

Sen PK (1999) Some remarks on Simes-type multiple tests of significance. J Stat Plan Inference 82:139–145

Simes RJ (1986) An improved bonferroni procedure for multiple tests of significance. Biometrika 73:751–754

Steel RGD, Torrie JH (1980) Principles and procedures of statistics: a biometrical approach. McGraw-Hill, New York

Storey JD, Taylor JE, Siegmund D (2004) Strong control, conservative point estimation and simultaneous conservative consistency of false discovery rates: a unified approach. J R Stat Soc Series B Stat Methodol 66:187–205

Tang D, Geller NC, Pocock SJ (1993) On the design and analysis of randomized clinical trials with multiple endpoints. Biometrics 49:23–30

van der Laan M Dudoit S Pollard K (2004) Augmentation procedures for control of the generalized family-wise error rate and tail probabilities for the proportion of false positives. Stat Appl Genet Mol Biol 3.doi:10.2202/1544–6115.1042

Westfall PH Young SS (1993) Resampling-based multiple testing: examples and methods for p-value adjustment. Wiley, New York

MIX
Papier aus verantwortungsvollen Quellen
Paper from responsible sources
FSC® C105338

If you have any concerns about our products,
you can contact us on
ProductSafety@springernature.com

In case Publisher is established outside the EU,
the EU authorized representative is:
Springer Nature Customer Service Center GmbH
Europaplatz 3, 69115 Heidelberg, Germany

Printed by Libri Plureos GmbH
in Hamburg, Germany